6811204
8205

FITTING GUIDE
FOR RIGID AND SOFT
CONTACT LENSES

A PRACTICAL APPROACH

FITTING GUIDE FOR RIGID AND SOFT CONTACT LENSES

A PRACTICAL APPROACH

HAROLD A. STEIN, M.D., M.Sc.(Ophth.), F.R.C.S.(C)

Professor of Ophthalmology, University of Toronto, Toronto;
Chief, Department of Ophthalmology, Scarborough General Hospital, Scarborough;
Attending Ophthalmologist, Mount Sinai Hospital, Toronto;
President Elect, Contact Lens Association of Ophthalmologists, New Orleans, Louisiana;
Secretary and Director, Joint Commission on Allied Health Personnel in
Ophthalmology, St. Paul, Minnesota;
Director of Professional Continuing Education,
Centennial College of Applied Arts, Toronto, Ontario;
Secretary, Canadian Ophthalmological Society

BERNARD J. SLATT, M.D., F.R.C.S.(C)

Associate Professor of Ophthalmology, University of Toronto, Toronto;
Consultant, Mt. Sinai Hospital, Toronto;
Attending Ophthalmologist, Scarborough General Hospital, Scarborough;
Director, Association of Ophthalmic Assistants of Ontario;
Board of Advisors, Toronto, Ontario

SECOND EDITION

with 610 illustrations, including 48
illustrations in full color and 15 in 2 color

The C. V. Mosby Company

ST. LOUIS • TORONTO • PRINCETON   1984

MOSBY

A TRADITION OF PUBLISHING EXCELLENCE

Editor: Eugenia Klein
Developmental editor: Kathryn H. Falk
Manuscript editor: Carl Masthay
Book design: Jeanne Bush
Production: Carol O'Leary, Barbara Merritt

SECOND EDITION

Previous edition copyrighted 1977

Printed in the United States of America

The C.V. Mosby Company
11830 Westline Industrial Drive
St. Louis, Missouri 63146

Library of Congress Cataloging in Publication Data

Stein, Harold A., 1929-
 Fitting guide for rigid and soft contact lenses.

 Rev. ed. of: Fitting guide for hard and soft lenses.
1977.
 Bibliography: p.
 Includes index.
 1. Contact lenses. I. Slatt, Bernard J., 1934-
II. Title.
RE977.C6S73 1983   617.7'523   83-692
ISBN 0-8016-4784-3

C/MV/MV 9 8 7 6 5 4 3 2   01/B/035

To ANNE and CAROL
our wives, who do not know the convex from
the concave side of a contact lens, but who
were good enough sports to keep us supplied
with free time and coffee while we were
working on this book

FOREWORD

Drs. Stein and Slatt should be congratulated for the success of their practical, clinical guide for the fitting of rigid and soft contact lenses, which is in its second edition. The major thrust of this book is to give a step-by-step, concise, clinical guide for contact lens fitting. This book is aimed at the clinician who wants to know how to fit a lens and deal with its problems without the theoretical and scientific background of corneal and lens physiology and biochemistry.

Practitioners will find this approach direct and clear. The visual emphasis on photographs and drawings and the well-illustrated instructions make this book easy to understand.

In this enriched second edition all aspects of rigid and soft lens fitting are covered meticulously, including the new modalities of gaspermeable lenses, extended-wear lenses, and silicone lenses. Controversial methods such as orthokeratology have also been dealt with.

Great care has been given to the strictly practical aspects of rigid and soft contact lens fitting. Without any doubt, this book should be profitable reading for the student learning contact lens fitting, as well as for the practitioner who needs help now and then with problem cases. The high standard of this book should be no surprise because Drs. Stein and Slatt are the authors of *The Ophthalmic Assistant*, which is in its fourth edition and has become a classic text in its field.

This book is a must on the bookshelf of every contact lens fitter. I consider it a privilege to recommend without reservation this most useful and practical fitting guide for rigid and soft contact lenses.

G. Peter Halberg, M.D., F.A.C.S.

Chairman, International Contact Lens Council of Ophthalmology; Professor of Clinical Ophthalmology, New York Medical College, New York, New York

We welcome the opportunity to bring out the second edition of the *Fitting Guide*. The first edition had been surpassed by so much advanced technology that it was on the verge of becoming a collector's item. Most new editions are strictly a matter of mending and pruning—correcting errors, updating materials, perhaps reorganizing, adding some tables, diagrams, and photographs here and there—the work of a dilettante. Not so with this new edition. It required so much work that the pruning knife was insufficient as a tool—it required an axe.

The soft lens section was literally redone. If we salvaged 20% of the old text, it was a lot. Care systems have totally changed. We now recognize the importance of cleaning and the potential toxic and hypersensitivity reactions of these supposedly innocuous solutions. Soft lenses have lost weight and become trimmer. It seems they can't get thin enough, especially in the quest for more oxygen permeability. The latter term has become such a buzz word that patients now request oxygen-permeable lenses.

There are so many companies now making soft lenses that we decided to go generic, using examples where indicated. Also the soft lens field has broadened immensely in the past years. Newer soft lenses come in a variety of polymers, with varying degrees of water content, tints, toric front and back surfaces, and variable central thickness. It meant new material and writing. Even the traditional sections of insertion and removal could not be salvaged because the newer hyperthin lenses easily collapse on a wet finger and the taco test for determining which side of the lens is right has fallen into the realm of being a quaint oddity. It doesn't work anymore with most of these newer lenses.

The section on extended wear lenses has been upgraded and expanded in deference to their new importance. They have penetrated the market, and contact lens fitters are now obliged to know them in detail. The current thrust is to develop lenses with the greatest comfort, convenience, and safety. We stress safety for obvious reasons but also for the fact that a patient may not know when these lenses are a hazard. The warning devices of reactive symptoms may be missing. Patients simply do not know when their corneas are slightly edematous and vascularized.

Gas-permeable lenses have been emphasized because these lenses have come out of adolescence into maturity. These lenses are now the prime lens of the rigid lens variety. In many areas of the world, gas-permeable lenses are preferred as first choice over soft lenses.

Silicone lenses, both in the resin and elastomer form, have made it to the present and are treated that way. No one is joking about silicone anymore. We added a fully developed chapter to bring it to its proper level of importance. We offer our thanks to Dr. John Morgan of Queen's University who wrote his usual organized, in-depth analysis for this chapter.

Polymethylmethacrylate is looking more like a lens of the past. Gas-permeable lenses do the same job but better. This discussion was pruned and reduced to indicate the material's shrinking prominence.

Bifocal lenses and the fitting of the presbyope have struggled along, but they now seem to be emerging as a practical reality.

The lid is off the age ceiling on the use of contact lenses. Children 1 day old are being fitted after cataract surgery as well as their grandmothers in their eighties. New instruments and techniques have been developed to adapt to the special needs of children.

This edition of the *Fitting Guide* is really a new book. Only the intent remains the same: to provide clear, useful information to assist the fitter in the practical management of a contact lens practice. It is not an academic reference book. We have our bias toward certain lens designs and our own ways of treating trouble. Our personal preferences are exposed because we make no attempt to hide in the name of impartiality what we think works best. This is our editorial license and our duty to show our experience.

Canada has a unique situation in North America in the contact lens area. Unhampered by restrictions imposed by the FDA, we serve as the center of cross winds blowing new and exciting products from Japan and Europe. In addition, our own Canadian contact lens industry coupled with the testing-ground status of American manufacturers has brought exciting new products to us for clinical evaluation long before their market introduction in the United States. We are thankful for our vantage point for being privy to this rich experience in the contact lens field.

New sections by Dr. John F. Morgan, Mr. Keith W. Harrison, and Jean-Pierre Chartrand have been added, in addition to revised chapters contributed by Dr. James Aquavella, Dr. J. Peter Halberg, and Penny Cook.

We are particularly indebted to the extensive critical review of the manuscript and the contribution of new concepts by Dr. Joshua Josephson. We are indebted to Dr. Richard Lembeck, Kenneth Swanson, and Keith Harrison for reviewing sections of the new manuscript.

We are grateful to Mr. Norman Deer for the illustrations and to Dr. Raymond Stein, who aided in the organization and research of the second edition.

Harold A. Stein
Bernard J. Slatt

CONTENTS

APPENDICES

COLOR ATLAS

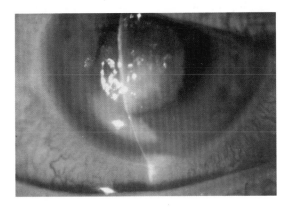

Plate 1. Corneal ulceration caused by *Pseudomonas aeruginosa.*

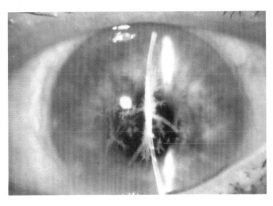

Plate 2. Granular corneal dystrophy.

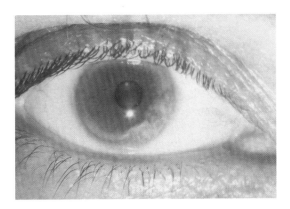

Plate 3. Terrien's marginal degeneration of the cornea.

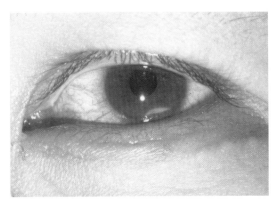

Plate 4. Marginal corneal erosion caused by *Staphylococcus aureus.*

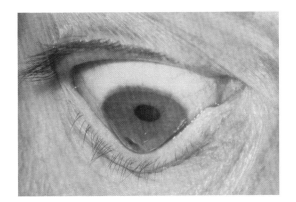

Plate 5. Advanced keratoconus. A cone-shaped deformity of the cornea with thinning of the cornea.

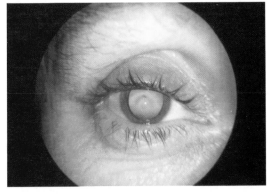

Plate 6. Keratoconus reflex. Retinal reflex as seen through a thin protruding cornea.

(**1** and **2,** Courtesy Mentor O & O Inc., Hingham, Mass.; **5** and **6,** Courtesy Dr. Dean Butcher, Australia.)

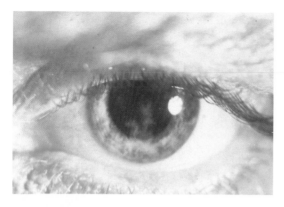

Plate 7. Herpes simplex dendritic ulcer. Fernlike projection on the epithelial surface of the cornea from herpes simplex of the cornea.

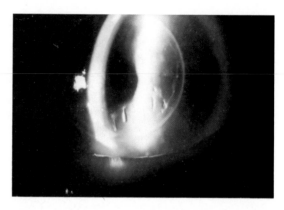

Plate 8. Filamentary keratitis covered by a therapeutic lens.

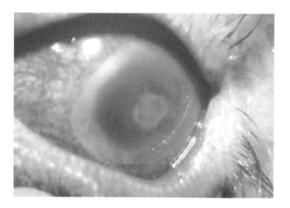

Plate 9. Fungal corneal ulcer leading to endophthalmitis.

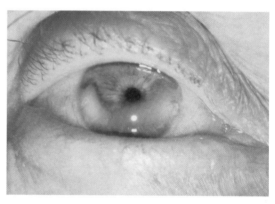

Plate 10. Band keratopathy of the cornea.

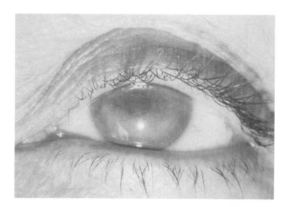

Plate 11. Fuchs' corneal dystrophy resulting in progressive decrease of vision and eventually bullous keratopathy.

(**7,** Courtesy Dr. Ira Abrahamson, Jr., Cincinnati, Ohio.)

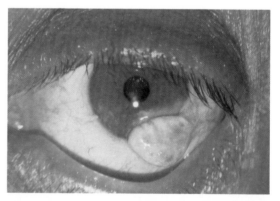

Plate 12. Large corneal dermoid requiring surgical removal before patient could wear contact lens.

II. EXTERNAL DISORDERS OF THE EYE AND EYELID

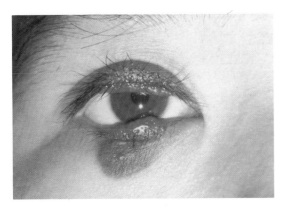

Plate 13. Kissing benign nevus of the upper and lower eyelid.

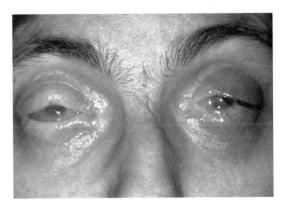

Plate 14. Advanced trachoma with diffuse scarring of the cornea and symblepharon and entropion.

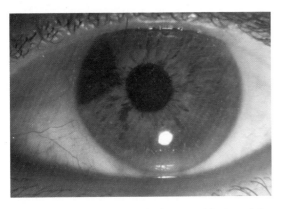

Plate 15. Melanoma of iris. A pigmented lesion of the iris.

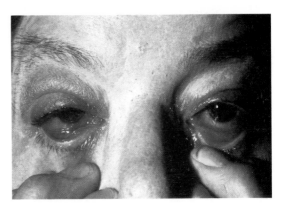

Plate 16. Acute bacterial conjunctivitis. Inflammation of the conjunctival lining caused by *Streptococcus.*

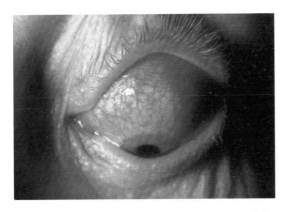

Plate 17. Scleritis. Nonbacterial inflammation of the sclera.

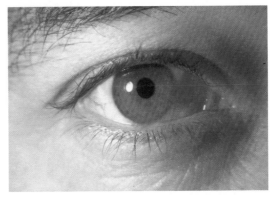

Plate 18. Pterygium. A triangular membrane extending from the conjunctiva over the cornea.

(**15** to **18** from Stein, H.A., and Slatt, B.J.: The ophthalmic assistant, ed. 4, St. Louis, 1983, The C.V. Mosby Co.)

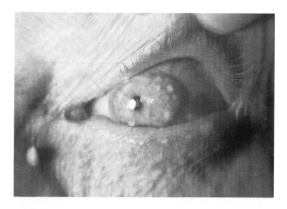

Plate 19. Squamous cell carcinoma of cornea. A cancer growth occurring at the limbus and invading the cornea.

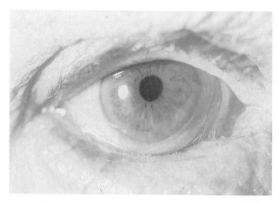

Plate 20. Spastic entropion. In-turning of the lower eyelid from spasm.

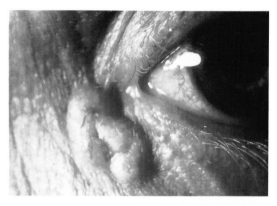

Plate 21. Basal cell carcinoma of eyelid (rodent ulcer), a neoplasm of the lower eyelid that is locally invasive.

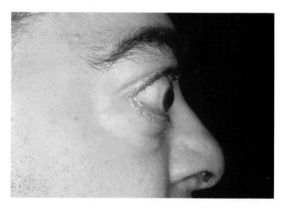

Plate 22. Thyroid exophthalmos. Note ocular protrusion and lid retraction.

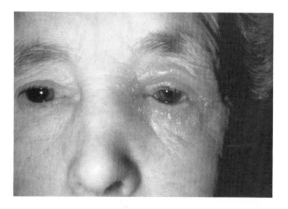

Plate 23. Allergic blepharodermatitis, a skin condition that resulted from atropine sensitivity.

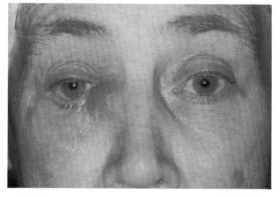

Plate 24. Acute dacryocystitis caused by obstruction of nasal lacrimal duct.

(**20,** Courtesy Dr. Ira Abrahamson, Jr., Cincinnati, Ohio; **19** and **21** to **23** from Stein, H.A., and Slatt, B.J.: The ophthalmic assistant, ed. 4, St. Louis, 1983, The C.V. Mosby Co.)

III. CONTACT LENS PROBLEMS

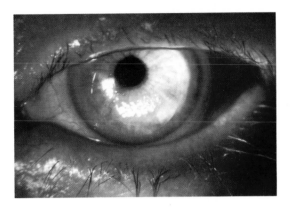

Plate 25. Plaque-like deposits on a soft lens.

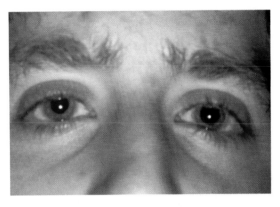

Plate 26. Allergic conjunctivitis occurring after the use of a soaking solution containing thimerosal.

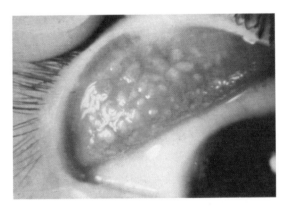

Plate 27. Giant papillary conjunctivitis in a patient wearing daily-wear soft contact lenses for 2 years.

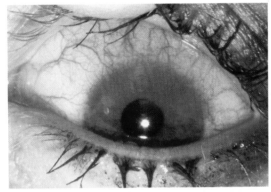

Plate 28. Vascular invasion superiorly in a patient wearing extended-wear contact lenses for 6 months without removal, cleaning, or monitoring.

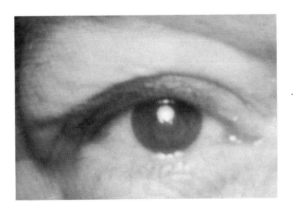

Plate 29. Overwear syndrome from acute corneal hypoxia after 12 hours of wear with PMMA rigid lenses. Denuding of the epithelium resulting in extreme pain, photophobia, and blurring of vision.

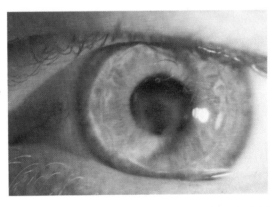

Plate 30. Keratoconus with central scarring. A rigid lens is shown partially decentered.

(**25,** Courtesy Dr. H. Jonathan Kersley, London, England.)

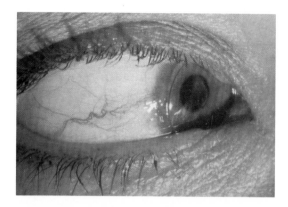

Plate 31. Staining at 3 and 9 o'clock positions in a patient wearing a small gas-permeable lens with thick edges. A large leash vessel has developed.

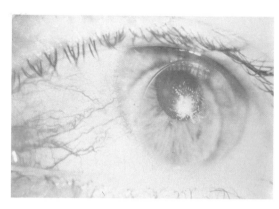

Plate 32. A partially decentered rigid lens leading to marginal erosion and vascularization.

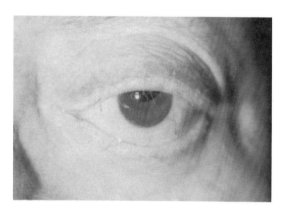

Plate 33. Scleral show below limbus caused by low-lying lower lid. This creates a dryness of the lower portion of a soft lens with resultant drying out of the lens and blurriness of vision.

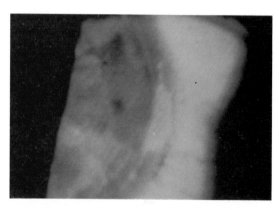

Plate 34. Marginal ulceration at the limbus caused by a decentered rigid lens on a toric cornea with constant indentation and necrosis of the underlying epithelium by the edge of the lens.

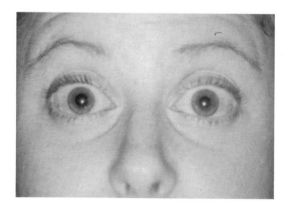

Plate 35. Staring effect of a new contact lens wearer. This may result in drying of the lens, blurring of vision, and 3 and 9 o'clock staining.

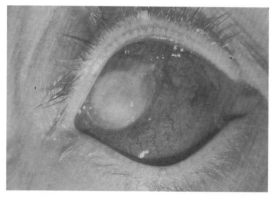

Plate 36. Endophthalmitis after finger-to-eye contamination of a daily soft lens wearer with *Pseudomonas aeruginosa*.

IV. SPECIAL INDICATIONS FOR CONTACT LENSES

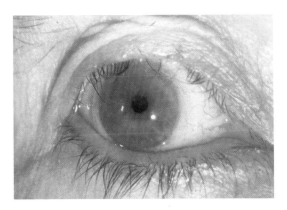

Plate 37. A plano high-water-content lens used for entropion after scarring from injury. The in-turned aberrant lashes are prevented from irritating the cornea.

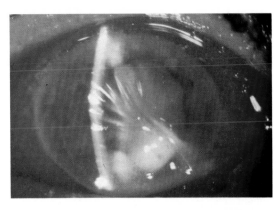

Plate 38. Penetrating corneal wound in which a therapeutic lens was used to restore integrity of the anterior chamber.

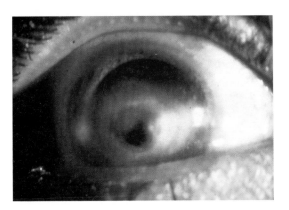

Plate 39. Lye burns with descemetocele. A therapeutic lens can prevent perforation.

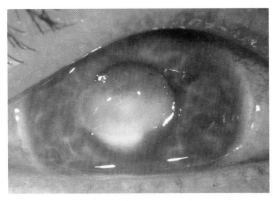

Plate 40. Necrotic metaherpetic corneal ulcer that failed to heal until a therapeutic lens was applied.

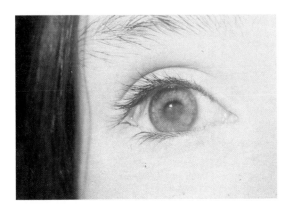

Plate 41. Riley-Day syndrome with necrotic corneal ulcer requiring a low-water-content, thin, extended-wear lens to maintain the corneal integrity.

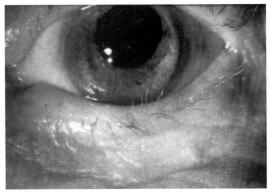

Plate 42. Aphakic extended-wear lens protecting against corneal irritation by trichiasis.

(**39,** Courtesy Dr. B. Bodner, Boston, and Syntex Ophthalmics, Inc., Phoenix, Arizona; **42,** courtesy Dr. H. Jonathan Kersley, London, England.)

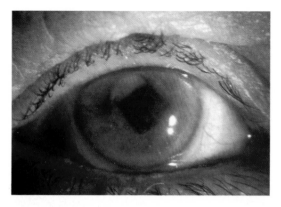

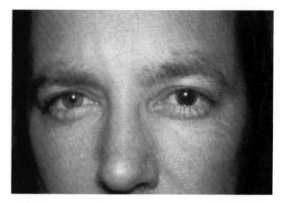

Plate 43. Bandage lens to give comfort to an eye with bullous keratopathy after intraocular lens insertion.

Plate 44. Red-dyed soft lens on one eye used to enhance color perception in a red-green–blind individual.

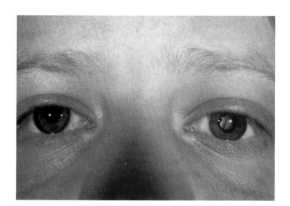

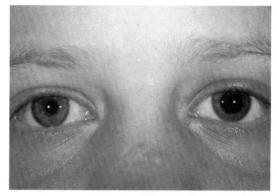

Plates 45 and 46. Inoperable cataract in which a colored therapeutic lens was applied for cosmetic advantage in a young child.

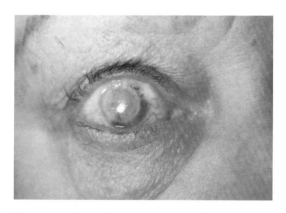

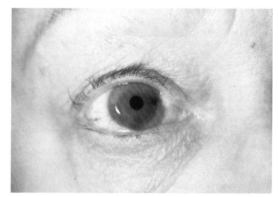

Plates 47 and 48. Cosmetic therapeutic lens used to cover a traumatic leukoma.

(**45** and **48**, Courtesy Narcissus Foundation, San Francisco, California.)

PART I

FUNDAMENTALS

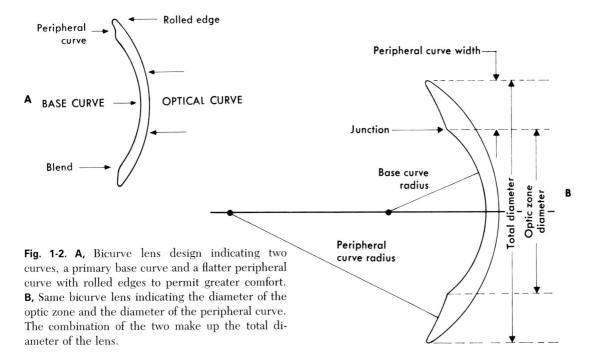

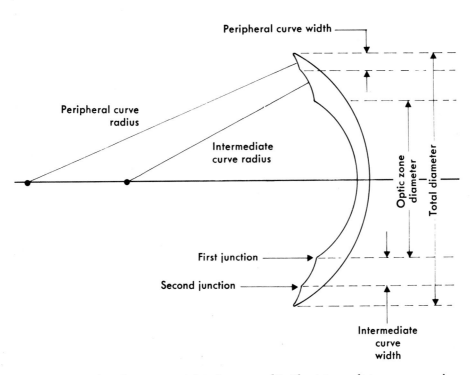

Fig. 1-2. A, Bicurve lens design indicating two curves, a primary base curve and a flatter peripheral curve with rolled edges to permit greater comfort. **B,** Same bicurve lens indicating the diameter of the optic zone and the diameter of the peripheral curve. The combination of the two make up the total diameter of the lens.

Fig. 1-3. A tricurve lens has two peripheral curve radii. The intermediate curve may be very narrow, as found in contour lenses. These lenses have large diameters—9.5 mm or greater—with an optic zone of 6.5 to 7.5 mm, which is just large enough to clear the maximum pupil diameter. The peripheral curves are slightly flatter than the base curves by 0.4 to 0.8 mm with a width of 1.3 mm. With a standard tricurve lens the intermediate curve is 1 mm flatter than the base curve. The peripheral curve is a standard 12.25 mm radius.

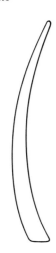

Fig. 1-4. Prism ballast to provide weight and stop rotation of a lens. (From Stein, H.A., and Slatt, B.J.: The ophthalmic assistant, ed. 4, St. Louis, 1983, The C.V. Mosby Co.)

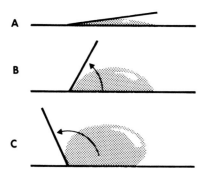

Fig. 1-5. The smaller the angle of contact (θ), the greater the spreading of a liquid over a solid. A hard lens is hydrophobic and has a 60-degree angle of contact with water. **A,** Low-wetting angle; **B,** wetting angle of polymethylmethacrylate rigid lens; **C,** large wetting angle with droplet of mercury.

cations have been used. Truncation is frequently employed to add stability to a soft toric lens.

The *back vertex power* of a lens refers to the effective power of lens measured from the back surface. The *wetting angle* of a lens is the angle that the edge of a bead of water makes with the surface of the plastic. The smaller the angle, the greater the wetting ability (Fig. 1-5).

Toric lenses or *toroid lenses*, derived from Latin *torus* meaning 'a bulge' or 'cushion,' are lenses with different radii of curvature in each meridian. The meridians of the shortest and longest radii are called the *principal meridians*

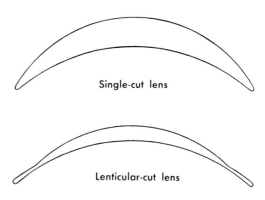

Fig. 1-6. Single-cut and lenticular-cut lenses. (From Stein, H.A., and Slatt, B.J.: The ophthalmic assistant, ed. 4, St. Louis, 1983, The C.V. Mosby Co.)

and differ by 90 degrees. These lenses are used to correct astigmatism.

A *front surface toric lens* has an anterior surface with two different radii but a posterior surface that is spheric. A *back surface toric* lens has a posterior surface that has two different radii and an anterior spheric surface. In a *bitoric* lens both the anterior and posterior surfaces have different radii.

Higher power plus lenses are often designed with a *lenticular bowl* or central area that has the appearance of an upside-down bowl-like lens sitting on the underlying lens (Fig. 1-6).

The *sagittal depth* or *height* of a lens is the distance between a flat surface and the back surface of the central portion of the lens. Thus for two lenses of the same diameter but of different sagittal depths, the lens of the greater sagittal depth would produce a greater "vaulting" of the lens and in effect would be steeper (Fig. 1-7). This is often referred to as the *sagittal vault*.

There are two important variables in understanding the mechanism of loosening or tightening a lens. These variables are the diameter and the radius of the lens. If the diameter is kept constant, with the radius being changed to a longer one, for example, from a 7.8 to an 8.4 mm radius, the sagittal vault or sagittal height of the lens becomes shorter and the lens becomes flatter. The converse is also true (Figs. 1-8 and 1-9).

If the radius of the lens remains the same but the diameter is made larger, for example, from 13 to 15 mm, as occurs with soft lenses, the sagittal vault or sagittal height of the lens is

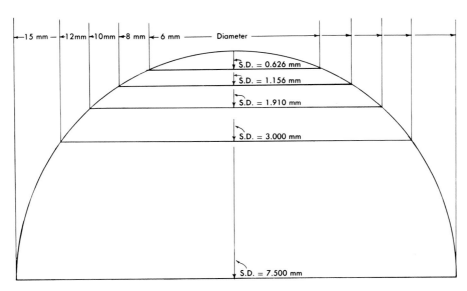

Fig. 1-7. A ball bearing is divided into five sections of different diameters. Compare the varying sagittal depths (S.D.) of one section to another. (From Soper, J.W., and Girard, L.J.: Designing the corneal lens. In Girard, L.J., Soper, J.W., and Sampson, W.G., editors: Corneal contact lenses, ed. 2, St. Louis, 1970, The C.V. Mosby Co.)

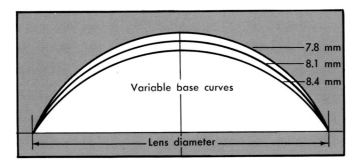

Fig. 1-8. If the diameter is held constant, when the radius of curvature is decreased from 8.4 to 7.8 mm, the sagittal height or vault of the lens is increased.

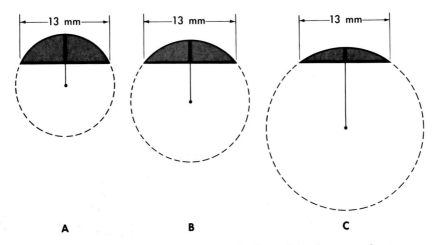

Fig. 1-9. A to **C,** Three circles of increasing length of radius. If the diameter of a given arc of the circle is kept constant, the sagittal height will decrease from **A** to **C.**

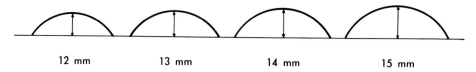

Fig. 1-10. When the radius is kept constant and the diameter increased, the sagittal height of the lens is increased and the lens becomes steeper.

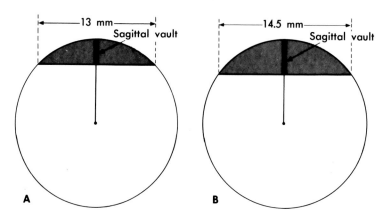

Fig. 1-11. If portions of two similar circles are cut off, each with a different diameter, portion **B**, with the larger 14.5 mm diameter will have a greater sagittal depth or vault than portion **A** with the smaller 13.0 mm diameter.

increased and the lens becomes steeper. The converse is also true (Fig. 1-10).

For example, if we consider the lens as being part of a similar circle (Fig. 1-11) and we take two parts of the circle with different diameters, the portion of the circle with the larger diameter will have a greater sagittal vault.

RIGID OR HARD LENSES

Rigid or hard lenses may have a *standard*, or *thin*, thickness. They may be composed of a material made of *polymethylmethacrylate*, sometimes referred to as *PMMA*, a hard transparent plastic with a long history of acceptance. They may also be composed of *cellulose acetate butyrate (CAB)*, of a combination of *silicone and PMMA*, or of a hard resin silicone. Both of these last two groups of materials transmit sufficient oxygen to be called *gas-permeable lenses*.

Rigid lenses may be modified by *fenestration*, which is the drilling of one or more holes through the plastic. The lens may be *polished* or the edges refinished by the *Con-Lish method* or the *rag-wheel method*, or by use of a *felt disc polisher*.

SOFT LENSES

Soft lenses are composed either of hydrogel material, a watery gel-like material, or of *silicone*. Soft lenses may be manufactured by the *spin-cast process*, utilizing liquid material revolving in a given mold at a controlled speed and temperature to produce the resultant curvature, design, and power. Silicone lenses are molded when the liquid form is placed into a metal or glass mold of known design and polymerized. Silicone lenses are more flexible than rigid lenses but still belong to the group of essentially rigid lenses. Many soft lenses are *lathe cut* by a machine lathe used to grind lens design, size, and power. Most hydrogel soft lenses are made with HEMA, which stands for *hydroxyethylmethacrylate*, as their basic ingredient but are often copolymerized with other materials.

CONTACT LENS PROBLEMS

When a lens or base curve is said to be made *steeper*, it means that the posterior radius of curvature is decreased. When a lens or base curve is said to be made *flatter*, it means the

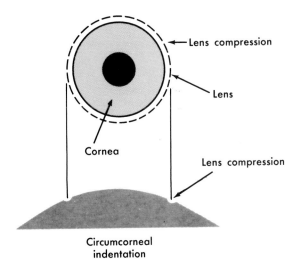

Fig. 1-12. The tight lens causes compression at the limbus.

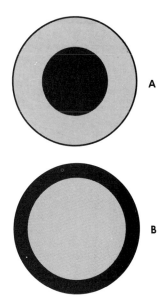

Fig. 1-13. A, Fluorescein pattern of a flat lens. Note absence of dye centrally. **B,** Fluorescein pattern of a steep lens. Note absence of dye at the periphery because of marginal touch. (From Stein, H.A., and Slatt, B.J.: The ophthalmic assistant, ed. 4, St. Louis, 1983, The C.V. Mosby Co.)

opposite, that the posterior radius of curvature is increased.

Decentration of a lens indicates that the lens is sliding off center and may give rise to poor vision or *arcuate staining*, or both. Arcuate staining is arc-like staining in the periphery of the cornea. *Vertical striae* are small vertical lines in the cornea caused by folds in Descemet's membrane and are an early sign of corneal hypoxia. *Limbal compression* occurs with soft lenses that are too tight and cause pressure at the periphery of the cornea (Fig. 1-12). *Fluorescein* is a dye used to analyze rigid lens problems because it mixes with the tear film and glows in the presence of ultraviolet light or cobalt blue light (Fig. 1-13).

Modulus is the resistance to change. The higher the modulus, the greater the resistance to change and the more likely the lens is to break, for example, the difference between a rubber lens and glass. A rubber lens is less likely to break than a glass lens, which has a higher modulus. On the other hand, a lens with greater modulus has less flexure and so provides greater optic performance.

INSTRUMENTATION

An *ophthalmometer* is an instrument designed to measure the radius of curvature of the cornea, using the mirror effect of the cornea's front surface (Fig. 1-14). This instrument is most commonly referred to as a *keratometer*,

the name originated by Bausch & Lomb from *kerato-*, meaning 'horn (cornea),' and *meter*, 'a measure.' The instrument measures a small portion of the *corneal cap* (Fig. 1-15), the central zone of the cornea, and the measurement is often called the *K reading*.

In *astigmatism with the rule* the vertical corneal meridian has the steepest curvature, whereas in *astigmatism against the rule* the horizontal meridian has the steepest curvature (Fig. 1-16).

In performing *keratometry* some authors record the flattest meridian first and the steepest meridian next so that a keratometer (K) value, for example, of 44.00 D × 46.00 D × 85, indicates that the horizontal meridian has a radius of 44.00 D and that the vertical meridian has a radius of 46.00 D with the axis at 85 degrees. Other authors prefer to always record the horizontal meridian first regardless of which is the flattest. This value may be expressed in either diopters or millimeters of radius. Table 1-1 gives a comparative value of the K reading in diopters and millimeters. Each 0.05 mm is equivalent to approximately 0.25

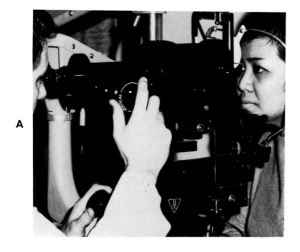

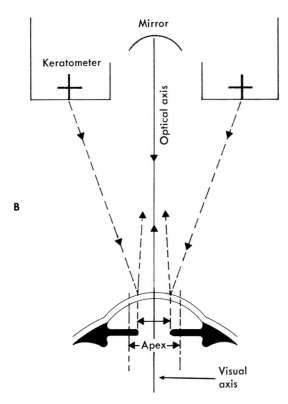

Fig. 1-14. A, Taking a K reading. **B,** The principle of the keratometer. The visual axis is aligned along the optic axis of the instrument so that the central front surface of the cornea reflects the mires of the keratometer. (**A** from Stein, H.A., and Slatt, B.J.: The ophthalmic assistant, ed. 4, St. Louis, 1983, The C.V. Mosby Co.)

D, so that a 0.5 mm radius equals approximately 2.50 D. Expressed another way, each 1.00 D change in the K reading equals approximately a 0.2 mm radius change.

In lens work one usually first considers the flattest K reading. If the back surface of the lens is to be the same radius as K, this is referred to as "fitting on K." One may fit "steeper than K" as in rigid lens design or "flatter than K" as in soft lens design. In the latter situation the lens will have a posterior radius flatter than the flattest K reading.

The size of the *corneal cap* measured varies with the instrument employed but is usually about 3.36 mm chord length. The *mires* of the ophthalmometer are the targets that are reflected back from the cornea (Fig. 1-17). The corneal cap is the central zone of the cornea and has a constant radius of curvature (Fig. 1-15) referred to as the *central posterior curve (CPC)*. The *peripheral* or *paracentral zone* of the cornea is the area surrounding the corneal cap and extending to the limbus. It has a much flatter curvature than does the central curve. The rate of flattening does not conform to a mathematical progression, that is, the cornea is not a true ellipse; it is generally described as being aspheric.

The *topogometer* is a keratometer attachment with a movable light designed to localize the apical zone or corneal cap of the cornea to be measured by the keratometer. The limiting margin of the apical zone is determined by the points on the corneal surface where the radius of curvature of the cornea begins to flatten. The average diameter of the apical zone is about 6 mm.

The *optic spherometer (Radiuscope*, a term coined by American Optical Co.; sometimes radius gauge) is an instrument that measures the radius of curvature of a rigid contact lens. A *dial thickness gauge* is used to measure the thickness of a rigid contact lens. A *profile analyzer* is an instrument utilized to assess the junctional zone blending of a hard lens (Fig. 1-18). A *shadowgraph* is an instrument that projects and magnifies a contact lens. It is used to examine defects in a lens and to determine measurements.

A *wet cell* or *hydrometric chamber* is used to retain a soft lens for evaluation and measurements of power and edge configuration (Fig. 1-19). *Templates* are small elevated plastic domes

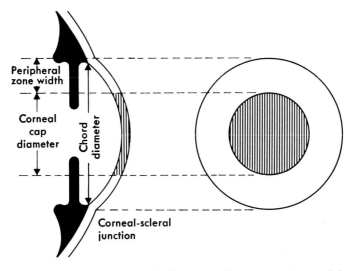

Fig. 1-15. Corneal cap, representing the theoretic spheric central zone of the cornea.

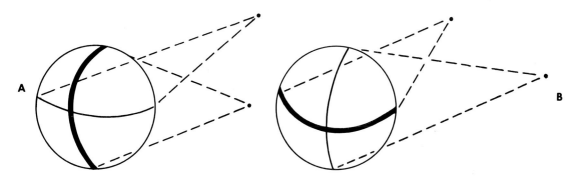

Fig. 1-16. A, Astigmatism with the rule. The vertical corneal meridian has the steepest curvature. **B,** Astigmatism against the rule. The horizontal meridian has the steepest curvature.

Table 1-1. Diopter-to-millimeter conversion

Keratometric reading (D)		Radius convex (mm)	Keratometric reading (D)		Radius convex (mm)	Keratometric reading (D)		Radius convex (mm)
47.75	=	7.07	45.00	=	7.50	42.25	=	8.00
47.50	=	7.11	44.75	=	7.55	42.00	=	8.04
47.25	=	7.14	44.50	=	7.59	41.75	=	8.08
47.00	=	7.18	44.25	=	7.63	41.50	=	8.13
46.75	=	7.22	44.00	=	7.67	41.25	=	8.18
46.50	=	7.26	43.75	=	7.72	41.00	=	8.23
46.25	=	7.30	43.50	=	7.76	40.75	=	8.28
46.00	=	7.34	43.25	=	7.80	40.50	=	8.33
45.75	=	7.38	43.00	=	7.85	40.25	=	8.39
45.50	=	7.42	42.75	=	7.90	40.00	=	8.44
45.25	=	7.46	42.50	=	7.95			

Courtesy Bausch & Lomb, Inc.

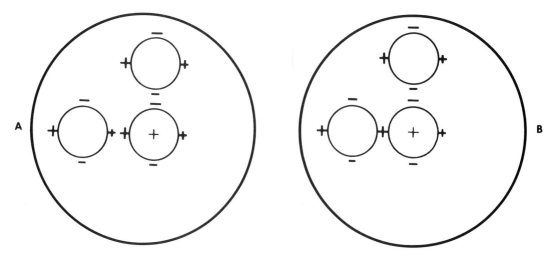

Fig. 1-17. Keratometer mires. **A,** Alignment of the mires for axis. **B,** Apposition of the plus mire to measure one meridian of corneal curvature. (From Stein, H.A., and Slatt, B.J.: The ophthalmic assistant, ed. 4, St. Louis, 1983, The C.V. Mosby Co.)

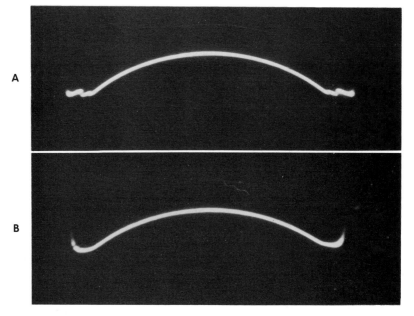

Fig. 1-18. A, Poorly finished transition zone as determined by the profile analyzer. **B,** Perfect transition zone with ski contour at its periphery.

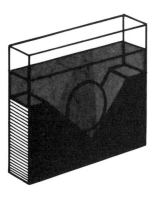

Fig. 1-19. Water cell used to measure power of a soft lens in the hydrated state. The soft lens is floated in normal saline solution and measured in a regular lensometer. (From Stein, H.A., Slatt, B.J., and Cook, P.: Manual of ophthalmic terminology, St. Louis, 1982, The C.V. Mosby Co.)

of known radius of curvature for evaluation of base curves of soft lenses in a number of existing soft lens analyzers.

The *photokeratoscope* is an instrument that photographs the front surface of the eye and provides a permanent record of a large corneal area.

ANATOMIC AND SURGICAL TERMINOLOGY OF CONTACT-RELATED AREAS
Cornea

The cornea is a clear, transparent structure with a brilliant, shiny surface. *Kerato-*, from Greek meaning 'horn,' is the prefix pertaining to the cornea. Ancient Greeks believed that the cornea resembled a thinly sliced horn of an animal.

When a cornea becomes cone shaped, the condition of *keratoconus*, or *conic cornea*, exists. If an inflammation *(-itis)* affects the cornea, it is called *keratitis*. A corneal transplant is referred to as a *keratoplasty*. A transplant may be penetrating, in which full-thickness layers of the cornea are replaced with a full-thickness layer from a donor, or a *lamellar section*, in which the outer two thirds of the cornea is replaced. *Refractive keratoplasty*, introduced by José Barraquer in 1949, refers to surgical procedures to modify corneal curvature and alter refractive errors. *Keratomileusis*, derived through Spanish from Greek words meaning 'cornea' and 'carving' *(mileusis)*, incorporates a lamellar section of the patient's own cornea layer in either a positive or negative fashion and used to correct either myopic or hyperopic refractive errors. *Keratophakia* is a surgical alteration of the alteration of the anterior radius of curvature of the cornea in which a positive lenticule *(phakos)* is cut from a fresh donor cornea and is incorporated within the patient's corneal stroma. This is presently being used to eliminate aphakic and hyperopic refractive errors. *Radial keratotomy* is a surgical procedure in which clocklike incisions are made into the cornea to flatten the cornea and correct myopic refractive errors. *Epikeratophakia* is a procedure designed and popularized by Kaufman and his co-workers in which a lenticule of donor cornea is sutured at the margins to a patient's cornea that is denuded for epithelium. *Keratoprosthesis* is an artificial synthetic cor-

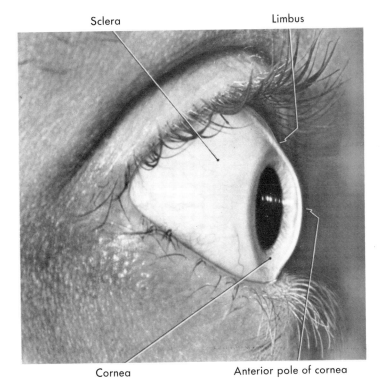

Sclera   Limbus

Cornea   Anterior pole of cornea

Fig. 1-20. The eye in side profile. (Courtesy Eastman Kodak Co., Rochester, N.Y.)

nea, which is implanted into the corneal substance for visual rehabilitation in severely scarred corneas in almost blind eyes. It is usually of a plastic material.

A surgical instrument used to open the anterior chamber by cutting the cornea is called a *keratome*, from *tomos* meaning 'a cutting.'

The *limbus* is the annular border between the clear cornea and the opaque scleral conjunctival area. Other anatomic areas of interest are depicted in Fig. 1-20.

Eyelids

The globe is covered externally by the eyelids to protect it from injury and excessive light and to spread a thin film of tears over the cornea. From *blepharo-*, Greek meaning 'eyelid,' we derive words such as *blepharoplasty*, referring to any plastic surgery performed on the

eyelid, and *blepharoptosis*, drooping eyelids. The muscle that elevates the eyelid is the *levator palpebrae superioris*, from Latin *levator*, 'one that raises,' *palpebra*, 'eyelid,' and *superioris*, 'upper.' The triangular spaces at the junction of the upper and lower lids are called *canthi* from Greek *kanthos*, meaning 'angle' (Fig. 1-21). These canthi are denoted by the terms *medial* or *lateral*, the former being close to the nasal bridge because it is toward the 'middle' of the head. A surgical procedure to correct defects in the canthus is called *canthoplasty*. To open the angle, the procedure of *canthotomy* is performed.

In the medial angle of the eyelids the *caruncle*, from Latin meaning 'little piece of flesh,' because this is a fleshy mound on the eye (Fig. 1-22). Adjacent to it lies a fold, the *plica semilunaris* from Latin *plica*, 'a fold' and *semilu-*

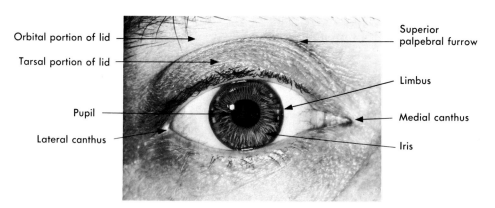

Orbital portion of lid
Tarsal portion of lid
Pupil
Lateral canthus

Superior palpebral furrow
Limbus
Medial canthus
Iris

Fig. 1-21. Surface anatomy of the eye. (From Stein, H.A., and Slatt, B.J.: The ophthalmic assistant, ed. 4, St. Louis, 1983, The C.V. Mosby Co.)

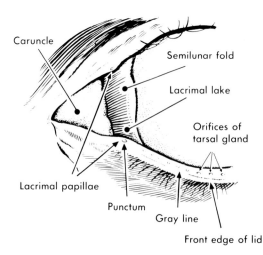

Caruncle
Semilunar fold
Lacrimal lake
Orifices of tarsal gland
Lacrimal papillae
Punctum
Gray line
Front edge of lid

Fig. 1-22. Inner canthus, showing the semilunar fold and the caruncle. Normally the punctum is not visible unless the lower lid is depressed. (From Stein, H.A., and Slatt, B.J.: The ophthalmic assistant, ed. 4, St. Louis, 1983, The C.V. Mosby Co.)

naris, 'half-moon shaped,' because the tissue is folded over like a half-moon and was originally a remnant of the third eyelid as found in lower animals.

The eyelids have as part of their structure hard plates called *tarsi* from Greek *tarsos,* a term used by the ancient Greeks for a wicker-work frame or various flattened objects such as a flat basket, the sole of a foot, the rudder of a ship, the blades of oars, the stretched-out wing, and edge of the eyelid. Because of the flatness of the eyelid, the term *tarsus* was applied to the fibrocartilaginous plate that is found in the eyelid, both upper and lower.

Within the tarsal plate of the eyelid lie the *meibomian glands* named after Heinrich Meibom (1638-1700), who published the first accurate description of these secreting glands. A disorder of the glands gives rise to a *chalazion,* a word derived from Greek meaning 'little lump' or 'little hailstone' because of the similarity of this lump in the eyelid to the appearance of a hailstone.

Oxygen studies

Terminology pertaining to oxygen studies have taken an increasing importance in the contact lens literature because of the development of extended wear lenses and gas-permeable contact lenses. Investigators such as Miguel Refojo, Irving Fatt, Robert Mandell, and Richard Hill have contributed significantly to our understanding in this area.

The oxygen transmission through a given material is a laboratory measurement, often referred to as the *DK value,* where D is the diffusion coefficient for oxygen movement in lens material and K is the solubility coefficient of oxygen in the material. It should be noted that a coefficient is a measure of a physical or chemical property that is constant for a system under specific conditions. The DK, or permeability, is characteristic of a given material obtained in a given condition at a given temperature in the laboratory only. The *oxygen flux* is the amount of oxygen that will pass through a given area of the material in a given amount of time driven by a given partial pressure difference of oxygen across the material. It is a function of the DK of the material, the lens thickness, and the pressure drop across the lens, ΔP.

$$\text{Oxygen flux} = \left(\frac{DK}{L}\right)\Delta P$$

L is the thickness of the central optical zone.
D is the diffusion coefficient for oxygen movement.
K is the solubility of oxygen in that material.
Low-flux materials. PMMA, HEMA, CAB, and some gas-permeable PMMA lenses.
Medium-flux plastics. Hard silicone, ultra-thin or high-water-content hydrogels, silicone-organic, copolymers.
High-flux materials. Pure silicone resins and elastomers, very high-water-content hydrogels.

When a lens is made thinner, more oxygen will pass through the material and so thickness becomes an important aspect of lens performance. The term *oxygen transmissibility* is used to indicate the oxygen permeability (DK) divided by the thickness of the lens, L, so that

$$DK/L = \text{oxygen transmissibility}$$

Of more meaningful and clinical importance is how much total oxygen passes through a lens and is permitted to reach the cornea. There are in vivo (in the living body) measurements. They involve the total lens and take into account not only the material but also the design of the lens. This measurement is called the EOP, or *equivalent oxygen performance.*

Comment. Water content alone does not ensure a high equivalent oxygen performance.

GLOSSARY

The following glossary provides some additional definitions and terms arranged alphabetically.

A

annular bifocal contact: a lens with distance portion ground into the center of the lens and near ground into the periphery.
anoxia: a diminished supply of oxygen.
aphakic lenses: lenses designed for postcataract fitting.
apical zone of cornea: area of the central portion of the cornea with a constant radius of curvature. Sometimes called the corneal cap.
artificial tears: wetting agents for the cornea to supplement the loss of tear formation (methylcellulose, Liquifilm, and so on).
aspheric lens: a continuous lens with an elliptic shape that has a peripheral curvature flatter than usual.

B

bactericide: a chemical that disinfects and kills pathogenic organisms.

benzalkonium chloride: a preservative used in contact lens solutions because of its germicidal qualities.

biomicroscopy: microscopic examination of the cornea, anterior chamber lens, and posterior chamber contents with a slitlamp (biomicroscope). The magnification is approximately 10 to 50 times.

bullous keratopathy: total swelling of the cornea with painful blister formation at the epithelial level; treated frequently with a therapeutic soft lens.

Burton lamp: an ultraviolet light used to excite the fluorescein dye that is used to analyze the fit of a rigid contact lens.

BUT: see *tear film breakup time* (BUT).

C

chord length: the straight-line measurement of the contact-lens diameter from edge to edge, distinguished from the slightly larger linear measurement of surface curvature.

chlorhexidine: a chemical used for disinfection.

chlorobutanol: an antimicrobial agent used in soaking solutions.

circumcorneal indentation: circular depression caused by lens (Fig. 1-23).

circumcorneal injection: redness around the limbus of the eyes surrounding the cornea (Fig. 1-23).

conjunctivitis, giant papillary: see *giant papillary hypertrophy* (GPH).

contact lens blank: a sheet or rod of plastic, which can be methylmethacrylate or hydroxyethylmethacrylate, used to make either hard or soft lenses.

contact lens wetting angle: the angle between the liquid and lens surface.

contour lens: a tricurve lens designed to conform to the curvature of the cornea, which flattens as it extends in the periphery.

copolymer: two or more chemicals that are combined to form a new chemical compound.

corneal cap: the apical zone or central zone of the cornea that has a constant area of curvature.

corneal diameter: the diameter of the cornea, usually taken along the horizontal meridian with a ruler, caliper, or reticule; see also *visible iris diameter*.

corneal edema: swelling of the cornea caused by hypoxia or insufficient oxygen.

D

dehydration: the drying out of a soft lens.

deturgescence, corneal: the state of relative dehydration maintained by the normal intact cornea that enables it to remain transparent.

diagnostic fitting set: a limited set of trial lenses used to gain a dynamic overview of the fit of a contact lens.

discoloration: a change in color of a contact lens.

disinfection: physical or chemical procedures that kill common pathogenic organisms but may permit some nonpathogenic organisms to survive.

DK value: a measure of the oxygen permeability through a given material where D is the diffusion coefficient for oxygen movement in the lens material and K is the solubility of oxygen in this material.

double slab-off lenses: sometimes called thick-thin lenses; the upper and lower portions of the lens

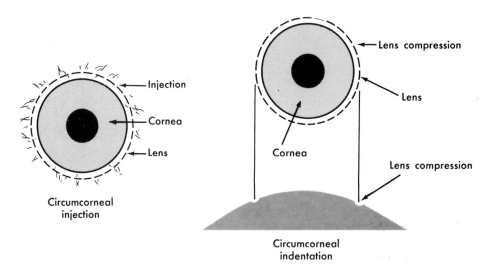

Fig. 1-23. Circumcorneal injection and circumcorneal indentation at the limbus. Notice considerable vascularity. (From Stein, H.A., and Slatt, B.J.: The ophthalmic assistant, ed. 4, St. Louis, 1983, The C.V. Mosby Co.)

are reduced in thickness so that when the lens is placed on the eye these portions lie under the upper and lower eyelids. The thin zones aid in stabilizing toric soft lenses.

dry spots: areas of drying as noted by absent areas of fluorescein-stained tear film on the cornea when the patient stares.

Dyer nomogram system of lens ordering: a simplified system of ordering rigid lenses based on clinical experience, corneal topogometry, and charts of associated lens parameters.

E

EDTA: see *ethylenediamine tetraacetate.*

elasticity: the ability of a lens to stretch and return to the same configuration; lens memory.

endophthalmitis: an inflammation of the entire eye including the outer coats.

enzyme cleaner: a cleaning agent that acts on a soft lens by a digestion of protein.

epithelial edema: edema of the superficial layer of the cornea.

esthesiometer (Cochet-Bonnet): a device used to evaluate corneal sensitivity, consisting essentially of a nylon thread mounted in a handle so that its length may be varied and calibrated in milligrams of weight necessary to bend a given length of the thread when pressed against the cornea.

ethylenediamine tetraacetate: a chemical used for disinfection.

eversion of the eyelid: the folding back of the eyelid on itself.

F

finished lens: a complete lens with anterior and posterior curves, a specified diameter, a designated peripheral curve, and edge design.

fitting set: a complete inventory of lenses of graduated powers and base curves.

flare: flutterings or fringing of lights, caused by a lens with an optic zone too small, a decentered lens, or an excessively loose lens.

flat cornea: a cornea with a K value less than 41 D.

fluid lens: power created by having a very convex or concave tear film; in most cases the power of the tear film is negligible because this layer is too thin (less than 0.02 mm) to have an appreciable effect on the power of the lens.

fluorescein: an organic compound that is inert and used to stain the tear film for contact lens fitting and to assess the integrity of the cornea.

G

galilean telescope: telescope with a minus ocular lens combined with a plus objective lens.

germicide: a chemical used for disinfection, such as chlorhexidine.

giant papillary hypertrophy (GPH): large elevated papules on the tarsal conjunctiva. Usually associated with soft lens wear but can occur with any contact lens. It is regarded as an autoimmune response to the patient's own protein. Also referred to as giant papillary conjunctivitis (GPC).

GPH: see *giant papillary hypertrophy.*

H

haptic: the part of a contact or intraocular lens that supports the optic portion and touches the peripheral or nonoptic portion of the cornea; the word indicates 'fastening, contact, sense of touch.'

Harrison-Stein nomogram: a series of lens specifications for prescribing a gas-permeable contact lens from silicone-PMMA material.

hydrogen peroxide: a bactericide used for soft lenses.

hypoxia: low in oxygen.

hysteresis: phenomenon in which a lens when subjected to stress slowly changes its form.

K

keratitis: inflammation of the cornea.

keratoconjunctivitis sicca: drying of the cornea and conjunctiva.

keratomalacia: softening of the cornea.

Korb lens: a PMMA lens that is fitted in a position on the superior portion of the cornea, regardless of weight or power, and designed to move vertically over the cornea when blinking as if attached to the upper eyelid.

L

LD + 2: the longest diameter (LD) of the optic zone plus 2 mm (for the intermediate and peripheral curves) yields the diameter of a lens; determined by use of the topogometer.

lenticular lens: relatively large lens most suitable for large, flat eyes; consists of a central optic zone and a surrounding nonoptic flange.

limbal zone: junction between the periphery of the cornea with the sclera.

loose lens: a contact lens with excessive movement; it can be caused by a lens that is too small in diameter, too thick, or too flat.

M

magnification: the ratio of image size to object size.

methylcellulose: a wetting agent.

microthin lens: a lens less than 0.10 mm in thickness.

minus carrier: a lens designed with an edge configuration similar to that of a minus lens that is thicker at its periphery; often used with high-plus lenses such as aphakic lenses.

monovision: single-vision contact lenses used for presbyopic people for whom the power of the lenses is such that one eye is used for distance vision and the other is used for near vision.

Morgan's dots: small discrete subepithelial corneal opacities resulting from corneal hypoxia.

N

nomogram: a table of precalculated mathematical values used to arrive at the specifications of a rigid lens design.

O

orthokeratology: the technique of flattening the cornea and thus correcting refractive errors by the use of a series of progressively flatter contact lenses.

overwearing syndrome: a misnomer for acute corneal hypoxia characterized by a latent interval after removal of the lens; extreme pain and congestion of lids, cornea, and conjunctiva are experienced. It is more common with rigid lenses.

oxygen flux: a measure of the amount of oxygen that will pass through a given area of material in a given unit of time.

oxygen permeability: the degree to which a lens permits the passage of oxygen across it. It depends on composition of the plastic (that is, silicone has excellent permeability, whereas PMMA has no permeability), the thickness of the lens, and its water content. It is often expressed as the DK value.

P

pachometer, pachymeter: an instrument used to measure the thickness of the cornea and depth of the anterior chamber; the spelling "pachometer" is etymologically preferable to "pachymeter," a frequent usage.

photokeratoscope: an instrument designed to photograph annular rings of the cornea and to aid in making a contact lens that will contour to the cornea. The data are often fed to a computer for a readout for a lens design.

photophobia: sensitivity to light.

Placido's disc: a disc with concentric rings to determine the regularity of the cornea when its reflection is revealed on the corneal surface.

plano lens: a lens with zero power.

polymer: a chain of linked molecular units of dimension greater than 5 monomer units.

polymerization: the union of molecules of a compound to form larger molecules and a new compound.

polyvinyl alcohol: a wetting agent.

polyvinylpyrrolidone (PVP): a polymer often copolymerized with other plastics in hydrogel lenses.

prism ballast lens: contact lens with based-down prism added inferiorly to improve the stability of the lens. Usually 1 to 1.5 D of prism is added.

PVP: see *polyvinylpyrrolidone.*

R

residual astigmatism: the astigmatism present after the corneal astigmatism has been nullified by a contact lens. It is the astigmatism usually created by the lens of the eye.

retroillumination: light is focused on deeper structures such as the iris, while the microscope is adjusted to study the cornea; best method of showing fine corneal edema.

S

Schirmer test: measures normal tear secretion; the ability of the eye to wet in 5 minutes 15 mm of a 5 × 35 mm strip of filter paper.

scratched lens: a defect in the lens surface consisting of a groove and ridge.

semifinished blank: a contact lens blank in which the posterior curve of the contact lens has been fabricated.

semifinished lens: a polished lens with an anterior and a posterior curvature.

soaking solution: a solution designed to keep a lens moist and free from contamination.

Soper lens: a rigid lens designed by Joseph Soper with a steep central posterior curve to accommodate large cones of keratoconus (Fig. 1-24).

spectacle blur: blurred vision that lasts for 30 minutes or longer after a rigid lens is removed and spectacles are employed.

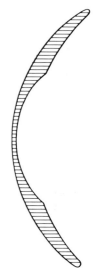

Fig. 1-24. Soper cone lens for keratoconus. There is a steep central posterior curve and a much flatter flange surrounding it. (From Stein, H.A., and Slatt, B.J.: The ophthalmic assistant, ed. 4, St. Louis, 1983, The C.V. Mosby Co.)

specular reflection: a reflection from a mirror surface, such as the back of the cornea.

spheric equivalent: It is the spheric power of the lens plus half the cylindric power. It represents the dioptric power of a cylindric or spherocylindric lens from the vertex to the plane of the circle of least confusion (the midpoint of the interval of Sturm).

SPK: see *superficial punctate keratitis.*

stable vision: visual acuity that does not fluctuate.

sterilization: a method to ensure the complete death of all forms of bacteria, fungi, and spores.

stippling: dotlike staining of the cornea.

superficial punctate keratitis (SPK): diffuse stippling of the cornea.

surfactant: a cleaner that acts on the surface of a contact lens.

T

taco test: a test whereby one can determine that a soft contact lens is not inside out by grasping the lens near its apex and folding it so that the edge will roll in like a Mexican taco if it is not everted. The test is not effective with ultrathin hydrogel lenses.

tear film breakup time (BUT): an evaluation of tear

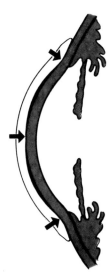

Fig. 1-25. Three-point touch—a normally fitting soft lens will rest lightly at the apex and at the periphery of the cornea.

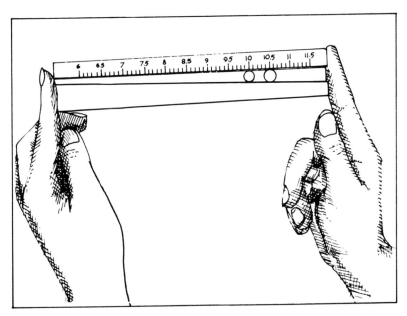

Fig. 1-26. V-groove diameter gauge. The lens is inserted at the widest opening and allowed to slide to its position of rest, where the diameter reading is obtained.

quality; the tear film will normally break up in 10 to 30 seconds and show dry spots. Any dry spot that appears in less than 10 seconds is pathologic.

tears: a composite of secretions from lacrimal glands, accessory glands of Kraus and Wolfring, mucin-secreting goblet cells of the conjunctiva, meibomian-secreting tarsal glands, and oil-secreting glands of Teis.

thermal disinfection: disinfection of a lens by heat.

thickness of a lens: the measurement of the center of a lens; a variable that depends on the posterior vertex power, the central base curve, the index of refraction of the lens material, and the lens diameter.

thimerosal (Merthiolate): a mercurial agent used for disinfection.

three and nine o'clock staining: erosion of the cornea at the 3 and 9 o'clock position; seen usually in patients wearing rigid lenses.

three-point touch: a lens that rests on the sclera and on the center of the cornea (Fig. 1-25).

tight lens: a lens that has minimal or no movement.

transitional zone: that area of the cornea between the apical zone and the limbal zone.

Trantas's dots: small peripheral limbal infiltrations caused by delayed hypersensitivity, as seen in vernal conjunctivitis.

truncation: a design feature used in toric lenses to reduce lens rotation by the cutting off of a peripheral portion of the lens to conform with the lower lid border.

U

ulceration of the cornea: a large defect in the cornea which may be caused by hypoxia, trauma, or infection.

V

V-groove gauge: a ruler measure with a groove to measure the diameter of a rigid lens (Fig. 1-26).

vascularization: increased blood vessels occurring in a cornea.

VID: see *visible iris diameter.*

visible iris diameter (VID): a term that represents the iris diameter and aids in selecting the initial lens; often used in place of the corneal diameter.

W

warpage: a permanent bending of a rigid lens. May also refer to a semipermanent altering of the corneal curvature.

wet storage: the use of soaking solution to store rigid contact lenses.

wetting solution: solutions that increase the spreading or wettability of liquids on the plastic contact lens by converting the surface of a lens from a hydrophobic to a hydrophilic surface.

X

X-CHROM lens: a red contact lens designed to aid the person with partial red-green color blindness.

xerophthalmia: a state of dryness of the eyes; conjunctivitis with atrophy and absent fluid discharge that produces a dry, lusterless condition of the eyeball.

xerosis: dying and keratinization of the tissues, usually the conjunctiva, seen most clearly when stained with rose bengal stain.

PATIENT SELECTION: FINDING THE RIGHT LENS FOR THE RIGHT PATIENT

Currently there is an extraordinarily large number of types of contact lenses. In addition to the now classic rigid (PMMA) lenses and hydrogel (soft) lenses, there are gas-permeable lenses made with the addition of silicone (polyorganosiloxane), called the silicone acrylates, silicone resins, silicone elastomers, and cellulose acetate butyrate and styrene derivatives.

New soft lens designs have also increased. There are soft lenses for the presbyope, toric lenses for the astigmatic person, tinted lenses, and lenses that can be retained in the eye for over 24 hours without removal (extended-wear lenses). With this variety, the choice becomes more difficult. Soft lens usage, which grew exponentially during the 1970s at the expense of the hard lens, is now being challenged by the gas-permeable rigid lenses.

The patient must be fitted with the appropriate lens. The question of which lens to choose is perhaps the fitter's most important decision. Does one go for the short-term reward and choose a soft lens because it meets with early and rapid patient acceptance or does one consider a rigid gas-permeable lens, which may over the years be superior in the long term? Questions to be answered in this chapter include the following:

Is the PMMA hard lens obsolete?
Do the newer soft lens designs and materials yield satisfactory visual performance?
Is gas permeability a feature that should be part of any lens—rigid or soft?
Which lenses are more likely to get dislodged from the eye, spoiled, or damaged?
Are contact lenses dangerous in some occupations?

SAFETY OF CONTACT LENSES

Safety is a most important consideration. A properly fitting individually biocompatible contact lens should not cause any damage to the cornea regardless of the lens choice. However, in the real world there are many instances of transient corneal damage ranging from induced acute hypoxia to corneal abrasions. Loss of corneal regularity, asymmetric astigmatism, corneal vascularization, and endophthalmitis have been previously reported with rigid and soft lenses.

Many occupations preclude the wearing of any type of contact lens. These involve welders, miners, construction workers, and people engaged in sand blasting or drilling. These are jobs in which the environment is inimical to the integrity of the cornea because of radiation, dust, high-velocity foreign bodies, vapors, or fumes.

The patient's hands may offer clues for their suitability for lenses. Many workers such as plumbers, furniture dyers, and automobile mechanics never get their hands clean. Their hands, palms, and nails at the best of times are etched with dirt and oil. The skin is tough and hard and could not ever handle a lens without damaging or contaminating it.

A patient with poor hygiene is a poor candidate. In most studies, the lack of hygiene by the patient has been the most common factor in injury to the eye by a contact lens. If the patient's teeth, hands, and face are dirty or his hair is unkempt, one can assume that the lenses will be carelessly maintained. A rigid lens can injure a cornea by either causing mechanical compression or creating erosions because of hypoxia. If the lens is contaminated, a portal of entry allows bacteria to penetrate the cornea and create a corneal ulcer or secondary iritis. The most common sources of contamination are dirty hands, wet, dirty cases, which permit *Pseudomonas aeruginosa* to grow, and the use of saliva as a wetting agent. These accidents are common. In 1 year, approximately 8000 eyes were damaged from improper rigid lens wear. Ninety percent of the damage was reversible, but there was some severe sequelae including total loss of the eye.

A soft lens cannot damage the cornea by abrasion because of its supple nature. However, it has a tendency to collect protein from the tear film. This protein is an excellent culture medium. Bacteria grow well on a lens coated with protein. It is particularly common to see these protein-based infections with aphakic soft lenses and extended wear lenses. Corneal ulcers and endophthalmitis have been shown to occur with the improper use of soft lenses.

In aphakic people the tears are not so abundant as with younger people, and so protein deposition is more likely to occur. Also, the decrease in the amount of lysozyme, a normal antibacterial enzyme in tears, raises the possibility of infections in people with a depleted tear function. In the elderly, because of changes in tear composition, there may be an increase in mineralization of the lens.

PATIENT SELECTION

The cosmetic lens patient with a healthy eye and intact adequate tear film has a 90% chance of being successfully fit with a contact lens (in regard to the full spectrum of lens designs, materials, and support systems). Patients with the best prognosis for successful fitting are those who fit the following criteria:

Best age group, 13 to 38 years of age.
Women > men.
Refractive error, > -1.50 D, > $+1.50$ D.
K reading, 41.00 to 46.00 D.
BUT's > 15 seconds.
Cornea with no significant sequential staining.
Good tear flow by Sherman test.
Regular corneas—no scarring or distortion of corneal mires.
Regular low astigmatism, < $+1.50$ D.
Good lid position with no scleral show.
Adequate manual dexterity.

Those patients with a reduced prognosis for successful fitting are the following:

Those who are going on a trip and need a lens in 7 days. Do not oblige unless you are prepared to handle an emergency call from Bermuda. In addition, this could be construed as professional negligence, since it is not ideally in the patient's best interest.
Smokers, who use pipes, cigars, or cigarettes.
Sloppy and careless persons.
Those who are chronically anxious or under anxiety during the time of the contact lens fit.
Those myopic patients who are about to become presbyopic.
Those who are poorly motivated:
  Spouse wants him or her to wear lenses
  Purchaser of a "party lens"
Those who have small refractive errors, less than -1.25 diopters.
Those who incur occupational hazards, such as hair dressers, truck drivers, mail carriers, factory workers in chemical environments.
Those with excessive fears, such as being terrified of having anything touch their eyes.
Patients with strabismus or ptosis because a contact lens may make them look worse.
Those with ocular allergies, chronic blepharitis, arthritis, and exophthalmos.
Those who work or live in an acid- or alkaline-fume environment.
Avoid the 5 D's—the dirty, the drunk, the diseased, the disabled, the dumb.

Medical factors that may reduce probability of wearing contact lenses

Skin disease. These particularly include seborrhea, psoriasis, and neurodermatitis, as well as chronic blepharitis from any atopic skin conditions. Swollen, inflamed lid margins significantly reduce progress for good patient comfort. The threshold for discomfort will be lower, and the debris from the lids will act as an irritant. In addition, the meibomian gland secretions become abnormal, thus affecting the stability of the tear film. The lens may be greasy and filmy, covered by sebaceous discharge from the irritated meibomian glands.

Dry eyes. This syndrome may include either individual dry spots or combinations of them on the cornea, aqueous deficiency, mucin deficiency, lipid deficiency, and extreme xerosis with conspicuous erosions of the cornea.

A Schirmer test should be done on each patient; the cornea should be observed for dry spots and a rose bengal test done to illustrate devitalized tissue.

Systemic drugs. Drugs for gastric ulcers (atropine-like drugs) may reduce tear flow and artificially create dry spots. Birth control pills may cause rigid lenses to be intolerable and soft lenses to be rapidly covered with protein debris. Diazepam (Valium) and other tranquilizers have no direct effect on the cornea or tear film. But anxious patients requiring medication of this nature may be difficult to fit.

Handling problems. Usually problems with handling are obvious. Patients with arthritis of the hands, a parkinsonian-like tremor, and psoriasis of skin or nails make poor contact lens candidates. However, patients with dirty fingernails should also be rejected. The most common cause of corneal ulcers with soft lens wearers is poor hygiene, specifically dirty lens cases that grow *Pseudomonas aeruginosa*.

Corneal disease. Recurrent corneal erosion, corneal dystrophy of any kind, corneal scarring with dry spots of the cornea, old vernal conjunctivitis or trachoma, and any disease that results in a vascularized cornea may contraindicate wearing contact lenses.

Allergies. Lesions of the limbus such as dermoid cysts may require surgical removal before lens wear (Fig. 2-1). A history of hay fever, drug reaction, or atopic skin reactions to cosmetics or perfumes may be a warning to a later sensitivity to preservatives in contact lens solutions or the formation of giant papillary conjunctivitis. Allergic reactions to the plastics of a contact lens have not been proved to be a factor in these atopic reactions.

Corneal warpage and corneal anesthesia. Some PMMA rigid lens wearers may develop corneal warpage because of corneal hypoxia. Before the development of the gas-permeable lenses, the fitter usually required the patient to abstain from wearing contact lenses until the warpage was corrected. The newer lenses make this abstinence period unnecessary because one can fit with gas-permeable lenses and provide functional restoration of vision while the keratometric mires are restored to their baseline measurements.

A patient may have 20/20 vision, comfort, and total freedom of any symptoms and still develop a toric cornea. Look at the cornea at least once a year without the lenses to ensure that an induced toricity has not occurred.

PMMA lenses usually will result in corneal desensitization. There is a linear relationship with wear. The sensitivity may be measured with the Cochet-Bonnet hair test (Fig. 2-2).

The monocular patient. The monocular patient should be treated with special concern. If the patient is a monocular lens wearer, that is, aphakia or anisometropia prevails, the person must be drilled about the ocular emergencies that can arise. A corneal abrasion in a monocular patient is a blinding event.

Pregnancy and menopause. Pregnancy, menopause, and birth-control medication cause a disruption in the normal hormonal balance. The sequelae are poorly understood, but the quality of the tear film and the integrity of the cornea is possibly altered during these states. Rigid lenses are rejected more easily than soft lenses, and it is certainly inadvisable to begin lens wearing during an endocrine flux.

Comment. We have observed a greater tendency for protein deposition on soft lenses during pregnancy and during the lactation period.

Diabetes. Stable diabetes may be fitted with contact lenses. Unstable diabetes, which are mainly juvenile in grouping, should not be fitted. With a volatile blood glucose, a stable refraction may be difficult to obtain. If a lens must be worn for optic purposes, a soft lens should be chosen.

Thyroid disease with exophthalmos. Only a soft lens should be considered because the retracted upper and lower lid will dislodge a smaller, rigid lens. However, even a soft lens may create variable vision if the blink rate is infrequent and the excursions of the lid are incomplete. Drying of the lens may occur, and the lens may become proteinized (Fig. 2-3).

Comment. Before fitting any thyroid patient, make sure the lids cover the cornea with light lid closure during blinking and sleep.

If there are dry spots of the cornea or inferior keratitis from exposure, a low-water-content soft lens may be attempted, supplemented with additional artificial tears. Low-water-content lenses create less water demand from the cornea than high-water-content lenses do and appear to perform better for dry eyes, but in dry environments the opposite is true.

These patients should be followed closely because 30% in our hands do poorly whatever lens or method is chosen. Contact lenses tend

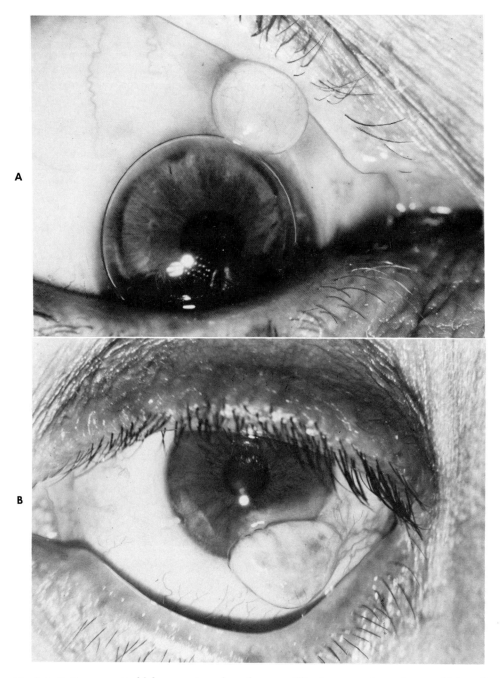

Fig. 2-1. A, Large cystic bleb occurring after glaucoma filtration procedure that would interfere with contact lens movement. **B,** Large limbal dermoid that should be surgically removed to permit the wearing of a contact lens.

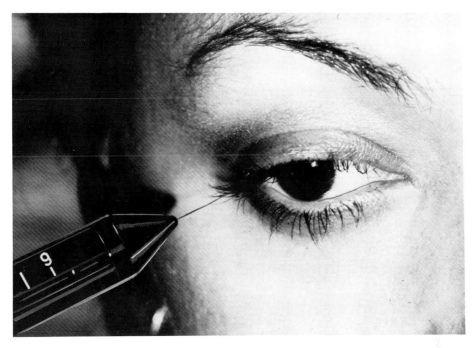

Fig. 2-2. The Cochet-Bonnet hair test for corneal sensitivity. Corneal sensation may decrease with oxygen deprivation after long-term use of rigid lenses that do not permit sufficient oxygen transfer.

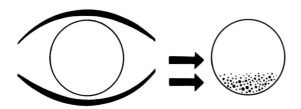

Fig. 2-3. Thyroid disease with exophthalmos. Incomplete blinking results in inferior keratopathy or drying of the surface of a soft contact lens because of exposure.

to dry because of incomplete or infrequent blinking.

Special indications

Nystagmus. Patients with congenital grade III nystagmus in which the eyes are oscillating all the time and patients with a significant refractive error with any congenital nystagmus may profit from contact lenses because the lenses move with the eye. Contact lenses may significantly improve visual acuity and also result in the lowering of the degree and amplitude of nystagmus.

Ocular albinism. A cosmetic contact lens with clear aperture but darkly tinted in the periphery may be very helpful against the glare effects that an albino suffers. The improvement in visual acuity is minimal because of the foveal aplasia found in this condition.

Aniridia. Most patients with aniridia have cataracts, gross nystagmus, and foveal aplasia. They are much more comfortable with tinted cosmetic contact lenses because they lack any iris development.

Previously fitted patient. It is always a challenge to fit a person who has failed in the past to wear lenses. However, the new fitter should attempt to obtain the history of the previous fits. It may conserve time because the same errors do not have to be repeated and it might yield some insight into the patient's personality and problems. A refitting may require only a change of solutions. Check the patient's method of handling, use of cleaners, and storage and rinsing solutions. If the problem is corneal edema go to a gas-permeable lens, rigid or soft. Try to solve the problem. It can be the fit, an inappropriate lens design, the wrong choice of plastics, or poor quality control from the laboratory. Resolve the technical problems before you attribute the poor fit to a lack of patient resolve.

Comment. Never speak in a derogatory way about another or previous fitter. The total circumstance may not be known, and the criticism may be unfair. Also, no one has complete success with all patients. Everyone can make an error or omission.

Psychiatric illness. The frequency of anxiety cannot be accurately gauged because there is no serum factor to reveal its presence. Seriously ill people are frequently on medications to control anxiety, depression, or manic-depressive states. Patients with psychiatric distress should be screened but not necessarily discouraged from wearing lenses. If contact lenses can significantly improve their vision or cosmetic appearance, the benefits to the patient must be assessed individually. If the mental health of the person is so marginal that the physician has to be concerned over the hygiene and consistency to regulations of contact lens care, this type of individual should be ruled out as a candidate.

In many instances, the distress of a person may be temporary and the fittings should be postponed. Postpartum depression, depression after a death of a spouse or after a divorce, anxiety about a new job or before examinations at school, or financial pressures may cause a temporary lowering of threshold to pain.

It is not within the scope of an ophthalmologist to ferret out a valid psychiatric assessment. But there are features to lend suspicion to a given case: history of taking mood-elevating or -depressing drugs; a history of admittance to a psychiatric institution; a desire to wear contact lenses that are perceived to be unreasonable; a person with a low refractive error -0.75 sphere and who barely uses spectacles; or a person who will not or cannot submit to an applanation tonometer test, a Schirmer test, or even a proper slitlamp examination. Such a person will show excessive blepharospasm or light sensitivity. Also any person who has unrealistic attitudes toward wearing lenses, such as a person who wants an extended wear lens because they are so easy to wear and require a cleaning only twice a year.

Comment. It is important to note that the initial wearing of contact lenses may be anxiety ridden. Many patients fear their dexterity will not be sufficient to get the lenses in or out, or the lenses will become trapped in or on the eye, or the pain will be excessive, or they are endeavoring to do something that can cause permanent damage to their eyes. These people are normal and rational and show the same fear as a novice skier who looking down from a hill asks himself, "Will I make it or not?" This is normal self-doubt. It is only when these normal, guarded feelings are excessive that a fitter has to be suspicious that he or she has embarked upon a task that will not be rewarding to both patient and physician.

RIGID LENS

The rigid PMMA lens still has a place in the contact lens fitter's armamentarium. It possesses the following qualities.

Durability. It is resistant to scratches and to breakage, especially at the edge; it does not become easily defaced with either lipids or protein adhering to its surface. As a result this lens lasts longer. Most types of PMMA lenses can be modified and blended, and their diameters can be reduced with office modification equipment. Surface scratches can be removed by polishing.

These durable lens features make them ideal starter lenses for high school students and teen-agers.

Comment. It is common to see rigid PMMA lenses survive 5 years or more, but rare for a soft lens.

High visual performance. The PMMA rigid lens and the gas-permeable rigid lens still offer the best visual performance (not necessarily true with toric corneas greater than 3.00 diopters when rigid PMMA lenses are used).

Good vision is constant and not subject to the variability of vision that often plagues the soft lens wearer. Qualitatively, the optics are better. Even though a rigid lens wearer and a soft lens wearer may achieve 20/20, the rigid lens wearer appears to "see better." Many rigid lens wearers who have been switched to soft lenses dislike the quality of soft lens vision, even though the visual numbers of both are 20/20. A reduction in contrast sensitivity is believed to be the factor for this discrepancy.

If vision is vital, a rigid lens with or without permeability may be the best choice. For architects, designers, and engineers, the rigid lens performance can be counted upon to give a consistent visual result.

Comment. Gas-permeable rigid lenses can cover up to 5 diopters of astigmatism when a large-diameter (>9.2 mm) spheric lens is used.

Ease in handling. For the bilateral aphake, a rigid lens may be the best choice. The aphakic person can feel the lens, a fact not true for one wearing a soft lens.

Lens removal is also easier for the aphakic person dealing with a rigid lens. One can remove the lens indirectly by using the lids or by a suction-cup device or in distress by a touch of honey on the fingertip.

Cost. Rigid lenses are less expensive than gas-permeable soft lenses, can be cleaned and polished easily, have a low maintenance cost, and can be modified in the office. Also rigid lenses last longer than other contact lenses and the replacement cost is less. On the other hand, a rigid lens is more likely to be lost because it is smaller, and it can be more readily dislodged from the eye because it is not a good lens when one is playing hockey.

Astigmatism correction. In lower spheric errors of refraction, a rigid lens is best. If the correction is -2.00 D $+1.00$ D $\times$ 90, a conventional soft lens will yield poor visual results. The ratio of cylinder to sphere should not be greater than 1:4 with an outside maximum of 1.50 diopters of astigmatism tolerated for a spheric soft lens.

Toric soft lenses are available, but they are more difficult to fit, do not give visual results comparable to a rigid lens, and are technically difficult in cases of oblique astigmatism or with patients with tight lids.

Gas-permeable lenses are very helpful with any kind of astigmatism, especially at high levels of 4 to 5 diopters, which can be covered with a spheric lens.

The PMMA lens has some serious faults. It has no permeability and can cause acute and chronic corneal hypoxia. It is the least comfortable lens and more prone to cause ocular irritation in the face of wind, sun, dust, and debris. It is inadequate for the poor blinker and the person who reads all day and whose blink rate deteriorates after hours of doing close work. The rigid lens is a tough lens for anyone who works outdoors. Finally, a PMMA lens in spheric form does not center well in conven-

tional diameters (7.8 to 8.2 mm) if significant corneal asigmatism is present (>2.00 diopters).

GAS-PERMEABLE LENS

Gas permeable lenses include the CAB lens, silicone-acrylate polymers, and polystyrene materials, and so on. These lenses do not depend entirely on blinking for oxygenation through the tear film because they transmit oxygen through the material itself to reach the cornea. Because of their oxygen permeability, they can be made larger, thus providing more stability and better centration. They can be made to rise high enough to allow the upper lid to cover the superior edge of the lens to prevent lid impact and blink inhibition. The ability of the lids to blink without engaging the upper edge of the lens also makes the lens more comfortable than any comparable PMMA lens.

A gas-permeable lens is preferred for the following situations.

Rigid lens dropouts. These people with either chronic corneal hypoxia or molding changes in the cornea induced by the wearing of a rigid lens can be *immediately fit* with gas-permeable lenses. The corneal edema will eventually disappear on wearing of such a lens. The old practice of wearing glasses until K readings stabilized or the refraction returned to normal is no longer necessary. The gas-permeable lens fills this void.

Keratoconus. The excellent optics of a gas-permeable lens and its ability to negate the effects of irregular corneal astigmatism make it the lens of choice for keratoconus.

The epithelium of the conic cornea is not likely to be healthy. It may be flattened, thinned, atrophic, or scarred. A gas-permeable lens provides sufficient oxygen to this atrophic layer of cells to keep it free of hypoxic complications.

Gas-permeable lenses require less frequent lens changes and are more comfortable for keratoconus patients. It should be the lens of choice. If it doesn't work, a soft lens carrier with a piggyback gas-permeable lens is the second best choice.

Comment. Gas permeability refers to physical properties of the plastic. Any lens design can be used.

Excessive spectacle blur. With gas-permeable lenses, spectacle blur is minimal because of

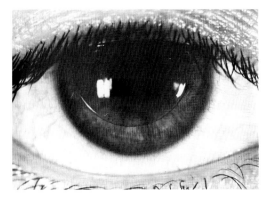

Fig. 2-4. The silicone-acrylate contact lens is gas permeable. It may be fitted larger than conventional rigid lenses. Notice that the upper eyelid margin is covering the upper portion of the contact lens. (From Stein, H.A., and Slatt, B.J.: The ophthalmic assistant, ed. 4, St. Louis, 1983, The C.V. Mosby Co.)

absence of central corneal hypoxia with resulting edema. With the patient who wants to read after the lenses have been removed for the night, this feature is very handy.

Comment. Spectacle blur caused by corneal edema is relieved with gas-permeable lenses. Spectacle blur caused by aberrations of a thick lens (about 6.00 D or greater) will not be altered with gas-permeable contact lenses.

Patients who are susceptible to flare. The optic zone of a standard PMMA lens is often too small to encompass the pupil. This is especially true for young blue-eyed myopic people with large pupils who drive in dim illumination. The small thin PMMA lenses are fitted tight but are not sufficient in size to counter the effects of a larger pupil.

The gas-permeable lens because of its larger size can have a larger optic zone than a PMMA lens has and is usually of sufficient size to eliminate flare, that is, the sunburst effect around a light.

Rigid lens discomfort. The gas-permeable lens is a remedy for people with rigid lens discomfort and who want rigid lens optics. (Fig. 2-4). The lens is more comfortable for several reasons.

The upper edge of the lens does not engage the upper lid.
The lens is stable and centers well.
The movement of the lens with blinking is less than that of a smaller PMMA rigid lens.

The cornea is well supplied with oxygen directly, and so the patient does not get burning of his eyes when the blink rate is likely to be reduced. This is likely to occur with prolonged reading, sewing, driving, and doing visual work that results in fatigue.

Soft lens dropouts. Some patients do not like a soft lens. The vision may not be crisp because of astigmatism, they may be more prone to giant papillary conjunctivitis, or they may not like the care systems of a soft lens.

The gas-permeable lens provides a good bridge to better vision.

SOFT LENS

A soft lens is preferred in the following situations and for the characteristics mentioned.

Rapid adaptation. A soft lens is recommended for people who require rapid adaptation; frequently a soft lens is comfortable 10 minutes after first being inserted and can be worn easily from the first day. Rapid adaptation is an important factor for people who are busy with work or study.

Comfort. For patients with a lowered threshold of discomfort, the soft lens is the only answer. Many who are rigid lens dropouts are quite content with soft lenses.

Low refractive errors. A soft lens is preferred for patients with low refractive errors of -1.50 diopters or less. With these persons the motivation to adapt to continuous daily wear of rigid lenses is not sufficient. As a result, the comfort of soft lenses combined with the ability to wear the lenses intermittently offers a distinct advantage.

Inability to wear rigid lenses. A soft lens is preferable for persons unable to wear rigid lenses for many reasons: (1) intolerance because of pregnancy, (2) a bad experience with an overwear reaction, (3) induced astigmatism and spectacle blur created by rigid lens corneal molding, (4) difficulty in maintaining a rigid wearing schedule, (5) excessive photophobia and glare, and (6) intolerance to sun, wind, and dust. A soft lens protects the eye and does not leave it vulnerable to exposure.

Athletes. Especially in body-contact sports such as hockey, basketball, and football a soft lens is less likely to be dislodged because it follows the eye closely on movement. In tennis the soft lens is less likely to drop when the eyes are raised for the serve, and in gymnastics the soft lens is less likely to pop out.

Safety. For the industrial worker who is working on dangerous machinery a soft lens is far less likely to be dislodged or decentered. The private pilot is better off with a soft lens, which is less likely to pop out of an eye or momentarily slide off the center of the eye.

Eye safety. The soft lens is less likely to cause a portal of entry in the cornea for bacteria or other pathogens by creating a cornea abrasion or ulcer. Corneal edema is minimal with an ill-fitting soft lens as compared to a hard lens.

Comment. Factory workers, patients who are working with chemicals, construction workers, furniture refinishers, and others are contraindicated for soft lens wear because of danger for toxic environmental vapors.

Children. Children who require contact lenses because of aniridia, amblyopia therapy, albinism, or congenital nystagmus should wear soft lenses. The soft lens is more comfortable and safer in these instances and, over the long haul, is less likely to abrade the eye. Also it is more suitable for sports or for play in a dusty atmosphere.

Swimming. There is less chance of loss in lake and pool water with a soft lens because the soft lens becomes hypotonic when exposed to ordinary water, and it forms a firm adherence to the cornea. The vision remains clear during swimming without the use of goggles. The effect of chlorine on the soft lens is minimal. It is important to splash water in the open eyes with contacts in place before swimming and not to remove the lenses for 30 minutes after swimming. Swimming in ocean water without masks or goggles is not recommended because of the high loss factor of the soft lenses in salt water. Also the lenses tend to become hypertonic and do not adhere to the cornea as they do in lake water.

Intermittent wear. Persons who wear contact lenses infrequently, such as public speakers, athletes, or actors, prefer a soft lens to a rigid lens. These individuals desire a lens only for social occasions, sports activities, or their work on stage. The soft lens can be used just for such purposes. The cornea adapts quickly to its presence and does not require a buildup of wearing time. Also, most soft lenses do not create significant corneal edema or spectacle blur, and as a result the shift back to glasses can be achieved smoothly and without any visual disability.

Nystagmus. Soft lenses may significantly improve vision in patients with nystagmus because the lens tracks with the eye of the patient. Vision is not distorted by the parallax effect that occurs when glasses are worn or by the disturbing movement of the rigid lens during blinking.

Wide palpebral fissures. In patients with thyroid disease or congenitally wide eyelids, the soft lens can be ordered in a larger size so that the margin of the lid is less likely to engage the edge of the lens.

COMMENT

As a practitioner you cannot select your patients, but you can select your lenses. Be realistic and flexible. If a patient has tight lids and oblique astigmatism and wants soft lenses, outline the pitfalls of such a choice. Do not let the patient dictate the lens you want to use. For sure, he or she will hold you responsible if the device does not work.

Also of importance is the quality control of the lenses. If a laboratory makes a poor gas-permeable lens with thick or fragile edges, it would be unadvisable to use them. Thick edges lead to lid gap, 3 to 9 o'clock staining, red eyes, symptoms of dryness, and an unhappy patient.

Patient selection is perhaps the most important aspect of effective successful contact lens fitting. The public perception of a given lens may be inaccurate; for example, soft lenses grow fungi when worn, rigid lenses are hard to wear, or gas-permeable lenses are semisoft. It is up to the fitter to educate the patients. It is most valuable to evert the eyelid and document for later comparison any changes in the tarsal plate before the lenses are shortened.

LENSES FOR SPECIAL SITUATIONS
Airline personnel

Commercial airlines generally frown upon the use of contact lenses for air-flight personnel, particularly the pilot and the copilot. Airline and commercial transport pilots are not allowed to wear lenses in case of a loss of lens from a windblast or from spontaneous ejection of the lenses. A soft lens can't be extruded easily, but it can be decentered or dehydrated in the dry environment of the plane's cabin. If vision was only momentarily lost, it would add risk to the safety of the plane and its crew and passengers. Also airplane air tends to be quite dry. When evaporation occurs, the soft lens loses its smooth contours and its surface becomes wavy.

At times exceptions are made and monocular aphakic pilots are allowed to wear a single contact lens.

Flight attendants are usually allowed to wear contact lenses if their unaided vision is 20/100. This proviso is added so that the attendant can function without contact lenses if need be. Anyone can get a foreign body under a lens from debris or a hard particle of mascara or whatever. The rule is wise. The other requirement is that the person must show an ability to wear the lenses for the duration of the flight intended.

Comment. Unfortunately, occasionally a contact lens scam occurs. Young men intent on being pilots have their eyes "normalized" by orthokeratology. The prospective pilot can pass the test and see 20/20 without glasses or contacts. He neglects telling anyone that he still needs a retainer lens to sustain his refractive status. We have seen a few cases of such a nature.

Athletes

Much has been said about the use of contact lenses for sports. They are certainly of value in tennis, squash, racquet ball, skiing, basketball, or football.

The contact lens offers no protection for the eye. If eye injury is a distinct possibility, eye guards must be used in addition to the contact lenses. Protection of this nature is mandatory for football, hockey, and squash where the incidence of ocular injury is high.

Most professional athletes are required to have a spare pair of lenses available in case of loss or displacement of lenses. The National Basketball Association frowns on 7-foot giants groping on the floor, feeling for a lost 8.5 mm lens.

Most eye professionals believe that the athlete is better served with contact lenses. Visual acuity for distance is better for the high myope, and the athlete does not have to endure restrictions of visual field and distortions of a thick lens system.

However, before becoming evangelic about the merits of contact lenses for athletes, let us remember that Reggie Jackson, Billie Jean King, and Arthur Ashe did quite well in their respective sports wearing spectacles.

Skiers at times can get epithelial edema while wearing their lenses. Because of the coldness of the environment, the oxygen needs of the corneal epithelium are low. The lenses feel quite comfortable. The tint on the lenses may make the skier feel well enough to go skiing without protective goggles. This can be a mistake because the skier may be exposed to an intense ultraviolet burn from the direct and reflected sun rays. Radiation burn from ultraviolet rays is still a hazard for the unprotected skier wearing tinted contact lenses.

Swimmers have to be careful with contact lenses. If swim goggles are used, they are rarely watertight and the lens may become dislodged or contaminated by the water.

Goggles for swimming do not handle the moisture well and "fog up."

Goggles do not offer protection against infection, inflammation, or decreased vision. They offer some protection against lens loss.

Lenses should not be worn for diving or water skiing because the risk of losing one's lenses are quite high.

PART II

BASIC FITTING:
AN APPROACH
TO LENS FITTING
FOR THE STUDENT
AND SMALL-VOLUME
FITTER

Soft lenses

CHAPTER 3

SOFT LENSES

CHARACTERISTICS, ADVANTAGES, AND DISADVANTAGES

There are two basic types of lenses considered to be soft lenses: (1) the hydrophilic (sometimes referred to as hydrogel) lens, which owes its softness to its ability to absorb and bind water, and (2) the silicone soft lens, which owes its softness to the intrinsic property of the rubbery material. The silicone lens is discussed under the heading "Advanced Fitting." In this chapter emphasis will be placed on the hydrophilic soft lenses, which have gained widespread popularity and are a readily available, reliable, and proved entity. Many comments, however, will apply to the silicone lens as well.

HISTORY

It is always interesting and informative to learn from the past, and so it is with soft hydrogel contact lenses, which have had a major impact in the world, not only for their correction of refractive errors for cosmetic purposes, but also for their contribution to the management of aphakia and the treatment of disease states of the eye by use of the bandage lens.

In 1960 two young New York lawyers established a company with a unique function of promoting patent exchanges between corporations. Their specialty was combing through the dusty corporate files for idle patents and setting up licensing agreements with other companies interested in putting the dormant ideas to use. They achieved a measure of success, and their clients included du Pont de Nemours, Chrysler Corporation, Swift & Co., and Thiocol Chemical Corporation.

In 1965 the men who had established the National Patent Development Corporation suddenly dissolved their patent law business. They had uncovered a patent with so many exciting possibilities that they decided to pick up a license themselves. In effect, they became their own client, squashing their role as middlemen.

The new material was a plastic, which they called "hydron." It was developed by Dr. Otto Wichterle, head of the Institute of Macromolecular Chemistry of the Czechoslovakian National Academy of Science and a leading expert on polymer chemistry, and by Dr. Drahoslav Lim. The new material appeared to be like other plastics in that it was a hard transparent substance that could be cut, ground, or molded into a variety of shapes. However, when placed in water or an aqueous solution, the tough, rigid plastic became soft and pliable. In the wet form it could be bent between the fingers until the edges met or could be easily turned inside out; yet it would snap back into its original shape quickly. When allowed to dry, the supple water-logged material became dry as a cornflake and crushed to a powdery dust if smashed. The substance was subjected to rigorous biologic tests and was found to be inert and fully compatible with human tissue. One of its spectacular properties was that although highly elastic when wet, it remained strong and able to hold its shape (Fig. 3-1).

The plastic is hydroxyethylmethacrylate (HEMA), a plastic polymer with the remarkable ability to absorb water molecules. Chemically, the polymer consists of a three-dimensional network of hydroxyethylmethacrylate chains cross-linked with ethylene glycol di-

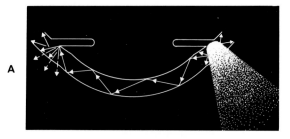

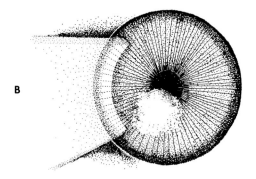

Fig. 3-1. A, Corneal edema can be detected grossly by angling the beam of the slitlamp 45 to 60 degrees at the limbus. **B,** Specular reflection. The internal reflection of light through the cornea makes the central edema stand out as a gray haze. The cornea is employed as a fiberoptic channel.

methacrylate molecules about once every 200 monomer units. As the water is introduced to the plastic, it swells into a soft mass with surprisingly good mechanical strength, complete transparency (97%), and the ability to retain its shape and dimensions when equilibrated in fluid.

Over the years, many modifications of the plastic were introduced, new polymers added, and new lens designs created. Five hard years of improvements and clinical trials were conducted on the soft lens before the Federal Drug Administration (which considered the lens a drug) approved the lens as a safe prosthetic device of good optic quality. The FDA's caution, after the thalidomide tragedies, was understandable. Both the public and the practitioner needed protection. In the first phase of research the soft lens was tested with laboratory animals to ensure that it was nontoxic; later it was given to selected practitioners and independent research workers for clinical trials on humans.

Many laboratories, most notably Griffin Laboratories, began experimenting with soft plas-

tics. Griffin's soft lens received its initial impetus as an optic bandage to be used over diseased corneas. Dr. Herbert Kaufman spearheaded the program. He found that many diseased and damaged corneas healed best under a soft lens, and thus it emerged as an exciting therapeutic device. As for tolerance, many of his patients wore their lenses 24 hours a day for months without any detrimental changes in their eyes.

It soon became apparent that the soft lens was an innovation of major importance with widespread application, not only as an instrument for treating diseased corneas, but also as a superior contact lens. In the early stages, however, the therapeutic possibilities of soft lenses overshadowed any other consideration, since it appeared that these lenses would replace many conventional treatments of external diseases of the eye.

As the number of soft lens companies expanded throughout the world, a search for newer and better lens designs and lens plastics resulted in some companies emphasizing and developing research activities directed toward correcting astigmatism with soft lenses, developing bifocal soft lenses, and tinting soft lenses for cosmetic purposes. Ultrathin and high-water-content lenses have opened up the realm of extended wear, which, though not without its shortcomings, is fast improving. In the manufacturing area, the emphasis has been on automated and semiautomated systems to produce a soft contact lens.

Comment. There are over 50 companies in North America making soft lenses. When one considers that the technology of the material and its application were developed in just over 20 years, it becomes evident that refinement of these lenses and their broad application has just begun.

CHARACTERISTICS

Durability. Many soft lenses can be stretched but are durable and have a "memory" to return to their original size and shape (Fig. 3-2). Some soft lenses, however, do not have a memory and will not go back; they can be ruined.

Size. The soft lens is tolerated in a size larger than the cornea for optimum centering and stability. Its large size lying under the eyelid margins permits the lid margins to glide over its surface (Fig. 3-3) without impinging on the

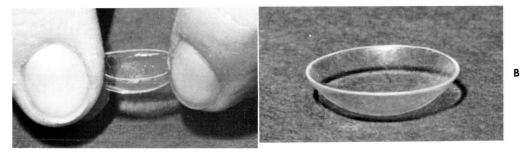

Fig. 3-2. A, The soft lens is sturdy despite its flexible quality. It can be stretched, dried, or crumpled and still retain its integrity. **B,** After stretching, the hydrophilic lens retains its "memory" and returns to its original shape. (From Stein, H.A., and Slatt, B.J.: The ophthalmic assistant, ed. 4, St. Louis, 1983, The C.V. Mosby Co.)

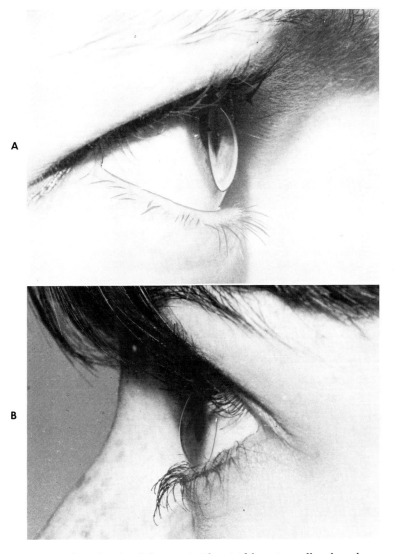

Fig. 3-3. Comparison of rigid and soft lenses. **A,** The rigid lens is smaller than the cornea and can be easily dislodged with the edge of the lid. **B,** The soft lens is larger than the cornea, hugs the eye tightly, and seldom is displaced even during body contact sports. (From Stein, H.A., and Slatt, B.J.: The ophthalmic assistant, ed. 4, St. Louis, 1983, The C.V. Mosby Co.)

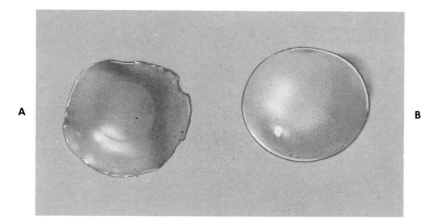

Fig. 3-4. A hydrophilic lens becomes hard and brittle like a cornflake when dry as in **A** but becomes soft and flexible when fully hydrated as in **B.** The great danger to the lens in the dry state is chipping.

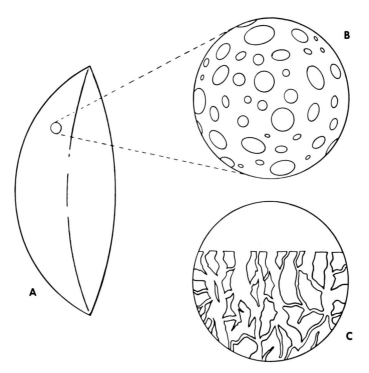

Fig. 3-5. A, Pore structure of a soft lens. **B** is an artist's drawing of a small section of a soft lens. **C** represents a single pore showing irregular size of each opening into the lens substance. The pore structure is sufficiently small to prevent penetration of bacteria. (Courtesy Barnes-Hind Pharmaceuticals, Inc., Sunnyvale, Calif.)

edges of the lens. This is one of the secrets of soft lens comfort. Interestingly enough, a small, 9 mm soft lens has all the initial discomfort of a hard lens because of the irritation of the edge against the lid margin.

Ability to contour to the eye. The softness of the lens permits the lens to contour itself to the shape of the eye. This is especially true of ultrathin lenses.

Composition. Soft lenses are made of different polymers but most are basically hydroxyethylmethacrylate (HEMA) cross-linked with ethylene glycol dimethacrylate (EDMA). These may be copolymerized with polyvinylpyrrolidone (PVP) to achieve a greater water absorption. A few soft lenses are made without HEMA as a constituent, and a few manufactured lenses have methyl methacrylate added for firmness. Glycerin combined with PMMA is also used.

Water absorption. These lenses absorb water in ranging degrees to provide a water content of 25% to 85%. The less water content, the more resistant the lens is to damage and the closer its behavior to the rigid lens. The higher the water content, generally the more fragile the lens, but there is a proportional increase in the oxygen transmission.

Flexibility. Hydrophilic lenses are hard and brittle when dry but become so soft and flexible when fully hydrated that they can be folded (Fig. 3-4).

Pore structure. Soft lenses have a very small pore structure with a variation in size of small openings. These pores are so small that they do not permit the larger molecules of bacteria or fungi to penetrate an intact lens (Fig. 3-5). They can, however, lodge on the surface of a soft lens. A damaged lens has a superficial abrasion may be contaminated by bacteria or fungi.

Wetting angle. The wetting angle in hydrophilic lenses can be grossly misleading because it depends a great deal on the technique of measurement and the type of hydrophilic material used. It does not appear to be dependent on the water content of the soft lens itself.

Oxygen transmission. A full discussion of soft lens oxygen transmission is covered in Chapter 28 concerning extended wear, in which oxygen transmission is more critical. Suffice it to say that if a lens is made one half as thick, the oxygen transmission will double. Also, if the water content of a lens is raised 10%, the oxygen transmission will double. There is little tear exchange under a soft lens with each blink (4% to 6%) as compared to a rigid lens (40% to 50%), and so one is dependent on through-the-lens oxygen transmission to prevent corneal hypoxia. Although these lenses are more fragile, the ultrathin type of high-water-content lenses provides better corneal physiologic performance.

Comment. The soft lens is much more comfortable than the rigid lens because of its soft qualities, its ability to flex on blinking, the minimal movement of the lens, and particularly its large size, which produces a fit with its edge lying under the upper and lower eyelids.

The pore structure of the soft lens is extremely small, being less than 3 nm, whereas the smallest bacterium is about 220 nm, and too large to invade the lens. Drugs, vapors, and chemicals, however, will penetrate the soft lens. This factor is important in the use of the soft lens in a smog environment and in fume-exposure industries. It may be important to discourage its use in persons who have occupations in which they are exposed to a high concentration of vapors.

ADVANTAGES

The soft lens has the following advantages:

Comfort. The soft lens is comfortable because the lens fits under the eyelid margins, flexes with each blink, and is soft (Fig. 3-6). It permits some oxygen to reach the cornea.

Rapid adaptation. It is easy for the wearer to build up an all-day wearing schedule.

Spectacle blur uncommon. After removal of the lenses the wearer can see as well with spectacles. Spectacle blur is uncommon because of the diffuse nature of any corneal edema, which spreads evenly over the entire cornea and does not alter its radius (Fig. 3-7).

Intermittent wear. The soft lens does not require a rigid daily wearing schedule. The individual can choose to wear the lens only at certain times, such as during the evening or during holiday periods.

Minimal lens loss. Because of the large size and minimal movement of the soft lens, lens loss is reduced considerably. The lens is not ejected by a blink because the lid margin does not touch the edge. Lens loss is further mini-

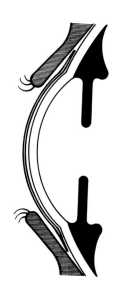

Fig. 3-6. Soft lens fits under the eyelid margins. This accounts for its comfort factor.

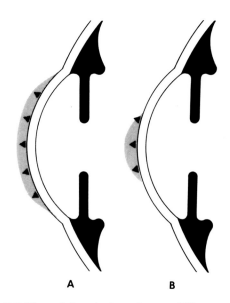

Fig. 3-7. The soft lens in **A** produces a diffuse area of corneal edema that does not alter the radius of curvature of the cornea and does not cause spectacle blur. In **B** the rigid lens produces a discrete type of corneal edema, confined to the corneal cap, which does cause spectacle blur because it produces a radical steepening of the corneal curvature.

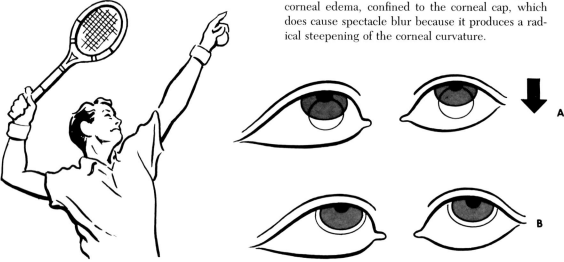

Fig. 3-8. A, With rigid lenses the lenses drop when the tennis player moves his eyes up to hit the ball. **B,** Soft lenses move with the eye and show only minimal lag.

mized on lens removal because one pinches and holds the lens rather than pops it out as in the removal of a rigid lens. The soft lens is difficult to dislodge and makes an ideal sports lens (Fig. 3-8).

Comment. Although lens loss is reduced, the wear and tear on the soft lens are considerably increased; consequently statistics show a much higher replacement requirement for the soft lens.

Minimal overwear reaction. Because of its soft nature and the ability to create an oxygen-tear pump mechanism by flexing with each blink, this lens has minimal overwear reactions (Fig. 3-9). In addition, oxygen can permeate through the soft lens, particularly if the lens is made very thin.

Less flare and photophobia. Because only minimal movement on the cornea occurs, there is less irritation of the corneal epithelium. The

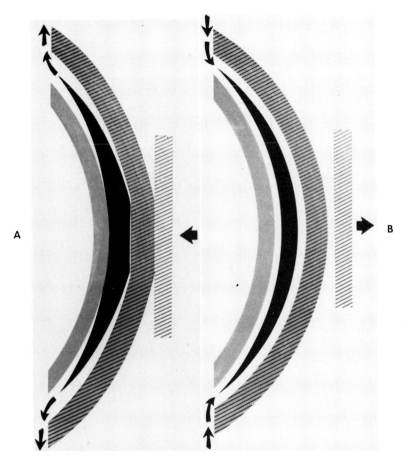

Fig. 3-9. A, Diagram showing pressure of upper lid being transmitted to soft lens with collapse of interface area. **B,** Diagram showing reformation of interface area after removal of upper lid pressure. (From Aquavella, J.V.: In Gasset, A.R., and Kaufman, H.E., editors: Soft contact lens, St. Louis, 1972, The C.V. Mosby Co.)

soft material of hydrophilic lenses is more compatible with the delicate tissues of the cornea. The generous size of the optic zone because of the large diameters of the soft lenses means that the pupil is always covered, a situation that minimizes flare.

Corneal protection. Because of its large size, the soft lens can protect the entire cornea from exposure and from debris getting under the lens (Fig. 3-10).

Alternative for rigid lens dropouts. Sensitive persons who are unable to tolerate the rigid lens can often find comfort with the soft lens.

Excellent cosmetic lens. These lenses are virtually invisible to the observer, particularly the smaller diameter sizes of the soft lens.

Ideal for infants and children. Because of the comfort feature and the larger sizes available with soft lenses, the lens loss factor can be min-

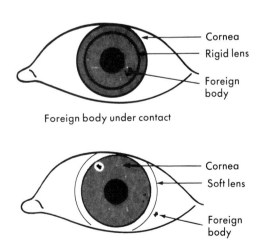

Fig. 3-10. The rigid lens permits foreign particles to enter under the lens, whereas the soft lens tends to prevent the tracking of foreign bodies under it by its scleral impingement and minimum movement.

imized. Thus soft lenses are ideal for small infants and children.

DISADVANTAGES

The soft lens has the following disadvantages:

Astigmatism. Astigmatism is not readily corrected or covered by conventional soft lenses and even less with ultrathin lenses. The soft lens contours itself to the eye, and corneal astigmatism frequently remains uncorrected. This feature becomes clinically more significant in the lower powers but is not significant in the higher refractive powers. For example, -3.00 D -2.50 D $\times$ 180 is difficult to mask with the soft lens, whereas in the higher powers, for example, -9.00 D -2.50 D $\times$ 180, the astigmatic error may be less significant and better tolerated, even though left uncorrected by the soft lens. The reason is that patients with high refractive errors, that is, -8.00 or more diopters, have macular problems and many see only 20/25 at best. A drop of one or two lines on the chart in these cases is tolerated.

Many optical firms claim that their soft lens masks a certain amount of astigmatism. Depending on the lens thickness only about one third to one half of the corneal astigmatism is corrected. We have found that this is highly unpredictable and that often none of the astigmatism is obliterated. However, there is a variety of toric soft lenses now being manufactured to provide the fitter an opportunity to correct both corneal and residual astigmatism. These lenses are discussed in Chapter 24.

Poor vision. In addition to faulty vision because of uncorrected astigmatic errors, poor vision may result from an improperly fitted soft lens. Fluctuating vision may result if the lens is fitted too steeply so that it vaults the central cornea, because as the patient blinks the center of the lens is compressed by the eyelid and so it "irons out" the lens on the cornea. If the lens is fitted too flat, it may become decentered or have excessive movement during a blink, resulting in faulty vision.

The soft lens may become partially dehydrated under certain conditions of low humidity such as indoors during the heating season and in air-conditioned rooms, especially for patients who are partial or infrequent blinkers or who produce an inadequate volume of tears.

Patients with insufficient tears are not good candidates for soft lenses. The hydrophilic lens demands water, and if it is not satisfied by adequate tears, the thickness and consequently the optic properties of the lens will change. Patients with excess tears may also have faulty vision because the lens may move about excessively.

Proper respiration is provided to the cornea through the tears by the pumping action created during blinking. This is a two-stage action: (1) During blinking the lens flexes inward, pumping the tears from the small vaulted areas in the intermediate areas across the cornea and out under the lens edge. (2) As the blink is completed, the lens recovers its shape, creating a lowered pressure area under the vault of the lens and thus sucking in fresh tears under the lens. This pumping action produces tear exchange so that proper oxygen is provided to the cornea. This is the most important reason for obtaining a proper fit with a proper cornea-lens relationship.

Allergic patients with excess mucus production will quickly form tacky deposits on the front surface of the lens, resulting in excessive blink-induced lens excursions.

Comment. The drier the eye, the harder the lens should be to offset the shift of tears into the lens to provide osmotic balance.

Lack of durability. Frequent handling may cause the soft lens to form a tiny crack and eventually to split. Rough handling or improper removal with a sharp fingernail can also cause a tear or scratch in the lens (Fig. 3-11). The edges may become roughened or damaged with time; occasionally the lenses become yellow and rigid with time. At times yellowing

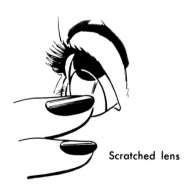

Scratched lens

Fig. 3-11. Scratch in a soft lens from a sharp fingernail.

may be a result of aging from boiling or disinfecting, or it may be a result of epinephrine-like compounds, protein, or impurities gathering in its substance. There is a life-span of a daily wear lens, even with the best of care. On the average, this has been about 2 years for most of our patients. Annual or biannual replacement of all lenses would greatly reduce lens wear–related problems.

Comment. Nasal sprays frequently contain epinephrine-like drugs, which can discolor a lens. Hair sprays cause vacuoles and punctate opacities in the lens.

Faulty duplication. Quality control on replacement of a lens is most important. Manufacturing processes for lenses must be extremely rigidly controlled so that if a lens is lost, it can be replaced with an exact duplicate. This exact duplication is dependent on the reliability of the manufacturer both in fabricating the lens and in checking its quality. Unlike those for rigid lenses, many parameters such as water content and edge design cannot be verified by the practitioner.

Comment. Spin-cast lenses as a group provide better quality control than lathe-cut lenses do.

Precipitates and protein buildup. With long-term wear precipitates occur in the lens and protein and lipids accumulate on the surface (Fig. 3-12). Although special cleaning and protein-removing agents are available, one must rigidly adhere to their use to eliminate precipitates and protein buildup and preserve the life of the lens. If protein is left present in the lens, fine stippling and even microcystic changes can occur in the cornea. Lens solution preservatives will cling readily and build up on the lens surface inducing a toxic reaction.

Comment. Protein precipitates can make the lens uncomfortable, make it lose some permeability features, change its shape to become steeper with resultant pseudomyopia, form a nidus for infection or hypersensitivity reactions, and add weight to it or alter its fitting. A happy lens wearer is a person with no protein on the lenses.

Impossible modifications. Although a soft lens can be dehydrated to the dry state, it does not form a regular shape in the dry state and modifications are not possible.

Lens disinfection. The routine of disinfecting must be rigidly adhered to, or infection may occur. This applies whether the lenses sit in the drawer during illness or vacations or when there is a respite back to glasses.

Both the boiling method and chemical method of disinfection have their advantages and drawbacks. In any event rigid adherence to disinfection procedures is most important both for the practitioner who keeps an inventory and for the patient who wears the lenses only occasionally. Fungus growth has been re-

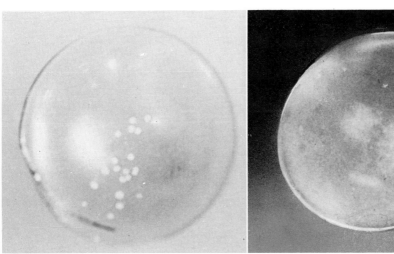
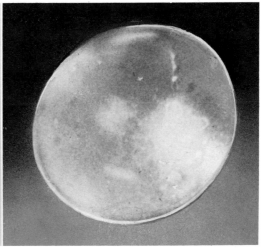

Fig. 3-12. A, Deposits on a soft lens. **B,** Protein buildup on a soft lens will vary with the duration of wear, the method of sterilization, and the tear composition and concentration of individual patients. (**A** from Stein, H.A., and Slatt, B.J.: The ophthalmic assistant, ed. 4, St. Louis, 1983, The C.V. Mosby Co.)

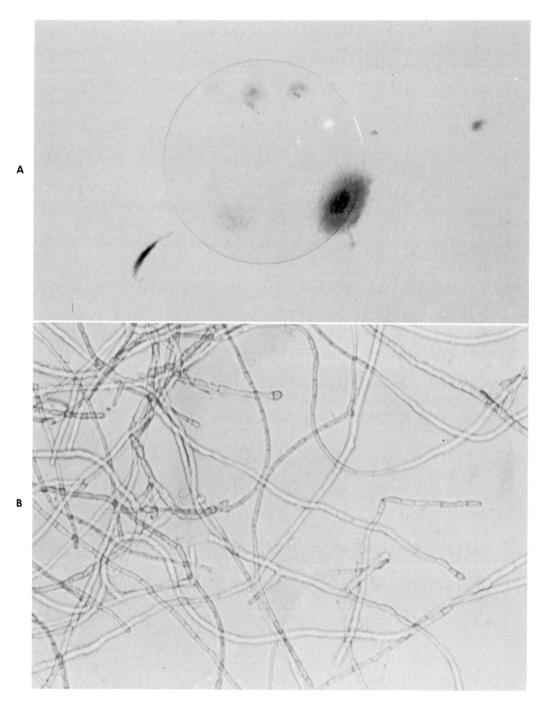

Fig. 3-13. A, Soft lens contaminated by fungus from improper daily sterilization routine. **B,** My-celium of *Cladosporium* identified from soft lens in **A.**

Table 3-1. Thin and ultrathin soft lenses

Advantages	Disadvantages
1. Initial comfort and rapid adaptation	1. Exaggerated dehydrating in a dry environment
2. Higher oxygen permeability	2. More difficult to handle
3. Decreased incidence of overwear	3. More easily damaged
4. Can be fitted tighter for stable vision during sport activities	4. Less masking of corneal astigmatism resulting in poorer quality of vision
5. Alternative for highly sensitive individuals	5. More difficult to manufacture and thus higher costs
6. Reduced risk of corneal warpage	

ported occasionally, as well as bacterial contamination of the lenses. However, widespread infection of the eye is clinically rare. Because soft lenses can be scratched and damaged more easily and consequently can be penetrated by infectious organisms, they are theoretically more dangerous than hard lenses. In clinical practice, however, this does not seem to be a real problem, and patients with soft lenses do not seem to have any higher incidence of corneal or conjunctival inflammatory conditions than people wearing rigid lenses do. One source of soft lens contamination results from human neglect. Patients neglect to boil their lenses as instructed or neglect to use fresh solutions daily for disinfection. Unlike that for rigid lenses, it is unwise to recommend a duplicate pair of soft lenses because the patient usually neglects the disinfection routine required of soft lenses. If the spare set is not opened and the vial is intact, there is no risk of infection. Once the vial is opened, fungus contamination will occur if the storage solutions are not changed regularly. As a result, fungus contamination may occur (Fig. 3-13).

THIN AND ULTRATHIN SOFT LENSES

A major technologic change in soft lens manufacture has been the development of the thin and ultrathin soft lenses with center thicknesses of less than 0.1 mm and even as thin as 0.025 mm for conventional lenses and 0.0005 mm for special lenses.

The advantages and disadvantages of these thinner soft lenses are outlined in Table 3-1. Of importance is the fact that these lenses provide exceptional initial comfort. Being thin, these lenses provide some diffusion of oxygen and minimize corneal edema formation from hypoxia. Because of their oxygen permeability characteristics, these lenses may be fitted slightly tighter than regular soft lenses and hence produce more stable vision and thus are useful for sporting activities.

On the disadvantage side of thin and ultrathin lenses is the fact that they are harder to handle and require more patience by the fitter and patient in instruction. They also have an exaggerated dehydration effect in dry environments. These lenses may become damaged more easily and may also not mask as much astigmatism as regular soft lenses do and thus may give a poor quality of vision in those with corneal astigmatism.

Comment. The advantages of the soft lens are its excellent comfort, rapid adaptation, and the ability of the wearer to wear the lens intermittently without adhering to a rigid wearing schedule. We have found the soft lens ideal for men and women who are active in sports, for the elderly, and for many persons who are not strongly motivated to persist with a rigorous daily wearing schedule often required of hard lenses. On the other hand, soft lenses are not so durable, require more care and attention to cleaning and disinfecting and a greater maintenance cost factor.

OFFICE EVALUATION AND VERIFICATION OF SOFT LENSES

What type of lens verification should be performed on soft lenses in the office of the average fitter? Unlike rigid lenses, soft lenses have a somewhat limited verification procedure insofar as parameters such as water content, base curve, and peripheral curve measurements cannot be easily obtained by the average fitter. In this situation the fitter must trust the manufacturer.

However, there are certain minimum procedures that we have found worthwhile in evaluating a soft contact lens to ensure a high standard of quality. The exercise is most helpful not only in ensuring the continuing quality of the manufacturers but also in explaining some of the contact lens problems that too often we assume is a poorly selected lens clinically when in reality it is a poorly manufactured lens. Also there are occasions when one reviews patients fitted elsewhere in which files are unobtainable and one wishes to have as much of the contact lens specifications on hand as possible.

GENERAL INSPECTION

Using a monocular magnifying lens or the slitlamp (biomicroscope), the lens should be evaluated for discoloration, protein buildup, and nicks and ruffled edges on the lens. The lens should be viewed against a black background in which the light beam of the slitlamp can be gradually spread over the lens surface. Dr. Hershel Boyd, an authority in the field, uses a Leitz slide projector to project the soft lens for inspection.

DIAMETER

Viewing the lens with the monocular magnifier with a reticule or gauge, the overall diameter and the optic zone as well can be measured (Figs. 4-1 and 4-2). There is available a special monocular magnifier with gauge that permits the soft lens to contour itself to the magnifier. One edge of the lens is placed along the base arch of the grid and the opposite arch is used to measure the diameter.

BASE CURVE

The base curve may be measured on plastic templates of known radius (Fig. 4-3). A central bubble indicates that the lens is too steep for the template and that the lens must be moved to a flatter template (Fig. 4-4). If there is edge stand-off, the lens should be moved to a steeper template of known radius. We have not found the template method to be a truly exact measure of the base curve because the lens will often accommodate to two or more of the templates of different radii and seem to be a good fit in each instance.

The template method is also dependent on the relationship of the diameter of the lens and the diameter of the template that corresponds to the sagittal height of the lens.

Template measurement is even less accurate when one is measuring ultrathin lenses.

One instrument, the Soft Lens Analyzer (Hydrovue, Inc., Richmond, California) was developed to measure the base curve of hydrogel lenses. In addition, it measures diameter and center thickness and provides close surface

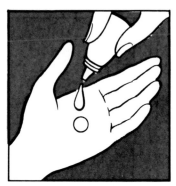 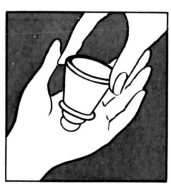 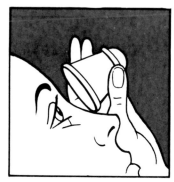

Fill lens with saline   Touch loupe to lens, forcing out excess saline   Look toward light source for inspection

Fig. 4-1. Viewing the soft lens with a monocular magnifier.

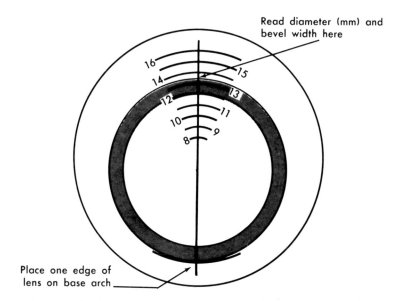

Read diameter (mm) and bevel width here

Place one edge of lens on base arch

Fig. 4-2. Obtaining the diameter measurement of a soft lens with a monocular magnifier.

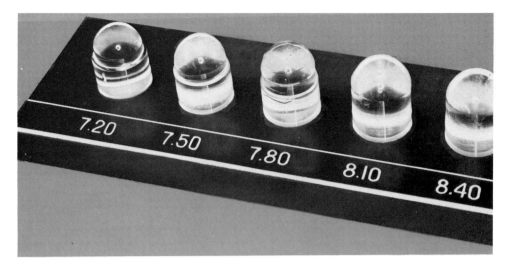

Fig. 4-3. Plastic templates of known radii can be used to determine the base curve of a lathe-cut soft lens.

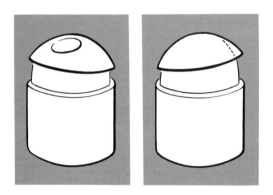

Fig. 4-4. Use of the template to measure the base curve of a soft lens. The lens on the left has a bubble under the center, indicating that the lens is too steep for the template. The lens on the right has edge stand-off, indicating that the lens is too flat for the template. (From Stein, H.A., and Slatt, B.J.: The ophthalmic assistant, ed. 4, St. Louis, 1983, The C.V. Mosby Co.)

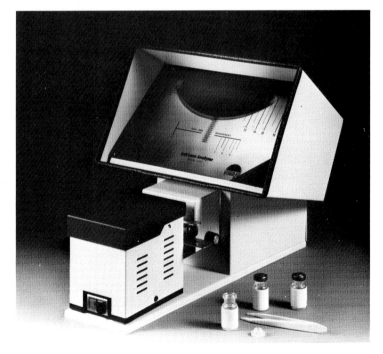

Fig. 4-5. The Soft Lens Analyzer. (Courtesy Hydrovue, Inc., Richmond, Calif.) (From Stein, H.A., and Slatt, B.J.: The ophthalmic assistant, ed. 4, St. Louis, 1983, The C.V. Mosby Co.

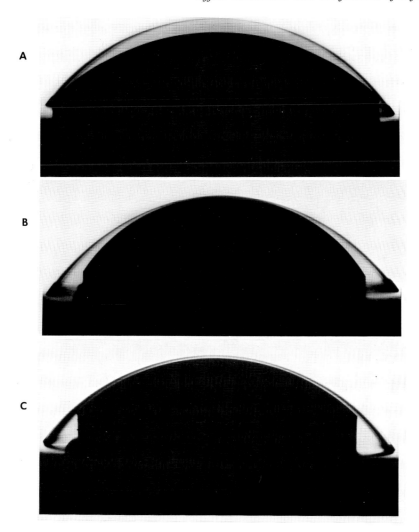

Fig. 4-6. A, Peripheral touch and apical vault or lens too steep. **B,** Apical touch and peripheral flare or lens too flat. **C,** Alignment: proper fit for accurate base-curve determination. (Courtesy Hydrovue, Inc., Richmond, Calif.) (From Stein, H.A., and Slatt, B.J.: The ophthalmic assistant, ed. 4, St. Louis, 1983, The C.V. Mosby Co.)

and edge inspection on soft lenses and on rigid lenses (Fig. 4-5). It may be used to show patients some problems with existing lenses such as surface defects.

Because hydrogel lenses all contain some percentage of water, accurate measurement is best attained in the hydrated state. This instrument provides a wet cell in which the lens is immersed in saline solution. The lens is then measured against a series of hemispheric standards with known radii from 7.6 to 9.8 mm in 0.2 mm increments. A beam of light is projected through and around the lens positioned on the standard. This image is projected onto a small built-in screen at 15 magnification. The operator determines the base curve based on the lens-bearing relationship to the standard on which it is centered (Fig. 4-6). This system for measuring the base curve of a lens is applicable to all lathed lenses. It fails to take into consideration the diameter of the lens in relation to the diameter of the template. There is no reliable office system for measuring the base curve of spin-cast lenses because of their thinness and asphericity.

There is available a soft lens radius gauge that measures the central posterior radius of a soft lens in the hydrated state. Other sophis-

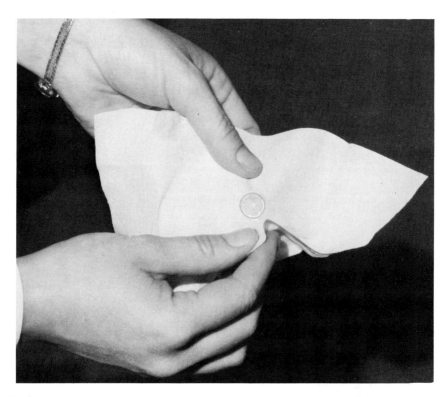

Fig. 4-7. To measure the power of a soft lens, clean and gently blot the lens dry with lint-free tissue before evaluating the power with a lensometer.

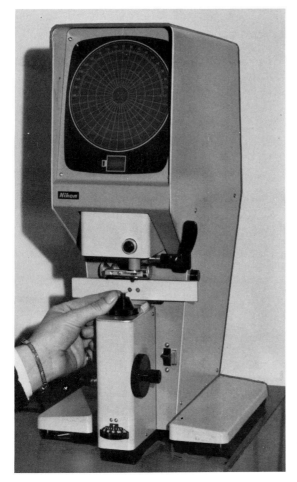

Fig. 4-8. Nikon lensometer used to measure the power of a soft lens.

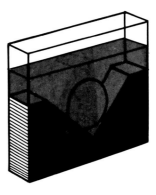

Fig. 4-9. Water cell used to measure power of a soft lens in the hydrated state. The soft lens is floated in normal saline and measured in a lensometer.

ticated wet cell radiuscopes are available, but these are fairly expensive for the average fitter.

POWER

To measure the refractive power of the lens, one should clean and gently blot the lens dry for a few seconds with lint-free tissue or chamois (Fig. 4-7) and then hold the lens in the lensometer with the concave surface against the lens stop. Care must be taken when the lens is being blotted. If it is too dry, the power reading will be less accurate.

The Nikon lensometer is ideal because it is able to measure the lens by resting it rather than pinching it because of the horizontal positioning of the lens (Fig. 4-8). One may use a water cell described by Maurice Poster to which normal saline has been added (Fig. 4-9). The lens floats freely with the finger held over the opening of the water cell. The water cell is placed in the lensometer with the concave side of the lens away from the observer and the lens power measured. By multiplying the lensometer reading by the factor four, one can compute the refractive power of the lens. This is a somewhat cumbersome and not totally reliable method, since there is considerable error in the water-cell method of determining power. The power can vary with the thickness of the plastic, which varies from high plus to low minus. In our experience the lensometer method has been faster and more reliable than the water-cell method.

OPTIC QUALITIES OF THE PLASTIC

Occasionally soft lenses are manufactured with stress lines in the lens or with an irregular anterior surface. The quality can be assessed with a hand magnifier or with the retinoscope. In a lens with poor surface optic properties the retinoscopy reflex appears either irregular or decentered. In many cases the faulty or irregular reflex is caused by improper fitting. This is most commonly seen with lenses that are too tight and are stretched out on the eye.

Comment. An important aspect of having the equipment and being able to verify soft contact lenses is that the practitioner will be in a better position to evaluate lens changes that may occur with time and thus solve clinical contact lens problems of the patient. Not uncommonly chips and nicks will appear, deposits will accumulate, or the lens may change its parameter and become steeper or occasionally flatter. We have seen lenses steepen with aging and deposit formation. We have seen lenses flatten in shape from too vigorous hand cleaning with loss of the material's shape retention.

It is important to note that verification of a soft lens is not up to the standards of a rigid lens. One must accept the water content as an article of faith. Base-curve measurement is not precise. The blend on a lathe-cut lens defies projection. A thickness gauge that is reliable still needs an inventor, and flexibility and tensile strength (durometer factor) cannot be gauged by the practitioner.

GENERAL GUIDELINES FOR FITTING SOFT LENSES

General principles
Basic guidelines for fitting
Evaluating a properly fitting lens
Inventory versus diagnostic
lenses

This chapter is written to provide basic principles and guidelines in the fitting of soft contact lenses. Manufacturers' specific instructions should be followed for any particular lens because each manufacturer has its own base curves and diameters. Companies for economic reasons have standardized dimensions that are available from that company. Individual custom-ordered soft lenses have not been so commercially workable an undertaking as they have been with rigid lenses that are manufactured by small laboratories. There are, however, small laboratories designing and manufacturing soft lenses to order.

This chapter provides guidelines in principles for considering small-diameter versus large-diameter lens, thin versus standard-thickness lenses, spheric lenses versus toric-designed soft lenses, and the fitting principles required for aphakia. We shall provide some rationale for what manufacturers have incorporated in their individual manuals.

GENERAL PRINCIPLES

All soft lenses, regardless of power, size, or manufacturer, are ideally theoretically fitted to obtain three-point touch. They should parallel the superior and inferior sclera and the corneal apex (Fig. 5-1). Rigid polymethylmethacrylate (PMMA) lenses, of small diameter, are usually fitted either on K, flatter than K, or steeper than K to increase tear exchange, minimize the bearing area, and still permit tear exchange. In contrast, soft hydrophilic lenses are usually fitted as large as or larger than the corneal diameter to maintain centration and stability. Be-

cause of the large diameter of these soft lenses, they should be fitted appreciably flatter than the flattest K of the cornea. Lens diameter and base curve are directly related. To arrive at essentially the same fit, the base curve of the lens selected should be flattened as the lens diameter is increased, for example, a 12 to 13 mm diameter lens is usually fitted approximately 2.00 to 3.00 D flatter than K, whereas a 14 to 15 mm diameter lens will have to be fitted approximately 3.00 to 5.00 D flatter than K. Expressed another way, if the diameter of a soft lens is increased, the lens becomes tighter, and one may lengthen the base curve to make the lens flatter.

Differences in lens design and in the properties of the various polymers from which soft lenses are made may affect the way in which they have to be fitted. Some differences that should be considered include the following.

Material considerations. Most hydrogel lenses consist of HEMA (hydroxyethylmethacrylate) or HEMA combined with PVP (polyvinylpyrrolidone). When PVP is added, it enhances the water-carrying component of the plastic but may cause some yellowing with repeated boiling or age. A few manufacturers add methyl methacrylate (MMA), which gives more firmness. Those that have this property are often slightly more rigid and perhaps more durable than the other materials.

Soft lenses that contain methyl methacrylate as part of their material composition, such as Aquaflex or AOsoft, have some firmness to the material and will usually vault over the elliptic periphery of the cornea (Fig. 5-2). This vaulting may create a minus tear layer and result in slightly more plus power required in the final prescription.

Type of posterior curvature. All lathe-cut lenses have spheric posterior curves in contrast to the Bausch & Lomb spin-cast lens, which utilizes an elliptic posterior curve.

Posterior peripheral curve width. For lenses of the same diameter and the same base curve,

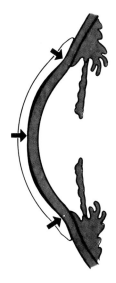

Fig. 5-1. Three-point touch—a normally fitting soft lens will rest lightly at the apex and at the periphery of the cornea.

the wider the peripheral curve, the looser the lens will fit.

Anterior surface construction. Single-cut lenses may fit differently from those with a lenticular construction because of the effects of lid action on the anterior periphery of the lenses. The carrier radius and carrier width of lenticular lenses also affect the fit of the lens.

Water content. Lenses of appreciably higher water content are usually less durable than those of lower water content but permit greater oxygen diffusion through the plastic than standard lenses of similar thickness.

In general, the lower the water content, the more durable the lens. The water content of various polymers will vary with the manufacturer of the lens. However, lenses of the same water content from different manufacturers may be more or less durable, depending on the properties of the polymers from which the lenses are made.

Lens thickness. Soft hydrogel lenses may be divided into standard-thickness, thin, and ultrathin lenses. The thinner the lens, the more oxygen is transferred across the lens material and consequently the tighter the lens may be fit because tear exchange and lens movement are not so critical.

Oxygen permeability. The thinner the lens, the greater the oxygen transmissibility. Also, for lenses of equal thickness, the higher the

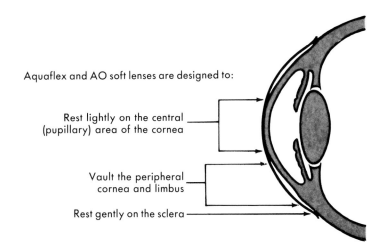

Aquaflex and AO soft lenses are designed to:

Rest lightly on the central (pupillary) area of the cornea

Vault the peripheral cornea and limbus

Rest gently on the sclera

Fig. 5-2. Lenses containing polymethylmethacrylate wrap around entire central pupillary area of the cornea and vault the peripheral area of the cornea.

water content, the greater the oxygen transmissibility. Hazy vision may arise from wearing a soft lens that is too thick, in that it does not provide sufficient oxygen to the cornea.

Many lens-design and polymer variations mentioned previously are interrelated. Some of these relationships include the following.

Lens weight. The lens weight is influenced by its thickness and water content. Polymers with higher water content are usually structurally weaker than those of lower water content and require lenses of greater thickness. The increased gravitational pull on a heavier lens such as an aphakic lens has to be offset by the use of a larger diameter.

Lens rigidity. The rigidity or stiffness of a lens is a function of its thickness, its water content, and the unique properties of the polymer from which it is made. (One way to understand the concept of rigidity is to visualize a very large rigid lens fitted much flatter than K. This lens would tend to rock excessively on the corneal apex because of its excessive rigidity, whereas a soft lens would tend to wrap itself around the corneal apex to varying degrees, depending on the degree of rigidity that it possesses.) Soft lenses of greater rigidity have to be fitted more precisely (and flatter) than those possessing a lesser amount of rigidity.

Edge considerations. The comfort of a soft lens is dependent on the manufacturing quality of the edge and the edge design. If the edge is too thick, it will cause discomfort, and if too thin, it will cause nicking and tearing. A fine balance between these two extremes is arrived at for each manufacturer and will vary with the durability of the material.

BASIC GUIDELINES FOR FITTING

Because of the many variables and interrelationships involved, the fit achieved with a certain diameter and base curve from one lens manufacturer may be considerably different from the fit that results from a lens with the same parameters obtained from another manufacturer. Therefore it is strongly recommended that the fitting guidelines supplied by each manufacturer be followed in the fitting of its lenses.

The following basic guidelines, however, apply to the fitting of all soft lenses:

1. A normal-fitting soft lens theoretically should show three-point touch, with touch at the corneal apex and the periphery. This is ideal but difficult to demonstrate insofar as fluorescein is usually not used.

2. Hydrogel lenses are usually fitted as large as or larger than the diameter of the cornea and the diameter ranges in size from 12 to 15 mm.

3. Small eyes often require smaller diameters and consequently steeper base curves, whereas larger eyes are fitted with larger lenses and flatter base curves. Certain racial characteristics may apply. For example, the Oriental eye usually has a smaller palpebral fissure and is a smaller eye than the Caucasian eye and will often require a smaller lens.

4. Soft lenses are generally fitted flatter than the flattest K; usually about 2.00 to 3.00 D flatter (approximately 0.4 to 0.6 mm) for the smaller lenses and 3.00 to 5.00 D flatter (approximately 0.6 to 1.0 mm) for the larger lenses.

5. Lens diameter and lens radius are inversely related. If one increases the diameter of the lens, one increases the sagittal height of a contact lens and so the lens will be tighter on a given cornea. If one decreases the radius or base curve of a contact lens, one also increases the sagittal height and so the lens will be tighter on the same cornea (Fig. 5-3). Thus some manufacturers maintain a constant diameter of their lenses but change the base-curve radius, whereas others feature a change in the diameter but keep the radius controlled. One should understand this relationship of sagittal height to both radius and diameter.

6. One may change the fit of a lathe-cut lens by varying the lens diameter, lens radius, or both (Fig. 5-4). It has been mathematically established that the change in lens vault (sagittal-height difference) for a 0.3 mm change in lens radius is approximately equal to a change of 0.5 mm in lens diameter (Fig. 5-5). Knowledge of this relationship (0.3 mm radius change = 0.5 mm diameter change) permits maintenance of the same vault through selective changes of either lens radius, lens diameter, or both.

The system of fitting lenses is designed to reduce the complications inherent in having so many different lens diameter/lens radius combinations by standardization of the lens diameter.

7. One may determine increased steepness

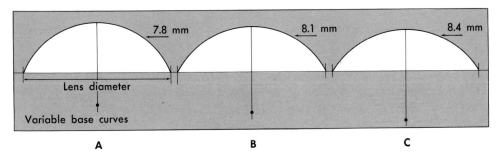

Fig. 5-3. All three lenses have a constant diameter. The radii of lenses **B** and **C** have been increased by 0.3 mm so that the lenses have a smaller sagittal height and are therefore flatter.

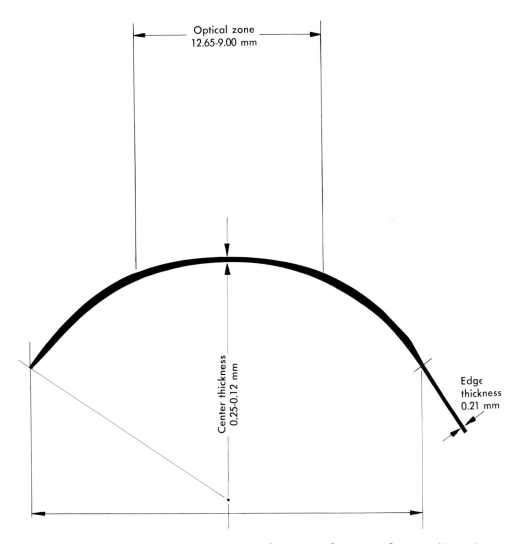

Fig. 5-4. TC 75 minus lens design with 14 mm diameter and wet specifications. (From Stein, H.A., and Harrison, K.W.: In Hartstein, J., editor: Extended wear contact lenses for aphakia and myopia, St. Louis, 1982, The C.V. Mosby Co.)

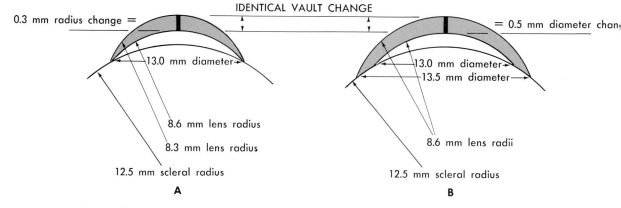

Fig. 5-5. By decreasing the radius 0.3 mm as in **A** or by increasing the diameter 0.5 mm as in **B**, there is an identical change in the vault of the lens.

Table 5-1. Sagittal relationship of various base curves and diameters

Diameter	Radius	Diameter	Radius
Flatter		14.0	8.1
12.0	8.7	13.0	7.2
12.0	8.1	14.5	8.4
12.5	8.7	13.5	7.5
12.0	8.4	15.0	8.7
12.5	8.4	14.0	7.8
12.5	8.1	14.5	8.1
12.5	7.8	15.0	8.4
12.0	7.8	15.5	8.7
13.0	8.7	13.5	7.2
13.0	8.4	14.0	7.5
13.5	8.7	14.5	7.8
13.0	8.1	15.0	8.1
13.5	8.4	15.5	8.4
14.0	8.7	14.0	7.2
13.0	7.8	14.5	7.5
13.5	8.1	15.0	7.8
14.0	8.4	15.5	8.1
13.0	7.5	15.0	7.5
14.5	8.7	15.5	7.8
13.5	7.8	**Steeper**	

or flatness from a table showing relationship of diameter to radius (sagittal values) (Table 5-1). To loosen a lathe-cut lens, one may fit smaller diameters in 0.5 mm steps or increase the radius in 0.2 to 0.3 mm steps.

8. Bausch & Lomb spin-cast lenses are fitted from two diameters, 13.6 mm and 14.5 mm. The selected diameter and series depend on the corneal diameter. The exception to this is the plano T bandage lens, which is a 14 mm diameter.

9. The lower the water content of the lens, the more durable the lens becomes. The higher the water content, the more fragile the lens.

10. With low-water-content soft lenses we have seen the painful overwear syndrome with corneal epithelial loss that is seen with rigid lenses. One must guard against advising a too rapid acceleration of the wearing schedule for the initial few weeks with low-water-content soft lenses.

11. The thinner the lens, the greater the oxygen transmission to the cornea.

12. Ultrathin lenses provide greater initial comfort than standard-thickness lenses.

13. Thin and ultrathin lenses can be fitted tighter and with less movement than standard-thickness lenses. This eliminates wrinkling of the lens, which may result in fluctuating vision.

14. Hazy vision caused by oxygen deprivation may occur from wearing a thick lens either centrally as in the case of high plus or in the periphery as in the case of high minus lenses.

15. Contact lens decentration can be caused by tight eyelids, large corneas, against-the-rule astigmatism, or asymmetric corneal topography.

16. Spheric soft lenses will not mask large amounts of corneal astigmatism. In general, astigmatism over 1.00 to 1.5 D requires correction by toric soft lenses, rigid lenses, or even spectacles.

17. With soft lenses, conventional fluorescein cannot be used to study tear exchange because it permeates the lens. High molecular

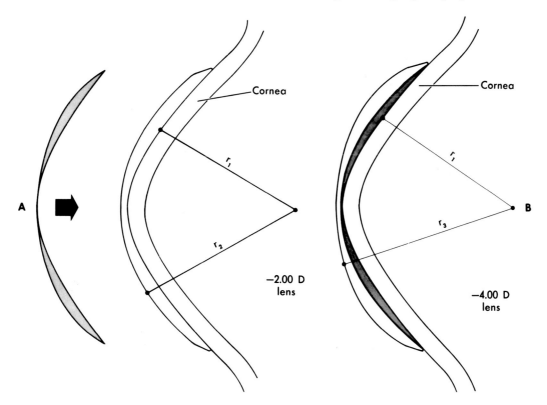

Fig. 5-6. A, r_1 = corneal radius; r_2 = new anterior surface radius, which has a flatter curve than that of the cornea. **B,** When additional plastic is added to the periphery to create a −4.00 D power lens, the new anterior radius r_3 has a still flatter curve because of the flexible nature of the material that is placed in the periphery. The fit will vary with the power of the lens. (Courtesy Bausch & Lomb, Inc.)

weight fluorescein can be used. but it is no more effective than an evaluation of tear exchange by noting the movement of the lens.

18. Heavier lenses usually have to be fitted larger than usual. The lens weight is influenced by its thickness and water content. Higher water content polymers are usually weaker than those of lower water content and require lenses of greater thickness. The increased gravitational pull on a heavier lens has to be offset by the use of a larger diameter.

19. The rigidity of a lens is a function of its thickness, its water content, and the unique properties of the polymer that it is made of.

20. When fitting soft lenses, one should aim at fitting the flattest possible lens that will provide good clear vision, center well, and have no effect on the corneal integrity.

21. With all soft lenses the practitioner is buying blindly, since there are no convenient and reliable inexpensive office measures available of lens thickness, water content, lens

weight, lens rigidity, and peripheral and base curves. Also faults in the plastic may be impossible to detect on first examination and may only appear as problems occur with the lens.

22. It should be noted that for the Bausch & Lomb spin-cast series the inside posterior apical radius (PAR) changes as the power becomes steeper in units approximately 0.05 mm for a 0.25 D increase in minus power. Thus large changes in power will change the fitting characteristics (Fig. 5-6). This is not true of lathe-cut lenses.

23. The less material on the eye, the better. Fit the smallest, thinnest lens that will provide a good fit, good comfort, and a good physiologic response.

24. The flatter the cornea, the larger the diameter of the lens required to give the lens a stable fit and prevent decentration.

25. Boyd has suggested that the dryer the eye, the lower the water content of the lens required.

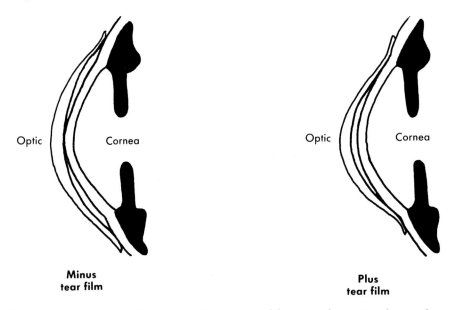

Fig. 5-7. Minus and plus tear film. A tear film is created between the contact lens and cornea. This tear film may balance as either a minus lens or a plus lens and may alter the end point of the refractive change.

26. The pore structure of a soft lens is 4 nm. The smallest size structure visible today is the herpes simplex virus, which is 15 nm.

27. There is only half the tear film thickness behind the thin and ultrathin lenses as compared to standard-thickness lenses; hence there is less opportunity for tear exchange with metabolic products and debris and there is more chance for red eyes to occur.

28. In fitting larger lenses, there is less movement because of (a) greater surface adhesion of a larger lens and (b) less lid impact with larger lenses and thus less movement.

Comment

Because there are no effective quality controls for soft lenses, the lens on the cornea becomes the best too for a fitting guide, albeit a pragmatic one. Some fitters do not even bother with K readings. The fitting is then based on centration, visual acuity, lens movement, and lens stability with eye movement. K readings do not add much science to the art of fitting a soft lens. They are merely a guide.

EVALUATING A PROPERLY FITTING LENS

Criteria for evaluating a properly fitting soft lens include the following (see also pp. 61 to 68 for more detail).

Movement. An acceptable fitting lens should

show about 0.5 to 1 mm of lag as the eye is turned up or to the side. Subtle differences in movements are best detected by having the patient look up and blink. The amplitude of movement depends on the lens size and the average thickness. A soft lens that moves excessively (more than 1 mm with each blink) is too flat; a soft lens that moves less than 0.5 mm with each blink is too steep and will limit tear exchange. Ultrathin lenses may be fit with less movement because some oxygen passes through the lens.

Position. A normal-fitting lens should completely cover the cornea. If a lens is slightly decentered, the fit is acceptable provided that the edge of the lens opposite the direction of decentration continues to cover the cornea. Uncovered corneal areas will often show corneal irritation and staining.

A soft lens that becomes decentered is usually too flat or too small. To correct this problem, select a lens with a larger diameter. It will usually reduce the flatness of the lens and improve corneal coverage.

Vision. For the fit to be acceptable, vision must be clear and constant before, during, and after blinking. Fluctuating vision is a symptom of a marginal or improper fit.

Relationship of lens power to refractive error. Soft lenses should rest on the corneal apex and may create a small minus-powered tear layer by standing away from the cornea peripheral to the apex (Fig. 5-7). This relationship has to be corrected by the addition of plus power to the final prescription (in the range from +0.12 to +0.50 D). This correction is in contrast to that of rigid lenses, which usually vault the corneal apex and create a plus tear layer, requiring the addition of −0.25 to −0.50 D to the final prescription of a hard lens. Therefore one way to determine whether a soft lens is seated properly on or is vaulting the corneal apex is to compare the refractive error to the final lens prescription.

The following simple rules are presented for hydrogel lenses for myopic refractive errors: (1) If the final lens prescription is more myopic than (or at least the same as) the refractive error, apical contact is being made and vision will probably be satisfactory. (2) If the final lens prescription is not as strong as (more plus than) the refractive error, the lens is probably vaulting the corneal apex and creating a plus tear film, and the patient will probably demonstrate variable vision (Fig. 5-7).

Aphakic lenticular lenses, because they are thick, may touch at the apex of the cornea but stand away paracentrally and thus create a minus tear film. Hence an aphakic lens may require an increase in plus power to what one would expect.

Fitting. When fitting soft lenses, one should aim at fitting the flattest possible lens that will provide good clear vision, center well, and have no effect on the corneal integrity.

Comment. "The best way to fit a contact lens is to use a given lens." Place a lens of known parameters on the eye evaluate the fit, and when the correct fit is achieved over-refract to determine the final lens power.

INVENTORY VERSUS DIAGNOSTIC LENSES

Soft lenses may be fitted in one of two ways: (1) from an inventory of lenses by selection of the proper lens that gives the best fit and the best visual acuity or (2) from a diagnostic trial set of standard diameters and base curves to obtain the proper fitting dimensions. One can then over-refract to obtain the correct lens power and order the final lens. This requires the fitter to be able not only to fit a lens but also to refract over the trial lens. It is almost impossible to predict how a soft lens will perform on an eye until it has been tested. The only indispensable method for the fitting of a soft lens is to apply a contact lens to the eye for evaluation of its performance.

With rigid lenses most practitioners know that the effects of lid action on the front surface and lens periphery may be different on lenses of greatly different powers. Most of us have had the experience of determining the fit of a person with high myopia with a −3.00 D diagnostic lens and then finding that the higher-powered minus lens that was ordered rode high or moved excessively. The same principle applies to soft lenses, though to a somewhat lesser degree. Therefore to ensure that the soft lens ordered will fit in the same manner as the diagnostic lens used, it is desirable that the lens power of the diagnostic lens be reasonably close (within 2.00 or at most 3.00 D) of the refractive error. Thus the inventory method is a more desirable method of fitting.

If one fits from inventory, it is important to set up some form of inventory control system so that when a lens is dispensed from stock it will be marked off on the master list and a replacement lens ordered to fill the depleted inventory. A number of systems are available from the manufacturers. It is important however to reorder a lens to the inventory set once it is dispensed out to keep the inventory intact.

Of great importance is the care and disinfection of the inventory set of soft lenses. At least once weekly, the lenses should be disinfected to prevent not only bacterial contamination but also fungal contamination.

Comment. For an inventory a high-volume practice is required. With the ever-changing advances in contact-lens technology, one should not be married to a single laboratory or given lens. It is important to be able to change one's entire inventory every 3 months just to be flexible and current. For low-volume practices a small diagnostic fitting set is the best choice. Do not accumulate obsolete lenses.

BASIC FITTING METHOD FOR SOFT LENSES

There is really no formula that can predict in advance that a certain lens will give a tight fit and another will give a loose fit. In our guidelines for fitting we have had to fall back on generalizations and hope that these will not be taken as dogma to be followed without deviation. The topography of each cornea, even with standard measurements, will often vary. The quality control check by the manufacturer of soft lenses is almost impossible to assess by the fitter. Factors such as lid adherence and thickness of the tear film cannot be quantitatively evaluated. Each point we have tried to make must be viewed and analyzed in reference to one's own fitting experience.

Standard fluorescein cannot be used with soft lenses. Early corneal edema may be not only too small but also too diffuse to detect. Consequently the evaluation of the fit of a soft lens is dependent largely on certain characteristics of lens behavior, determined by its positioning and movement on the eye and by the final vision obtained.

Fitters today are in a fortunate position because they can choose from among a variety of materials with different amounts of hydration, thickness, durability, size, design, and cost. As a result they can provide the lens that performs best for an individual patient.

Lens selection may be based on one of three methods: (1) selection of soft lenses based on probable corneoscleral profiles in which one may select a lens diameter based on the horizontal iris diameter and observe how the lens performs on a given eye, (2) selection of a soft lens with a posterior radius of curvature based on K readings of the cornea determined by actual measurement of the cornea, and (3) selection of a soft lens based on the sagittal value of the lens, which requires the K reading of the cornea and takes into account not only the posterior radius of the lens curvature but also the diameter of the lens.

Each manufacturer has its own fitting method depending on the diameter and base curves that the company makes available. The following is an outline of a universal system appearing applicable to most soft lens fitting. Specialized types of fitting for aphakia, toric soft lenses, and silicone lenses are discussed in the chapters specific to these areas (Chapters 27, 24, and 21).

BASIC FITTING METHOD

1. Record the K readings and convert to millimeters.

2. Measure the corneal diameter in millimeters. The initial lens diameter to be selected should be 0.5 to 2 mm larger than this measurement. There is no set rule. This is a judgment decision based on clinical experience combined with the diameters made available by the manufacturers.

3. Determine the spheric power required: Change the refraction prescription to minus cylinders and use the spheric equivalent of the cylinder if the cylinder is greater than 0.50 D. Add this to the sphere to determine the initial lens power. Compensate this for vertex distance; for example:

$$-5.50 +1.00 \times 90$$
$$\text{change to } -4.50 -1.00 \times 180$$

Add ½ of cylinder (0.50) to sphere so that power = −5.00. Look up in the vertex table; so −5.00 at a spectacle vertex of 12 mm becomes −4.75 at the corneal plane. Power selection is −4.75.

4. If using a trial set, select a suitable trial lens with a base curve of 0.4 to 0.6 mm (2.00 to 3.00 D) flatter than the flattest K in the smaller diameter lenses (12 to 13 mm) and 0.6 to 1 mm (3.00 to 5.00 D) flatter in the large diameter lenses (14 to 15 mm).

Evaluate the fit of the lens according to the criteria just outlined for a normal fit (see below).

Perform an over-refraction on a properly fitted lens.

Order the lens of appropriate power, base curve, and diameter or select it from the lens inventory.

Reevaluate the fit and the vision.

5. If using an inventory set, repeat steps 1, 2, and 3 above. Over-refract with ± 0.25 sphere lenses to refine the power requirements after the lens has become stabilized.

Helpful hints to fitting. Keratometric readings should always be made primarily (a) to compare at a later date in case the corneal measurements change, (b) to detect whether any astigmatic error is corneal or lenticular in origin, and (c) to use as a guideline for selecting the initial base curve of the lens.

One should measure the visible iris diameter (VID) by using a number of methods such as a pupillary gauge, a reticule in a slitlamp objective lens, a rule held toward the cornea, or a draftsman's caliper with blunted points, or by the application and centering of a trial soft lens of known chord diameter. The P-D Gauge manufactured by Essilor (Paris, France) is an excellent instrument for measuring the visible iris diameter.

The best method of all is by a contact lens of known diameter. Place the lens on the eye and allow to settle for 15 to 20 minutes to equilibrate with tears. Then check the diameter on the slitlamp so that the lens fully covers the cornea, centers well, and shows satisfactory movement.

Soft lenses are best fitted from a complete inventory set where an instant fit can be achieved and the patient instructed and able to wear the lenses that day. Alternatively, for those with low-volume practices, diagnostic

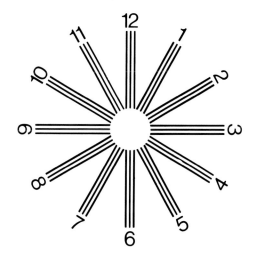

Fig. 6-1. Astigmatic clock, which can be used to determine poor vision caused by residual astigmatism. Once detected, a different type of lens can be selected. This test can save considerable chair time.

trial lens sets may be used to determine the optimum lens diameter.

Our usual procedure for standard thickness lenses is to use as flat a base curve as possible and satisfy our previously mentioned criteria. Ultrathin lenses can be fitted slightly steeper because of their oxygen-transmission properties.

Decentration of a lens may be caused by tight eyelids, large corneas, astigmatism against the rule, or asymmetric cornea topography.

The astigmatic clock is helpful in lens fitting (Fig. 6-1). After the patient has the initial or second-choice lens fitted, he or she is asked to look at the clock. If some lines are considerably more predominant, this indicates that the problem is residual astigmatism, which cannot be overcome with changes in soft lenses. A considerable amount of chair time can be saved if one switches to the central type of lenses.

FITTING EVALUATION
Normal fit

A soft lens should be fitted with what is known as three-point touch. The lens should parallel the superior and inferior sclera as well as the corneal apex. When the lens rests only on the superior and inferior sclera and vaults the corneal apex, the lens is too steep (Fig. 6-2). If the lens rests on the corneal apex and the

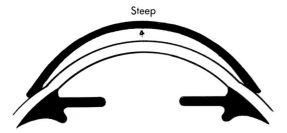

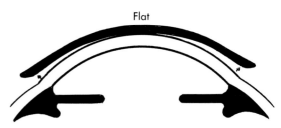

Fig. 6-2. Cross section of a steep lens showing absent touch centrally.

Fig. 6-3. Cross section demonstrating a flat lens with edge stand-off.

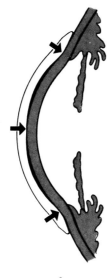

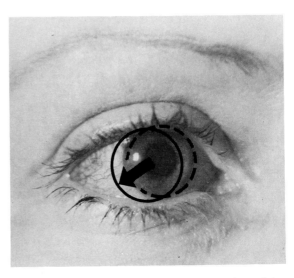

Fig. 6-4. Three-point touch—a normally fitting soft lens will rest lightly at the apex and at the periphery of the cornea.

Fig. 6-5. Decentration of a soft lens. The lens slides temporally and down.

edges stand off from the sclera, the lens is too flat (Fig. 6-3).

All soft lenses, regardless of power, size, or manufacturer, should be fitted to obtain this three-point touch (Fig. 6-4).

A well-fitted lens will show five basic qualities: good centration, adequate movement, stable vision, a crisp retinoscopic reflex, clear undistorted keratometry mires, and clear endpoint over-refraction.

Good centration. The lens will center itself well easily after insertion in the eye. After the patient blinks, it will not show more rim of lens on one side of the cornea than on the other side. Lens decentration requires refitting with either a steeper base curve or a larger diameter (Fig. 6-5). In some cases a shift to a flatter lens will be necessary.

A decentered spin-cast lens that persists in decentering after trial with a different and larger series will necessitate a change either to a thinner spin-cast lens or to a lathe-cut lens for stabilization and proper fit. Spin-cast lenses result in more centering difficulties than do lathe-cut lenses because of either the smaller size, the shape of the lens, or the design of the lens periphery.

Adequate movement. A standard-thickness lens may show movement of 0.5 to 1 mm on upward gaze after a blink, and it should show no greater movement on lateral gaze. If the lens is equilibrated with tears and does not move, the person should be switched to a lens with a flatter base curve (Fig. 6-6, *A*). If the lens moves excessively, a lens with a steeper base curve (Fig. 6-7) series or one with a larger diameter should be substituted (Fig. 6-6, *C* and *D*).

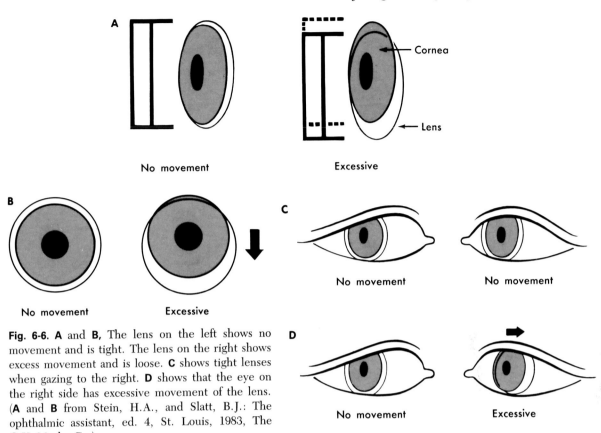

Fig. 6-6. A and B, The lens on the left shows no movement and is tight. The lens on the right shows excess movement and is loose. C shows tight lenses when gazing to the right. D shows that the eye on the right side has excessive movement of the lens. (A and B from Stein, H.A., and Slatt, B.J.: The ophthalmic assistant, ed. 4, St. Louis, 1983, The C.V. Mosby Co.)

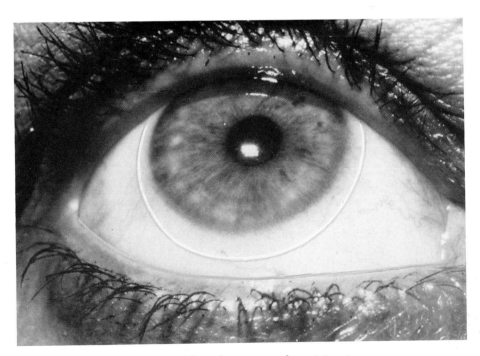

Fig. 6-7. Normal fit with excursion about 0.5 to 1 mm.

Vision

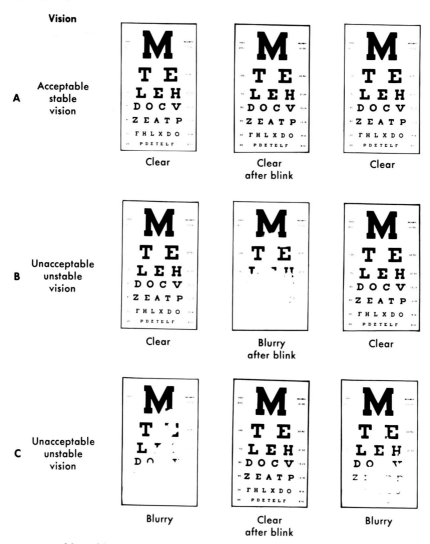

A Acceptable stable vision

Clear   Clear after blink   Clear

B Unacceptable unstable vision

Clear   Blurry after blink   Clear

C Unacceptable unstable vision

Blurry   Clear after blink   Blurry

Fig. 6-8. A, Acceptable stable vision. Vision is clear at first, clears immediately after blinking, and remains clear when not blinking. **B,** Unacceptable unstable vision that occurs when a lens is too loose because of the sliding effect of the lens after blinking. **C,** Unacceptable unstable vision that occurs when a lens is too tight. Vision is unclear at first but clears after blinking because of the flattening effect of the eyelids on a steep lens at the apex of the cornea.

The thinner series of soft lenses are fitted with slightly less movement than a standard-thickness lens needs. Thus lenses of a thinner series may be fitted with 0.5 mm movements or less. This prevents a wrinkling effect that can be produced by looser thin lens. Also one may successfully fit these lenses slightly tighter than standard-thickness lenses because thin lenses provide sufficient oxygen transmission through thin lenses to ensure corneal integrity.

The slitlamp is invaluable for evaluation of proper movement. Fit should be evaluated while the patient looks straight ahead, upward,

and laterally. The patient should be asked to blink under slitlamp observation. Evaluation should then be made clinically as to whether the movement is excessive, negligible, or adequate.

Stable vision. When the patient blinks, the vision should remain equally clear before and during the blink and visual acuity should be as sharp as possible (Fig. 6-8). If trial-set lenses are used for fit evaluation, an over-refraction should be performed.

If visual acuity is not adequately sharp after changing the lenses or holding over low-plus or

Retinoscope reflexes

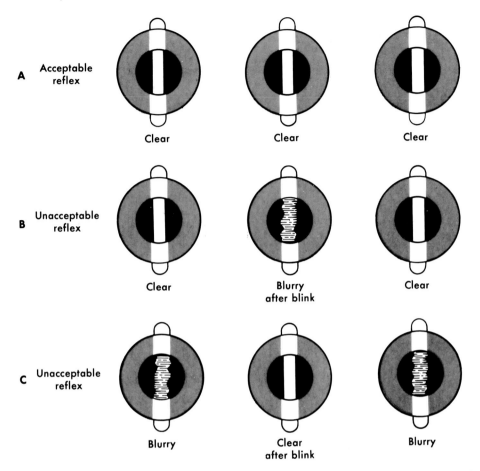

A Acceptable reflex — Clear / Clear / Clear

B Unacceptable reflex — Clear / Blurry after blink / Clear

C Unacceptable reflex — Blurry / Clear after blink / Blurry

Fig. 6-9. A, Acceptable retinoscopic reflex when lens fits well. **B,** Unacceptable retinoscopic reflex when lens is too loose. **C,** Unacceptable retinoscopic reflex when lens is too tight.

low-minus lenses, we have found it useful to have the patient view an astigmatic clock. If some of the clock lines are significantly blurred, residual astigmatism is present and vision cannot be improved any further with conventional soft lenses. Variable vision initially may be caused by a lens that is either too loose or too tight. If the fit is found to be adequate and the patient still complains of fluctuating vision, such factors as dryness of the eye or from the environment, lack of blinking, or excess mucus secretions must be considered as causative factors.

Comment. Normally, blinking may be reduced with driving and reading. The patient should be warned of soft lens variable vision. It is easily reduced by a series of blinks or artificial tears.

Crisp retinoscopic reflex. As confirmatory evidence of a good fit, the retinoscope, streak, or spot, is flashed in all meridians while the patient blinks. When the patient is adequately fitted, the retinoscopic reflex will be sharp and crisp as if no lens were in place, both before and after blinking (Fig. 6-9, *A*). If the lens is steep, there will be a spreading of the streak centrally in the rest position, which will clear after a blink because of ironing out of the apical vault (Fig. 6-9, *C*). If the lens is flat, it may ride low, a position that can be detected by retinoscopy, or the retinoscopic shadow may be blurry immediately after a blink (Fig. 6-9, *B*).

Even though residual astigmatism may be detected, if the fit is adequate the reflexes will remain sharp and clear when there is an adequate fit.

Comment. Occasionally the lens may have a poor surface optic figure and, even though the

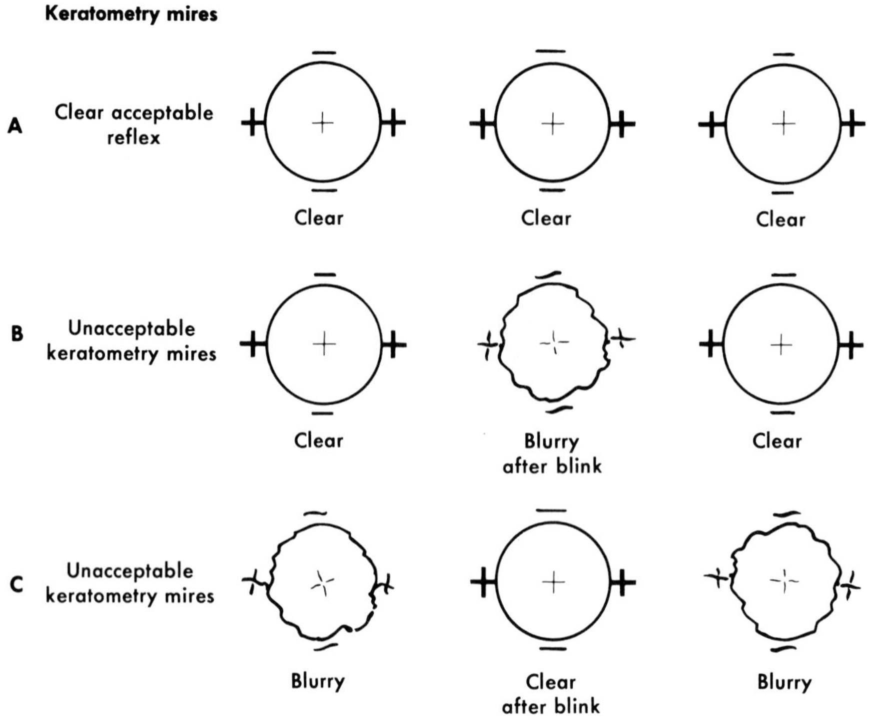

Keratometry mires

Fig. 6-10. **A,** Clear mire reflexes when the lens fits well. **B,** Unacceptable mire reflexes when the lens is loose. **C,** Unacceptable mire reflexes when the lens is tight.

fit is adequate, the retinoscopic reflex will not be sharp. A poor surface optic figure in a new lens is caused by uneven hydration, flaws in the plastic, or poor polishing. In a worn lens this may be a result of protein, lipid, or mineral deposits.

Clear, undistorted keratometry mires. The mires that are reflected from the keratometer while the person is wearing the soft lens will often indicate if the fit is adequate. With the correct fit, the mires of the keratometer should not be distorted either before or after a blink (Fig. 6-8, *A*). If the mires are blurred, the patient should blink several times; if the mires are still distorted, the lens should be changed (Fig. 6-10, *B* and *C*).

Comment. Keratometry is a valuable and simple test to perform for final evaluation after centration, vision, and movement have been analyzed. It will act as a check on the other parameters that have been evaluated. Occasionally the mires will be blurred because of surface mucous or dehydration. When this occurs, blinking will usually restore the anterior surface to a normal luster if the problem is not one of fitting. Any blurring of the mires or ir-

regular patterns are indicative of a poorly fitted lens, which may give rise to potential fitting problems. Occasionally blurring may be caused by a poor surface figure in the lens, a drying out of the lens surface, or mucous debris.

Dr. Josh Josephson has pointed out an additional method of evaluating the fit of a soft lens. While viewing the eye with the slitlamp, one can press gently on the lower lid toward the globe and against the edge of the lens. The lens, if an acceptable fit, will show a slight edge lift-off after it is digitally moved across the limbus. If the lift-off is excessive, the lens is too flat. If the lens does not lift off from the globe at all, it is probably too tight. This is referred to as the edge-lift effect.

Loose fit

Symptoms and signs of a loose lens. The following indicate that the fit of a lens is loose:
1. Variable vision, clear at first but poor after blinking (Fig. 6-8, *B*)
2. Excess awareness of the lens
3. Poor centering
4. Excess movement (Fig. 6-6, *A, B,* and *D,* and 6-11)

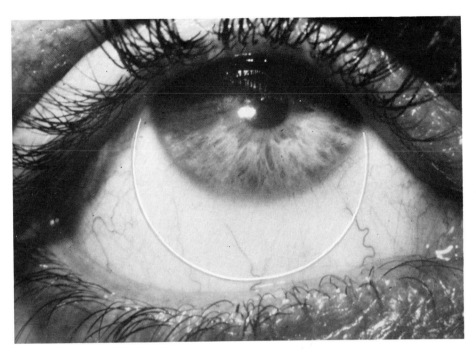

Fig. 6-11. Loose lens indicated by lag on upward gaze.

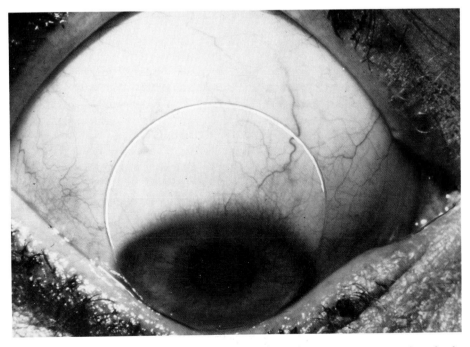

Fig. 6-12. Loose lens. On downward gaze the lens rides high. A valuable test to confirm the fitting of a soft lens.

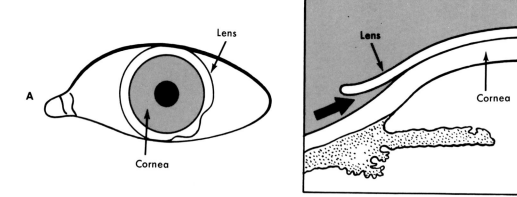

Fig. 6-13. Loose lens with edge stand-off. **A,** Edge lifting off the scleral rim; **B,** Schematic side view interpretation of the edge lift-off of a loose lens.

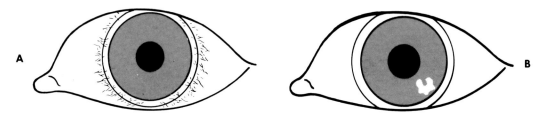

Fig. 6-14. A, Circumcorneal injection; **B,** bubble under a loose soft lens.

5. Edge stand-off (Fig. 6-13)
6. Lens falling out of the eye
7. Bubble under the lens edge (Fig. 6-14, *B*)
8. Keratometry showing clear mires at first that blur after a blink and then clear (Fig. 6-10, *B*)
9. Retinoscopy that is clear at first but blurs after blinking (Fig. 6-9, *B*)

A loose lens may show movement of 2 to 4 mm on downward excursions and may even slide off the cornea entirely on lateral movement (Fig. 6-6, *B*). The vision is often clear at first but may decrease two or three lines after a blink, though it may recover quickly. In an extremely loose lens the edge may roll out the so-called edge stand-off and the lens may fall out of the eye on a blink because of contact of the lids with the rolled-out edge. Because it may require a few minutes before edge stand-off appears in a loose lens, it is best to allow 15 to 20 minutes before completion of the evaluation of fit.

Comment. A valuable test for a loose lens is to have the patient look down. If the lens floats

high, it should be considered as loose (Fig. 6-12).

Correction of a loose lens. The following steps should be taken to correct a loose lens:
1. For a lathe-cut lens, switch to a lens with a steeper base curve or a larger lens diameter.
2. For Bausch & Lomb spin-cast lenses, switch to a series of a larger diameter.

Comment. It is therefore necessary because of the thinness and asphericity of the Bausch & Lomb lenses that they be fitted according to the horizontal visible iris diameter (HVID). The initial lens chosen should be 1 mm larger than the HVID.

With lathe-cut lenses one can switch to a radius steeper in 0.2 to 0.3 mm steps or increase the diameter 0.5 mm up to a lens size of 15 mm in diameter. Both methods will tighten the lens and decrease lens movement. It is preferable to fit initially with a loose lens and make it tighter until the lens of choice is determined. This should be the flattest lens possible that fulfills all the criteria of a good fit.

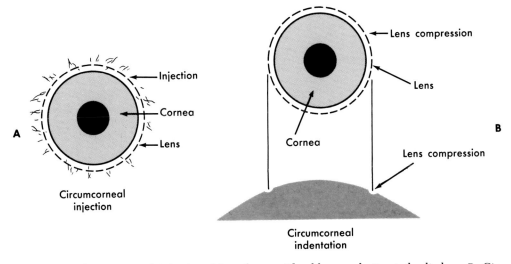

Fig. 6-15. A, Circumcorneal injection. Note the considerable vascularity at the limbus. **B,** Circumcorneal indentation. The tight lens compresses the peripheral limbal tissues.

Tight fit

Symptoms and signs of a tight lens. The following indicate a tight fitting for a lens:

1. Fluctuating vision that clears immediately after blinking (Fig. 6-8, *C*)
2. Initially comfortable but increasingly uncomfortable as the day progresses
3. Circumcorneal injection, or redness around the circumference of the cornea (Fig. 6-15, *A*)
4. Circumcorneal indentation—the conjunctiva is compressed at the limbus and there is a ditchlike depression that obstructs the normal flow of the vessels (Fig. 6-15, *B*)
5. Absent or minimal movement after a blink (Figs. 6-2 and 6-16)
6. Keratometry with lens in place that shows distorted mires before a blink, which clear immediately after blinking (Fig. 6-10, *C*)
7. Retinoscope reflex that may be fuzzy at first and may clear momentarily after a blink (Fig. 6-9, *C*)

If the lens is too steep, there is no touch at the apex because of apical vaulting. Vision is improved immediately after a blink because the eyelid on a blink "irons out" the soft lens and compresses the lens against the apex of the cornea. The patient's only complaint may be fluctuating vision, which may be momentary but annoying.

It may take several days of wearing time before circumlimbal injection and indentation occurs. This is a late sign of a tight lens. Lenses, however, should be changed before this has had a chance to occur. Complaints of a burning sensation may precede limbal compression and are a forewarning sign of a tight lens. The uncomfortable feeling of a tight lens may take several hours or days to appear.

We have noted that some lenses that are well fitted at the beginning gradually change their parameters and tighten up months later. This may be caused in part by alteration in the plastic by the chemical disinfection process or by the accumulation of denatured protein. This should be taken into consideration at every examination.

If the lens is very tight, the patient or the practitioner may have difficulty in removing the lens. There have been instances of denuding the epithelium on removal. If removal is difficult, saline drops should be added before removal.

Exceptions to the rule. A tight lens may show excessive movement and may ride low and behave like a loose lens. When the lens is made tighter, it may move even more than initially. There reason is that there is no longer three-point touch (apex and periphery) but only touch at the periphery so that the lens loses some of its normal capillary attraction to the cornea. Thus the degree of movement alone is

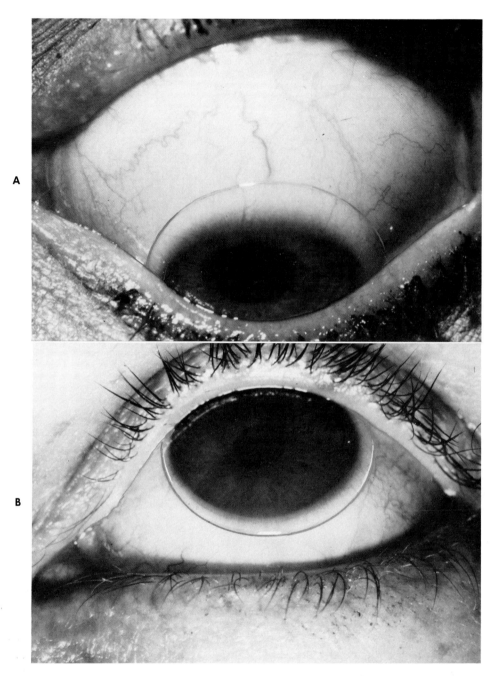

Fig. 6-16. A, Slightly tight lens as indicated by minimal movement up on downward gaze. **B,** Tight soft lens. Note the lack of lag on upward gaze and indentation in perilimbal area.

not sufficient to determine whether the lens is loose or tight.

A steep lens, like a flat lens, may decenter low because of increased lid action on blinking resulting from lack of touch of the lens at the apex of the cornea. A steep lens frequently decenters downward and nasally because of the direction of the lid action and because peripheral scleral flattening does not come into play.

Correction of tight lens situation. The following steps should be taken to correct a tight lens:

1. Switch to a flatter lens.
2. For spin-cast Bausch & Lomb series lenses, switch to a smaller diameter series or a thinner lens.
3. For lathed lenses, switch to a flatter base curve or reduce the diameter of the lens.

A reduction in the diameter of a lens or flattening the base curve will reduce the apical vault of the lens; as a result the lens apex will be closer to and will rest lightly on the apex of the cornea. Unlike with rigid lenses, fenestration is not a solution for soft lenses because bacteria and fungus invasion can occur when a portal of entry is created in the lens substance. Although it is theoretically possible to dehydrate carefully an existing soft lens for modification, it is not practical from a financial point of view. It is easier and less expensive to fabricate a new lens.

A lens may behave as a tight lens if blinking is infrequent or incomplete.

HELPFUL HINTS ON FITTING

1. If rigid methyl methacrylate lenses have been worn, it is essential that stabilization of the keratometry mires occurs before a soft lens evaluation is made. The cornea may require several weeks or even months to resume a stable topography. This can be shown by two repeatable refractions and K readings.

    A thin, oxygen-permeable soft lens should be used as a temporary lens until the refraction or K readings are stable.

2. Peripheral arcuate abrasion of the cornea, which can cause moderate to severe discomfort, may be caused by an eccentrically positioned, small soft lens. It can be overcome by choosing a larger or steeper lens.

    At times the problem of decentration is best handled if one switches to a lathe-cut lens.

3. If a particular lens appears too loose and the next lens is too steep, try another lens of the same specification as the original lens. Occasionally lenses have been found to be incorrectly labeled.

4. The importance of blinking, especially while one is reading and driving, should be stressed.

    Alteration in the blink rate is the most common cause of late afternoon variable vision. This is especially true if one has to read a great deal in his job and works in a relatively dry office environment.

5. A measure of the visible iris diameter with a gauge or ruler may be helpful in selecting a lens of the proper diameter, particularly if the cornea is unusually large.

6. Keratometer mires should be rechecked over the lens to make sure that they are not distorted.

7. When a lens is applied to the eye, it may take a few minutes before edge stand-off occurs and the lens shows characteristics of appearing loose. Always wait 15 to 20 minutes before completing an evaluation of the fit.

8. The configuration of the lids and the size of the palpebral aperture are very important in determining the size of the lens required. Wide palpebral fissures such as those that may occur with lid retraction of hyperthyroidism or congenitally prominent eyes may require larger lenses. The small palpebral fissure of Orientals and the small corneal diameters usually require smaller diameter lenses than normal.

    Tight lids can cause traction and make the lens move excessively with a blink. It can ruin a good toric lens fit.

9. The elliptic curve of the back surface of the Bausch & Lomb spin-cast lens, however, makes it more difficult to predict the initial performance of a Bausch & Lomb spin-cast lens.

10. Clinically it is important to work always in the same direction from looser to tighter fit, starting with a loose lens and working toward a lens of proper fit. As previously indicated, one may tighten lathe-cut lenses

by steepening the base curve in 0.3 mm steps or by increasing the diameter in 0.5 mm steps. Alternatively one may loosen lenses by flattening the base curve in 0.3 mm steps or by decreasing the diameter in 0.5 mm steps.

11. In those instances where larger or smaller diameter lenses are not readily available and changing the base curve does not produce the desired effect, it may be necessary to switch to a manufacturer that can custom grind the desired lens.

12. With the low-water-content soft lenses, an acceptable fit is one that has considerable movement compared to that of other soft lens materials. Even a soft lens fit that would normally appear sloppy is acceptable with a low-water-content lens.

13. Because the posterior surface of a spin-cast lens is aspheric, the traditional K readings and their relationship to base curve do not apply with spin-cast lenses. The basic fitting system depends on measurement of the horizontal visible iris diameter and selection of a suitable diameter of lens with proper power. The numerical suffix on the label denotes the lens diameter. A label ending in 4 is 14.5 mm, a 3 is a 13.5 diameter, and the absence of a number is 12.5 mm in diameter.

Minus-power contact lenses are available in nine primary series. The O series lens is the thinnest lens presently available having a thickness of 0.035 mm.

14. The slitlamp is invaluable in detecting many of the foregoing criteria for a good fit. Attention should be paid to bubbles under the lens or scleral indentation indicating a steep fit and one in which a flatter base curve should be selected.

15. Drs. Hikaru Hamano and Hideaki Kawabe of Japan have shown that the base curve of a lens decreases within 5 to 10 minutes after a lens is worn and then becomes stable. Thus one should always permit the patient to wait beyond that period, that is, at least 15 to 20 minutes before assessing the fit.

A thick soft lens can cause changes in the endothelium in 1 day. If the vision is impaired, switch to a much thinner lens to avoid minimal corneal edema.

16. Discomfort can arise even with thin soft lenses. They may be too low so that movement with a blink is excessive. They may be slightly decentered so that a rim of cornea is exposed. The eyes may be moderately dry, and the thin lens exaggerates the condition to become symptomatic. The lens may be turned inside out, and that position not be recognized.

CHAPTER 7

HANDLING OF SOFT LENSES

INSERTION, REMOVAL, AND WEARING SCHEDULE

Insertion and removal technique
Taco test
Helpful hints on patient instruction
Wearing schedule and follow-up

INSERTION AND REMOVAL TECHNIQUE

The technique for insertion and removal of soft lenses is different from that of conventional rigid lenses. The soft lens is inserted onto the lower part of the sclera and gently pushed onto the cornea with the lower eyelid. When soft lenses are being removed, it is generally recommended to slide the lens down with the index finger to the lower part of the sclera and then pinch off the lens.

Insertion by the practitioner

The following technique is used for lens insertion by the practitioner:

1. Keep fingernails short at all times.
2. Wash hands and rinse thoroughly to remove all traces of soap. Dry with a lint-free towel. Avoid using oils and hand creams on hands before handling the lens.
3. Remove the right lens from the vial or case. Lenses that have been soaked in a germicide must be rinsed thoroughly with normal saline solution. Do not touch the inside lens surface after rinsing.
4. Place the lens on the tip of the index finger, concave side up. Have the patient look straight ahead. Stand to the right of the patient and retract the lower lid with your middle finger (Fig. 7-1).
5. Have the patient look up and stare at a point on the ceiling. Be sure that the head is held firmly against a head rest. Roll the lens onto the lower white of the eye and express the air bubble. Swirling the lens momentarily on the lateral part

of the sclera also helps to make the lens comfortable by introducing tears under the lens and thereby replacing the saline along the lens with the patient's own tears.

6. Have the patient close his or her eyes and lightly massage the closed lid to help center the lens.
7. Repeat the same procedure for the left lens.

Comment. If the eye feels irritable after insertion of the lens on the cornea, slide the lens on the conjunctiva and swirl it around to permit tears to flow under the lens and take on the tonicity of the tears before centering again on the more sensitive cornea.

If the patient is a squeezer, it may be easier to fold the lens and insert it on the temporal conjunctiva rather than on the lower part of the eye.

With thin lenses, permit the lens to dry on the finger for a moment before insertion. Be sure the finger itself is kept relatively dry or the lens will stick to the finger (Fig. 7-2).

Removal by the practitioner

The following technique is used for lens removal by the practitioner:

1. Wash hands before removal as before insertion.
2. Be sure that the lens is on the cornea before attempting removal.
3. Have the patient look up. Place the middle finger on the lower eyelid, and touch the edge of the lens with the forefinger.
4. While the patient is looking up, slide the

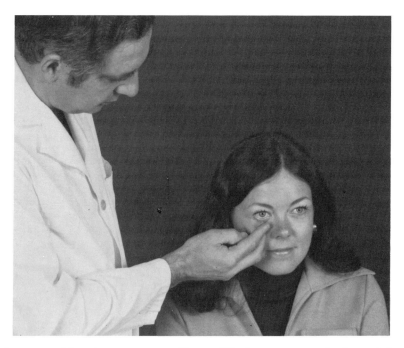

Fig. 7-1. Insertion of lens by practitioner. The middle finger retracts the lower lid while the contact lens is gently applied with the index finger to the lower conjunctiva.

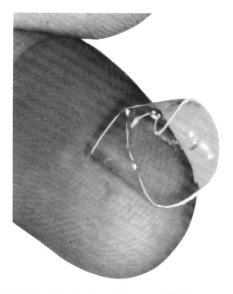

Fig. 7-2. An ultrathin lens is more difficult to insert unless permitted to dehydrate.

lens down onto the lower conjunctiva of the eye. Bring the thumb over and compress the lens lightly between the thumb and the index finger so that the lens folds and comes off easily.

Comment. If the patient is apprehensive and makes the application of a lens difficult because of blepharospasm, have him open his mouth. It is difficult to squeeze the lids shut with the mouth wide open.

Insertion by the patient

The following technique is used for lens insertion by the patient:

1. Keep fingernails short. Wash hands carefully with soap that does not contain cold cream and dry them. (It is important that the hands be carefully scrubbed and that all traces of makeup or nicotine be removed; otherwise, these will be transferred onto the lens.)
2. Take the lens out of the vial preferably by pouring the contents of the vial into the palm of the hand. Alternately one can use forceps but lenses are often damaged by this manner. Shake any excess fluid off the lens.

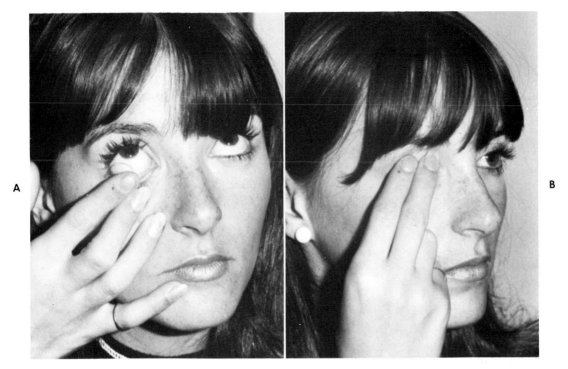

Fig. 7-3. A, Inserting the soft lens. **B,** Centering the lens through the closed eyelid. (From Stein, H.A., and Slatt, B.J.: The ophthalmic assistant, ed. 4, St. Louis, 1983, The C.V. Mosby Co.)

3. Place the lens on the tip of the index finger of the dominant hand.
4. While looking up, retract the lower lid with the middle finger, and while gazing upward, apply the lens to the lower part of the eye (Fig. 7-3, *A*).
5. Express any air, remove the index finger, and then slowly release the lower lid.
6. Close the eyes and gently massage the lids to help center the lens (Fig. 7-3, *B*).
7. Cover the other eye and focus to make sure that the lens is centered.
8. Repeat the same procedure for the left lens.

Comment. The ultrathin transparent lenses are difficult to see and feel. A tinted lens aids in the visual identification of the lens.

Clinical experience has shown that the thin edge of a high-plus lenticular lens, an ultrathin lens or a high water content lens may sometimes tend to fold over while it is being placed on the patient's eye. This difficulty may be reduced if the lens is held on the patient's finger for about 60 seconds before placement, thus allowing drying to occur and the edge to stabilize.

Removal by the patient

The following technique is used for lens removal by the patient:
1. Check each vision separately by covering the opposite eye to be sure that the lens is in place on the cornea.
2. Wash hands and rinse thoroughly.
3. Look upward. Retract the lower lid with the middle finger and place the index fingertip on the lower half of the lens.
4. Slide the lens down to the white of the eye.
5. Compress the lens between the thumb and the index finger so that air breaks the suction under the lens. Remove the lens from the eye (Fig. 7-4).
6. Prepare the lens for cleaning and sterilizing according to the recommendation of the manufacturer and the practitioner.
7. Alternative methods of removal: (1) Look nasally and slide the lens to the outermost portion of the eye before removal (Fig. 7-5), and (2) use the thumb to press the lower lid up and the index finger against the upper lid edge. By flexing the edges and blinking, one can make the lens come

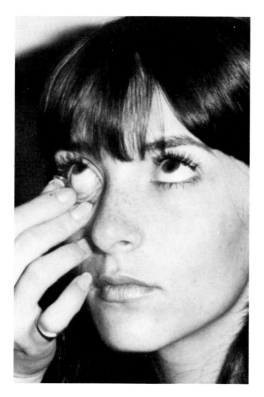

Fig. 7-4. Removing the lens. The lens is gently pinched between the thumb and forefinger. (From Stein, H.A., and Slatt, B.J.: The ophthalmic assistant, ed. 4, St. Louis, 1983, The C.V. Mosby Co.)

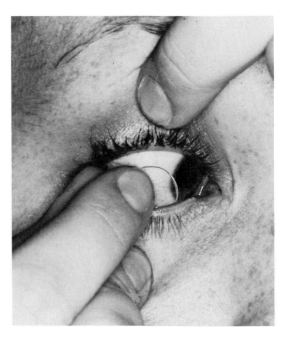

Fig. 7-5. An alternate method of removal is to slide the lens to the temporal portion of the globe and fold it off or else use light pressure on the lids at the upper and lower edges of the lens to flex the lens to permit the eyelids to blink the lens out.

out and can grasp it by the thumb and forefinger.

Elderly patients may have difficulty in placing, removing, and handling lenses. Normally if this problem cannot be overcome by in-office training, the patient should not receive the lens. Often, however, another person—a spouse, daughter, or son—may be taught to place, remove, and handle the lenses for the patient. The same is true with children who are being fitted with hydrophilic lenses. Insertion devices are available for the soft lens, but we have not found them to be very helpful on a prolonged basis. The patient must learn to handle his own lenses directly. See Fig. 7-6.

For those females who resist cutting their nails or who constantly damage lenses, we have occasionally resorted to the use of rubber finger cots in the insertion and removal procedure (Fig. 7-7).

Dr. Thomas Spring of Melbourne, Australia, has suggested the use of a sterile finger cot to minimize contamination from fingers. Finger

contamination in America has not been a serious problem, but it may apply in other parts of the world.

Comment. One of the advantages of extended-wear lenses is that lens handling is drastically reduced. But persons who wear such lenses do not have a lesser frequency of infection. Lens handling is probably overrated as a cause of infection in contact lens wearers.

TACO TEST

Before insertion of lenses by either practitioner or patient, one should be sure that the lens is not inside out. One can verify this by gently folding the lens between the thumb and forefinger. The edges should point inward and look like a Mexican taco with the edges touching. When the edges roll out rather than in, like an inverted wartime helmet, the lens is inside out and must be reversed (Fig. 7-8).

It is important that the lens be grasped and folded near the apex of the lens rather than at its edges. Grasping the lens near the edges may give a false and unreliable result. This test does not appear to work well with the very large lathe-cut lenses.

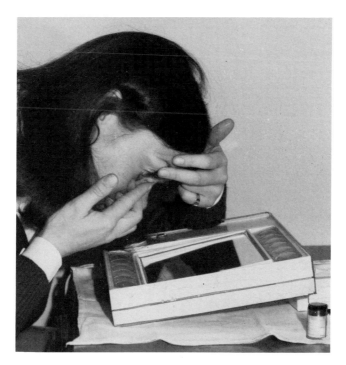

Fig. 7-6. A large mirror is a helpful adjunct in insertion of a lens.

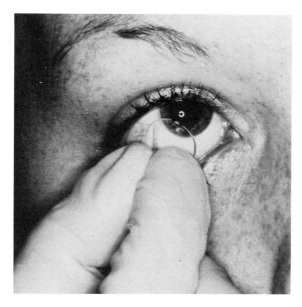

Fig. 7-7. Finger cots can be used for those who persistently scratch their lenses or who resist cutting their fingernails.

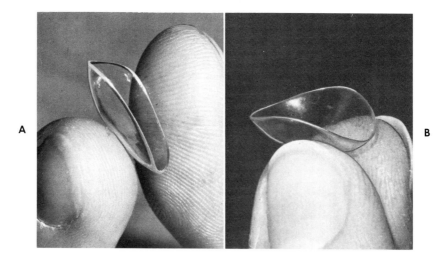

Fig. 7-8. Taco test to determine correct side of the lens. **A,** Correct side. Edge is erect and points slightly inward. **B,** Edge appears to fold back on the fingers, indicating that the lens is inside out and must be reversed. (From Stein, H.A., and Slatt, B.J.: The ophthalmic assistant, ed. 4, St. Louis, 1983, The C.V. Mosby Co.)

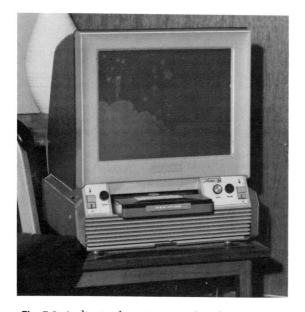

Fig. 7-9. Audiovisual equipment is helpful in patient instruction.

HELPFUL HINTS ON PATIENT INSTRUCTION

1. Show an audiovisual training film and give instruction booklets to patients before instruction (Fig. 7-9).
2. Do not rush patients. They have spent their lives keeping things out of their eyes, and it is a worrisome experience to put anything in them.
3. Be patient with instruction. Do not go beyond a 1-hour session.
4. If patients cannot master insertion and removal on the first day, do not keep them there until they can; otherwise, they will become nervous and tense and the eye irritated. Have them return another day for further instruction. If they are allowed to take their lenses home before they feel confident in their handling, a high percentage of these patients stop wearing their lenses.
5. Carefully explain the importance of hygiene and care. Patients who have received good instructions in the beginning will have fewer problems.
6. Explain that lenses may be extremely difficult to find in the bottle or lens container and that the container should be emptied into the palm of the hand (Fig. 7-10).
7. Emphasize that great care should be observed by the patients to avoid switching lenses by placing them in the wrong container.
8. When applying the lenses for the first time, have the patients rest their heads on the headrest. Nervous patients will back away as the practitioner comes close to the eye.
9. If patients are extremely nervous, pull the lids apart without inserting the lens to re-

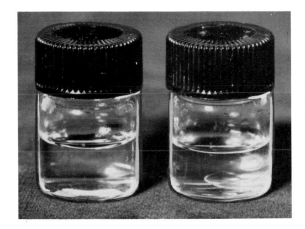

Fig. 7-10. Two bottles. The bottle on the right contains a soft lens. It is often impossible for the patient to identify the presence of the lens in the bottle. The bottle should be emptied in the palm of the hand.

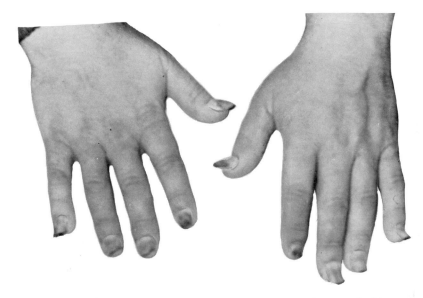

Fig. 7-11. Onychogryposis of fingernails, which makes insertion and removal of lenses virtually impossible.

lax the patients and get them used to the feel of the lids being pulled apart. Tell patients than lens awareness may be present initially on the lower lids but will disappear shortly.

10. When the soft lens is applied and stings, it is helpful to slide the lens from the cornea onto the outer part of the sclera and rub gently to get patient's own tears under the lens. This makes the lens isotonic with the tears, resulting in a more comfortable lens. We have called this technique the "scleral swirl."

11. If a patient's eyes are red while wearing soft lenses, remove lenses and stain the eye with fluorescein, checking for staining,

stippling, or any interference with corneal metabolism or breaks in the corneal epithelium. Do not reinsert lenses for at least 1 hour after fluorescein is used because the residual fluorescein may stain the lens.

12. Always remember that problems of corneal irritation are usually caused by a sensitivity to the cleaning, storing, saline solutions used, and, in particular, thimerosal, which is used as a preservative in contact lens solutions.

13. Outline a conservative wearing schedule for the patient to follow.

14. Explain the various systems available for disinfecting lenses and explain why a particular one is being recommended and the

reasons why patients should not change systems on their own.

15. Carefully instruct patients (1) not to use any over-the-counter eye medication or lens cleansing solutions and (2) not to switch from disinfecting by chemicals to boiling without advice from the practitioner.

16. Avoid fitting patients with any abnormal hand or fingernail problems (Fig. 7-11).

17. Avoid moist heat disinfection with anything but the recommended saline solution. Some preserved saline solutions have an adverse effect on lenses.

WEARING SCHEDULE AND FOLLOW-UP

Soft lenses that are well manufactured, are polished, and have good edge design can be worn for a considerably longer period the first day than was initially realized. Each manufacturer outlines its own protocol, which usually tends to be somewhat conservative. As new lens designs and new soft lenses appear, with better oxygen performance, routines will naturally have to be modified. We can only offer as a guideline our present protocol for standard-thickness and toric soft lenses. The wearing time may be increased considerably for ultra-thin and higher water content lenses.

The first day the patient may wear the soft lenses for 4 hours. The wearing time may be increased 2 hours daily until an all-day wearing schedule is achieved. Persons with hyperopia, including those with aphakia, should have a somewhat reduced initial wearing time on the first day because of the greater central thickness of the lens. Three hours is a safe initial wearing time for these persons.

Many practitioners recommend a more rapid wearing schedule in which the patient wears the lenses 4 or more hours the first day, removes the lenses for 1 hour, and then wears the lenses again for 4 or more hours. The wearing time increases by 2 hours daily with a 1-hour break period. Occasionally we have found patients whose cornea has not tolerated such a lengthy contact the first few days with standard-thickness and low water content lenses. Also, inexperienced lens wearers sometimes have difficulty with the extra insertion and re-moval procedure that is required for this schedule.

Full wearing time is an individual variation, and some persons may develop diffuse corneal edema in 10 to 12 hours or sooner. They may not be able to tolerate a soft lens beyond this time even when extremely thin lenses are provided.

Acquired astigmatism has been noted with changes in K values in over 80% of soft lens wearers who wear their standard lenses continuously for more than 12 hours daily.

The degree of astigmatism induced is minor, and most fitters do not limit their soft lens wearing time to 12 hours a day. In the fully adapted lens wearer, full daily wearing time is advocated especially with the newer oxygen-permeable soft lenses. Induced astigmatism should and can be monitored with follow-up K readings. One has to pay attention to the quality of the mires and to the change in the radius of curvature. The mires may be blurred or distorted and the valves unchanged. This condition would indicate the start of alterations in corneal topography.

The patient should return to the office for follow-up in 1 week and then at 2-week intervals for three visits. During these visits the fit of the lenses should be evaluated and lens changes made if required. This follow-up procedure is usually adequate for the majority of myopic soft lens wearers.

The appearance of any constriction at the limbus or vessels that begins to invade deeply into the cornea, or any reduction in movement, should be noted and the lens changed to a flatter lens.

Conventional standard-thickness soft lenses should not be worn during sleep. The absence of blinking results in absent tear exchange, insufficient oxygen, and consequently corneal anoxia (see Chapter 26).

With the development of more oxygen-permeable soft contact lens of either the higher water content, the silicone polymers, or the considerable reduction in thickness of the lens, we may be more permissive in letting patients wear their lenses all day right from the beginning, provided that the cornea does not respond adversely.

CARE SYSTEMS FOR SOFT LENSES

A wide variety of products are presently available for contact lens care. This large number of available products frequently results in confusion by the practitioner and the public. This section discusses some basic principles and the rationale for the various cleaning, disinfecting, and rinsing solutions. Whenever changes are made in the care system, one must be fully aware of the interactions of products and the nature of possible adverse reactions. One must also keep in mind the efficacy of the product as to both cleaning the lens and its ability to disinfect. Thus there must be some guidelines for a systematic method of selecting an appropriate effective hydrogel care system for a given person or type of material.

Available care products fall into four categories:

1. Cleaning agents
2. Disinfecting solutions—chemical and thermal
3. Rinsing solutions
4. Lubricating-rewetting-cleaning eye drops

There is a variety of available products to be discussed. Although reference may be made to specific trade names, this has been done to illustrate and clarify and does not necessarily reflect their endorsement by us.

CLEANING AGENTS

Soft lenses worn over a period of time become gradually coated and cloudy. This cloudiness not only interferes with the clarity of vision but also acts as an irritant, making the patient uncomfortable. The coating may also cause adverse tissue responses. The cloudiness is usually related to surface debris consisting of protein, inorganic films, mucin, lipids, and minerals (Fig. 8-1).

Surface debris on the lens may be diffuse, mottled, or concentrated in one area. It may be a mixture of protein with lipid or calcium deposits. It is more common in persons with relative tear deficiency or with high serum cholesterol levels. Microorganisms usually adhere tenaciously to the surface; the most common

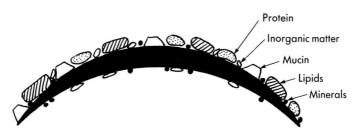

Fig. 8-1. Common deposits on the surface of a contact lens.

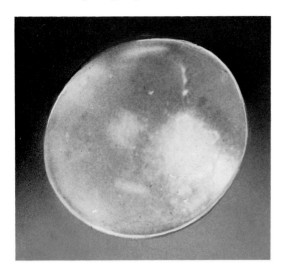

Fig. 8-2. Protein buildup on a soft lens will vary with the duration of wear, the method of disinfection, and the nature of the tears of the wearer.

deposits are protein and lipids (Fig. 8-2). However, there are many extrinsic factors that contribute to lens spoilage. Unclean fingers may transfer grease, dirt, mascara, eyeliner, nicotine, or lipstick. Face powder or environmental dust as well as toxic fumes may affect the lens surface. Blinking causes the palpebral conjunctiva to rub over the deposit up to 15,000 to 25,000 times per day, releasing mucin from the goblet cells and perhaps exposing the tarsal conjunctiva to an immunologic response to the coating on the surface of the lens.

The buildup of protein, lipids, and minerals on the lens may result in the following:

1. A decrease in vision
2. A red and irritable eye
3. An increase in the mass of the lens, which may affect the fit of the lens
4. A change in the parameter of the lens, which may cause the lens to tighten.
5. Decrease in the oxygen transmission of the lens
6. An increase in the protein antigen factor on the lens, which may in turn cause:
   a. Giant papillary hypertrophy of the conjunctiva
   b. Corneal and bulbar conjunctival inflammatory response

The net effect of these changes is to make the lens uncomfortable and the vision blurry.

Allansmith and Fowler have shown that surface deposits extend over 50% of a hydrogel lens within 5 minutes after the soft lens is worn and over 90% of the lens in 8 hours.

Because some coating occurs within 30 minutes, it is quite likely that it may be necessary for coating to occur. Perhaps mucinous coating is necessary to reduce the wetting angle of the plastic and to permit greater comfort and vision. With time, however, the coating becomes plaque-like and produces problems as described above.

Kleist has demonstrated that the thermal method of disinfection produced an incidence higher than usual of most deposits except calcium, which appeared higher with chemical disinfection (Table 8-1).

We have also found deposits to be more frequent with the thermal method of disinfection than with chemical disinfection. The heat tends to denature or coagulate the proteinaceous material on the surface of the lens. Josephson, in a retrospective study, found that the rate of replacement almost doubled in switching patients from chemical to thermal disinfection. The exception to this rule is white crystalline deposits, which occur less frequently with the thermal system.

Protein buildup is now believed to be a form of denatured lysozyme, a normal antibacterial enzyme found in tears (Fig. 8-3). Almost all soft-lens wearers eventually will develop this protein build-up, but it will vary with the type of soft-lens material, the duration of time that the lenses are worn, the nature of the tears of each individual, and the method and efficiency of cleaning.

Small amounts of protein buildup can be detected more easily if the lens is removed from the eye, allowed to partially dehydrate, and then held against a black background with oblique light from a slitlamp. If the protein buildup is excessive, a reasonable assessment can be obtained when one examines the lens on the eye with the slitlamp. Even modest amounts may be detected by intense scrutiny.

Unfortunately there are no methods to ensure that an adequate cleaning has been done by the patients when they take their lenses home.

Another excellent method of lens inspection is a slitlamp attachment called the "View All" (Optical Science Group, Inc., Petaluma, Calif.).

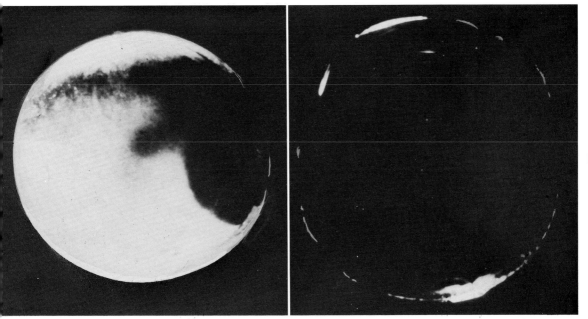

B

Fig. 8-3. A, Soft lens with protein accumulation on the surface. **B,** Soft lens that has been routinely cleaned with cleaning agents.

Table 8-1. Incidence of common deposits on 370 lenses with deposits

	Incidence		
Type of deposit	*Overall (%)*	*Cold regimen (%)*	*Heat regimen (%)*
Abrasions	25	28	22
Protein films	19	14	24
Pigment	25	9	38
Microorganisms	10	4	28, unpreserved saline
			11, preserved saline
Inorganic films	10.5	5.9	14.4
Rust-colored spots	13	7	18
Lens calculi	13	13	13
Calcium carbonate	9.5	16	4
Calcium phosphate	4.6	9	1
Mercurial origin	10.5	5	21, preserved saline

From Kleist, F.: Deposits, International Contact Lens Clinics, May-June 1979.

The View All snaps into the right part of the slit-lamp so as to position its two spheres (one 42.00 D, the other 35.00 D) in front of the slit beam. By using this method one can carry out a fast and comprehensive lens inspection with the slitlamp (Fig. 8-4). Surface haze and hydrophobicity are indicative of small amounts of coating.

Allansmith and Fowler have shown that the deposits on daily wear soft lenses show peaks and valleys whereas the deposits on extended wear lenses are diffusely coated with a relatively even smooth surface (Fig. 8-5). In effect, these deposits on extended wear lenses may be more innocuous because they provide a smooth refracting surface on the lens, which may be less traumatic for the tarsal conjunctiva. Allansmith believes that the peaks and valley coating on daily wear soft contact lenses are attributable to repeated dripping away of a portion of the plaques on the surface of the contact lenses whereas with extended wear soft lenses the deposits are not cleaned frequently and build up as a flat coating.

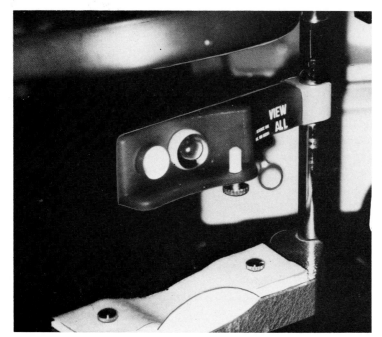

Fig. 8-4. System for viewing a soft contact lens with the biomicroscope. (Courtesy Optical Science Group, Inc., Petaluma, Calif.)

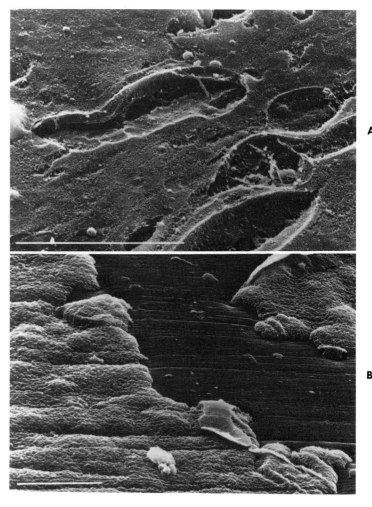

A

B

Fig. 8-5. A, Electron microscopy photograph showing coating on an extended-wear lens being relatively flat. **B,** Coating on a daily-wear lens revealing large valleys and bare areas of a contact lens after cleaning. (Courtesy Mathea Allansmith and Sherry Fowler, Boston.)

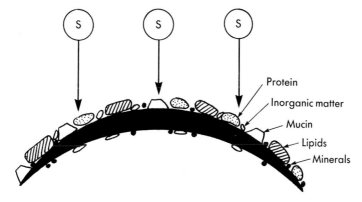

Fig. 8-6. Action of surfactant on a lens surface is to mobilize, emulsify, and solubilize the deposits on a lens.

METHODS OF CLEANING

There are three distinct types of soft lens cleaners—surface-acting, oxidative, and enzyme cleaners. Added to this is the use of ultrasound, which can help speed up the cleaning process.

Surface-acting (surfactant) cleaners

Surfactants mobilize, emulsify, and solubilize the adhered accumulation of proteins, lipids, and minerals from the surface of a lens during a day of wear (Fig. 8-6). Bacteria adhere to the surface of lens deposits, and surfactants facilitate disinfection by reducing microbial contamination on the lens surface.

The surfactant agent is usually of high molecular weight to prevent molecules from entering the pores of the lens. Surfactants act to lower surface tension of the lens-water interface. Surfactant-cleaner formulations also contain a chelating agent that binds metal ions. Some surfactant cleaners are hypertonic with the purpose of drawing out or absorbing material from within the lens. Other surfactant formulations lower or raise pH so as to maximize protein removal. Examples of these are Softmate and Pliagel. Miraflow incorporates isopropryl alcohol added to Pliagel to remove lipids and protein. The isopropryl alcohol is both a disinfectant and solvent that solubilizes lipids and protein.

Some surfactants are anionic or negatively charged, which means that they react with cations such as magnesium or calcium and precipitate these ions out. These cleaners can be used for any type of soft lens, rigid lens, CAB, gas-permeable rigid lens, or silicone lens. One cleaner, Opti-Clean (Polyclens), contains large molecule beads that shear the deposits from the lens surface without any adverse effects on the surface.

Comment. All surfactants should be thoroughly rinsed. Otherwise stinging, burning, conjunctival hyperemia and keratoconjunctivitis may occur.

We have found the use of Miraflow, which is 20% isopropyl alcohol added to Pliagel, a better surfactant cleaner than Pliagel alone. It must be washed off by thorough rinsing and the lens soaked or the residual alcohol on the lens surface can cause corneal insult.

Boyd and Korb have advocated the use of commercial salt made into a paste and used twice weekly for cleaning of a hydrogel lens. This salt mush has an excellent abrasive effect in removing surface coating. Others practitioners have suggested baby shampoo diluted with water and used on the lens surface for at least 20 seconds. Allansmith believes that the mechanical action of rubbing a lens is just as effective as the surfactant.

Method of use of surfactants. The hands are carefully washed with a soap without cream, oils, or perfume and rinsed well. A drop of two of a surface-acting solution is placed on the lens, which is held concave side up in the palm of the hand (Fig. 8-7). The lens is rubbed lightly with the ball of the finger for at least 20 seconds. The palm should be fully open so that the skin is stretched firm. The patient should

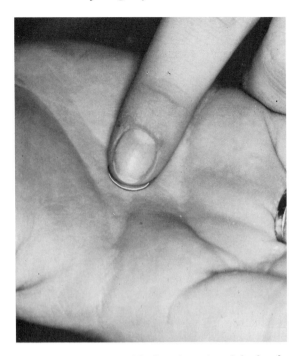

Fig. 8-7. The lens is rubbed in the palm of the hand with a surfacting soft lens cleaner.

press the lens into the palm while rubbing so that the palm begins to blanch. The lens is inverted and cleaned in the same manner. The lens is rinsed well with preserved saline solution or distilled water. While rinsing, the patient rubs the lens until it feels clean. This should be a daily routine. Any unrinsed residue can produce a film by itself, and so careful rinsing of the surfactant cleaner is important.

LC 65 (Allergan). This chemical compound was initially introduced as a rigid lens cleaner. It has been modified to act as a surface acting agent for both soft and rigid lenses.

Opti-Clean (Polyclens). Opti-Clean (Alcon/ BP, Fort Worth, Texas) is a broad-spectrum universal contact lens cleaner that may be used to reduce deposit formation on all rigid and soft contact lenses. This cleaner is composed of a surfactant with high molecular weight polymer beads. These beads act by actually shearing off many deposits from the contact lens surface without damage to the lens surface. The cleaner is a milky suspension preserved with thimerosal and EDTA. It is compatible with both heat and chemical disinfecting regimens. It is effective in action when used for 20 seconds on each side and minimizes the necessity

for using enzyme cleaners or weekly cleaners.

Comment. Clinical studies that we have performed indicate that Opti-Clean (Polyclens) can effectively remove protein as well as lipids and minerals in most instances. It is the first cleaner in which a high molecular weight polymeric bead has been introduced in a surfactant for mechanical shearing of surface bonds of protein and lipids. In our detailed study of 25 patients (49 eyes) followed for 1 year, 95% to 97% of the lenses remained clear. Most of them did not require the use of an enzyme cleaner. The product has a milky color and a slight texture to it that aids the patient in thorough rinsing of the cleaner before lens insertion. However, during clinical studies, one patient inserted the lens daily without rinsing and suffered no corneal insult except a mild stinging and feeling of grittiness. All individuals found this product comfortable when used as directed.

Oxidative agents

The oxidative agents are used to remove bound deposits. By a combination of heat, oxidation, and large swings in the pH and osmolarity, these agents degrade pigment and discolor lenses. A large shift in pH and osmolarity stresses the lens. This may crack some deposits from the lens surface. They may irreversibly damage the lens by oxidation of the hydroxyl group. This may result in an alteration of the lens parameters and the fitting characteristics of the lens. Monoclens, Ren-O-Gel, Lipofrin, and hydrogen peroxide fall into this group.

Lipofrin. Although not available in North America, Lipofrin is used in many parts of the world. It is an inorganic electrolyte with oxygen-releasing action. The released oxygen breaks down organic material by oxidation into smaller components, which become readily soluble. Dr. John DeCarle has described a modified use in which one sixth of a packet is dissolved in 120 ml of water and the lens in a basket is boiled in this solution for 10 minutes. Lipofrin works best between 45° and 60° C. It then remains in the solution for 1½ hours and is removed and disinfected in a disinfecting solution for 2 hours before the lens is worn. Lipofrin was originally used for Permalens when the lens became uncomfortable. It has been shown to have germicidal and viricidal activity as well as cleaning ability.

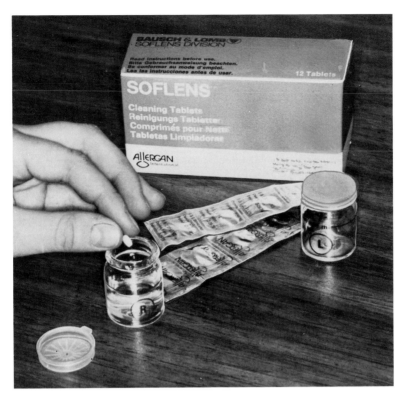

Fig. 8-8. Use of the enzyme cleaning tablet to clean soft lenses. This is available as either Soflens Cleaning Tablet or Allergan Protein Cleaning Tablet.

Hydrogen peroxide. In our hands hydrogen peroxide (3%) is an effective oxidative agent to clean a soft lens. Because hydrogen peroxide is also a disinfectant, its use is covered later in this chapter when disinfection is discussed.

Enzyme cleaners

The forerunner of the enzyme cleaner group has been papain, a proteolytic enzyme used in meat tenderizers and derived from the fruit of the tropical melon tree. Papain acts on peptide linkages in protein. When used properly and regularly, it retards protein deposit formation on the lens and removes some previously formed protein deposits from the surface of a lens. Unfortunately papain has no action against lipids, oils, cosmetics, or minerals. The enzyme cleaner has a larger molecular size than the lens itself and penetrates only slightly below the surface of a hydrogel contact lens of low water content. It will however build up within a lens of high water content and may leave residual enzymatic activity within the lens matrix, which may be toxic to the cornea.

Other enzyme cleaners that contain not only a proteinase compound but also a lipase and a mucinase are available.

Comment. Papain is retained in the superficial pores of HEMA lenses and may cause adverse reactions such as burning, stinging, photophobia, redness, and superficial punctate keratitis. Thorough rinsing of enzyme cleaner is important. It is also useful to clean the lens between forefinger and thumb with a surfactant and rinse thoroughly.

Method of use of Hydrocare tablets. The lens is placed with the cleaning tablet and distilled water in a vial (Fig. 8-8). The vial is shaken until the tablet is dissolved. The lens should be left in the vial for a minimum of 2 hours, or it may be left overnight. The lens is then removed, rinsed, and disinfected by the recommended procedure. The lens should remain in the disinfectant solution for a minimum of 8 hours.

We have found that this method of cleaning is the most effective and practical and that it adds considerably to the preservation of the clarity and comfort of a lens. It should be used once weekly by those patients who use thermal disinfection or lay down protein regularly. This can be reduced to only twice monthly for those using a chemical disinfecting system.

We have found that with higher water content lenses (more than 60%), the lens should not be left a lengthy time in the enzyme solution. The higher the water content, the more retention in the lens.

Comment. Check the source of your distilled water. Up to 50% of the random samples of distilled water obtained through pharmacies were contaminated.

Ultrasound

An effective way of cleaning a soft lens is the use of ultrasound, especially biphasic ultrasound. An ultrasound bath in which the lens is placed in a cleaning solution, such as any of the surfactants, enzyme cleaners, or hydrogen peroxide, will aid in cleaning a very soiled lens. In addition to the ultrasound waves, heat is generated and the combination of heat with ultrasound reinforces the cleaning action of the compound (Fig. 8-9). As a final action, one can place the lenses in the ultrasound bath in a vial filled with preserved or unit dosage saline solution.

Ultrasound units are presently becoming available for home use.

Comment. Ultrasound may effectively clean the lens. However, protein may recur more rapidly after an ultrasound bath. If this occurs, replacing the lens is the best recourse.

DISINFECTION OF SOFT LENSES

Sterilization implies the complete death of all bacteria, fungi, and spores. Disinfection refers to either physical or chemical procedures that kill common pathogenic organisms but may permit some nonpathogenic organisms to survive. Lens care involves disinfection, which is adequate for soft lenses.

Disinfection of lenses is important to prevent the growth of common organisms that may be present in the environment and cause serious eye trouble. Examples are *Staphylococcus aureus*, *Pseudomonas aeruginosa*, *Candida albicans*, and *Herpes simplex* virus. Disinfection procedures are aimed at removing the presence of the organisms. Both hands and contaminated cosmetics may represent potential sources of a high number of these organisms. Normally, the conjunctiva and conjunctival cul-de-sac have nonpathogenic normal flora, but this may be significantly altered by the presence of new bacteria not related to soft lens wear. These may in turn contaminate the surface of soft lenses. Disinfection is practical and clinically effective, if proper hygiene and care are used. Soft lenses are usually supplied in

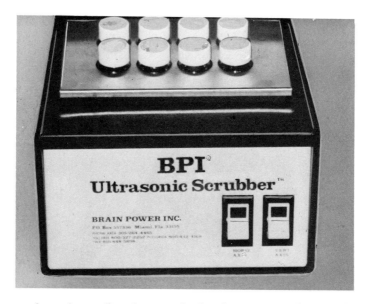

Fig. 8-9. Ultrasound unit for in-office cleaning of soft and rigid contact lenses. This unit provides ultrasound in two directions.

a sterile state from the manufacturer. Most lenses with water content below 50% can withstand temperatures of up to 260° F (127° C); therefore the packaged lens can be autoclaved before shipping. Once the vial is opened, however, the lens is no longer sterile and both the practitioner and the patient must maintain a high level of cleanliness and must follow proper disinfection procedures between usage.

There are basically two methods of disinfection available commercially for soft lenses:

Thermal disinfection

Chemical disinfection

Both procedures require the use of a cleaning agent and should be followed by thorough rinsing. Ideally, thermal disinfection should be accompanied by regular use of an enzyme cleaner.

Thermal disinfection

Boiling method (100° C). With the boiling thermal method, practitioners have the option of prescribing preserved saline or nonpreserved saline solution. The latter is made by the patient who adds a salt tablet to a measured amount of distilled water. Sterile disposable units of preservative-free buffered salt solutions are also available.

The pharmaceutically prepared saline solution considerably reduces the effect of contaminants in the distilled water and the errors of users who put the salt tablet in tap water. In the latter situation, there is a fundamental error that clear water is pure and free of chemicals and metals, which may in turn have a deleterious effect on the lens.

Heat method. These steps are followed in the heat method of disinfection of soft lenses:

1. Lenses are cleaned in the palm of the hand with a surface-acting cleaning agent.
2. Lenses are rinsed well with a saline solution.
3. Lenses are placed in the lens container, which is filled with saline solution.
4. The container is placed in the heating unit.
5. The unit is turned on; it will heat up and cool down in approximately 45 to 60 minutes and shut off automatically. The time cycle will vary from one manufacturer to another. Lenses are now ready for use.

There are four main advantages to boiling: (1) Many consider it to be more effective for

disinfection, (2) it is unquestionably cheaper in the long run, (3) about 30% of persons develop adverse reactions to chemicals, and (4) the thermal method is shorter in duration to achieve disinfection, whereas chemical disinfection requires 4 to 6 hours.

Boiling is used chiefly for soft lenses with a water content below 60%. Laboratory tests have shown that repeated boiling and cooling of the lens over hundreds of hours has minimal deleterious effect on the plastic itself. However, degradation of the plastic does occur with repeated exposures to temperatures above the normal boiling point of water. This may cause slow degradation of the plastic and may lead to loss of the original parameters, such as base curve, with a change in the fitting characteristic of the lens. This may be more noticeable with one lens material than with another. Many high-water-content lenses are adversely affected with repeated heating. Extended-wear soft lenses of high water content should not be disinfected with the autoclave or heating method.

The system depends on making fresh saline from salt tablets and distilled water. The lens material and the wearability factor may be affected if the patient substitutes tap or spring water, which often contains undesirable impurities, especially unwanted minerals. In addition, the wrong amount of water or the wrong number of salt tablets used may result in a lens that is uncomfortable.

Another problem with the thermal disinfection system is the coagulation of protein on the lens surface and the baking on of this protein with repeated heating. This results in lack of clarity, mass increase, and an increase in the adherance of immunoglobulin A. This last may be responsible for giant papillary conjunctivitis. There also may be a resultant change in parameters and fitting characteristics.

Dry heat method (80° C). The new miniature dry heat units that are available do not require water added to the unit and subject the lens, in its carrying case, to a minimum of 80° C for 10 to 20 minutes. This time-temperature cycle has been demonstrated to be effective in accomplishing disinfection of the lens. It has been demonstrated that a variety of bacteria, mold spores, yeast, and the virus *Herpes simplex* are all killed in these units (Fig. 8-10).

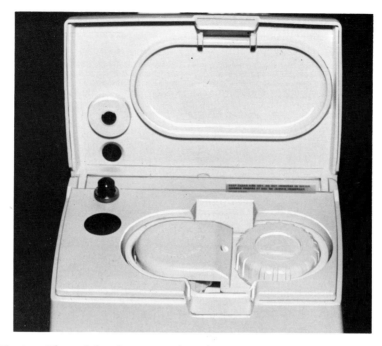

Fig. 8-10. Thermal disinfection unit for soft contact lenses. Dry-heat method.

Table 8-2. Chemicals used for soft lens disinfection

Chemicals	Example
Thimerosal	Preserved saline
Chlorhexidine	MiraSoak
Chlorhexidine-thimerosal	Combiflex, Flexsol, Flexcare, Barnes-Hind Storage Solution, Hydrosoak
Thimerosal–sorbic acid products	Permasol
Alkytriethanol ammonium chloride –thimerosal product	Hydrocare/Allergan Soft Lens Solution and Soflens
Hydrogen peroxide	Lensept
Iodine	Pliacide, Transoft
Dichloroisocyanurate	Soft Tab
Nipastat-thimerosal	Sterisoft

Chemical disinfection

Chemical solutions containing combinations of chlorhexidine, thimerosal, and EDTA have been shown to be effective in killing organisms. A number of companies have introduced into the Canadian, European, and Asian markets soft lens disinfecting agents that have shown adequate clinical effectiveness.

One major problem in developing adequate soft lens accessory products is the binding of preservatives by the soft lenses. Preservatives like chlorobutanol, benzalkonium chloride, phenylmercuric acetate, phenylethyl alcohol, methylparaben, and benzyl alcohol may con-

centrate in the lenses and cause corneal changes. Thus one cannot use conventional rigid lens solutions on soft lenses. Benzalkonium chloride notoriously binds with the soft lens material and can cause severe corneal damage.

Chemicals commonly used for soft lens disinfection are shown in Table 8-2.

For each manufacturer the percentage of each chemical may vary.

Four of the more common systems for disinfection will be reviewed.

Chlorhexidine-thimerosal system (such as Flexsol, Flexcare, and Normol). Flexsol, which

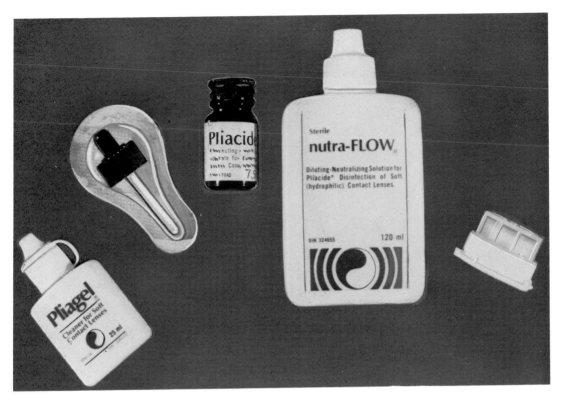

Fig. 8-11. Pliacide solution used with nutra-FLOW to disinfect soft lenses.

was the first approved chemical for disinfection, is formulated with EDTA, thimerosal, chlorhexidine, and borate buffers along with normal saline. It is permitted to remain in contact with the lens overnight and is then carefully rinsed off with saline solution before the lens is inserted in the eye.

The following are the steps in disinfection:

1. Remove the lens from the eye.
2. Place the lens in the palm of the hand.
3. Pour a few drops of a surfactant cleaner on the lens and rub the lens gently for 20 to 30 seconds.
4. Rinse the lens with saline solution.
5. Place the lens in the container and add disinfecting solution, such as Flexsol, until the lens is well immersed.
6. Store the lens for a minimum of 4 hours before insertion.

On inserting the lens:

1. Remove the lens from the case.
2. Rinse the lens well with saline solution.
3. Insert the lens in the eye.
4. Empty the case and rinse with warm tap water; air-dry the case.

Comment. Rinsing the contact lens after using this solution is most important. Chlorhexidine or thimerosal is mildly irritating to the cornea if any remains in the lens or on the lens surface. Fresh disinfection solution must be used daily. Flexcare was introduced as different from Flexsol because the absence of the adsorbable polymer permits the solution to be used as a rinsing solution as well as a disinfecting solution.

Iodine solutions (such as Pliacide). Pliacide is an iodine compound containing 0.1% iodine. Lenses are placed in 2 to 4 drops of the codeine solution diluted with a neutralizing solution to a colorless normal saline solution (Fig. 8-11). Heat and light speed up the neutralization process. The end point of disinfection is reached when the brown solution has turned clear. The lenses are stored overnight in this solution. These iodine solutions can only be used with soft lenses of water content less than 45%.

Quaternary ammonium solutions. Hydrocare or Allergan Cleaning and Disinfecting Solution and B&L Soaking Solution are used as cleaner and storage solutions. Their main germicide is alkytriethanol ammonium chloride combined with some surfactant agents and buffering solutions. This is a quaternary ammonium compound that binds with surface-acting molecules of the solution and becomes large enough that it does not penetrate into the soft lens matrix. In this way the solution does not become eluted from the lens while in the eye and produce chemical insult to the cornea.

The steps in disinfection are similar to the chlorhexidine-thimerosal routine.

Comment. Although the lenses can be worn directly after removal from this quaternary ammonium germicide solution, Morgan has pointed out that 15% of persons will develop small intraepithelial microcystic changes in the corneal epithelium after prolonged use. This is eliminated if the solution is thoroughly rinsed off with preserved saline before use.

We have performed clinical and comparative studies with this solution for over 1 year and have found greater comfort, fewer protein deposits on the lenses, and fewer discontinuances with this disinfectant than with a chlorhexidine-based solution.

We also found that some patients who were unsuccessful with a chlorhexidine system such as Flexsol were successful with a quaternary ammonium system and vice versa.

Because chemical systems are easy to use and portable, the system is a definite convenience for patients when traveling.

Hydrogen peroxide (such as Lensept, Septicon System). This system acts as a cleaning agent and as a good disinfectant for all soft lenses. The excellent performance of 3% hydrogen peroxide is marred only by the fact that patients may fail to neutralize the hydrogen peroxide adequately and a chemical burn of the cornea results. In Canada, a neutralizing disc is used to break down any residual peroxide to oxygen and water. Ongoing product developments will eventually resolve and simplify care management with hydrogen peroxide.

The lens is gently rubbed with a surfactant cleaner and then placed in a specially designed lens container. The container is then filled to a line with 3% hydrogen peroxide (Lensept) and soaked for 10 minutes. It is then transferred to the second container, containing preserved normal saline (Lensrins) or unit-dosage nonpreserved saline solution and a catalyst that breaks down any peroxide into free oxygen and

water. The lens is allowed to remain overnight, or for 6 hours or more. It is then shaken and rinsed once again in fresh saline for 3 minutes, after which the lenses are ready to be worn.

Hydrogen peroxide 3% has the ability to penetrate the entire matrix of the soft contact lens in 30 seconds. It kills many organisms quickly.

In clinical experience the lenses containing polyvinylpyrrolidone may become discolored and yellow in time. The use of hydrogen peroxide has a whitening or bleaching effect on the lens.

Comment. Hydrogen peroxide is easily decomposed. Light accelerates this decomposition, and hence the hydrogen peroxide should be kept away from direct light. The Septicon disc has been practical and effective in neutralizing the hydrogen peroxide and preventing ocular irritation and corneal damage. The present system is somewhat cumbersome for the patient. However, a newly evolved version of this system promises a simple one-step automatic procedure.

About 27 parts per million of hydrogen peroxide may remain after storage overnight. If any adverse effects are experienced by some patients, one may eliminate these effects by spilling out the saline solution, filling the case with fresh saline, and letting this stand for 5 to 10 minutes before insertion.

Useful hints on disinfection and cleaning

1. All remarks previously made and those made by the manufacturer are made on the basis of an intact soft lens. If a lens has a slight crack or roughened edge, bacteria or fungi may penetrate the lens substance and may not be adequately disinfected by some of the techniques of disinfection.

2. Whatever system of disinfection the patient has been instructed in, he or she should continue with that system rather than switch to newer or different systems unless indicated. Some of the different chemicals may react with each other or accumulate and cause irritative problems to the cornea.

3. If a patient is using one chemical system and switches to another, it is important that the lenses be purged in fresh distilled water three or four times to leach out the previous chemical. The lenses should then be disinfected. Al-

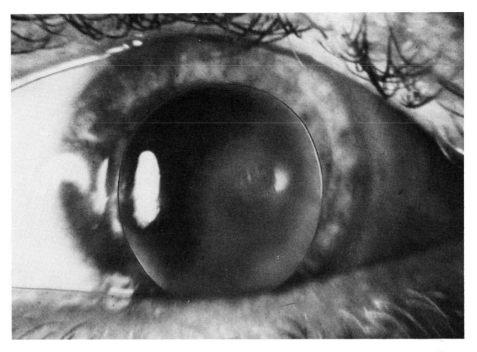

Fig. 8-12. Protein deposit on a contact lens. It is considered moderate to advanced when seen grossly with the slitlamp.

ternately, the lenses may be soaked or even shaken for 15 minutes in distilled water with three or four changes of distilled water to leach out the chemical. This osmotically removes the chemical. Lenses are then placed in the new disinfecting solution.

4. If protein deposits on the surface of a soft lens are not removed, they lead to reduced visual acuity, interference with oxygenation to the cornea, giant papillary conjunctivitis, and binding of preservatives to the lens. Bound preservatives may produce a burning sensation (Fig. 8-12).

5. Adverse ocular response to disinfecting agents may occur and is manifested by (1) red and itchy eyes, (2) a burning sensation, and (3) diffuse corneal stippling. One may correct this by switching to a boiling system or else by boiling the lenses several times in distilled water followed by boiling them in saline to leach out accumulated chemicals.

6. To be effective, the disinfecting solution must be changed daily in the lens-storage case.

7. The friction of rubbing the finger on the lens against the palm with surfactant cleaners tends to shorten the life of soft lenses by causing scratches, particularly if the skin of the fingers or palm is rough.

8. Nonpreserved unit doses of pharmaceutically prepared saline is preferred over salt tablets mixed with distilled water. Chemical impurities have been found in the distilled water and may vary from area to area. The distilled water has been shown to contain 20 times the amount of impurities than triply distilled and deionized water.

9. If an enzyme tablet has turned brown, it has lost its effectiveness and should not be used (Fig. 8-13).

10. Lens cases should periodically be scrubbed clean.

11. Once a lens container is unsealed, spare lenses or lenses not used regularly should be disinfected at least weekly either thermally or by a change of the disinfecting solution. We have seen both bacterial and fungal contamination of these lenses when this disinfection procedure is not followed.

12. Studies we have undertaken with Opti-Clean (Polyclens) (Alcon/BP, Fort Worth, Texas) surfactant cleaner show that it can remove protein, lipids, and inorganic matter

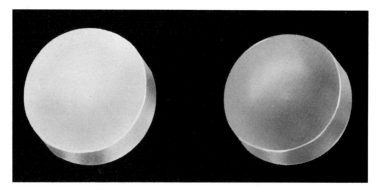

Fig. 8-13. The enzyme tablet on the right has become discolored because of oxidation and has lost its effectiveness.

without the use of enzyme tablets in at least 80% of patients.

13. Strong oxidizing agents should be used only infrequently or never with HEMA lenses because they degrade the plastic.

14. Patients with dry eyes as suggested by an abnormal Shirmer test or a very thin tear meniscus or a poor BUT (tear film breakup time) often develop deposits more frequently.

15. Tears may be deficient in mucin as indicated by a low BUT or by vital staining with rose bengal. This altered tear state may promote deposit formation.

16. When a soft lens has heavy white calcium deposits and is professionally cleaned, the lens is more likely to develop deposits much sooner with each succeeding use.

17. In some persons the lens may become coated in a few weeks, whereas in others it may take a year before any significant deposits develop.

18. There are some problems associated with patient preparation of salt tablets: possibility of contamination, use of water that does not conform to distilled or purified standards, use of the wrong type of salt tablets, and patient error in mixing.

19. Kleist has shown that there is an increase in inorganic and organic deposits on lenses that use the thermal disinfection system as compared to those lenses that are chemically disinfected.

RINSING SOLUTIONS

A large variety of rinsing solutions are available. These solutions may be used to rinse

some debris from the lens after cleaning. They are also used to rinse the lens after disinfection by chemicals to reduce the degree of adverse reactions to these chemicals. A toxic reaction may result initially in tiny microcysts of the epithelium, which may break down and lead to find punctate corneal staining.

A list of rinsing solutions may be divided into unpreserved and preserved saline as well as distilled water. Unpreserved saline rinsing solutions may be saline freshly made from salt tablets or individual unit doses of saline available commercially such as Unisol. A number of manufacturers of purified salt tablets have reentered the market since the withdrawal of such tablets a few years ago. The freshly prepared solutions must be discarded after individual use or they may become contaminated and result in infection. One problem with salt tablets is that patients often do not comply and instead of using distilled water will use tap water, the quality of which may vary for different areas of the country.

Preserved saline solutions contain either thimerosal alone in concentration of 0.001% or sorbic acid 0.1% or combinations of either of these preservatives with EDTA (0.1% or 0.01%) or sodium borate 0.22%.

Josephson and Caffrey found that 14% of their patients presented with an adverse ocular response to saline preserved with thimerosal. Changing to the use of nonpreserved saline solution eliminated this reaction. Symptoms included stinging, burning, itching, and blurry vision. Signs include punctate keratitis, edema, staining, chemosis, hyperemia, infiltrates, and a granular appearance to the bulbar conjunctiva.

Comment. The incidence of ocular toxicity, hypersensitivity, and corneal precipitates attributable to solutions is far greater than the frequency of ocular infection. The iatrogenic effect of antibacterial devices is considerable. We rarely see contact lens–induced infections, but inflammatory side effects of antibacterial solutions are common.

LUBRICATING/REWETTING SOLUTIONS
(such as Adapettes, Clerz, and Comfort)

Minor degrees of ocular discomfort result from prolonged exposure to environmental conditions such as tobacco, smog, pollution, and dust. In addition, areas of low humidity will dry out soft hydrogel lens producing discomfort. Those persons exposed to heaters or air conditioners, either in a car or in their work environment, may have dehydration of the soft lenses.

Comment. Dehydration of a lens makes it uncomfortable and reduces the clarity of vision. The anterior surface of the lens instead of being regular and spheric becomes irregular and wavy.

Inadequate tear production is another cause for lenses to dry, requiring special eye drops. There are also persons who are heavy mucus secretors, and the mechanical cleansing of their lenses by a lubricating solution will be helpful. The use of a sterile fluid to rehydrate the lens while it is being worn can be helpful in providing comfort and clarity of vision. Fluids today that are manufactured primarily for this purpose also contain a detergent that helps clean the lenses by loosening and dispersing any mucous and inorganic accumulations on the lens surface.

Comment. For those who have symptoms of fluctuating vision or discomfort, from dryness, it is helpful to add a lubricating drop two or three times daily to their routines.

Ultrathin lenses are more subject to drying because of their thin substance. Persons wearing these lenses are often benefited from lubricating drops.

Persons wearing extended-wear lenses may be helped with lubricating drops that contain a cleaning agent in addition to the rewetting agent.

ROLE OF PRESERVATIVES

Preservatives provide protection against chance contamination. Preservatives frequently used are thimerosal, sorbic acid, EDTA, and chlorhexidine. The chlorhexidine binds to the lens, and protein of the tears binds to the chlorhexidine. Laboratory data contrasted with clinical experience frequently provide conflicting results in the efficacy of any one preservative. Many preservatives in rigid lens solutions cannot be used in soft lens solutions because of penetration into the lens resulting in toxic reactions to the eye. However, the same preservatives, when used in therapeutic eye drops such as pilocarpine and used with soft lenses are permissible because of the total lower concentrations.

The agent in soft lenses that is most likely to induce hypersensitivity is the mercurial thimerosal, which is the active preservative in the majority of soft lens solutions. A search for less allergenic types of preservatives is ongoing. In some countries thimerosal has been omitted from the solutions to eliminate the red eye and irritability syndrome that develops in those persons sensitive to thimerosal.

Comment. We are presently working with a new preservative other than thimerosal. If the work is successful, eventually thimerosal may be eliminated from soft contact lens care systems.

To purge lenses, it has been reported one can use a denture cleaner containing sodium perborate. One fills a small soft lens vial with distilled water about halfway and adds one eighth teaspoon of this cleaner. Run this through moist sterilizer, drain the solution, and refill with plain distilled water and run through unpreserved saline. The use of sodium perborate has been shown to effectively purge thimerosal.

SELECTING THE CORRECT CARE SYSTEM

The initial step in selecting the correct care system is to decide on the disinfection method. One has to decide between the thermal or chemical method. If the lens is not compatible with heat, one must make a decision from among the list of chemical solutions. Those who have any allergic tendencies should be placed on an unpreserved saline storage system. Those who have abnormal tear chemical

Table 8-3. Interchangeable products

Hydrocare Tablets	=	Soflens Cleaning Tablets
Hydrocare Cleaning and Soaking Solution	=	Soflens Soaking Solution
Allergan Saline Solution	=	B&L Saline Solution
Hydron Comfort Drops	=	Hydrosol
Hydron Cleaning Solution	=	Hydroclean
Hydron Soaking Solution	=	Hydrosoak
B&L Daily Cleaner	=	Preflex
B&L Lens Lubricant	=	Adapettes
Flexcare	=	Normol

From Lum, V.J., and Lyle, W.: Chemical components of contact lens solution, Can. J. Optom. **43**(4), Dec. 1981.

patterns or who are more likely to be deposit formers should be placed on a chemical disinfection system to reduce the tendency for deposit formation.

Comment. Any allergic tendency, such as a history of hay fever or allergies to drugs or cosmetics, should be a warning to use unpreserved saline solution.

We arbitrarily consider some individuals as requiring conventional cleaning routines and others as requiring maximum cleaning routines. Maximum cleaning routines are for those who use the thermal method and are deposit formers. They should use the strongest surfactant cleaner available. Supplementary enzyme cleaning on a weekly basis should be used. Patients with incomplete blinking may have increased deposit tendencies and may require maximum cleaning routines.

One should be aware that some products made by different manufacturers are identical in chemical composition. Some of these interchangeable products are listed in Table 8-3.

Manufacturers today are constantly researching new and better cleaning agents for soft contact lens. At the time of this writing, no firm recommendation can be offered because technologic changes are proliferating so rapidly in this area that anything written today becomes obsolete tomorrow.

In addition to the selection of the individual system and the individual specific pharmaceutical vehicle, one should consider the cost factors. The thermal systems may provide for some an initial cost factor but in the years of use may reduce the cost of maintenance. However, the replacement lens cost is increased with the thermal method, which offsets the cost savings of avoiding chemicals. For some the life-style may be more suitable to chemical disinfection or perhaps to conversion to the minimal care routine of extended-wear lenses. Product availability in some local geographic areas and in some parts of the world may predetermine the care system selected.

SWITCHING FROM ONE SYSTEM TO ANOTHER

The beginner fitter can easily become confused with the large variety of care systems that are available for the choices that he may have. Added to the confusion of the fitter is the dilemma of the patient who enters his local drug store and views the special bargains that may entice him to deviate from the solution he is using and to try a new brand. In addition, color coding of care systems for rigid lenses, gas-permeable lenses, soft lenses, and silicone lenses has not reached the sophisticated level that now identifies red-topped bottles as mydriatic solutions and green-topped bottles as miotic solutions.

The responsibility of the fitter is not only to be acquainted with as many care systems as he can but also to understand two important aspects: (1) when he should change from one type of system to another and (2) which types can be mixed and still be compatible.

Josephson and Caffrey have outlined one system of care selection (Fig. 8-14). Essentially this view is in agreement with ours in that a history of lens wear and problem analysis is critical to determine when to change and just how to change.

Our method is to divide new patients into two groups: those with previous problems related to allergic reactions and those with no history of difficulty. For the first group, a thermal system usually with unpreserved saline is recommended. For the second group, any one

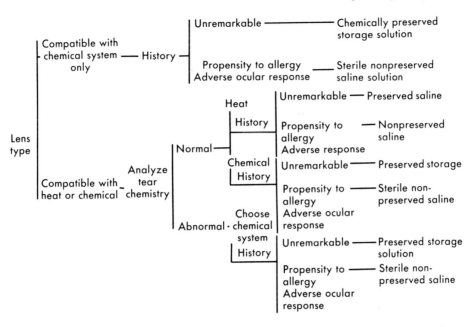

Fig. 8-14. Selection of care system. (From Josephson, J., and Caffrey, B.: Selecting an appropriate hydrogel lens care system, Am. J. Optom. Physiol. Opt. **52**(3): 227-233, March 1981.)

Table 8-4. Products for use with soft contact lenses

Proprietary name	Manufacturer	Preservative	Other ingredients	Sizes
Cleaning products				
Soflens Enzymatic Cleaner Tablets	Allergan Pharmaceuticals Inc. (Irvine, Calif.)	None	Papain, stabilizers	12s, 24s, 48s
Bausch & Lomb Daily Cleaner	Bausch & Lomb Inc.	Thimerosal 0.004%	Edetate disodium, sodium phosphate, sodium chloride, tyloxapol, hydroxyethylcellulose, polyvinyl alcohol	45 ml
Pliagel	CooperVision Pharmaceuticals Inc.	Sorbic acid 0.1%	Edetate trisodium, Poloxamer 407, sodium chloride, potassium chloride	25 ml
Preflex	Alcon/BP (Fort Worth, Texas)	Thimerosal 0.004%	Edetate disodium, sodium phosphate, sodium chloride, tyloxapol, hydroxyethylcellulose, polyvinyl alcohol	45 ml
Soft Mate	Barnes-Hind Pharmaceuticals Inc. (Sunnyvale, Calif.)	Thimerosal 0.004%	Edetate disodium, sodium chloride, tyloxapol, hydroxyethylcellulose	30 ml
Barnes-Hind Weekly Cleaner	Barnes-Hind Pharmaceuticals Inc.	None	Detergents	

Continued.

Table 8-4. Products for use with soft contact lenses—cont'd

Proprietary name	Manufacturer	Preservative	Other ingredients	Sizes
Miraflow	CooperVision Pharmaceuticals Inc.	None	Poloxamer 407, amphoteric detergent, isopropyl alcohol	25 ml
Hydroclean	Contactosol Ltd.	Thimerosal 0.001%	Detergents	
Softcon Lens Cleaner	Softcon	Thimerosal 0.001%	Detergents	
Ren-O-Gel	CooperVision Pharmaceuticals Inc.	None	Acidic and basic inorganic peroxy compounds	
Monoclens	Medical Optics Center	None		
Lipofrin	Alcon/BP	None	Sodium perborate	
Clean-O-Gel	Alcon/BP	None	Enzymes	
Opti-Clean (Polyclens)	Alcon/BP	Thimerosal 0.001%	High molecular weight polymer beads	
LC 65	Allergan Pharmaceuticals Inc.			

Thermal disinfecting and rinsing products

Allergan Saline Solution	Allergan Pharmaceuticals Inc.	Thimerosal 0.001%	A sequestering agent, boric acid, sodium borate, edetate disodium	8 oz
Bausch & Lomb Preserved Saline Solution	Bausch & Lomb Inc.	Thimerosal 0.001%	Boric acid, sodium borate, sodium chloride, edetate disodium	8 oz
Bausch & Lomb Saline Solution	Bausch & Lomb Inc.	None	Sodium chloride	14 × 10 ml
Blairex Salt Tablets	Blairex Laboratories Inc.	None	Sodium chloride	135 mg
BoilnSoak	Alcon/BP	Thimerosal 0.001%	Boric acid, sodium borate, sodium chloride, edetate disodium	8 oz
Unpreserved Saline Solution	Alcon/BP	None	Boric acid, sodium borate, sodium chloride	15 ml
Lensrins	Allergan Pharmaceuticals Inc.	Thimerosal 0.001%	Sodium phosphate, sodium chloride, edetate disodium	8 oz
Salette	Medical Optics Center	None	Sodium chloride and buffer	10 ml
Buffered Salt Tablets	Barnes-Hind Pharmaceuticals Inc.	None	Sodium chloride, sodium bicarbonate, edetate disodium	
Pliasol	CooperVision Pharmaceuticals Inc.	Sorbic acid 0.1%	Sodium chloride, edetate disodium, sodium borate, boric acid	4 & 8 oz
Steri-sal	Medical Optics Center	Nipastat 0.01%	Sodium chloride, edetate disodium	
Soft Therm	Barnes-Hind Pharmaceuticals Inc.	Thimerosal 0.001%	Boric acid, sodium borate, sodium chloride, edetate disodium	8 oz
Mirasol	CooperVision Pharmaceuticals Inc.	Sorbic acid 0.1% Thimerosal 0.001%	Poloxamer 407, edetate disodium, boric acid, sodium borate, sodium chloride, potassium chloride	8 oz
Unisol	CooperVision Pharmaceuticals Inc.	None	Sodium chloride, boric acid, sodium borate	25 × 15 ml

Table 8-4. Products for use with soft contact lenses—cont'd

Proprietary name	Manufacturer	Preservative	Other ingredients	Sizes
Chemical disinfecting solutions				
Allergan Cleaning and Disinfecting Solution	Allergan Pharmaceuticals Inc.	Thimerosal 0.002% Tris (2-hydroxyethyl) tallow ammonium chloride 0.013%	Sodium bicarbonate, sodium phosphate, propyleneglycol, polysorbate 80, soluble polyHEMA	8 oz
Bausch & Lomb Disinfecting Solution	Bausch & Lomb Inc.	Thimerosal 0.001% Chlorhexidine 0.005%	Sodium chloride, sodium borate, boric acid, edetate disodium	8 oz
Normol	Alcon/BP	Thimerosal 0.001% Chlorhexidine 0.005%	Sodium chloride, sodium borate, boric acid, edetate disodium	8 oz
Flexsol	Alcon/BP	Thimerosal 0.001% Chlorhexidine 0.005%	Edetate sodium, polyoxyethylene, polyvinylpyrrolidone, sodium chloride, boric acid, sodium borate	6 oz
Flexcare	Alcon/BP	Thimerosal 0.001% Chlorhexidine 0.005%	Sodium chloride, sodium borate, boric acid, edetate disodium	12 oz
Soft Mate	Barnes-Hind Pharmaceuticals Inc.	Thimerosal 0.001% Chlorhexidine 0.005%	Edetate disodium, conditioning and buffering agents	8 oz
MiraSoak	CooperVision Pharmaceuticals Inc.	Thimerosal 0.001% Chlorhexidine 0.005%	Sodium chloride, boric acid, sodium borate, edetate disodium, Poloxamer 407	4 oz
Pliacide	CooperVision Pharmaceuticals Inc.	Iodine 0.1%	Stabilizing agents	5 ml
nutra-Flow	CooperVision Pharmaceuticals Inc.	Sorbic acid 0.1%	Sodium chloride, potassium chloride, edetate disodium, sodium borate	4 oz
Lensept	Softcon	Hydrogen peroxide 3%		4 oz
Hydrosoak	Contactosol Ltd.	Thimerosal 0.001% Chlorhexidine 0.001%	Salts and buffers	
Sterisoft	Medical Optics Center	Thimerosal 0.001% Chlorhexidine 0.001%	Sodium chloride, edetate disodium	
Lubricating/rewetting eye drops				
Adapettes	Alcon/BP	Thimerosal 0.004%	Povidone, polyoxyethylene, edetate disodium, sodium chloride, and buffering agents	15 ml
Bausch & Lomb	Bausch & Lomb Inc.	Thimerosal 0.004%	Povidone, polyoxyethylene, edetate disodium, sodium chloride, and buffering agents	15 ml
Clerz	CooperVision Pharmaceuticals Inc.	Sorbic acid 0.1%	Hydroxyethylcellulose, Poloxamer 407, edetate disodium, sodium chloride, potassium chloride, sodium borate	25 ml
Comfort Drops	Barnes-Hind Pharmaceuticals Inc.	Thimerosal 0.004%	Tyloxapol, sodium chloride, edetate disodium, borate buffer	

of the disinfectants is recommended combined with a surfactant cleaner and usually the enzyme cleaner as well. If an adverse reaction develops, as in red eyes or irritation, one may reduce enzyme-active agents, switch to another nonthimerosal type of disinfectant, or just switch to the thermal system with unpreserved saline.

The most innocuous system to use for persons who are highly allergic is to clean the lenses with a nonthimerosal surfactant and to just soak the lenses at night in fresh unpreserved saline.

CONCLUSION

New and better products are fast appearing on the market. Table 8-4 indicates some of the available products at this time. This is a multimillion dollar industry as more and more people turn to contact lenses. This era of increasing contact lens wear has been brought about not only by the explosion of new developments in soft and rigid contact lens that make lenses more comfortable and more reliable for visual performance than before, but also by a wider variety of effective care products. New-product development in care systems not only allows lenses to be cleaned and disinfected better, but also tends to simplify the care of contact lenses. The next advance may be an in vivo type of drop that cleans a lens perfectly while one is wearing it, and a disinfecting system that works quickly and leaves no sensitizing or toxic products in or on the contact lenses.

PROBLEMS ASSOCIATED WITH SOFT LENSES

Patient-related problems
Problems related to ocular response
Lens-related problems
Helpful hints on problem solving

When a patient has been wearing soft lenses comfortably but returns with abnormal symptoms, the problems presented must be carefully analyzed and corrected. Because contact lenses now represent a significant proportion of an eye practice, even practitioners who do not fit contact lenses must be aware of the problems associated with contact lenses so that they may provide a proper examination and evaluation of their patients and thus be able to make a professional diagnosis of the underlying problem. Only then will practitioners be able to construct a treatment plan to remedy the situation.

We have arbitrarily divided up the encountered soft lens problems according to their main sources, recognizing that areas of overlap of causation do occur. We shall consider the problems from soft lenses as those related to the patient, to the eye itself, to the contact lens, and to the care systems involved.

PATIENT-RELATED PROBLEMS

Selection of patients for soft lens is by far the most valuable single act that will result in a happy and successful wearer of soft contact lenses. Selecting poor candidates, such as the highly nervous person, the patient with high degrees of astigmatism, or someone who works in a dusty and dirty environment will only result in troublesome visual problems. One should eliminate, where possible, the 5 Ds— the dirty, the dumb, the drunk, the disabled, and the diseased eye.

In evaluating patients one should consider the following specific ocular factors that influence success.

Corneas

Corneas that are flat require a large-diameter lens to maintain stability and centration. Orientals as a group have smaller corneal diameters than Caucasians do, and so a 13.5 mm lens may be optimum for Oriental eyes whereas a 14.5 mm lens may be optimum for Caucasian eyes.

Large-diameter corneas require large lenses to cover the cornea.

Lid abnormalities

Lid abnormalities and size of the eye should be taken into account in selecting the correct diameter for the lens. When faced with a clinical problem, keep in mind that small palpebral fissures require small-diameter lenses. Lid tension may influence one in selecting a small-diameter lens.

Large eyes or eyes with lax or depressed lower lids that exhibit "scleral show," in which a rim of sclera is exposed below the limbus, may lead to dehydration of the lower portion of the contact lens and subsequent edge lift and ejection of the lens by the lower eyelid.

Astigmatic eyes

Astigmatic eyes may require special toric lenses (see Chapter 24). Without these special lenses or rigid lenses, the conventional soft lenses in an eye with astigmatism may result in fluctuating and blurred vision.

Lens discoloration

Lens discoloration may be produced after the patient has used over-the-counter proprietary decongestant drops procured at the local

101

drug store. Such drops contain epinephrine-like compounds. Epinephrine has a tendency to yellow a soft contact lens when used over a prolonged time. Also nicotine from a smoker's fingers may be transferred to soft contact lenses.

Environmental factors

Environmental factors play a considerable role in the quality of vision with a contact lens. In a dry atmosphere or in an atmosphere in which the wearer is near an air conditioner or behind the heater-blower of a car, the front surface of a soft lens may become dehydrated and rippled and result in blurred vision. This is more exaggerated with thin and ultrathin lenses, which lose their small reserve of water faster than standard lenses do. The blurring may be reported as fluctuating or variable, rather than steady because each blink restores the surface smoothness of the contact lens and restores clarity of vision. It has been reported that hydrogel lenses can become contaminated by chemical vapors coming from the environment.

Aphakia

In aphakia, the rupture of the wound is a potential threat from the stress of insertion and removal of a contact lens. Thus daily-wear lenses should be postponed until the wound has healed. Extended-wear lenses are a safer alternative because the tensile strength of a wound is acquired over a long period from the time of surgery. Dr. Linsy Farris has reported on hypopyon induced after contact lens wear in aphakia from an iridectomy site.

PROBLEMS RELATED TO OCULAR RESPONSE
Epithelial corneal edema

Epithelial corneal edema results from hypoxia of the cornea. Unlike rigid contact lenses, in which the epithelial edema is confined to the central portion of the cornea, the edema of the epithelial layer of the cornea is diffuse and confined to the entire cornea.

Edema can be detected clinically with the slitlamp by retroillumination. Edema is often an indication that the lens is too tight and a looser lens is required, one with either a flatter base curve or a smaller diameter. The pa-

chometer attachment to the slitlamp can be used to determine an increase in corneal thickness resulting from corneal edema.

Comment. If you do not own a pachometer, the following simple test will do:

1. Placido's disc. The reflection will be irregular.
2. Retinoscopy. The central reflex will be fractured and irregular.
3. K readings. The mires will be distorted and the K readings steep.
4. Retroillumination. A gray central area appears.

Corneas of patients wearing soft lenses 12 hours or more will generally show a 6% to 8% increase in thickness as a measure of an adverse effect. Edema at this level may be difficult to detect on slitlamp examination. For the most part, patients can tolerate this well with no early or late complications. If the resulting edema is so great that slitlamp edema is detectable, the patient should be instructed to remove his lenses for 2 hours after 8 hours of lens wear in the early stages of adaptation. If this persists, he should be switched to extremely thin contact lenses or high water content lenses that are more oxygen permeable.

In patients living in altitudes over 8000 feet above sea level, mild oxygen deprivation of the cornea may occur with soft lenses if they are worn for too long a period.

Vertical striae in cornea

Sarver was the first to observe vertical striae appearing in the posterior portion of the corneas of soft lens wearers. The striae may be seen with the slitlamp with direct focal illumination. They represent an indicator of early corneal edema, occurring in some cases before clinical corneal edema can be seen. They are probably a slight wrinkling in Descemet's membrane brought on by some corneal anoxia. When they are first seen, lenses should be replaced with flatter lenses, and the striae will disappear.

Fixed folds in Descemet's membrane

Fixed folds in Descemet's membrane have been noted after prolonged wear of a soft lens. In particular, they arise in patients who sleep overnight with their soft lenses and so cause corneal anoxia of a severe nature.

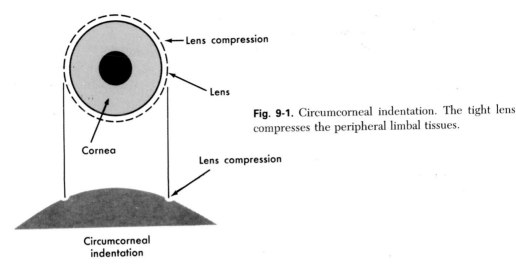

Fig. 9-1. Circumcorneal indentation. The tight lens compresses the peripheral limbal tissues.

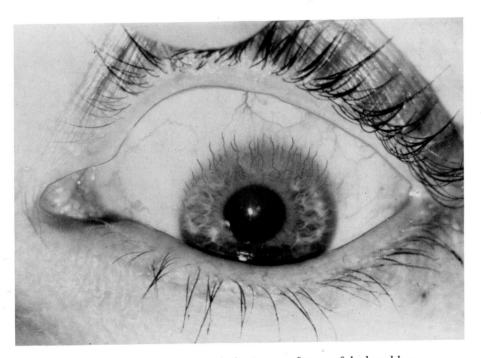

Fig. 9-2. Vascularization superiorly from a poor-fitting soft hydrogel lens.

Compression

An indentation near the area of the limbus is an indication that the lens is too tight. Depending on the size of the lens, it may occur at the periphral cornea, limbus, or sclera. When it occurs at the limbus or sclera, it is often noted by a blanching of the blood vessels followed later by an indentation (Fig. 9-1).

Vascularization at limbus

Limbic vascularization indicates a gradual anoxia to the cornea caused by an adverse reaction to a tight fit. A looser lens, a reduction in the total wearing time, or even discontinuance of the lens may be required (Fig. 9-2).

Epithelial edema, limbal compression, and vascularization are symptoms significantly important to require a change in the lens to a looser lens fit or to a more gas-permeable soft lens, either ultrathin or of a high water content.

Photophobia

Sensitivity to light may be the result of a poorly fitting flat lens that irritates the cornea by friction. It also may be caused by a dirty lens, the chemicals used in sterilization, or the lack of proper isotonicity of prepared or preserved saline solution.

Excess tearing

Tearing may be a result of a poorly fitting, a dirty, or a damaged soft lens. It also may be caused by a foreign body under the lens or in some cases local allergy to chemicals.

Induced myopia and astigmatism

Wearing conventional standard-thickness soft lenses for a prolonged period greater than 12 hours per day has been shown to produce changes in keratometric readings of the cornea. In some instances there has been an increase in steepness of the cornea; in other instances there has been the development of significant irregular astigmatic error that required several months to subside. For some patients there has developed a permanent form of acquired keratoconus, resulting from chronic oxygen starvation to the cornea. Many of these problems have been remedied with the use of thin and ultrathin lenses or high-water-content soft contact lenses, which permit better oxygenation of the cornea, even for marginal corneas.

Epithelial and subepithelial infiltrates

Small nummular lesions from infiltrates occur in the periphery with soft contact lenses result in localized redness. Some believe that they are caused by chronic anoxia. The majority of corneal cells lie in the peripheral ring of the cornea, and hence cellular reaction is more vulnerable here. Some observers such as Falasca believe that these subepithelial infiltrates are antigen-antibody reactions brought about by something adhering to the contact lens. The treatment may require steroid drops combined with antibiotics for 2 or 3 days to clear up the reaction. Either new lenses or maximum cleaning of the existing lenses is required. If the

condition recurs, one may switch to more gas-permeable lenses such as ultrathin lenses, along with a maximum cleaning regimen.

Josephson and Caffrey reported on epithelial and subepithelial infiltrates in contact lens wearers. Lens-solution infiltrates had an average recovery time of 2½ months after the lens was discontinued, whereas virus-induced infiltrates took an average of 5½ months to disappear.

Staining

Although 2% fluorescein should not be used with a soft lens, it may be important that on reexamination the soft lens be removed and the eye stained with fluorescein. The lens should not be reinserted for 1 hour after fluorescein has been used. If the eye is flushed, the lens may be reinserted after 20 minutes.

High molecular weight fluorescein is available and can be used with low and medium water content lenses. Usually, however, defects in the epithelium can be detected without fluorescein by someone trained with the slitlamp.

An area of staining in the periphery of the cornea is often indicative of a dry area or an irritated epithelial area from the edge of the lens that occurs because the lens does not center well (Fig. 9-3, *A*). A new lens with better centering properties should be provided. This may involve substitution of a larger diameter lens or a change in the base curve to permit better centering. A peripheral staining area may also be caused by poor edge design, and a new lens may be required.

Arcuate staining in a spotty fashion in the periphery may be a result of poor blending at the junctions of a lathe-cut soft lens (Fig. 9-3, *B*).

Decentration of a lens (Fig. 9-3, *C*) may cause chafing at the edges of the cornea.

Scattered stippled staining of the cornea is often a result of a dirty lens or a lens that builds up particles of protein material and creates anoxia of the cornea (Fig. 9-3, *D*). This lens should be carefully cleaned or replaced.

Generalized stippling of the cornea, often diffuse over the whole cornea, is indicative of environmental toxicity, such as chemicals, oils, or grease. It is most commonly caused by thimerosal, a preservative widely used in the care of soft contact lenses. It may be remedied if one changes the chemical solution used for dis-

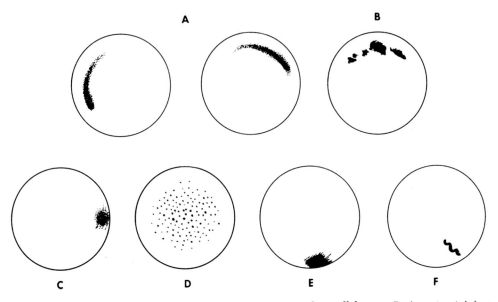

Fig. 9-3. A, Peripheral arcuate staining caused by decentered, small lenses. **B,** Arcuate staining as a result of poor blend at the junctions of a lathe-cut soft lens. **C,** Chafing at the edge of the cornea because of decentration of a soft lens. **D,** Generalized stippling of the cornea caused by environmental contamination or protein buildup on the lens. **E,** Inferior staining of the cornea resulting from trauma on removal of the lens. **F,** Foreign body stain occurring when a small foreign body finds its way under a soft lens.

infection or changes to the boiling method of disinfecting the lens with preservative-free saline (see Chapter 8). Occasionally it may represent an infectious element and should be treated accordingly.

John Morgan has pointed out small microcystic dot formation in the corneal epithelium that precedes stippling. He found this as a result of germicide toxicity to the cornea, but it may occur with any toxic influence on the cornea.

Foreign-body stains are similar in nature to those seen with persons wearing hard lenses who have linear or curved staining areas on the cornea (Fig. 9-3, *F*).

Inferior staining at the 6 o'clock position of the cornea usually indicates trauma arising from an improper removal technique (Fig. 9-3, *E*). To avoid this, one should keep the fingernails short.

Staining of the cornea is a cause of concern, since these stains represent portals of bacterial entry. Even though the patient is comfortable and not complaining, the problem must be solved and, if specific remedies fail, the lens changed.

Comment. Corneal erosion with soft lenses also occurs with the following:

1. Decentration of the lens.
2. Lid gap especially if the lens edges are bulky and thick.
3. Truncated lenses, especially if the truncation has not been beveled.
4. Lens too small in diameter to cover fully the lens with blinking.

Allergy versus toxicity

With the widespread use of chemical preservatives associated with soft contact lenses, it is important to differentiate allergy from toxicity (Table 9-1). *Allergy* represents a reaction of the body to a large molecule, usually protein, lipoproteins, and occasionally polysaccharides. These are referred to as *antigens*. There then results a complex series of events in which the body reacts to the foreign substance and produces an *antibody* resulting in an *antigen-antibody reaction*. A *toxic reaction* is a reaction that a person will show to some applied substance, whether it is a chemical or just a protein molecule. This reaction is a direct insult to the cell. A *toxic idiosyncrasy* is a specialized form of toxicity that occurs to just a few persons. The history becomes important. With *toxicity* there is usually a cumulative progressive irritation with usage of any chemical with time. With *allergy*, such as to thimerosal, the history is one in which the patient suddenly develops a red eye and no longer is comfortable with contacts, or the eyes clear even with with reduced amounts of the agent in question. In our experience differentiation of allergy from toxicity may be noted not only by the medical history, but also by the target that is involved. With allergy, the conjunctiva participates more with conjunctival chemosis and giant follicles. With toxicity the cornea participates more with corneal epithelial punctate changes, beginning with small microcysts to epithelial erosions. When faced with red eyes and suspicion of allergy, one should use Table 9-2 as a guide.

Table 9-1. Differentiation from an allergic response and a toxic response to a solution used for soft lenses

Allergy	Toxicity
Conjunctival response equal to or greater than corneal response	Corneal response equal to or greater than conjunctival response
Chemosis	Punctate keratitis
Giant follicles	Microcysts

Table 9-2. Signs and symptoms of allergy

Symptoms	Signs
Itching	Chemosis
Burning	Limbal injection
Blurred vision	Conjunctival redness
	Mucous discharge
	Tearing

LENS-RELATED PROBLEMS
Tear resistance

Splitting of the lenses has not been a major problem with the newer materials available. However, one must use proper instruction in regard to lens handling to avoid damaging lenses. Needless to say delicacy is required in the handling of the material and care of the fingernails, which must be kept short. The higher the water content or the thinner the lenses are made, the more fragile they are. Today's models however are within acceptable guidelines for wear and tear. When looking with a slit-lamp, it is often the edges that are first to show nicks, which gradually enlarge into a split (Fig. 9-4).

Comment. A split lens should be replaced regardless of whether there is discomfort or irritation with it. Once the seal of the lens is broken, the lens itself can permit bacteria to enter the plastic.

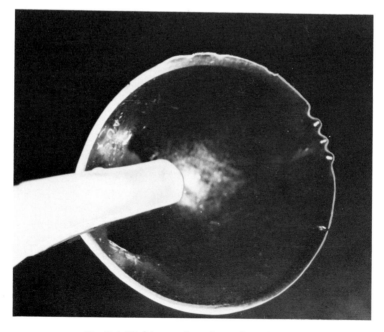

Fig. 9-4. Nicking at the edges of a soft lens.

Hazy or variable vision

If the vision is poor, the easiest way to determine if this is a result of a loose lens is to manually manipulate the lens with the eyelid on the patient's eye so that it is objectively centered. If vision clears, chances are the lens is loose and has been gradually slipping off center. If, on the other hand, vision is not improved, some factor other than a loose lens is accounting for poor vision. In that case this procedure should be followed:

1. Examine the patient with the slitlamp.
2. Reevaluate the fit—the lens may have changed its parameter over time and become tighter or looser, either of which will affect vision.
3. Check that the lens is not inverted.
4. Check the power of the lenses to be sure that the lenses have not been switched between the right and left eye.
5. Check for deposits on the lens.
6. Check protein buildup and the clarity of the lenses.

The most common cause of deterioration in vision with soft lenses is caused by deposit buildup. These deposits are protein, lipids, and inorganic matter. Prophylactic cleaning must be reemphasized to the patient. Lenses often can be restored to normal clarity, but if not, lens replacement is necessary.

Comment. When in doubt, replace the lens and do not change the parameters.

Vision may deteriorate because of drying of the lens (Fig. 9-5). Such environmental conditions as dry rooms or dry climates (Arizona) with low humidity may cause drying of the lens with reduction in the visual acuity. Patients who read a great deal, particularly when tired, will have a reduced blink reflex, which in turn will result in drying of the lens. In addition physical and mental fatigue decrease tear formation; consequently patients will experience irritation with their lenses at the end of a busy day.

Patients should be warned against driving with air-conditioned or heated air blowing in their eyes, since this will dehydrate the lens and cause visual blurring during driving. The blink reflex is also reduced during driving. When a lens dehydrates, a rippling effect occurs on the front surface and causes blurring.

Occasionally we have found that selecting a lens identical to the one the patient is wearing will significantly improve vision. The initial poor vision is probably caused by defective optics in the first lens.

Cellular debris under a lens may occur if the lens becomes too tight. When viewed with a slitlamp, the lens shows inadequate clearing centrally after each blink, and the patient notes blurring of vision. One may see trapped mucoid particles. The remedy is to make the lens flatter for better tear exchange and removal of waste products. Some extended wear lenses exhibit this trapped-debris phenomenon. This is cleared by either scleral swish or removal for cleaning.

Lens-power changes

In myopia, there may be a tightening of the lens with time, resulting in an increase in minus power. This occurs because a plus tear film becomes present in the central portion of the cornea, which no longer touches centrally resulting in a pseudomyopia and more minus power required to correct vision (Fig. 9-6, A). The important factor here is that when one is overrefracting a myope who is wearing soft contact lenses and one finds an increase minus power this may be pseudomyopia and not true

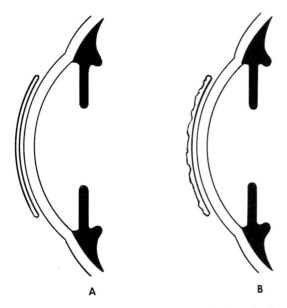

A   **B**

Fig. 9-5. A, Normal contact lens. **B,** Dehydrated soft contact lens after exposure to a dry environment causing blurring of vision.

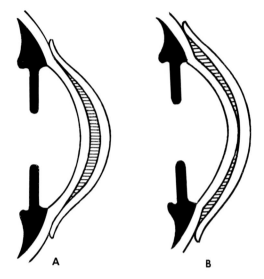

Fig. 9-6. A, Plus tear film created by a tight lens behaves as a plus lens requiring more minus power in order for the patient to see. **B,** Minus tear film. In aphakia, thick plus lenses may fall away from the periphery and thereby form a minus-lens tear film and thus require more plus to correct vision.

myopic change. If the lens has changed in fit, simply replacing the lens with the same-power lens with a correct fit will usually correct the problem.

In aphakia, the opposite holds true. The thicker aphakic lens with aging or with dehydration may become more rigid and stand away from the peripheral cornea and permit tears to fill the interface between lens and cornea. This creates a minus tear layer so that an increase in plus power is required (Fig. 9-6, *B*).

Optic zone

The larger the diameter of soft lenses, the larger the optic zone that permits improved vision. In aphakia a small optic zone can be a real problem because when the manufacturers attempt to reduce thickness a smaller optic zone results. This problem is more prevalent in the higher plus powers and results in fluctuating blurred vision. Some manufacturers hold the optic zone as a constant regardless of power increases.

Edges

Each manufacturer of soft lenses designs edges that are specific for that company. It is a compromise to design an edge that is very thin and well rounded and will provide optimum comfort and tear exchange, and yet be sufficiently durable to withstand the wear and tear of handling. If one manufacturer's products do not result in sufficient patient comfort, one should try another manufacturer's lens, which may provide comfort because of better edge design for that patient.

Thin and ultrathin lenses

Thin and ultrathin lenses, though showing increasing popularity, are more prone to damage by poor handlers. They are also more time consuming for the average person to insert; thus one should assess the individual personality, hygiene, work habits, and motivation of the patient to determine whether he is a suitable candidate for thin and ultrathin lenses. Certainly the person who gets up in a hurry and rushes off to work early in the morning may find the handling problem with these thin lenses a frustration.

We have found thin lenses wrinkle more easily on the eye causing blurring of vision (Fig. 9-7). They should be fit tighter than conventional lenses with only minimal movement to overcome this effect and provide stable vision. Generally we initially fit conventional soft lenses 3 to 4.5 D flatter than K, whereas we fit the thinner lenses only 2 to 3.5 D flatter than K. The tighter thin-lens fitting is possible because of the greater oxygen transmission of the lenses.

If a patient reports initial discomfort with an ultrathin lens on the eye, it is likely that either a particle of debris is on the back surface of the lens or the lens is inside out. An everted or inside-out ultrathin lens generally does not affect vision the way an everted standard-thickness lens does, but it will cause greater lens awareness because of the anterior bevel.

Falling out of lens

If lenses continue to fall out, the reason may be that the lens diameter chosen is too small in relation to the palpebral fissure. This may also occur if the lens fits too flatly resulting in edge stand-off, with the lid catching on the everted lid during blinking action. Inadequate tear production may cause drying of the edges and ejection of the lens by the lower eyelid. The

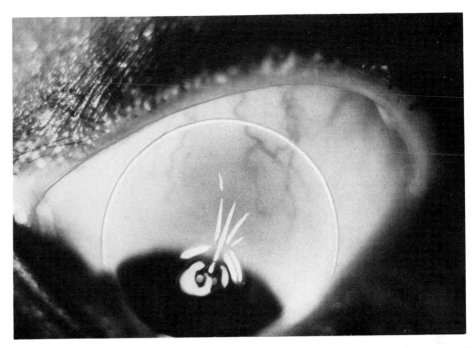

Fig. 9-7. Wrinkling of an ultrathin lens demonstrated on looking up when it is on the cornea. This effect results in a degradation of visual acuity. (Courtesy Lester Yanoff, American Optical Corp., Southbridge, Mass.)

accumulation of excess surface deposits may reduce lens hydration and cause dehydration of the lens.

Care-related problems

Deposits. Deposits are found more frequently in the aphakic patient. Electron microscopy has shown these spots to be compatible with derivatives of the tear film such as denatured lysozyme, albumin, gamma globulin, and lipids. Often calcium is present. These spots act to irritate the eye and make the lens uncomfortable to wear and may contribute to poor fitting with decentration (Fig. 9-8). If the spots increase in size and number, vision will be affected and a replacement lens will be required. Lens-cleaning procedures should be reviewed with the patient. If deposits continue to recur, the patient should be switched to rigid lenses.

Clinically the deposits may be seen with the slitlamp while the patient is wearing the lens. However, early deposit formation cannot clearly be seen unless the lens is removed, permitted to partially dehydrate, and viewed through the slitlamp or a magnifying lens against a dark background.

Comment. Heavy deposit formation can be seen after 3 weeks of wear. If this occurs, switch to a gas-permeable lens.

Thimerosal sensitivity. Thimerosal is sodium ethylmercurithiosalicylate, a compound of organic mercury and thiosalicylic acid. Thimerosal has a broad range of antibacterial activity. A 0.01% solution inhibits the growth of *Pseudomonas aeruginosa, Escherichia coli,* and *Staphylococcus aureus.* Clinically it is often used in 0.01% or 0.001% concentrations.

Thimerosal has been the chief component responsible for delayed hypersensitivity of the eye. Patients have had patch tests along with intradermal tests to prove the sensitivity to thimerosal. Typical ocular symptoms are redness, foreign body sensation, and lacrimation. Ocular examination reveals conjunctival hyperemia, conjunctival folliculitis, and corneal epithelial opacities or punctate keratopathy. Studies have reported about 6% to 8% sensitivity to thimerosal.

Fungus growth. Fungi will occasionally seed on a soft lens and burrow deep into the plastic (Fig. 9-9). Fungi should be clinically recognized and differentiated from protein buildup on a soft lens.

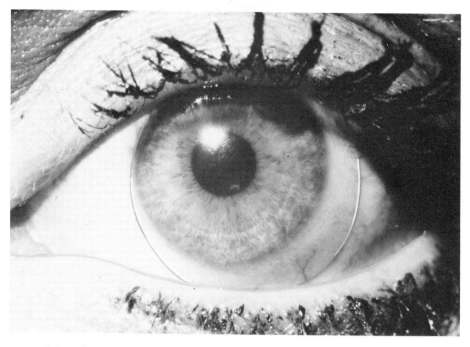

Fig. 9-8. Soft lens decentered inferonasally because of a flat lens. Mascara eventually may contribute to clouding, particle discomfort, and decentration.

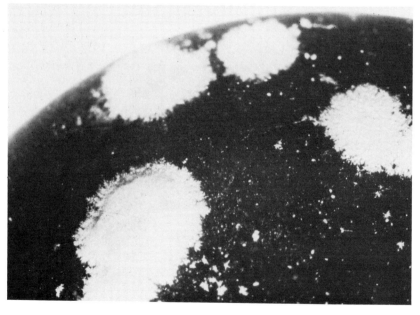

Fig. 9-9. Fungus colonies identified as *Penicillium* growing on a hydrophilic lens in a patient wearing a soft lens. (Courtesy Dr. John F. Morgan, Kingston, Ont.)

Fungus growth develops on lenses that have not been used for some time and during this time have been stored in unpreserved saline solution. It is important that lenses be continually disinfected both by the practitioner for the inventory or diagnostic set and by patients who wear their soft lenses only occasionally. The problem of fungus growth with stored lenses is one of the major obstacles to the patient requiring a spare pair of lenses. Unfortunately the solutions in which the spare lenses are kept are not changed frequently and boiling is neglected.

Infection. There have been several cases of contamination of soft lenses or their containers. Bacteria have been shown to enter fissures in the plastic, whereas fungus has been reported to invade the intact soft lens. However, despite these reports of lens or lens-container contamination, there have been few reports of widespread clinical infection to either the cornea or conjunctiva. We have found only one case of serious inflammatory condition of the cornea as a result of soft lens wear in a series of a few thousand daily soft lens wearers.

Comment. Our low incidence of infection may not be widespread. We are compulsive with regard to teaching our patients hygiene, lens care, and proper storage techniques. Also we have a hot line for any problems.

Red eye in contact lens wearers. The most frequent cause of red eyes in contact lens wearers is allergy to thimerosal, an organic mercurial found as a preservative in many soft lens solutions (Fig. 9-10). Thimerosal causes allergy in 4% to 8% of patients. Although red eyes is a major problem in clinical practice, there is a variety of possible causes other than thimerosal sensitivity that should be considered (Table 9-3).

Giant papillary hypertrophy of tarsal conjunctiva (cobblestone conjunctivitis). Spring first drew our attention to this entity and Allansmith and her co-workers have shown that although giant cobblestones appear in 0.5% of normal individuals it occurs in 10% of rigid lens wearers and a significant amount in 50% of soft contact lens wearers who wear contact lenses for any length of time. It also occurs in persons wearing an ocular prosthesis. There appears to be some direct relationship to individual sensitivity, to the duration the person is

Table 9-3. Causes of red eye in soft contact lens wearers

Allergy	to thimerosol to solutions to environment
Infection	bacterial viral chlamydial
Toxicity	to retained enzyme to finger debris to cleaning agents poorly rinsed
Tears	quality quantity
Tight lens syndrome	
Glued-on lens syndrome	
Incomplete blinking	
Lens thickness	too thick too thin (dehydra- tion effect)
Lens changes	deposits change in fit
Abrasion	foreign body fingernail from decentration
Lids	in-turned lashes blepharitis scleral show and dehydration
Anterior membrane dystrophies	
Lens inside out	

wearing the contact lenses, and to the type of care routine followed. The larger-diameter soft lenses appear to produce an increased incidence over the smaller-diameter soft lenses.

When this sensitivity occurs, there is often an associated redness, itchiness, and shorter wearing time of the lenses though in many cases it is asymptomatic until the advanced stages. It is important to evert the eyelid under slitlamp examination to detect early stages of this condition. When the eyelid is everted, a typical vernal type of papillary hypertrophy of the conjunctiva can be seen (Fig. 9-11). Occasionally a large papillary hypertrophy of the conjunctiva may be seen.

The causation of giant papillary conjunctivitis appears to be a combination of allergy (antigen-antibody) reaction and foreign-body mechanical irritation.

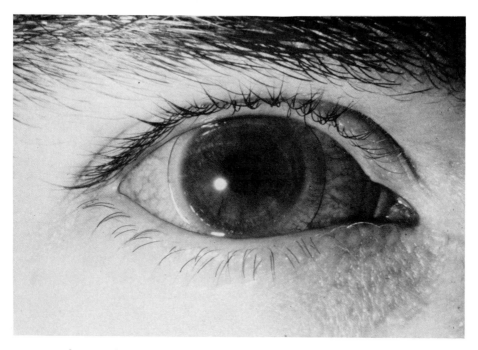

Fig. 9-10. Thimerosol sensitivity resulting in a red eye with punctate staining of the cornea.

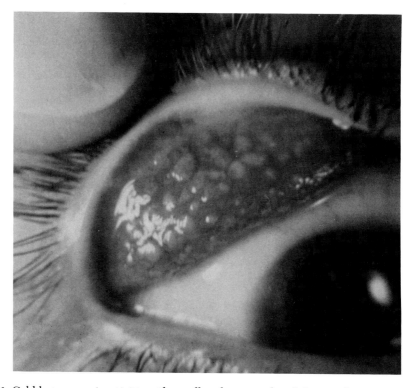

Fig. 9-11. Cobblestone conjunctivitis with papillary hypertrophy of the tarsal conjunctiva seen in a patient who has worn soft lenses for 2 years with chemical disinfection.

Fluorescein should be instilled. If the top of the papule stains, this staining indicates the presence of acute inflammation, and steps should be taken to either clean the lenses more completely, switch to new and smaller diameter lenses or one of a different material, or discontinue lens wear.

HELPFUL HINTS ON PROBLEM SOLVING

1. Impaired reading may occur with soft lens wearers for the following reasons: (a) because of lid-induced flexion of the soft lens when the eyes are rotated downward (this may be improved by instructing the patient to hold the reading material in a higher position), (b) after prolonged reading because of fatigue and the lack of blinking, which leads to excessive drying of the front surface of the lens, or (c) an optic zone that is too small.

2. Discomfort may result from deposit accumulation. This may be overcome by the routine use of an enzyme-cleaning tablet and attention to more careful surfactant cleaning.

3. If peripheral erosions or fine peripheral staining occurs with a soft lens, it may be the result of a decentering of the lens or poor edge finishing.

4. Induced astigmatism and steepening of the K measurement is occasionally found with soft lens wearers who wear their lenses for prolonged times. This is particularly exaggerated if the fit is inadequate. An improvement in fit and a reduction in total daily wearing may be required. A 12-hour wearing time would appear to be optimal for conventional soft lenses. A switch to ultrathin lenses may be required for better corneal performance.

5. A burning sensation along with conjunctival redness may be the result of chemical contamination. This may be transferred from the patient's hands or be caused by the germicide used in asepsis. It may be a chemical allergy to the soaking solution, particularly if thimerosal is used, because mercury can be sensitizing. Occasionally a viral keratoconjunctivitis may cause this, and scattered small gray intraepithelial nonstaining corneal infiltrates may be seen on slitlamp examination. One must be aware of possible environmental toxic fumes that can produce these symptoms.

6. In those patients with naturally dry eyes or poor tear formation who are being fitted with soft hydrophilic lenses, a soft lens of low water content should be selected to reduce water demand by the soft lens.

7. Epithelial edema in soft lens wearers is more common with lenses with low water content because they may behave like hard PMMA lenses. A switch to ultrathin or higher water content lenses may be required.

8. Some patients wearing soft lenses, either lathe cut or spin cast, develop an increase in myopia with steepening of K readings or develop astigmatism. Lenses should be discontinued for a short while or switched to a flatter lens or an ultrathin lens.

9. Small bubbles of oxygen or debris trapped under the lens and seen on the slitlamp may be indicative of a steep lens, resulting in a poor exchange of tears under the lens.

10. When lenses fit well at first and then become very loose and decentered, this process may be caused by a loss of shape retention ("memory") of the plastic with time.

11. Repeated blurring of vision resulting from drying of the soft lens, either from environmental factors or from the staring effect caused by fatigue after prolonged reading, may be minimized by the use of Comfort eye drops. This solution hydrates, wets, and cleans the soft lens while the patient is wearing the lens. Other hydrating drops, such as artificial tears, may be helpful.

12. Farris has pointed out that in some eye conditions, particularly in the elderly, the tears may become hypertonic and result in corneal irritation from a contact lens. There is value in diluting the salt concentration in the eyes of some persons by the use of Hypotears, a hypotonic tear substitute. This may be used along with soft contact lenses.

13. We have seen falling out of well-fitted lenses when patients are subject to low humidity conditions, as when in climates similar to that of Arizona or when driving a car with heated or air-conditioned air blowing directly onto their eyes. The lens dries out, the edge everts, and the lid edge expresses the lens from the eye.

14. One should also be aware that glaucoma can occur in soft contact lens wearers. One can slide the lens temporally onto the sclera and perform applanation tonometry without fluorescein using the white light of the slitlamp.

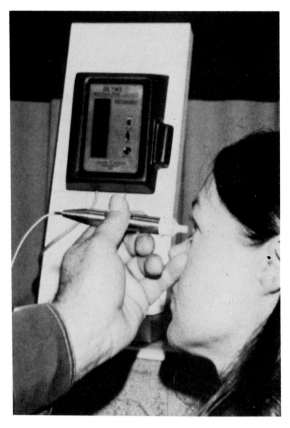

Fig. 9-12. Applanation tonometry may be performed over a soft lens without fluorescein or anesthesia by use of the Electro Medical Technology digital applanation tonometer.

Alternately one can use an electronic applanation tonometer (Fig. 9-12) or the Shiøtz tonometer, if the lens is removed or shifted.

Comment. Applanation readings are still more precise without the lens present. For the patient with glaucoma, the lens should be removed. Also there is no indication that soft lenses cause glaucoma.

15. In patients with a high incidence of lens deposits, one should reassess the care system and be sure there is compliance. A new system may be required. One should also reassess the fit because loose lenses tend to reduce any cleansing action by the tarsal conjunctiva.

16. Professional cleaning in the office, aided by an ultrasound unit, may be helpful in increasing the longevity of the soft lens. Ultrasound aids in increasing the action of many chemical agents on the lens and increasing the speed of the cleaning process.

Comment. Although ultrasound can yield an almost new soft lens, the rate of recurrent deposit formation is accelerated over that of a new lens.

17. Thin and ultrathin lenses may be fitted tighter and with less movement than standard lenses. Fitting these lenses in this way minimizes wrinkling of the lens that may result in fluctuating vision.

18. Ultrathin lenses have an exaggerated dehydration effect in dry environments and may produce symptoms of poor vision. With these lenses you are often exchanging corneal problems with patient problems.

19. Avoid ultrathin lens for patients who are poor handlers.

20. A deficient tear state may be present in the elderly, the aphakic, or the arthritic. This may result in chronic irritation, red eyes, recurrent infection, and corneal ulcers. Liberal use of artificial tears combined with a reduced schedule of contact lens wear can help in correcting the problem.

21. The aphakic eye is particularly reduced in corneal sensation, and a wearer may have a lens problem or foreign body under the lens and not recognize it sufficiently early.

22. The aphakic eye that is dry and has excessive mineral concentrations may cause excessive deposit buildup. This may be minimized by daily rinsing of the lens in the eye either by a stream of saline or balanced salt solution in the eye or with saline solution in an eyecup as an eyewash. If the lens is to be removed daily, you might as well switch to a gaspermeable lens.

Rigid lenses

CHAPTER 10

HISTORY OF RIGID LENSES

The development of contact lenses is an old story dating back to 1508. The first insight into the concept of covering the optical defects of a cornea with a device is credited by most people to Leonardo da Vinci. Da Vinci made glass water cups that were placed on the eye. He also had a contact lens with a funnel on one side for water to be poured in.

The first corneal lens was described by René Descartes. Descartes in a treatise called *Ways of Perfecting Vision* published his findings in 1636. He also used the water principle to neutralize the front surface of the cornea. In the seventeenth century the concept of the cornea as an instrument of vision was already known. Descartes also made from glass a crude elongated corneal contact lens.

In 1801, Thomas Young appreciated the change of a water-filled lens on his eye. He was aware of the change in power (in his case he became presbyopic) within the eye and knew how to fix it. He noted: "The addition of another lens . . . restores my eye to its natural state."

Sir John F.W. Herschel in 1823 had great insights into irregular astigmatism. He wrote: "Should any very bad cases of irregular corneas be found . . . vision could be improved . . . by taking an actual mould of the cornea and employing some transparent medium."

The scientific design of a contact lens was really evolved by A. Eugene Fick. His lenses had refractive power and were actually tried. He worked on rabbits to obtain correct molds made of glass for the eye. Then from a cadaver's eye he did the same thing to correct prob-

lems such as irregular astigmatism. His intent was to replace the scarred cornea by a regular surface made of glass. His first lenses consisted of a thin sphere of glass of about an 8 mm radius of curvature. He also experimented with a scleral lens with not much success. All his lenses were made with glass, which is about twice the weight of plastic lenses.

E. Kalt, using techniques similar to Fick's, in 1888 made a glass lens to treat keratoconus with the idea of apical touch and flattening of the cornea. Kalt actually saw considerable clinical visual improvement in some of the cases upon which his lens was tried.

From the beginning of the twentieth century to 1948, only scleral lenses made of glass were made. Some of these lens were blown, whereas others were ground and polished. These lenses were mostly applied to eyes with keratoconus, and the wearing time was limited to only a few hours during the day.

The major breakthrough into a useful contact lens occurred in 1947 when Kevin Tuohy began making contact lenses out of plastic rather than glass. The initial lenses caused corneal edema after hours of wear because the diameters were very large, ranging from 10.8 to 12.5 mm. In reality these were scleral lenses.

The next landmark in the history of the hard or rigid lens occurred in Germany in 1952. Wilhelm Söhnges began to use a smaller-diameter strictly corneal lens that was less than half the mass and weight of the Tuohy lens. After this achievement the contact lens finally emerged from being a research tool of limited use to become a real challenge in substituting

117

for glasses as a commercial practical device.

The technology of rigid lenses is still evolving. There are changes in design characteristics and materials. Gas-permeable lenses are crowding out the hard lens field, and lenses once more are becoming larger in size.

The search for better, more comfortable, safer lenses still persists. However, looking to the future, we may find that both glasses and contact lenses as we know them will disappear. Surgery for the correction of common refractive errors is now a reality. Other solutions to present issues may not be resolved with optical devices but rather through genetic engineering.

SYSTEMS FOR LENS ORDERING

Many different philosophies of rigid lens fitting have been developed in recent years. Fitters who believe that the thickness of the lens is of prime importance fit the majority of their patients with microthin lenses. Others believe that the diameter of the lens is the key to good technique. There are fitters who primarily fit large lenses and those who prefer small lenses. Some, who reject thickness and diameter as the ultimate factors, keep both constant and fit their patients largely by altering the primary base curve of the lens. The measurement of the corneal topography is believed by others to be the basis of fit of a lens. In this group some fitters use only the keratometer, whreas others prefer to topogometer. Still other groups reject them both, claiming that the photokeratoscope is the only means of measuring the true dimensions of all areas of the cornea. Despite the bewildering variety of approaches, each group appears to be honest, sincere, and forthright in its belief that its particular method offers the best and most rational approach to rigid lens fitting. How should a person view these claims? Which is best? Should the K readings be taken and mailed to a laboratory with the hope that a decent pair of lenses will be returned 2 days later? Should trial lenses be used because of the often repeated statement that the best device for fitting a contact lens is a contact lens? If this is true, perhaps an inventory of lenses is a little better.

There is no doubt that the neophyte lens fitter must be confused by the claims and counterclaims of many who teach lens philosophy. Obviously there is not one but a number of answers, all of which seem to work. In fact almost any given technique can work, since the relative success or failure of a particular method rests largely with the skill and experience of the practitioner. Which to choose? That is the question.

We have used all the systems, and our conclusion is that no system works all the time for everybody. One needs a steady, reliable approach plus alternatives if the customary method fails.

The success of good fitters is not how well they fit lenses but how they deal with any resulting problem.

Special reference has to be made to gas-permeable lenses. Although rigid lens techniques are applicable to gas-permeable lenses, the approach is different because of the unique facility of this lens. One can take advantage of large-diameter lenses and their improved stability and centration without worrying about hypoxia of the corneal epithelium. Also the fitting of a high-riding lens, satisfactory for gas-permeable lenses, is not consistent with rigid PMMA lens objectives. Although PMMA lens trial sets are satisfactory for gas-permeable lenses, the diameter of the lenses must be appropriate and the fitting criteria taken into account. What is desirable for a PMMA lens fitting is not satisfactory for gas-permeable lenses. The amount of movement of a gas-permeable lens need not be as great as that of a PMMA lens, which entirely depends on tear exchange for oxygenation. Although gas-permeable lenses belong to the general family of rigid lenses, their application, objectives, and complications are quite different.

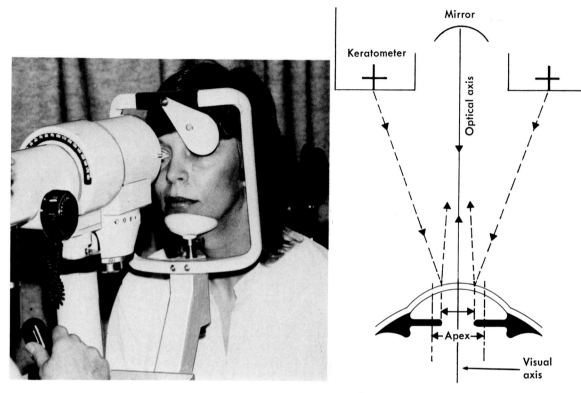

Fig. 11-1. A, Taking a K reading. **B,** The principle of the keratometer. The visual axis is aligned along the optic axis of the instrument so that the central front surface of the cornea reflects the mires of the keratometer. (**A** from Stein, H.A., and Slatt, B.J.: The ophthalmic assistant, ed. 4, St. Louis, 1983, The C.V. Mosby Co.)

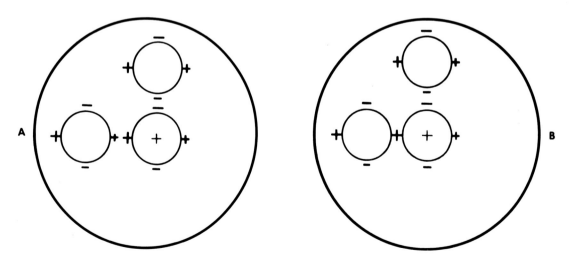

Fig. 11-2. Keratometer mires. **A,** Alignment of the mires for axis. **B,** Apposition of the plus-sign mire to measure one meridian of corneal curvature. (From Stein, H.A., and Slatt, B.J.: The ophthalmic assistant, ed. 4, St. Louis, 1983, The C.V. Mosby Co.)

SYSTEMS BASED ON CORNEAL TOPOGRAPHY
Keratometer method

The keratometer method is probably the most commonly employed method and is simple to perform. K, the measurement that parallels the steepest zone of the flattest primary meridian, is measured (Figs. 11-1 and 11-2). The steepest zone relates to the apex of the cornea, which is steeper than the peripheral portion.

Method. K readings are taken. The spectacle prescription is recorded in minus cylinder form and the cylinder reading is dropped. If the lens is fitted on K, the power is not changed. If the lens is fitted steeper than K, the plus power of the lens is decreased 0.25 D for each 0.25 D steeper fit. The added steepness causes the lens to vault the cornea centrally and creates a

tear lens of plus power. This is the reason that a slight reduction in power is made to compensate. On the other hand, the minus power is increased 0.25 D for each 0.25 D of steeper fit.

The keratometer is designed to measure a spheric surface with the cornea acting as a front-surface convex mirror (Fig. 11-3). However, frequently the cornea is aspheric and is steeper inferiorly and temporally (Fig. 11-4). The keratometer measures a limited circular area of the cornea, 2 to 4 mm apart, and if one mire is on the steeper side, the result given will be an average. The keratometer reflects only a small segment of the cornea (Fig 11-5). Each instrument makes an assumption as to the index of refraction of the cornea. The Bausch & Lomb keratometer is calculated for an index of refraction of 1.3375 mm, whereas others are set for 1.332 to 1.336 mm.

Guide for lens system

System	Comment	Rating
Keratometer	Strictly for beginners; a one-measurement system with faults in the single measurement	*
Topogometer	Attempts to define the topography of the cornea by outlining the corneal cap; rather inflexible; works well, possibly because most of the lenses come out small and thin	**
Nomogram	The number game in disguise; still a one-measurement system; works better than keratometry; good for the novice	*
Photokeratoscopy	Like the topogometer method except that it adds a permanent photographic record; more polish but practically the same thing	**
Microthin lens	A very thin lens must be a small-diameter lens; too limited as a first-choice lens; good for rigid lens problems or dropouts	**
Large-diameter lens	Good for special situations; requires too much skill for the fitter and the laboratory; complications can be gross	*
Hartstein	Simple and practical; takes into account pupil diameter and corneal dimensions; despite the use of arbitrary calculations, the system works	**
Custom	No particular philosophy attached to this method; takes into account palpebral fissure size, corneal diameter, pupil size, and corneal topography, which are measured; from this information fitter determines lens size, size of optic zone, type of edge, and thickness; not for beginners	***
Diagnostic lens	Probably the best approach to lens fitting; provides a dynamic overview of the lens-cornea relationship; requires few modifications for a custom-fit lens that can be universally applied; problems such as effect of power additions to the lens and exact base curves can be immediately determined; trial set does not require a major financial commitment and can easily be replaced if lenses become obsolete	****
Inventory	Its simplicity is its greatest asset; not economic for the occasional fitter, good for the large-volume practice; the system works like a fast-food restaurant outlet—the lens waits for the patient to arrive	***

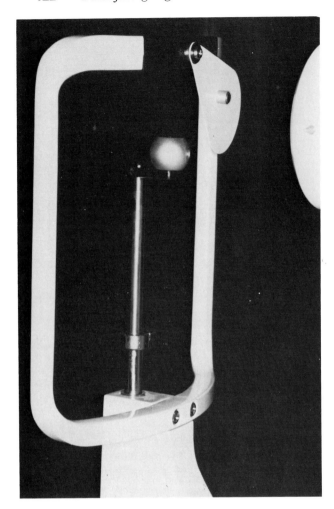

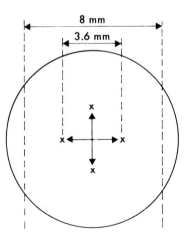

Fig. 11-3. Test ball is used to calibrate the keratometer for a given radius of curvature.

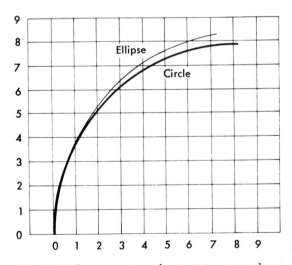

Fig. 11-4. The cornea is aspheric; it is not a sphere or a true ellipse. The rate of flattening in its periphery is not symmetric. The keratometer is a limited instrument, designed only for spheric surfaces.

Fig. 11-5. The chord diameter (3.6 mm) of the corneal cap spans the linear distance between two points of the cornea. The chord diameter of the corneal cap is usually between 4 and 5 mm, whereas the radius of the corneal cap (8 mm), which measures the curvature of the cornea, is frequently between 6 and 8 mm. The keratometer, which measures a chord area of 3 to 3.6 mm, reflects only a small segment of the cornea.

Comment. Since this method depends on one measurement, it would be reassuring if that measurement were precise. Unfortunately it is not, and even if it were it would be inadequate.

Despite the fact that keratometry works in a majority of cases, it is probably the least desirable method of lens fitting. The laboratory is left with the awesome responsibility of determining the peripheral curves, the design of the edge, the diameter of the lens, the thickness of the lens, and the size of the optic zone. This method also precludes any assessment of lid aherence, centration of the lens, and the effect of power on the fit. Its simplicity is its only attractive feature.

Topogometer method

The topogometer is an attachment to the keratometer that contains a movable light source so that the visual axis can be decentered from the optical axis of the instrument (Figs. 11-6 and 11-7). One takes K readings across the surface of the cornea by changing the angle of the fixation light. The fixation light is quite handy because it steadies fixation in eyes with poor acuity. Flattening of the cornea is indicated by a change in the radius of curvature.

The topogometer may also be employed to scan the corneal cap to detect a steeper zone away from the visual axis. If allowances are not made for such a variation in corneal contour, a lens will fit flat. The topogometer method assists in measuring the size of the corneal cap.

This approach to keratometery is quite helpful for patients with poor vision, aphakia, and keratoconus, where the change of radius of curvature from the apex of the corneal cap to the peripheray is great. For ordinary lens patients this method is certainly superior to the K reading method because the optic zone of the lens can at least be ordered so that it coincides with the radius of curvature of the corneal cap.

This technique is also quite popular because most corneas have an optic zone between 5.8 and 6.2 mm, which results in thin, small, steep lenses that have many attractive features. These are discussed more fully under microthin lenses (p. 127).

This approach to lens fitting is also arbitrary. Once the horizontal and vertical meridians of the corneal cap are plotted, a lens is chosen with a diameter 2 mm greater than the corneal cap diameter. One millimeter is added for stability and movements, and 1 mm is added for proper edge design and secondary curves. The formula is commonly abbreviated to read the LD + 2 method (Fig. 11-8).

The topogometer approach was introduced by Louis Girard, Joseph Soper, and Whitney Sampson.

Photokeratoscopy

The photokeratoscope also depends on the cornea acting as a convex mirror to produce a virtual image (Fig. 11-9). Its advantage is that its image reflects the curvature of a larger corneal area than does the keratometer (Fig. 11-10).

The better photokeratoscopes have aspheric targets with an aperture at the center. Behind the aperture a Polaroid camera is mounted to photograph the corneal image for a permanent record.

The annular radius of curvature is derived from assessment of the separation of the target rings in the corneal photograph. In fact the precise margin of the ring may be difficult to identify because of blurring from the film grain. Variability may also be introduced from differences in the photosensitive material on the film. The photokeratoscope does not have any greater accuracy than the keratometer. However it measures more of the cornea, providing information on the periphery as well as the central corneal cap.

The major disadvantage of the system is the expense, which is marginally justified. It is really a variant of an approach to fitting lenses based on a more accurate assessment of corneal topography. It ignores many important considerations, despite the scientific sophistication of having a computer analyze the data regarding corneal topography. No allowance is made for the weight of the lens, the effect of lid lift, the correct lens diameter, or the centration of the lens. These factors can only be judged by a diagnostic lens. On the plus side the photokeratoscope is extremely versatile, being applicable for very flat corneas less than 40.00 D to very steep corneas greater than 50.00 D. Also one can feed into the computer any desired requirements such as diameter thickness and base curve, and the computer will then design

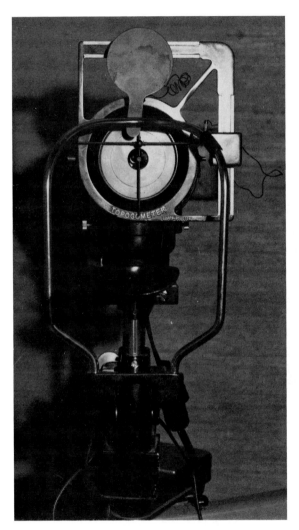

Fig. 11-6. The topogometer.

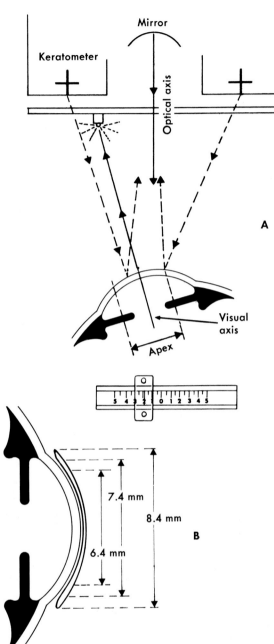

Fig. 11-7. A, The topogometer. The visual axis is displaced by the fixation light of the topogometer. The mires are now reflected from a paracentral arc of the cornea. A change in the radius of curvature as the eye is decentered indicates the limits of the corneal cap. **B,** The final diameter of a lens as determined by the formula LD + 2 where LD indicates the longest apical diameter and 2 refers to a 2 mm greater lens size than the longest apical diameter. In this case the longest apical diameter is 6.4 mm; thus the total lens diameter is 8.4 mm.

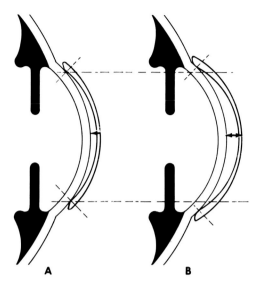

Fig. 11-8. A, The power of the lens is influenced by the apical vault. **B,** As the vaulting of the cornea is increased, the plus power of the tear film is increased.

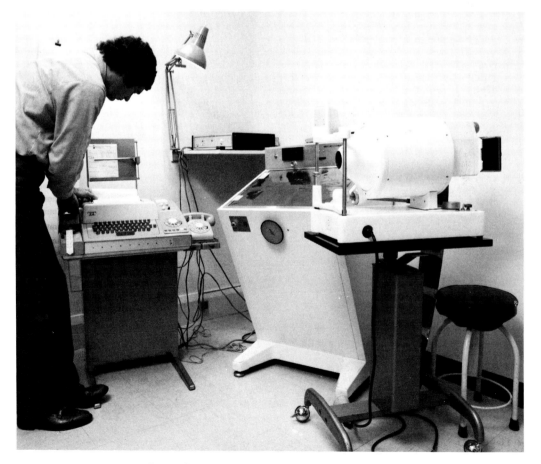

Fig. 11-9. System 2000 Photo-Electronic Keratoscope with Telex relay to computer. (From Stein, H.A., and Slatt, B.J.: The ophthalmic assistant, ed. 3, St. Louis, 1976, The C.V. Mosby Co.)

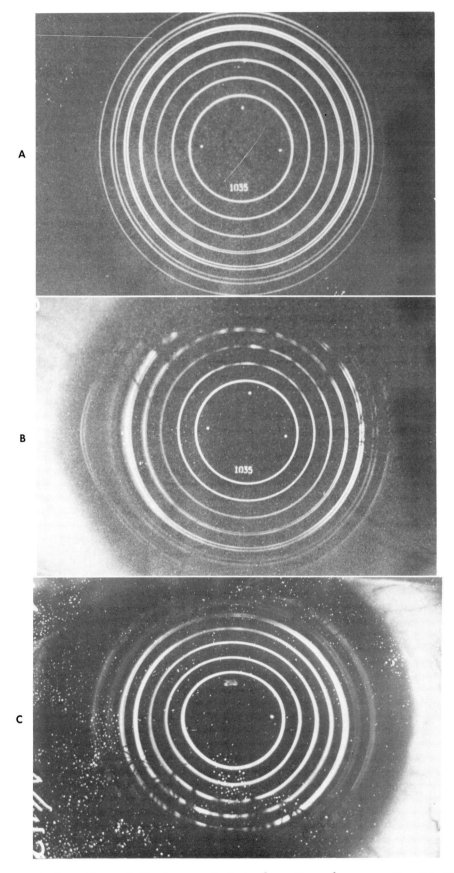

Fig. 11-10. Photo-Electronic Keratoscope. **A,** Test sphere; **B,** regular cornea; **C,** astigmatic eye (approximately 4.00 D).

the balance of the lens from its memory bank. This can be done as often as one wishes.

Comment. The computer computes well, but the bulk of the information must come from the fitter.

How to fit with the photokeratoscope (based on system 2000)

The practitioner supplies keratograms of patients' corneas and specific diameter sizes, tear layer thicknesses, and Cycon limits. The Cycon limit is the astigmatic difference in K readings that is tolerated before a toric lens is required.

Failure to assign a diameter will result in the computer program specifying a lens diameter of 8.2 mm for a cornea with a base curve of 44.00 D. Steeper corneas result in smaller diameters, and flatter corneas receive larger diameters; the typical range is 7.9 to 8.5 mm for PMMA lenses. Unless specified a tear layer thickness of 0.025 mm is assigned by the computer.

Cycon limit is exceeded when the difference in base curves exceeds 0.35 mm; when this happens a toric posterior surface is designed. The toric difference is calculated by the difference between the base curves calculated for the flattest meridian and the meridian at right angles to the flattest meridian.

When a lens of spheric design is ordered for a toric cornea, large diameter lenses, 9.9 mm, are used. The other lens dimensions are assigned. The optic zone is 1.2 mm less than the diameter. The intermediate curve is always 0.3 mm wide, the peripheral curve is always 0.3 mm wide, the the minimum center thickness is always 0.1 mm.

SYSTEMS BASED ON TYPES OF LENSES
Microthin lenses

The core of this fitting system is that the lenses must be thin and lightweight so that they are less likely to mold the cornea and mechanically abrade it. These lenses are small in diameter, usually between 7.8 and 8.6 mm. A reduction in diameter is an inevitable consequence with thin lenses (Fig. 11-11). In fact it is difficult to make a large, thin lens. The center thickness is between 0.08 and 0.12 mm. The peripheral curves are relatively steep with a width of 0.3 to 0.6 mm. The steep narrow edge along with other features in the design of the lens allows the lens to center properly (Fig. 11-12). Also the thin edge does not jar the upper lid, and so blinking is likely to be comfortable and regular in frequency. The thinness of the lens causes some flexure with blinking, which helps tear exchange by creating a tear pump. The excellent tear exchange with the lightness of the lens usually results in minimal corneal edema after a day's wear, and, as a result, spectacle blur is frequently no more than 15 minutes in duration.

Bending or flexure of this lens may result in the introduction of some astigmatism with the rule to the cornea, and so it is ideally suited for corneas that have astigmatism against the rule.

Eye movement is free from lid irritation when microthin lenses are worn because the lens is usually smaller than the palpebral fissures. These lenses bend slightly on nonspheric corneas because of the capillary forces involved, creating better alignment between the lens and the cornea. For many fitters this is the lens of choice.

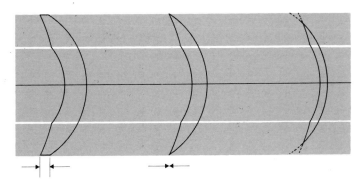

Fig. 11-11. Diameter reductions. As the thickness of a lens is reduced, the edge of the lens becomes thinner. Finally, as further reductions in thickness occur, the edge disappears so that a small-diameter, thin lens results.

A light, thin lens may be a good solution to some conventional rigid lens problems. For instance, these thin lenses are more comfortable than conventional lenses and can be employed as an alternative to soft lenses in cases of rigid lens dropouts (Fig. 11-13). In those cases in which significant astigmatism is present they may be the best alternative. In situations where a lens rides low a microthin lens offers less gravitational pull and more lift from the upper lid. At times a large, high-riding lens problem may be solved with small, microthin lenses that may center better. Because of their thinness and small diameter they are useful in those wearers who have a limited wearing time

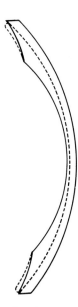

Fig. 11-12. The peripheral curves are made steep to allow the lens to center properly. This thin, steep edge provides minimal obstruction to the lid, which adds to the comfort of the lens.

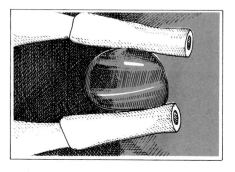

Fig. 11-13. Microthin lens, though a rigid lens made of polymethylmethacrylate, is flexible.

resulting from the presence of corneal edema. Those patients who have induced corneal astigmatism caused by the molding effect of large lenses may be helped with a microthin lens. They cannot see with spectacles, and the time lag in waiting for their corneas to assume their natural shape may be intolerable. The soft lens is a poor substitute in such cases, since it does little to correct the induced astigmatic error.

How to fit

The following steps are used to fit microthin lenses:

1. Fit either with K readings as a base or by the diagnostic trial lens procedure. The base curve is usually fitted slightly steeper than K by 0.25 to 0.50 D (Table 11-1). Fit the least steep lens that provides satisfactory lens position and lens movement. The diameter and optic zone vary with the base curve and are selected from tables (Table 11-2). The general rules still apply. A flat cornea (42.00 D or less) requires a larger lens (8.6 mm), whereas a steep cornea (45.00 D) requires a smaller lens (8.0 mm).
2. Normally the fit should have slight apical clearance; 1 mm lens movement with blinking is optimal. Minimal lag in ocular rotation is desirable. Central touch can be tolerated because of the thinness of the lens (Fig. 11-14).
3. The fluorescein pattern appears uniform under the lens. Because of the steep peripheral curves a narrower than normal band of fluorescein is found at the periphery (Fig. 11-15).
4. With astigmatism from 1.00 to 2.00 D, fit 0.50 D steeper than K. For astigmatism between 2.00 and 3.00 D, fit one third the value of K. These lenses are superior to toric base curve lenses in correcting astigmatism less than 4.00 D.

The microthin lenses seem too good to be true. They have the comfort and rapid adaptability of a soft lens and the optic properties of a rigid lens. There are, however, disadvantages.

Disadvantages. Microthin lenses have the following disadvantages:

1. Microthin lenses frequently cannot be used with some lenses that are likely to

Table 11-1. Diameter selection*

Palpebral fissure	Horizontal corneal diameter				
	12.5	12.0	11.5	11.0	10.5
Large	9.2	9.0	8.8	8.6	8.4
Normal	9.0	8.8	8.6	8.4	8.2
Small	8.8	8.4	8.2	8.0	7.8
Very small	8.2 or smaller	8.0 or smaller	7.8 or smaller	7.6 or smaller	7.4 or smaller

*Initial lens diameter in mm.

Table 11-2. Base-curve selection*

Lens diameter (mm)	9.0	8.8	8.6	8.4	8.2	8.0	7.8	7.6	7.4	7.2	7.0
Optic zone diameter (mm)	7.8	7.6	7.4	7.2	7.0	7.0	7.0	6.8	6.8	6.6	6.6
Peripheral curve width (mm)	0.4	0.4	0.4	0.4	0.4	0.4	0.3	0.3	0.2	0.2	0.1
Peripheral curve radius (mm)	Should be flatter than base curve by:										
Minus lenses	1.5	1.5	1.5	1.5	1.5	1.5	2.0	2.0	2.5	2.5	3.0
Plus lenses	1.0	1.0	1.0	1.0	1.0	1.0	1.5	1.5	2.0	2.0	2.5
Blend curve width (mm)	0.2	0.2	0.2	0.2	0.2	0.1	0.1	0.1	0.1	0.1	0.1
Blend curve radius (mm)	Should be flatter than base curve by:										
All lenses	0.7	0.7	0.7	0.7	0.7	0.7	1.0	1.0	1.0	1.0	1.0
Fit steeper than K by (D)	0.12	0.25	0.37	0.50	0.62	0.62	0.75	0.87	0.87	1.0	1.0
	plus 25% of the corneal cylinder (difference between K readings)										

*Minus lenses from −6.00 to −8.00 D should be fitted 0.12 D steeper than shown; beyond −8.00 D they should be fitted 0.25 D steeper.

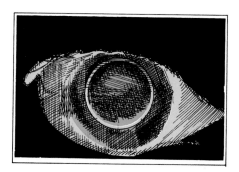

Fig. 11-14. Microthin lens fitted on K. The fluorescein pattern shows some central touch and pooling at the periphery of the lens because of the steep peripheral curves.

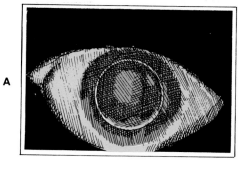
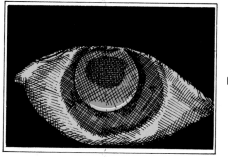

Fig. 11-15. A, Microthin lens fitted steeper than K. The ring of fluorescein around the lens is indicative of the very steep fit. **B,** Microthin lens fitted flatter than K. Large area of apical touch with pooling of fluorescein elsewhere is typical of a flat lens-cornea relationship.

be high riding, as in severe myopia. Their extreme thinness can carry the lens higher.

2. They are especially hard to remove. That nice, thin edge makes it difficult for the upper lid to dislodge the lens. Also the tightness of the fit makes removal awkward.
3. They do not center well in certain patients with high astigmatic corrections.
4. They are difficult lenses to modify in the office because of their size and flexibility. These lenses cannot be held in place with a suction cup. If they are modified, they must be stabilized using a holder with a wax mounting.
5. They warp easily.
6. The base curve may not be stable.
7. Patients with large pupils complain of flare.
8. Because of their thinness, it is easier to damage and break these lenses in handling.

Base-curve selection. The smaller the lens diameter, the more corneal cylinder present, and the smaller the optic zone, the steeper the base curve should be.

Lens thickness (Table 11-3). The key to proper performance of ultrathin lenses lies in

making them extremely thin. Small lenses of conventional thickness tend to stay down because of their excess weight in relation to their small size. A conventional lens fitted steeper than K will have poor tear exchange, whereas an ultrathin lens tends to flex with each blink. This pumping action provides movement of tears under the lens.

Comment. Microthin lenses are particularly useful as starter lenses in patients with small palpebral fissures, tight upper lids, or corneas steeper than 46.00 D. They also provide an alternative to soft lenses for rigid lens dropouts. Microthin lenses are useful for residual astigmatism against the rule, since they flex in the opposite meridian.

Some authors attempt to identify flexible lenses as a separate entity. We believe that all rigid lenses can be made flexible or semiflexible, depending not only on their thickness, but also on their material composition. We consider flexible lenses as a subtype of a rigid lens.

The comfort of the lens is largely related to its relatively steep peripheral curves and thin edges, which provide only a minimal obstruction to the lid margin. The comfort is not a function of its size. Even a hydrophilic lens that is reduced in size so that the lid makes contact with its edge, will be uncomfortable.

Table 11-3. Recommended thicknesses for minus and plus power lenses

Lens powers (D)	Diameter (mm)				
	9.0	8.5	8.0	7.5	7.0
Minus power					
Plano to −0.62	0.18	0.17	0.16	0.15	0.14
−0.75 to −1.37	0.17	0.16	0.15	0.14	0.13
−1.50 to −2.12	0.16	0.15	0.14	0.13	0.12
−2.25 to −2.87	0.15	0.14	0.13	0.12	0.11
−3.00 to −3.62	0.14	0.13	0.12	0.11	0.10
−3.75 to −4.37	0.13	0.12	0.11	0.10	0.10
−4.50 to −5.12	0.12	0.11	0.10	0.10	0.10
−5.25 to −5.87	0.11	0.10	0.10	0.10	0.10
−6.00 & over	0.10	0.10	0.10	0.10	0.10
Plus power					
+0.12 to +0.75	0.20	0.18	0.17	0.16	0.15
+0.87 to +1.50	0.22	0.20	0.19	0.18	0.16
+1.62 to +2.25	0.24	0.22	0.21	0.20	0.18
+2.37 to +3.00	0.26	0.24	0.23	0.21	0.20
+3.12 to +3.75	0.28	0.26	0.25	0.23	0.22
+3.87 to +4.50	0.30	0.28	0.27	0.25	0.24
+4.62 to +5.25	0.32	0.30	0.29	0.27	0.25

Table supplied with permission of Dr. Stanley Gordon, Rochester, N.Y.

Large lenses with wide peripheral curves

Unless a fitter is committed by tradition to a given lens diameter, there should be some rationale for arriving at a given lens diameter.

Generally a flat cornea is a large cornea and requires a large lens, whereas if a cornea is small, less than 11 mm, or steep, greater than 44.00 D, a small-diameter lens should be considered. The range of diameters considered is between 8.3 and 9 mm.

Generally a large palpebral aperture, 10 mm or greater, requires a larger lens, whereas a small palpebral aperture, 10 mm or less, should have a smaller lens. Despite these general rules, however, there are fitters who prefer primarily the large-diameter lens as their lens of choice.

Design. These lenses are between 9 and 10 mm in diameter. They have an intermediate curve that is 1 mm flatter than the base curve and a peripheral curve that is 1 mm flatter than the intermediate curve. The optic zone is large, varying from a high normal size of 7 mm to a generous size of 8 mm. This large size would of course eliminate the annoying flare of small lenses. The diameter of the optic zone is usually 1.5 mm less than the corneal diameter.

If fitted properly, these lenses are very comfortable. The large size enables the edge of the lens to remain under the upper lid during blinking.

The wide peripheral curves hold a large reservoir of tear fluid that cushions the lens and assists in tear exchange.

Advantages. This is a good lens for a high-riding lens. The extra weight adds gravitational force to bring it down especially with single-cut plus lenses. This feature is not so relevant with minus lenses. Spheric lenses can be employed for corneal astigmatism up to a range of 3.00 to 4.00 D. The lenses are stable, center well, and are easy to handle. They are more comfortable than a smaller lens of similar edge design.

Disadvantages. A large lens has its place in overcoming many fitting problems but as a lens of first choice it has too many drawbacks. There is greater corneal molding because of its bulk. If a lens is reduced from 10 to 8 mm, the entire area of the lens is reduced by 36%. Molding of a cornea can induce serious astigmatic errors of the cornea of 5.00 to 6.00 D in magnitude, which in some cases can be permanent.

This is a difficult lens to handle with small palpebral fissures.

The large lens is poor for steep and for small corneas.

The peripheral curves are complex but must be fashioned precisely. If they do not become contoured to the cornea, the lenses will become very loose.

Comment. The disadvantages of a large PMMA lens has been counteracted with gas-permeable material. The positive features still stand.

HARTSTEIN MODIFICATION

This method, popularized by Jack Hartstein, utilizes two basic parameters—corneal diameter and pupillary size—to arrive at the dimensions of a lens.

The corneal diameter is measured with the ophthalmoscope with a +10.00 D lens for magnification and a millimeter ruler. With the patient fixating in the distance and the ruler covering half the pupil, the pupillary size is similarly measured. The illumination of the ophthalmoscope is dimmed to prevent any pupillary constriction (Fig. 11-16). A pupillometer may also be used (Fig. 11-17).

The lens diameter is determined when 4 mm are added to the pupillary diameter; for example, a pupil of 4.2 mm will require a lens size of 8.2 mm.

The optic zone is an arbitrary figure and is simply 1.5 mm less than the lens diameter. The total lens diameter is influenced by the corneal diameter. If the corneal diameter is 12 mm or more, 0.5 mm should be added to the lens diameter. If it is 10 mm or less, the lens size should be reduced 0.5 mm.

Despite these calculations, arbitrary limits are placed on lens size, the minimum being 7.5 and the maximum 9.5 mm.

The secondary curve is 0.75 mm wide and 5.00 D flatter than the primary base curve.

The standard thickness for a plano lens is 0.16 mm. For each diopter of minus power, 0.01 mm is subtracted. For plus lenses 0.02 mm is added for each diopter of plus power. Again, there are limits, because a lens with a thickness of less than 0.12 mm will begin to flex and will require a reduction in diameter.

The primary base curve is 0.25 to 0.50 D steeper than the K reading. With astigmatism

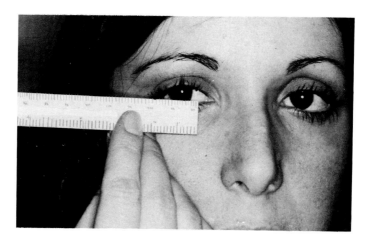

Fig. 11-16. Measuring the pupillary and corneal diameter with a ruler. (From Stein, H.A., and Slatt, B.J.: The ophthalamic assistant, ed. 3, St. Louis, 1976, The C.V. Mosby Co.)

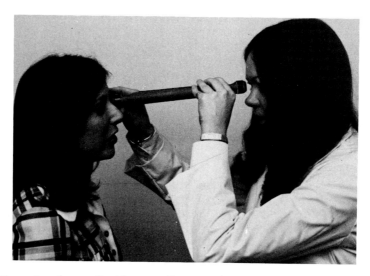

Fig. 11-17. Measuring the pupil with a pupillometer. (From Stein, H.A., and Slatt, B.J.: The ophthalmic assistant, ed. 3, St. Louis, 1976, The C.V. Mosby Co.)

between 0.50 and 2.00 D a spheric lens is ordered parallel to the flattest corneal meridian. Astigmatism between 2.00 and 3.00 D requires a lens 0.50 D steeper than the flattest corneal meridian. A toric lens is required for astigmatism greater than 3.00 D.

Comment. Obviously this method works; however, it is not any better than other techniques mentioned such as the topogometer approach or the microthin lens method.

This method is important because it stresses the value of making measurements of pupillary size and corneal diameter, which should influ-

ence the final dimensions of a lens. In patients with large pupil sizes and large corneas, an adjustment in lens dimension must be made and the lens made larger.

GENERAL RULES FOR CUSTOM-DESIGNED LENSES
Primary base curve

Slight apical clearance over the cornea is desirable as long as it is adequate. Up to 3.00 D of astigmatism can be corrected with a spheric lens. As the degree of astigmatism increases, the base curve must be made steeper. The following is a general guide showing the relationship between the amount of corneal astigmatism and the lens base curve.

Cornea	Base curve
To 0.50 D astigmatism	0.25 D steeper than K reading
0.50 to 2.00 D of astigmatism	0.50 D steeper than K reading
2.00 to 3.00 D of astigmatism	0.50 to 0.75 D steeper than K reading
More than 3.00 D of astigmatism	Bitoric or inside toric lens

The primary base curve may be ordered in diopters or millimeters radius of curvature.

Corneal diameter

The corneal diameter is obtained when one measures the visible iris diameter with a ruler. The most accurate way is to use calipers to determine the limbus-to-limbus diameter after a topical anesthetic is placed on the cornea. Although the cornea is slightly larger, for clinical purposes this amount can be ignored. The diameter of the cornea in the horizontal meridian usually ranges between 10.5 and 12 mm.

Lens diameter

The lens diameter may be determined in various ways. With the microthin lenses the lens diameter must be small, usually less than 8.5 mm.

Lenses over 4.00 D power usually need a diameter of 8.5 mm or more to avoid a high-riding lens. The greater the minus power, the larger the lens.

If the topogometer is employed, the lens will be 2 mm larger than the corneal cap, which varies from 5.8 to 6.2 mm. One may calculate the lens diameter in relation to the pupillary size by adding 4 mm to the pupillary diameter.

Generally, large, flat corneas require a large lens, that is, a corneal diameter greater than 11.5 mm and flatter than 44.00 D. Conversely a small, steep cornea, for example, less than 11.5 mm and steeper than 44.00 D, requires a small lens. Without going to extremes the acceptable range of minus-powered lens diameters is between 8 and 9 mm. A large palpebral aperture accommodates a large lens, whereas a small fissure demands a small lens.

Another aid to determining lens diameter is to flash a light into the other eye blurred with a plus lens. This maneuver creates a consensually smaller pupil in the other eye. If the vision is improved by the small pupil, a larger lens is needed.

Increasing the lens diameter with concomitant increase in optic zone without altering the base curve has the same effect as making the lens tighter. It increases apical vaulting. Conversely reducing the lens size serves to decrease the apical vaulting effect. A change in the clearance of the cornea can affect the shape of the tear film layer and consequently can also affect the power of the lens (Figs. 11-18 and 11-21). Smaller lenses can be fitted steeper than larger lenses. A lens of 7.5 to 8.5 mm diameter can be fitted 1.50 to 2.50 D steeper than K, whereas a 9.5 to 10 mm diameter lens should be fitted on K or perhaps 0.25 D steeper.

Optic zone diameter

The optic zone diameter varies with the pupillary size, the lens diameter, and the palpebral fissure size.

If the optic zone is too small for the size of the pupil, the person will experience flare in dim illumination when the pupillary aperture increases. This person is annoyed by the streaming of lights and may also be subject to fluctuation in visual acuity because at times the pupil is partially covered by the peripheral curve of the lens. Flare occurs as a result of the flatter peripheral curve, creating a prismatic deflection of light passing through it.

For large pupils (5 to 7 mm), that is, for persons with blue eyes, myopia, or anxiety, the size of the optic zone should be increased 0.5 mm. For small pupils (less than 4 mm) for example, for persons who have brown eyes or who are middle aged, the optic zone can be reduced by 0.5 mm.

The optic zone usually varies with the size of the lens. In large, flat eyes with K readings of 42.00 D or under, the optic zone should be larger.

Lens diameter (mm)	Optic zone
9 or greater	1.5 mm less than lens diameter
8.2 to 8.8	1 to 1.3 mm less than lens diameter
8	1 mm less than lens diameter

When in doubt about the correct size of the optic zone diameter, a lens on the large rather than small side should be selected. The optic

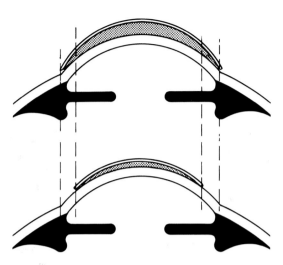

Fig. 11-18. As the diameter of the lens is increased, the lens becomes steeper, the apical clearance of the cornea becomes greater, and the shape of the tear film becomes more convex in shape, which adds plus power. Both lenses have the same radius of curvature.

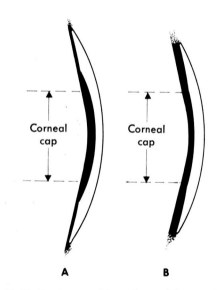

A   B

Fig. 11-19. Optic zone. Two identical lenses placed on corneas with the same K readings. **A,** The size of the optic zone is too large for the corneal cap, and the lens vaults the cornea. The net effect is the same as if the lens was made too steep. **B,** The size of the optic zone is compatible with the size of the corneal cap, and the lens is comfortable. If the optic zone is too small, flare is frequently experienced.

zone of a lens can be made smaller by modification of the lens but cannot be made larger unless a new lens is made.

The lens diameter and consequently the optic zone vary directly with the palpebral fissure size. A small palpebral fissure requires a smaller-diameter lens and hence a smaller optic zone. Decreasing the optic zone (base curve) radius of a lens has the effect of making the fit tighter, whereas decreasing the optic zone diameter or increasing the optic zone radius (making it flatter) will loosen the rigid lens. A decrease in optic zone diameter is the same as an increase in the width of the intermediate curve. Reduction of the size of the optic zone is done in 0.1 or 0.2 mm steps.

The size of optic zone should bear a close relationship to the size of the corneal cap (Fig. 11-19), which can be determined by either the topogometer method or by photokeratoscopy.

Sometimes the optic zone seems too small because the person experiences halos or fringes around lights. Flare can frequently indicate a flat fit if the lens moves excessively displacing a peripheral portion of the lens onto the pupillary area.

Comment. The factors affecting the size of the optic zone are frequently ignored and its size determined arbitrarily from a nomogram or indirectly from corneal diameter measurements. It is surprising how well a system without any scientific rationale really works. Few practitioners actually measure the size of the corneal cap or concern themselves with the dimensions of the optic zone of a lens.

Thickness of lens

The thickness of a lens varies directly with the power and the lens diameter.

The greater the plus power, the greater the central thickness must be. An aphakic lens is frequently 0.35 to 0.4 mm thick, whereas a myopic lens of −4.00 D is often no thicker than 0.13 to 0.15 mm. If a lens is reduced to less than 0.10 mm, bending or flexure of the lens may become extreme and result in variable vision. A plano lens should have a central thickness of 0.15 mm. For every 2.00 D of minus power 0.01 mm should be subtracted from 0.15 mm. For every 1.00 D of plus power 0.025 mm should be added. The minimum thickness should be 0.10 mm.

If a lens is reduced in thickness, the periphery of the lens disappears, and its diameter must correspondingly be made smaller.

The comfort of a lens depends not on its thickness but rather on the edge treatment. A thick lens, however, is likely to ride low and mold the cornea and is less capable of producing tear exchange because of the absence of flex.

If a lens is relatively thin, it will have a tendency to fit tightly, whereas a thick lens may tend to fit loosely and move excessively.

Peripheral curves

The width and the curvature usually vary with the size of the lens, its thickness, and the base curve. For any specified lens diameter the width of the peripheral curve determines the size of the optic zone. A lens can be made looser by widening the peripheral curves or by flattening them. The choice of which modification to make is often determined by the optic zone requirements: if the patient has a large pupil and the optic zone is already reasonably small, it might be wiser in this instance to flatten the peripheral curve than to reduce the optic zone.

Most practitioners rely upon the laboratory to specify the radius of curvatures of the peripheral curves. But any trial set employed should have the same peripheral curve as the lenses ordered. A typical posterior peripheral curve is 0.3 mm wide with a 12.25 mm radius. The intermediate peripheral curve is frequently 0.3 mm wide with a 9.0 mm radius.

The peripheral curves are always flatter than the base curve to comply with the flatter peripheral corneal contours.

Blend curves

Blend curves are used to remove the sharp junction of the peripheral and secondary curves and are also used at the secondary base curve junction. Blends can be light, medium, or heavy.

The No. 1 blend is that blend placed between the secondary and base curves. It is 0.5 mm longer in radius of curvature than the base curve.

The No. 3 blend is between the secondary and posterior curves, and its radius is halfway between the radius of the secondary and posterior curves.

Edges

The edges should be smooth, free of sharp areas, and contoured to slip under the eyelids during blinking. On thick edges of high myopic lenses −5.00 D or more, a bevel is added on the anterior surface to contour the lens edge. The lens edge should be contoured posteriorly, since an anterior lens design, though good for tear exchange, causes lid irritation and displacement of the lens.

Comment. Any lens over 5.00 D should have its edges beveled. The myopic lens should have that prism base effect trimmed similar in shape to a plus lens, whereas a high-plus lens requires a myopic profile to aid in comfort and lens lift.

Power calculation

The refraction must be expressed in minus cylinder. The cylinder is then dropped, and the sphere is retained as the refractive power. For example,

Spectacle lens power	*Contact lens power*
−3.00 D −2.00 D × 180	−3.00 D

If the spectacle lens power is greater than ±4.00 D an adjustment is required to make the accurate contact lens power. For myopia less minus power is required in the contact lens form as compared to the spectacle prescription. For example, a spectacle lens power of −5.00 D with 15 mm vertex power would result in a contact lens power of −4.65 D.

For hyperopia more effective power is needed in the contact lens form. For example, a spectacle lens power of +5.00 D with 15 mm vertex distance would result in a contact lens power of +5.41 D (Fig. 11-20).

If the contact lens is not fitted on K, a further modification of power must be made. When the base curve is steeper than the flattest central corneal curve (flattest K reading), a tear lens of plus power is formed (Fig. 11-21). To correct for this the contact lens should be made with less plus or more minus power.

For every 0.25 D that the base curve is steeper than the corneal curve, −0.25 D should be added to the contact lens. For each 0.25 D that the base curve is flatter than the corneal K reading, 0.25 D should be added to the power of the contact lens.

If a trial lens is used, the computation of power is relatively simple, since the spectacle

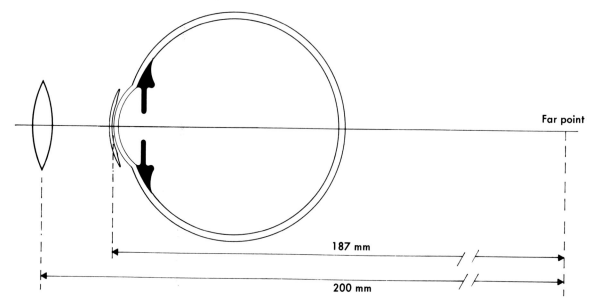

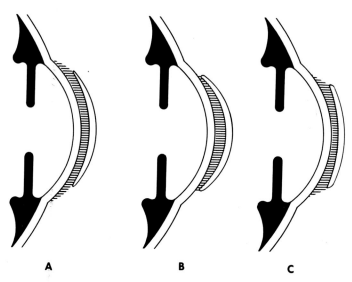

Fig. 11-20. Vertex power. The far point of a plus lens is reduced with the shift from a spectacle lens to a contact lens. To achieve the same power, added plus power must be incorporated into the contact lens as follows: 5.00 D hyperopia—in front of the cornea by 13 mm—far point = 200 mm. Far-point distance of contact lens = 187 mm. Power of contact lens = $\frac{1000}{187}$ = +5.34 mm.

Fig. 11-21. Tear power. **A,** Plano power of tear film when the lens is fitted parallel to K. **B,** Plus power of the tear film when the lens is fitted steeper than K. The tear film is convex. **C,** Minus power of the tear film when the lens is fitted flatter than K. The tear film is concave in shape. The tear film has an optic density of 1.336, whereas polymethylmethacrylate has an optic density of 1.488.

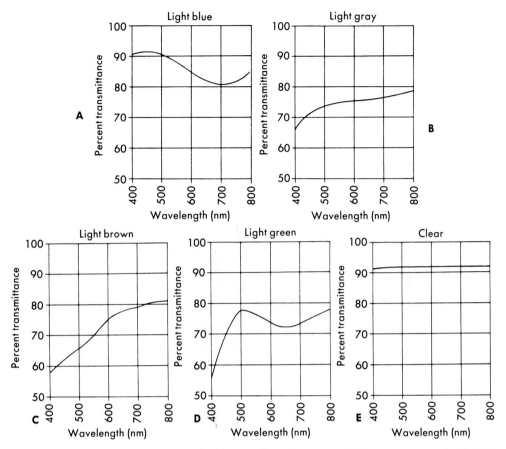

Fig. 11-22. Light transmittance. **A,** Light blue tint has the greatest light transmittance in the 500 nm area (91%) and the lowest in the 700 nm area (80%). The wavelength of maximum retinal sensitivity for the scotopic eye is between 500 and 510 nm and, for the photopic eye, around 550 nm. **B,** Light gray tint has less than 80% light transmittance anywhere on the spectrum. **C,** Light brown tint has only 65% transmittance in the 500 nm area. **D,** Light green tint has a maximum light transmittance of 75% in the 500 nm area. **E,** Clear lenses show slightly greater light transmittance than do blue-tinted lenses in the area of greatest retinal sensitivity. (Courtesy American Optical Corp., Southbridge, Mass.)

over-refraction is merely added to the power of the contact lens.

A power change of ±0.50 D can be made on an original contact lens. With a microthin lens no practical power change can be made.

Tint

The tint of a lens is used to assist the patient in finding a dropped lens or in retrieving a lens displaced on the sclera. Tinted lenses are not a substitute for sunglasses, regardless of the density of the tint. The cosmetic aspects are really slight because the diameter of most lenses is substantially smaller than the size of the visible iris. At times the color of a pale blue, gray, or green iris can be enriched with an appropri-

ately tinted lens, but a change of color, for example, from brown to blue, cannot be done.

A light blue tint is the most practical. Light blue transmits more light under scotopic and photopic conditions than does any other tint (Fig. 11-22). Activities such as night driving are much safer and more enjoyable for a lens patient with a light blue tint. Blue lenses are easy to locate when dropped on the floor.

One practical advantage to making all the lenses one color is that lost lenses can be replaced easier from an office that maintains a supply of lenses.

Comment. The tint of a lens should be the prerogative of the fitter, not the patient. The tint should be selected on the basis of maximum retinal sensitivity under photopic and scotopic conditions. Green and brown solid pigments used in the plastic have been generally avoided because they were unstable in the plastic. However this problem has been rectified in recent years, and pigments employed for these colors are now virtually as stable as for other colors.

Good fit

A good fit is one in which the lens is centered and moves well and the underlying cornea is free of edematous changes.

The following are sample typical lens specifications for the laboratory and fitting information.

Ideally the geometric center of the lens should coincide with the line of fixation. However, a minus lens often rides 1 or 2 mm higher, whereas a plus lens rides slightly lower. A lens should not touch the limbus (Fig. 11-23), a situation that commonly occurs during the act of reading. With reading the eyes are lowered and the lenses may be pushed up by the lower lid. If this occurs, the diameter of the lens should be reduced. However reducing the diameter may make the lens looser, and so a steeper base curve may be required.

The lens should be stable when the patient looks straight ahead and should move with blinking, first downward with lid closure and then up as the lid elevates. When the lids are fully open, the lens gently drops. At times the bottom of the lens rotates nasally with blinking. If the upper lid is held, a normal lens will drop 1 to 2 mm in smooth motion, whereas a loose lens will take a rapid fall, often to the lower lid.

With version movements a lens will lag 1 or 2 mm in all directions. If the lens decenters more than this, it is too loose and will be uncomfortable.

During the adaptation period the contact-cornea relationship may change because of corneal edema. Some steepening in the area of 0.50 D is common. However, if it exceeds 1.00 D, there is need to reevaluate the fit.

Typical lens specifications for laboratory (gray-tinted lenses)

	Lens thickness (mm)	Lens diameter (mm)	Lens power (D)	Base curve (mm)	Optic zone (mm)	Blend curve	Peripheral curve Radius (mm)	Width (mm)
Right	0.13	8.2	−3.50	7.5	6.0	Light	11.5	0.3
Left	0.13	8.2	−4.00	7.52	6.0	Light	11.5	0.3

Fitting information

	Right	Left	Comment
K readings			Central readings only; peripheral readings only if topogometer is used
Refraction in minus cylinders			
Palpebral aperture size			Note shape of apertures, as in Orientals
Corneal diameter			Visible iris measurement adequate
Pupil size			Small < 3 mm Medium 3 to 6 mm Large > 6 mm
Corneal sensitivity with Cochet-Bonnet esthesiometer			Of little value
Visual acuity			Near measurements must be done
Slitlamp assessment			Note: corneal scarring or vascularization; history of corneal erosion is important

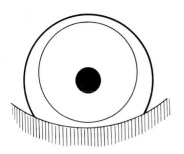

Fig. 11-23. Normal position of the lens lies 1 to 2 mm above the edge of the lower eyelid. (From Stein, H.A., and Slatt, B.J.: The ophthalmic assistant, ed. 4, St. Louis, 1983, The C.V. Mosby Co.)

The integrity of the cornea is best documented by slitlamp examination. The presence of central corneal clouding indicates that hypoxic changes are taking place because of either inadequacy of the tear pump or direct mechanical compression of the cornea.

TRIAL SET AND INVENTORY METHOD (Fig. 11-24)

A trial set system of fitting basically utilizes a lens as an instrument to detect a proper fit. A diagnostic lens will replace the front surface optics of a cornea and therefore can be em-

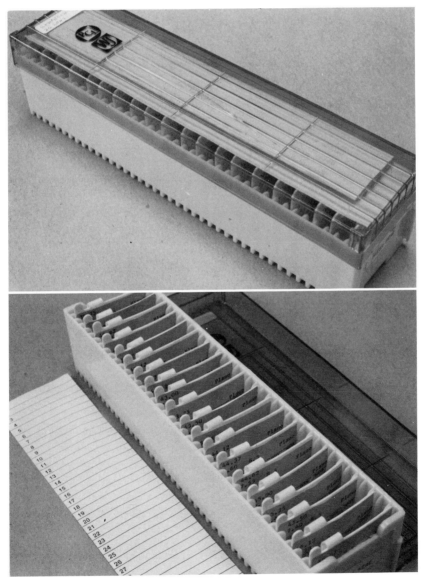

Fig. 11-24. Trial set. (Courtesy Plastic Contact Lens Co., Toronto, Canada.)

ployed to determine major and minor irregularities in the contour of the cornea. The procedure is not just trial and error. By observing the fitting characteristics of each lens one can judge the changes to give the best final fit. Many fitters deplore the connotations of the term "trial lens" and prefer the term "control lens" or "diagnostic lens."

Trial sets usually contain a small number of fitting lenses with a maximum of about 20. These sets can be stored either wet or dry. If wet storage is used, the solutions should be changed daily. An inventory system operates on a similar principle, but the precise lens can be tried and fitted at the time of examination. An inventory of lenses is basically a large trial set, and so both methods will be considered together.

Since any system is more or less dependent on the skill and experience of the fitter, the beauty of the inventory system is its absolute simplicity. It requires minimal sophistication in lens fitting because only one parameter is altered at a time and the changes can be made instantly. The base curve can be altered while the diameter is held constant, or the diameter can be varied while the base cuve remains constant.

Set

Most fitting sets contain 400 to 600 lenses with a power range between −1.00 and −7.00 D in 0.25 D steps. The base curve range is between 41.00 and 46.00 D in 0.25 D increments. The diameter choice, between 8.2 and 8.6 mm, is very limited (Table 11-4). The tints in the sets are restricted to a choice of blue or gray.

Fitting

The base curves are established by conventional keratometry. The diameter of the lens is selected by general principles, that is, small-diameter lenses are chosen for a small cornea with a base curve over 44.00 D.

A lens is selected that is the same as or slightly steeper than the K reading and placed on the eye. After the initial reaction to the lens has subsided, the fitter can assess the final visual acuity, the centration, the fluorescein pattern, and the movement of the lens without delay. If the lens is too loose, a steeper base

curve is selected. If the visual acuity is not up to par, an over-refraction is done and the power is adjusted.

There is nothing else to alter. Thickness, edge, peripheral curves, and optic zones are standardized.

Practical benefits

Seventy percent of rigid lens candidates can be fitted with a standard set of lenses. Modifications are unnecessary because the lens is simply replaced instead of modified. These lenses are usually of high quality because of the rigid specifications that lend themselves to quality mass production. A custom-designed lens requires more expertise; therefore it is more subject to error.

A fitting set eliminates an enormous amount of paperwork. No longer are ordering, notifying patients of arrival of lenses, sending major adjustments out, and ordering and billing for replacement lenses necessary. When a lens is used, reordering is done by a simple return of the lens case to the laboratory for replacement.

The cost of an inventory lens is less than that of a custom lens.

Patients can be refitted with a temporary lens without a period of being deprived of their lenses. This aspect of an inventory is very important for patients with high refractive errors who simply cannot function with a spectacle correction.

Finally a patient may be trial fitted with lenses that are precise for his or her eyes without anyone making a financial commitment to those lenses. Some fitters would regard this point as a drawback, considering a financial commitment to a set of lenses an aid to motivation.

Drawbacks

The blessing of cheaper lenses is offset by the cost of an expensive inventory. Unless there is a reasonable turnover of lenses the inventory can become a "white elephant." Also the set can become obsolete with new developments. Imagine owning a large inventory of scleral lenses or several hundred of the prototype soft lenses. The present generation of rigid lenses is now being eclipsed with newer, oxygen-permeable lenses.

Custom-designed lenses are still required for

Table 11-4. Master Control Method fitting chart

Flatter corneal curve	Lens diameter (mm)	Diopters of corneal toricity				
		0-0.50	0.75-1.25	1.50-2.00	2.25-2.75	3.00-3.75
41.00	8.2	*	*	*	*	*
	8.7	41.00	41.50	41.75	42.00	42.25
41.25	8.2	41.50	42.00	42.25	42.50	42.75
	8.7	41.25	41.75	42.00	42.25	42.50
41.50	8.2	41.75	42.25	42.50	42.75	43.00
	8.7	41.50	42.00	42.25	42.50	42.75
41.75	8.2	42.00	42.50	42.75	43.00	43.25
	8.7	41.75	42.25	42.50	42.75	43.00
42.00	8.2	42.25	42.75	43.00	43.25	43.50
	8.7	42.00	42.50	42.75	43.00	43.25
42.25	8.2	42.50	43.00	43.25	43.50	43.75
	8.7	42.25	42.75	43.00	43.25	43.50
42.50	8.2	42.75	43.25	43.50	43.75	44.00
	8.7	42.50	43.00	43.25	43.50	43.75
42.75	8.2	43.00	43.50	43.75	44.00	44.25
	8.7	42.75	43.25	43.50	43.75	44.00
43.00	8.2	43.25	43.75	44.00	44.25	44.50
	8.7	43.00	43.50	43.75	44.00	44.25
43.25	8.2	43.50	44.00	44.25	44.50	44.75
	8.7	43.25	43.75	44.00	44.25	44.50
43.50	8.2	43.75	44.25	44.50	44.75	45.00
	8.7	43.50	44.00	44.25	44.50	44.75
43.75	8.2	44.00	44.50	44.75	45.00	45.25
	8.7	43.75	44.25	44.50	44.75	45.00
44.00	8.2	44.25	44.75	45.00	45.25	45.50
	8.7	44.00	44.50	44.75	45.00	45.25
44.25	8.2	44.50	45.00	45.25	45.50	45.75
	8.7	44.25	44.75	45.00	45.25	45.50
44.50	8.2	44.75	45.25	45.50	45.75	46.00
	8.7	44.50	45.00	45.25	45.50	45.75
44.75	8.2	45.00	45.50	45.75	46.00	46.25
	8.7	44.75	45.25	45.50	45.75	46.00
45.00	8.2	45.00	45.50	45.75	46.00	46.25
	8.7	44.75	45.25	45.50	45.75	46.00
45.25	8.2	45.25	45.75	46.00	46.25	46.50
	8.7	45.00	45.50	45.75	46.00	46.25
45.50	8.2	45.50	46.00	46.25	46.50	46.75
	8.7	45.25	45.75	46.00	46.25	46.50
45.75	8.2	45.75	46.25	46.50	46.75	47.00
	8.7	45.50	46.00	46.25	46.50	46.75
46.00	8.2	46.00	46.50	46.75	47.00	*
	8.7	45.75	46.25	46.50	46.75	*
46.25	8.2	46.25	46.75	47.00	*	*
	8.7	46.00	46.50	46.75	*	*
46.50	8.2	46.50	46.75	47.00	*	*
	8.7	46.25	46.75	*	*	*
46.75	8.2	46.75	47.00	47.25	*	*
	8.7	46.50	*	*	*	*

Courtesy American Optical Corp., Southbridge, Mass.
*This diameter lens not recommended.

special cases. This includes those patients with high refractive errors, residual astigmatism, keratoconus, and presbyopia, as well as those who require a toric fit.

Comment. For the busy practitioner an inventory of lenses can certainly streamline a practice. It is an efficient, fast system that reduces paperwork and the fitter's dependency on the laboratory. The lenses are of high quality and can be applied to a majority of conventional cases. For the occasional fitter a diagnostic set of lenses makes more sense.

The weakness of inventory is the commitment to use that inventory. One in effect marries a given laboratory.

The link to a laboratory may be attractive in a stable environment, but consider the recent technologic changes. There are new generations of plastics, such as silicone, elastomers and polymers, newly fabricated cellulose acetate butyrate (CAB), and various mixtures of plastics that combine PMMA, CAB, and silicone.

The designs of lenses are changing. Large-diameter lens are in because of permeability, stability, and centration.

Soft lenses have been changed. They have become hydrated and thinned to unbelievable levels to make them oxygen permeable. These are now commercially available as a toric lens, a bifocal lens, and as an extended wear lens.

There is talk of a disposable lens.

Do you really want to commit yourself to a large number of lenses that cannot be turned over rapidly? Unless your practice is a high-volume one, a better suggestion is a trial set or diagnostic fitting set.

DIFFICULT CASES TO FIT
Spheric corneas

A lens fitted to a spheric cornea may tend to slide off the cornea or create tight symptoms. An element of corneal toricity is desirable so that the lens is centered. In such cases it is advisable to make the diameter 1 mm larger than normal or large enough so that the lens slips under the upper lid.

Exophthalmic eye

A soft lens is preferable because it offers protection to the cornea and stability of position and does not offend the blinking lid with a hard edge.

Flat corneas (41.00 D or less)

Large, flat corneas provide a poor base for the lens to rest on. The lens tends to slide off, become decentered, or even pop out of the eye. A large-diameter lens is indicated here.

High refractive errors

They cause thick centers or thick edges, depending on whether the refractive error is high hyperopia or high myopia. Thicker lenses are heavier, harder to center, and more likely to cause corneal hypopia and compression.

Comment

Most of the difficulties with rigid PMMA lenses relate to corneal edema, lens centration, and lens stability on the moving eye. A gas-permeable lens of large diameter usually will remedy most of these complications.

INSERTION AND REMOVAL TECHNIQUES

Insertion by practitioner
Removal by practitioner
Insertion by patient
Removal by patient
Recentering a displaced lens
Wearing schedule

Basically the novice lens wearer worries more about the handling of a lens than any other consideration. It seems implausible that a large foreign body can sit comfortably on a naked eye. Normally when anything is brought before an eye, the head recoils, the eye looks away, and the lids close. Because these natural reactions must be suppressed when a lens is brought to the cornea, the patient is suspicious and fearful. There is the nagging fear that the determination and discipline will not be there and that the entire exercise will be a failure. There is also the worry that an unnatural marriage is taking place and that as a result a great deal of suffering will ensue.

The fitter must be gentle and reassuring at all times. The patient should be told what to expect so as to avoid the shock of any unpleasant feelings. The lens should be placed upon the cornea by the fitter initially. A smooth performance can only increase the confidence of an apprehensive patient. In a short time repressed fears are destroyed, for a lens can be tolerated by the cornea, which under usual circumstances will violently reject a cinder or any other tiny foreign body. The insertion and removal techniques are the same for the PMMA lenses and gas-permeable lenses. However, there are a few differences to bear in mind.

The *silicone elastomers*, that is, the Boston Lens material, are quite fragile and will split at the edges if handled roughly.

Microthin PMMA lenses are usually fit on K or on the tight side of K. These lenses are more difficult to eject from the eyes with conventional techniques. It may be neces-

sary to add a drop of artificial tears to loosen the lenses.

CAB (cellulose acetate butyrate) lenses may warp with time. The dimensional stability of these lenses is not so good as that of PMMA. They have to be handled with greater care.

Pure silicone lenses can become very tight and difficult to remove, that is, produce the sucked-on lens syndrome. The patient should be forewarned and taught emergency techniques for lens removal—eyecup, or dunking the head in a basin of water.

Aphakic lenses are difficult to remove. The manual dexterity of an elderly person may not be sufficient to remove a lens consistently. Also the lids may be lax, and so indirect techniques using the lids are hard to apply. It is important to teach a spouse, relative, or friend to remove the lens should the aphakic person become unable to do so and become agitated in the process.

Children's lenses. Children should be taught to insert and remove their lenses as soon as possible. Dependency in lens handling is not advisable.

Lenses that pop out. If the lens pops out spontaneously or springs forth with a small flick of the lid, it is too loose or too thick at the edges. *Removal should be controlled.* The lenses should not be ejected onto a basin or floor. They become contaminated and scratched that way.

Before the end of a lesson in insertion and removal, the patient should have a set of written or typed instructions regarding what to do if lenses cannot be removed. A few instructions may defuse a potential emergency. For example, a small pamphlet, outlining emergency procedures is helpful.

"What to do if you cannot get your lens out of your eye"

1. Add a few drops of tears, saline solution, Comfort drops, or anything that will loosen the lens from the eye.
2. Use an eyecup to wash out the lens.
3. Place the head in a basin of water with the drain closed and blink forcefully once or twice.
4. Add a touch of honey to your finger and once or twice touch it to the lens. This is useful for any rigid lens.
5. Have a friend or relative use a small rubber suction cup to remove the lens. If you have this rubber lens remover, do not apply it yourself.
6. Do not be afraid if the lens is on the white of the eye. It can stay on the white coat (the sclera) without being lost behind the eye or causing ocular damage.
7. Do not work excessively to get the lens out. You may cause a corneal abrasion or ulcer. If the techniques to remove the lens fail after one or two passes, call the doctor, the technician, or the emergency department of the hospital.
8. Do not sleep with the lens unless you have been told to do so.
9. Do not put any medication in the eye except the fluids to loosen the lens.

10. Do not panic. There is little likelihood you will do permanent damage to your eye no matter what happens.

INSERTION BY PRACTITIONER (Fig. 12-1)

Insertion by the practitioner should be done first to help patients dispel their fears. If this is done smoothly, patients not only experience a sense of relief and accomplishment but also develop more confidence in the ability of the fitter.

1. Have the person look down and cast his or her gaze away from the approaching lens.
2. Retract the upper lid, place the lens above or beside the cornea, and shift it centrally.
3. Let the lens remain in the eye for about 20 minutes. It is important to forewarn the person that the eye may feel irritated, be sensitive to light, and tear after the lens has been inserted. You may reduce some of this early unpleasant foreign-body sensation by asking the patient to keep his or her head up and gaze downward. It is the impact of the upper lid with the margin of the lens that leads to much of the irritation.

Some authorities will use a topical anesthetic when a trial lens is first employed to reduce reflex tearing. It enables a better assessment of the lens-cornea relationship, since a pool of tears can distort the secondary refraction over the lens and interfere with the normal movement of the lens. The major fault of this ap-

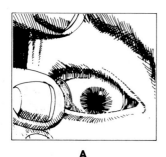 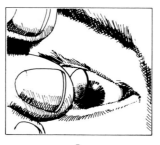 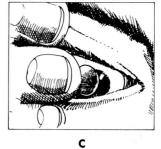

A   B   C

Fig. 12-1. Insertion by the fitter. **A,** The lens is placed on the index finger. **B,** The approach is to the side or above avoiding the line of fixation. The upper lid is retracted up and laterally. **C,** Once the lens is applied, the upper lid is used to center the lens.

proach is that it accustoms the patient to a false sense of comfort.

If topical anesthetics are used, they should be used only once, preferably under special circumstances, as with children, excessively nervous people, or people who tear excessively upon attempted insertion of a lens.

Helpful hints on insertion

1. The fitter should attempt to place the lens on the eye of a novice patient without blocking the line of sight. This avoids the menace response of the blink reflex.
2. The apprehensive patient should be asked to open the mouth during initial lens insertion. Forced closure of the lids is very difficult to do with the mouth open.
3. The patient should be given something to look at. Controlled fixation invariably makes insertion easy. Both eyes should be kept open.
4. Retraction of the upper lid should be gentle. A forceful maneuver invites a strong lid-closure response.

REMOVAL BY PRACTITIONER (Fig. 12-2)

Removal of the lens is easier for the practitioner, and the following method should be used:

1. Squeeze the lens off by the thumbs of each hand by applying pressure on the upper or lower lids, respectively.
2. Alternatively apply the fingers of one hand to the outer canthal region, resting on the upper and lower lids. The patient's eyes should be kept wide open so that the lid margin can engage the lens. A voluntary blink coupled with a lateral jerk of the lids to increase the lid tension is usually sufficient to dislodge the lens.

INSERTION BY PATIENT (Fig. 12-3)

There are two natural motions that the novice must overcome—a desire to look away and a desire to close the eyes as the lens is brought near. One can control the blink response by placing the free hand near the margin of the lid and retracting it. The position of the eye can be controlled by fixation. A mirror is most

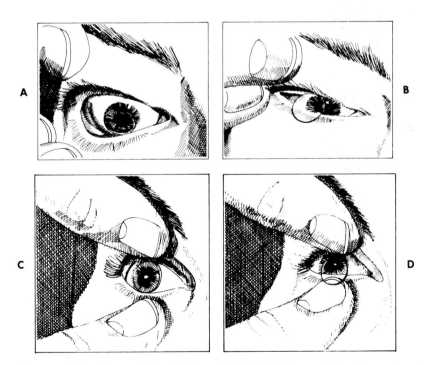

Fig. 12-2. Two methods of removal by the fitter: (1) **A,** The lids are held wide apart and pulled laterally. **B,** The lid margin catches the upper and lower edges of the lens and displaces it. A scissors movement by the lids ejects the lens. (2) **C,** The thumbs of both hands are placed on the upper and lower lids, respectively. **D,** The lids are brought together, squeezing the lens off the eye.

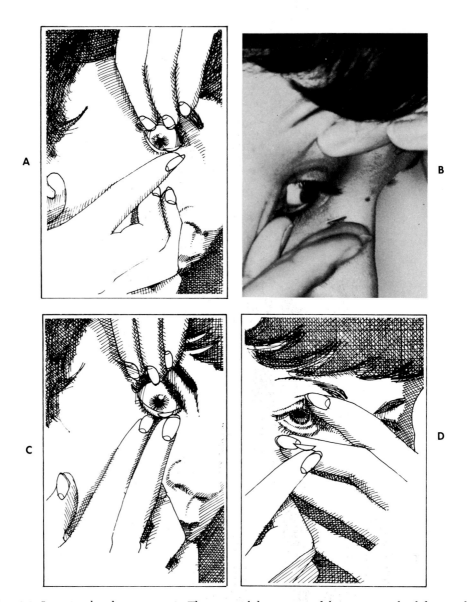

Fig. 12-3. Insertion by the patient. **A,** The upper lid is retracted by grasping the lid near the margin and retracting it. The left hand is used to elevate the right upper lid. The patient's gaze is directed downward, and the lens is carried to the eye by the index finger of the right hand. **B,** Incorrect method—the upper lid should be grasped near the lid margin, and the lens should rest on the tip of the finger. **C,** For the unsteady or tremulous patient, the middle finger carrying the lens rests on the index finger. **D,** The lids are separated by the index finger retracting the upper lid and the middle finger depressing the lower lid. The index finger of the free hand brings the lens to the eye. **E,** The lids are separated laterally between the index and middle fingers while the hand opposite the eye carries the lens. **F,** Use of a mirror for insertion of a lens.

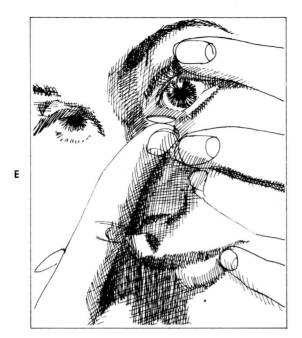 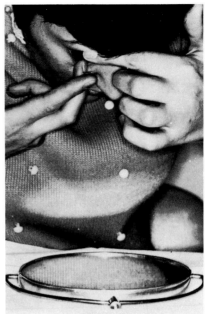

Fig. 12-3, cont'd. For legend see opposite page.

helpful so that the patient can watch his or her own eye.

1. Depress the lower lid by the middle finger while the index finger carrying the lens is gently applied to the cornea.
2. Slowly release the lids to avoid accidental ejection of the lens. Release the lower lid first and then the upper.

Alternate approaches

1. Retract the lids with the fingers of one hand, the index finger retracting the upper lid, the middle finger depressing the lower lid. Carry the lens on the index finger of the other hand.
2. For the nervous patient the lens-carrying finger is the middle one. It is supported by the fourth finger, upon which it rests as the lens is carried toward the cornea.

Helpful hints on insertion

1. Most lenses are lost or damaged in the first few months because of clumsy handling techniques. The novice should be extra careful with the lenses during this period. Drains should be closed before the lenses are rinsed with water. A good lens case should have a rinsing chamber so that the risk of accidental loss can be eliminated. A dropped lens should not be grasped directly between the thumb and forefinger; instead the finger should be moistened and the lens lifted. Insertion and removal should initially be done over a desk covered by a white towel so that the lens is easy to find if it falls and so that it can be cushioned by impact.
2. Suction-cup devices may be employed by an assistant in dealing with children or the elderly. They should not be given to a new lens patient. If the lens happens to be decentered upon removal, a suction cup may take off the corneal epithelium.
3. The patient should be told to be gentle and that the lens will adhere to the eye if brought close enough. Some patients will try to ram the lens on the cornea and will abrade it.

REMOVAL BY PATIENT (Fig. 12-4)

Removal of the lens may cause more apprehension than insertion does. Failure to insert a lens results in frustration. Failure to remove a lens creates a problem that can result in panic. Fear that the lens cannot be removed makes the exercise more difficult, and a vicious cycle can result. Furthermore, with the use of mi-

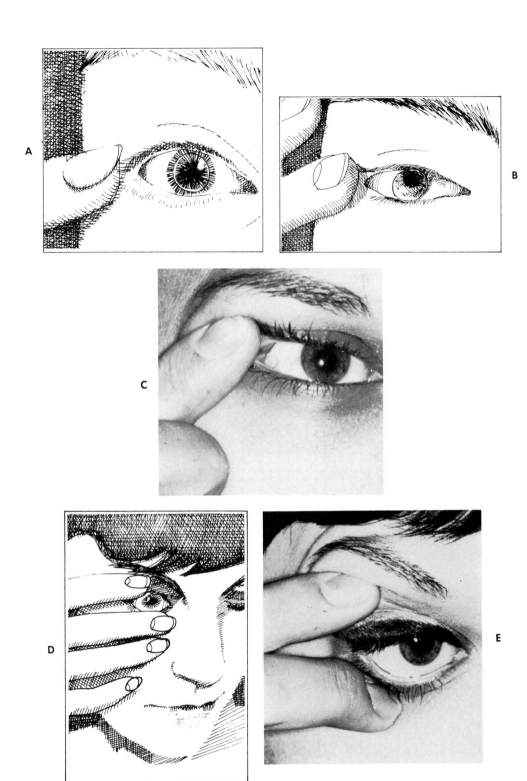

Fig. 12-4. Removal by the patient. **A** through **C,** The index finger tugs at the lateral canthus in an outward and upward direction. If the lids are held widely open, the edge of the lid margin should engage the lens and dislodge it. **D** and **E,** The open-handed scissors method. The lids are opened widely and the index and middle fingers are applied to the upper and lower lids to squeeze the lens off the eye. **F** and **G,** The two-handed scissors method. **H** and **I,** The use of a suction cup is best delegated to an assistant to avoid inadvertent application of the cup to the cornea.

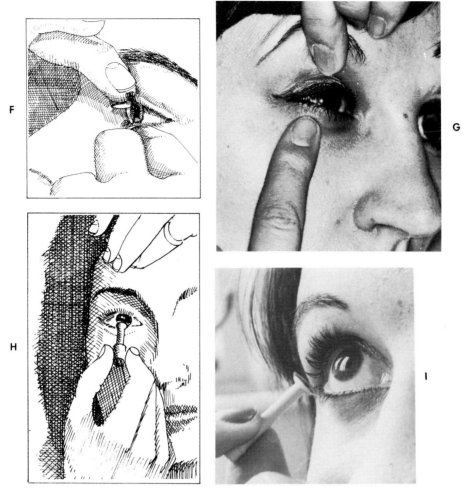

Fig. 12-4, cont'd. For legend see opposite page.

crothin lenses, removal of a lens is even more difficult without a thick edge for the lid to dislodge.

The simplest method is the following:

1. Look downward, open the lids wide so that the edge of the lid will engage the edge of the lens, draw the lid tight by a lateral pull of the index finger, and blink. The lid should dislodge the lens.
2. Cup the other hand under the eye to catch the lens.

Alternate approaches

One-handed method. Draw the upper lid up and out with the thumb while the same hand is cupped under the eye to catch the lens.

Scissors technique. Hold the upper lid by the index finger and the lower by the middle finger, apply lateral traction to the lids, and squeeze the lens off by a scissors motion.

RECENTERING A DISPLACED LENS
(Figs. 12-5 and 12-6)

The displaced lens must first be located. A lens that is decentered inferiorly, temporally, or nasally is usually easily seen. If the lens is displaced upward, assistance is often needed to find the lens in the superior cul-de-sac. The eye must be rotated downward and the lid retracted; under good illumination the lens can easily be located.

The following approaches may be successfully employed to replace the lens onto the surface of the cornea:

1. Manipulate the lens by the fingers through the closed lid until it is centered.

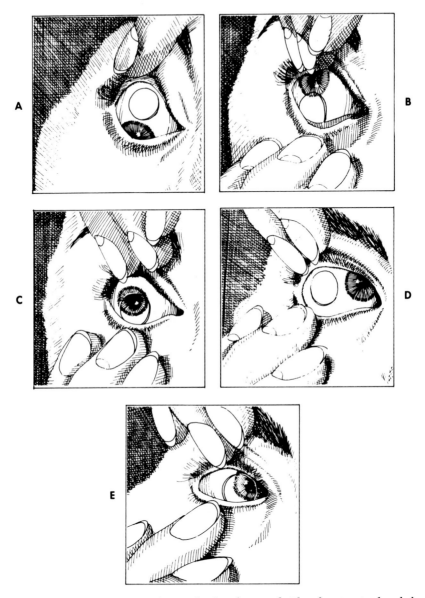

Fig. 12-5. Recentering a lens. **A,** The lens is displaced upward. The chin is raised and the eye is lowered while the edge of the upper lid is used to engage the lens and push it down. **B,** The lens is displaced downward. The eye is raised and the lower lid is depressed with the index finger. **C,** Through the lid, the lens is pushed up by an upward movement of the finger. At the same time, the eye is lowered. **D,** The lens is displaced laterally. The eye is moved medially while the index and middle fingers of each hand push the lens centrally. **E,** With the fingers exerting pressure through the lid, the eye is then rotated under the lens.

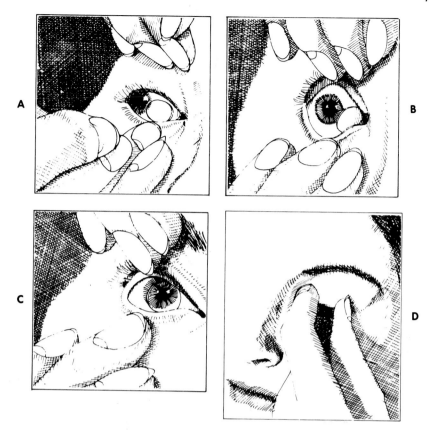

Fig. 12-6. The lens is displaced medially. The eye is rotated laterally. **A,** While the fingers are used to secure the lens, the lids are opened and the eye is rotated medially, **B. C,** The eye rotates under the fixed lens. **D,** The lens can frequently be palpated through the closed lid and moved centrally. While it is held there, the eye is rotated under it.

2. Move the eyes in a direction opposite to the position of the lens. The lens is centered by manipulation and held there; then the eye is rotated centrally, sliding under the held lens.
3. Push the lens into position by using the upper and lower lid margins. This method applies only to superiorly and inferiorly displaced lenses.
4. Pinion the lens by the index fingers of both hands by pressure through the closed lids and rotate the eye slowly and deliberately toward the lens until it moves under it.

Lost lenses

There have been reports of lost lenses found in the upper fornix and even embedded in the conjunctival tissue above the tarsus. A complete search includes eversion of the lids. At times the lost lens may become glued to its mate.

Helpful hints on recentering

1. The patient should manipulate the lens gently through the lids. If too much pressure is applied, the lens becomes more adherent to the conjunctiva and is almost impossible to dislodge. If such a contingency occurs, the patient is best advised to use a suction cup or to put some eye drops into the eye to relieve the suction effect of the lens upon the eye.
2. The lens must climb the limbal ridge to mount the cornea. If pushing movements are forceful, the edge of the lens can get caught on the limbus and cause irritation to the eye and corneal abrasions.
3. At times a practitioner will have difficulty in finding the lens. The most common hiding

place is the superior cul-de-sac. In this case the upper lid should be everted. Fluorescein stain will accent the presence of a lost lens.

FACTORS AFFECTING WEARING SCHEDULE

The rapid adaptation to the presence of a rigid lens depends on several factors:

1. Gas permeability. A gas-permeable lens will benefit the cornea because it reduces the shock of sudden corneal hypoxia. Also the lens has a large diameter and is slightly high riding. In ideal cases, the upper edge of the lens will be under the upper lid, a position thus eliminating lid impact, which is a major source of discomfort.

2. Edge treatment. If the edges are beveled on their anterior aspect especially for refractive errors greater than 4 diopters, an accelerated schedule may be tolerated, that is, a myopic contour on the periphery of an aphakic lens.

3. Good tear presence, which means a good aqueous tear flow, an intact mucin layer, and an anterior sebaceous film to prevent dehydration. Dry eyes or corneas with a short tear-film breakup time requires a longer period of adaptation and shortens the tolerance to full-time wear.

4. A normal blink response. If the patient blinks infrequently or incompletely without lenses, he or she will suffer a long time with the introduction of any kind of lens. The lens will drop to a low position and generally behave as though the lens fit were tight.

5. Favorable anatomic lid position. If the upper lids are retracted above the superior limbus or the lower lids are high, skirting the lower limbus, then lens displacement by the lids will be inevitable and the discomfort factor greater.

6. Tight lids as found with many Oriental lid configurations with strong lid adherence may make a good fit intolerable. The lens will be excessively raised by the action of the lids.

7. Large heavy lenses. Large heavy lenses are more likely to cause corneal edema and lid irritation. If the lenses are not permeable to oxygen, one must proceed very slowly. These lenses tend to ride low, do not rise adequately with a blink, and cause excessive 3 and 9 o'clock staining.

8. An excessive response to a lens. Some patients, especially fair-skinned people immediately tear, develop puffy lids, and complain immediately of pronounced photophobia. These persons are usually identified in the process of a trial fitting. These persons may become very apprehensive and show many compensatory reactions to the negative reception of the lens. To reduce lens movement and lid sensation, the person may tilt the head backwards. They may not move the eyes for fear of losing a lens. Their eyes are literally frozen with fear. This discomfort may be accentuated when they look up, a position that makes the lens drop low and strike the lower lids. The patient reacts by squinting the lids close together because of fear of any vertical lens motion. These patients suffer too much with any rigid lens and frequently are better off with a soft lens.

9. Corneal edema. Signs of clinical corneal edema in the initial fitting lenses would indicate a slower schedule. Corneal edema may be manifest with the slitlamp through direct or indirect illumination or retroillumination. It may become apparent through staining of the cornea with fluorescein, which may show central corneal epithelial stippling. A change in K readings, a change in pachometry, or an alteration of the quality of Placido's disc may indicate excessive corneal edema. If clinical corneal edema is clinically evident, the initial wearing schedule must be slowed.

10. The size of the refractive error may be important. With high hyperopes such as aphakic persons, the lenses are three times thicker in the center than that of a myope's lens.

A thick lens may negate the permeability features of lenses, drop low because of gravity, fail to ride up with blinking, and be more prone to cause corneal edema through hypoxia or compression.

The secret to large heavy lenses of high refractive errors is the treatment of the edges. If the edges are not thinned out, they will be bulky, engage the upper lid with blinking, and create considerable discomfort.

A high myope has his own problems except that the added thickness to the lens is at the edges. These lenses are frequently high riding, uncomfortable because of thickened edges, and more prone to cause peripheral corneal erosions. The wearing schedule should be simple and easy to remember. One schedule is to have persons wear their lenses 1 hour every morning, afternoon, and evening on the first day. On each subsequent day 1 hour is added to the schedule three times a day, so that by the third day the lenses are being worn 9 hours a day. The patient is seen on the fourth day after the lenses have been worn 8 hours. By the fifth day the breaks in lens wear can be obliterated. The lenses are first worn through the lunch break and then finally through the afternoon to the evening, so that by the seventh day the lenses are worn full time.

The wearing schedule is highly variable and should fit into the office pattern of the practitioner. Another approach is as follows:

Contact lens wearing schedule

First and second day	2 hours in, 1 hour out
Third and fourth day	3 hours in, 2 hours out
Fifth and sixth day	4 hours in, 2 hours out
Seventh and eighth day	5 hours in, 2 hours out
and so on	

Patients are reassessed at the end of 2 weeks for reinforcement sessions on handling of the lenses, office modifications if there are signs of poor fit, and appraisal of the corneal epithelium. Changes in the cornea should not be tolerated. These include staining of the cornea, corneal edema as viewed through retroillumination or specular reflection, changes in the K readings of 0.60 D or greater, or 0.50 D of spectacle blur.

The wearing schedule must be adjusted to the person's needs. If all systems are favorable, the patient may adapt in a week to the presence of a rigid lens. If there are clinical problems, a month may elapse before full-time wear is established.

Comment. With gas-permeable lenses, liberty can be taken in accelerating the adaptation cycle. Frequently we can "adapt" an eye in 4 or 5 days.

Some people can adapt to a rigid lens in a day. However, these people are impossible to define, and so it is risky to use this type of speedy schedule. For those fitters who wish to attempt this kind of fast fit, it is prudent to keep the patient in the office for the first day and check for corneal edema on the first, fourth, and eighth hour of wear. If there is no corneal edema, full-time wear can be attempted.

Basically we advocate a slower schedule because it reduces the chances of sudden hypoxic symptoms. In the beginning it is not wise to accentuate your patient's fears and anxieties about wearing lenses.

Patients who miss 2 or more days of wearing time should revert to their original wearing schedule. If only 1 day is missed, rest periods of 1 hour each at noon and at 6:00 PM are helpful to avoid an overwear reaction. One rest perid can be gradually collapsed after 2 days, and the other can be eliminated in 4 days.

When returning home, the patient should be instructed not to persevere with unsuccessful insertions or removals if the eye becomes red and painful. After the initial visit the patient should be seen in 1, 2, and 4 weeks.

Comment. Young teen-agers frequently have to be restrained when they first obtain lenses. They are anxious to demonstrate their new lenses and frequently will overwear them while attending a party or social function.

Some fitters advocate continuous wear of lenses during sleep. Although this is possible, especially for short naps and while one is wearing microthin lenses, the practice should be deplored. A little risk is too much. Even the device of pushing the lenses onto the sclera for sleep is not recommended. The lenses often become centered on the cornea again or develop such a heavy coating of mucus secretions that they must be removed for cleaning.

Liberties, such as short naps, can easily be taken with gas-permeable lenses. If the patient is not careful and wears gas-permeable lenses too long, too fast, corneal edema may occur, but not with the acute painful episode that characterizes PMMA overwear or more precisely acute hypoxic reaction.

CHAPTER 13

OFFICE MODIFICATION OF RIGID LENSES

Penny Cook*
Keith W. Harrison‡

Polishing compounds
Blending transition or junction zones
Reducing optic-zone diameter
Reducing overall lens diameter
Flattening intermediate curves
Adding minus power
Adding plus power
Removing scratches
Polishing and refinishing lens edges
Adjusting peripheral curves
Flattening the base curve
Identifying the lens
Fenestrating the lens

Some practitioners' disillusionment with soft lenses combined with the advent of new and better rigid lens materials has given cause for the "dusting off" of many a modification unit. Certainly oxygen-permeable materials and improved lens designs give sophistication in fitting, which lessens the need for modifications. However they may be necessary in some cases, and when this is so, a faster and better service can be given to the patient by having modification equipment available in the office.

An added advantage of in-office alteration is that the patient's wearing schedule is not disrupted. Rigid lenses should be worn for a consistent number of hours daily, and if such minor adjustments cannot be done in the office, the wearing schedule will be seriously affected. The patient may be willing to put up with such disruptions initially, but any repetitions that prolong this may culminate in a dissatisfied patient and some irritation with the fitter.

There are many types of modification units available ranging from the sophisticated and rather expensive to the simple and moderately priced. The simplest unit is recommended for the average lens office; if necessary more elaborate equipment can be added as the need arises (Fig. 13-1).

*Penny Cook, M.O.C.L.A. (Optician, Certified Contact Lens Fitter), Toronto, Canada.
‡Keith W. Harrison, M.O.C.L.A., Lecturer and Instructor, Contact Lens Certification Program, Seneca College of Applied Arts and Technology, Willowdale, Ontario.

The following is a list of in-office adjustments that can be made to rigid and rigid gas-permeable lenses.

1. Blending transition or junction zones
2. Reducing optic-zone diameter
3. Reducing overall lens diameter
4. Flattening intermediate curves
5. Adding minus power
6. Adding plus power
7. Removing scratches
8. Polishing and refinishing lens edges
9. Adjusting peripheral curves
10. Identifying the lens
11. Fenestrating the lens
12. Flattening the base curve

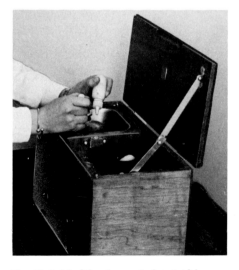

Fig. 13-1. Modification unit for rigid lenses.

All the adjustments that can be made to a lens will have the effect of loosening the fit or increasing tear flow between the lens and cornea. Any adjustments to tighten the fit of a lens necessitate the fabrication of a new lens.

POLISHING COMPOUNDS

Most polishing compounds used in lens modification are abrasive agents such as Silvo or Xpal mixed with oil or water. When one is working with gas-permeable materials, a fine compound such as Xpal is the most desirable. Silvo is coarser and lends itself to more scratching of the gas-permeable lenses. There are several commercially available polishing solutions for gas-permeable lenses. BPI of Miami, Florida, and Polymer Technology Corporation of Wilmington, Massachusetts, are two companies that market these solutions.

BLENDING TRANSITION OR JUNCTION ZONES

The junction zones between the central, intermediate, and peripheral posterior curves can be examined with an instrument called a "profile analyzer." If these junction zones are not smooth, they can interfere with the tear exchange under the lens, thus causing "tight-lens" symptoms. If the junction zones are extremely sharp, they may cause irritation in the same manner as a sharp lens edge (Fig. 13-2).

Fig. 13-2. A and **B,** Blending junction zones. **C,** Blending transition zones to eliminate sharpness of junction zones.

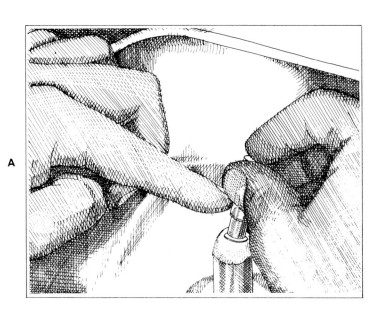

A

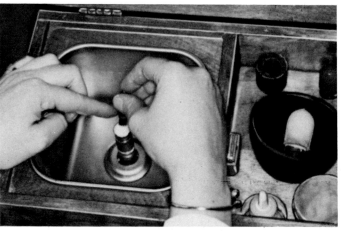

B

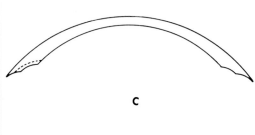

C

To blend the transition zones of a lens, a radius tool is used, the radius of curvature of which is halfway between either the central posterior curve (CPC) and the intermediate posterior curve (IPC) or the intermediate posterior curve and the peripheral posterior curve (PPC). The radius tool should be covered with a felt-surfaced polishing tape. This tape is usually 0.2 mm thick, and its thickness must be taken into consideration when the alteration is made. For example,

CPC	42.00 D or 8.04 mm
IPC	38.00 D or 8.88 mm
Halfway radius	40.00 D or 8.44 mm
Less allowance for tape	0.20 mm
Thus select tool	= 8.24 mm

Since tools are standardized and come in increments of 0.2 mm, ranging from 7.6 to 10.0 mm, an 8.2 mm tool should be used. The unit also has 11.0 and 12.0 mm tools.

Either the lens is held by a suction cup (convex side against the holder concave side against the tool), or it is mounted with double-sided adhesive tape on a small lens block. The lens block is supported against the rotating radius tool by a pencil or other pointed object inserted into a hole on the top of the lens block. This enables the lens to spin freely while the radius tool rotates. A polishing compound is used in blending to prevent scratching of the lens surface.

Blending a lens takes only a few minutes. Practice enables the fitter to estimate how long it will take to smooth out these transition zones.

Comment. Sometimes blending can make a fit tighter by bringing the lens closer to the cornea.

REDUCING OPTIC-ZONE DIAMETER

If blending a lens does not alleviate the problems of tight fit, the next modification would be to reduce the optic-zone diameter. The optic zone determines the stability of the lens, and the size and curvature of this zone determine how loose or tight the fit will be. This modification is similar to that of blending a lens. A tool is selected that has a radius of curvature halfway between that of the central posterior curve and the intermediate or peripheral posterior curve, allowing again 0.2 mm for the thickness of the tape. The length of time of

polishing will determine how much the optic zone needs to be reduced.

Another method of reducing the optic zone is to increase the width of the intermediate or peripheral curve. One does this by using a diamond-impregnated tool of the same radius as was used in the original grinding of the intermediate and peripheral zones with grinding maintained for a longer period. This type of tool should be soaked in water before use and should be kept moistened with water while the lens is being modified to avoid burn spots on the lens. Polishing compounds should not be used with this type of tool. After the diamond-impregnated tool is used, the surface of the lens will be quite rough, and so it must be polished with a regular tool covered with velveteen, with polishing compound being used.

REDUCING OVERALL LENS DIAMETER

The trend in fitting gas-permeable lenses is to use larger diameters than those with PMMA, as has been the practice. It is therefore important that a fitter be knowledgeable in the reduction of lens diameter. If blending, reduction of the optic zone, or flattening of the intermediate and peripheral curves does not solve the problem of a tight lens, reduction of the diameter may solve the problem. Again, with experience in lens fitting this may be the first modification done if the diameter of the lens appears too large. A good rule of thumb to follow in the reduction of diameter is, Reducing the overall diameter of a lens by 0.1 mm is the equivalent of blending the peripheral curves 0.2 mm. The diameter may be assessed on a V-groove diameter gauge (Fig. 13-3). There are several techniques available for reducing the diameter of a lens.

Razor-blade technique

The lens is centered and mounted on a spindle with double-sided adhesive tape, and the blade is contoured around the lens edge as the lens rotates. Accurate centering of the lens is of the utmost importance (Fig. 13-4). The blade must be kept wet or moist; otherwise the friction it creates will cause the lens to crack. After this the lens edge must be polished. Adjustments to the peripheral curves may then become necessary. Variations of this technique involve files or other grinding material (Fig. 13-5).

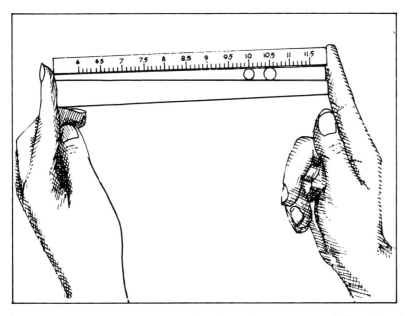

Fig. 13-3. Diameter gauge. The lens is inserted at the widest opening and allowed to slide to its position of rest.

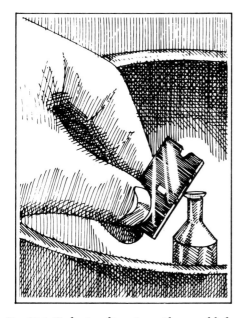

Fig. 13-4. Reducing diameter with razor blade.

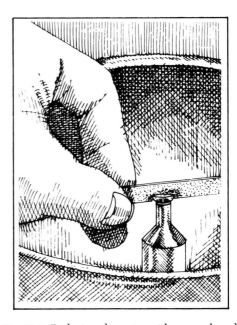

Fig. 13-5. Reducing diameter with emery board.

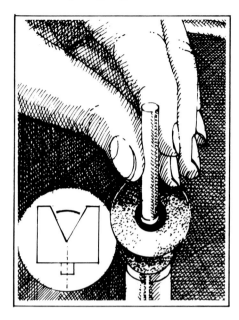

Fig. 13-6. Reducing diameter with conic stone.

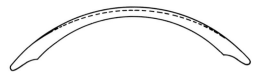

Fig. 13-7. Adding minus power.

Conic-stone technique

In this technique a diamond-impregnated 60- or 70-degree hollow stone is used. The lens is held convex side against the suction cup and gently rocked in the hollow tool (Fig. 13-6). Care must be taken to keep the tool wet during this procedure. Once the diameter of a lens is reduced, the peripheral and intermediate curves have to be reapplied and blended and the edge of the lens refinished. Therefore the diameter should be reduced to approximately 0.1 mm larger than the finished diameter. For example, a lens with a diameter of 9.5 mm that needs to be reduced to 9.0 mm should initially be reduced to 9.1 mm; the edge refinishing and polishing will yield a lens of 9.0 mm diameter.

Comment: Most laboratories work on a diameter tolerance of 0.1 mm.

FLATTENING INTERMEDIATE CURVES

The intermediate curve of a lens can be flattened when one blends the lens with a felt-covered tool of a flatter radius than the intermediate curve of the lens.

ADDING MINUS POWER

Up to −1.00 D can be added to a lens by use of a velveteen- or sponge-covered drum

tool (Fig. 13-7). The lens is held on a suction cup (concave side against the holder) away from the center of rotation of the drum tool. The lens is rotated a full 360 degrees against the rotation of the drum for one or two turns. The drum tool must be kept wet with polish during this procedure.

Another method of adding minus power is to use a velveteen cloth, which is placed on a thin foam backing. A 4- or 5-inch diameter circle of polish is put on the cloth. The lens is held against the cloth with the index finger, and the lens is rotated around the circle with the lens being kept free of any wobble. It should be rotated clockwise for three rotations and counterclockwise for three rotations, after which the power is inspected. Caution must be taken not to use excessive pressure because this will cause distortion in the optic figure.

ADDING PLUS POWER

Up to +1.00 D can be added to a lens. The procedure for adding plus power is similar to that for adding minus power, but the lens should be held slightly off the center of rotation of the drum tool and rotated so that the lens thickness is reduced more at the edge than at the center; thus the anterior curve is steepened.

REMOVING SCRATCHES

Scratches on the anterior surface of a lens will interfere with the wetting characteristics of the lens. In this age of gas-permeable rigid lenses, this can be an extensive problem. As a result of the "softness" of some of the gas-permeable materials and the difficulty in wetting them, the lenses may require regular polishing. The accumulation of mucus, oils, and fat lipids in the scratches causes poor wetting of the lens and thus foggy vision. In addition, there can be discomfort from the rough lens surface.

To remove scratches from the anterior surface of a lens, place the lens on a suction cup,

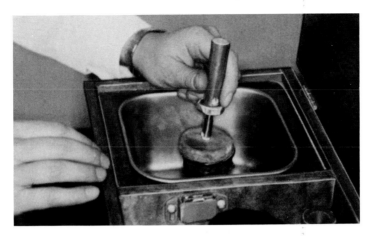

Fig. 13-8. Polishing lens on velveteen with Silvo polish to remove scratches.

concave side against the holder, and apply the front surface of the lens against a rotating felt-covered drum tool and gently buff and polish the front surface (Fig. 13-8).

To remove scratches from the posterior surface of a lens, a steep tool such as one with a 6.9 mm radius is used. The tool should be covered with a narrow strip of molefoam, approximately 1⅛ inches wide by 2 to 2½ inches long. The tool is wet with polish, and the concave side of the lens is placed on the tool using a suction cup while the tool spins. Scratches on the inside of a lens cannot easily be removed without causing changes in the curvature of the lens, which often necessitates replacement of the lens.

POLISHING AND REFINISHING LENS EDGES

There are several methods available to the fitter for polishing and refinishing lens edges, including the rag-wheel, felt-disc, and Con-Lish methods. Of these three, the one most often used is the felt-disc method because of its simplicity.

Rag-wheel method

The rag wheel is mounted on the spindle and the lens is held on a spinner. A suction cup or brass rod may be used, but one must take care to avoid burn spots by turning the tool by hand. Liberal use of a polishing compound is also recommended to reduce the incidence of surface burn caused by friction. The lens should be held against the rag wheel in three positions for equal time: (1) 45 degrees above horizontal, (2) horizontal, and (3) 45 degrees below horizontal.

Felt-disc method

A small, round disc covered with moleskin or velveteen is used in this method. The lens is fixed to a spinner with double-sided tape, and a polishing compound is used. The spinner is held at a 45-degree angle against the disc, midway between the center of rotation and the circumference of the disc. The lens should be gently pressed on the disc and moved toward the center while the angle is being simultaneously reduced to 10 degrees. This process is used for both sides of the lens and is an excellent method for in-office adjustments (Figs. 13-9 and 13-10).

Con-Lish method

Five separate tools are used in this method. Four tools have concave cones of different degrees—40, 60, 90, and 140—and the fifth tool is a flat tool. All the tools are lined with velveteen or moleskin, and the lens is held with double-sided adhesive tape on a rod or by a suction cup. The procedure is as follows:

1. Place lens convex side down on 60-degree tool for 10 seconds at 110 rpm.
2. Place lens convex side down on 40-degree tool for 5 seconds at 110 rpm.
3. Place lens concave side down on flat tool for 20 seconds at 110 rpm.
4. Place lens concave side down on 140-degree tool for 15 seconds at 110 rpm.

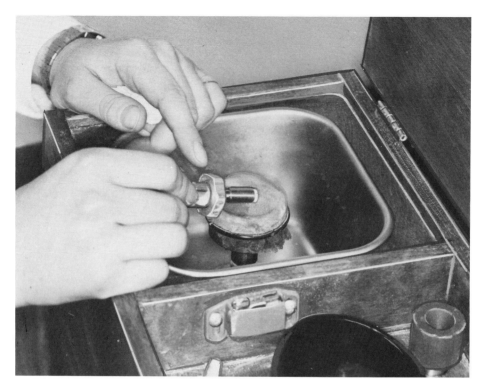

Fig. 13-9. Use of a felt disc in polishing edges of rigid lens.

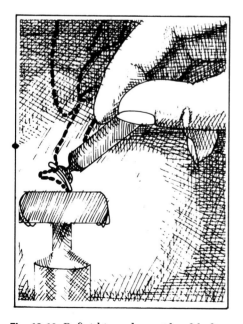

Fig. 13-10. Refinishing edges with a felt disc.

5. Place lens concave side down on 90-degree tool for 10 seconds at 110 rpm.
6. Place lens concave side down on 60-degree tool for 5 seconds at 110 rpm.
7. Place lens concave side down on 40-degree tool for 2 seconds at 110 rpm.

The advantage of this method is that is standardizes the lens edge shape and is therefore good for duplication. Another advantage is that it produces an edge with the outside shaped away from the eyelid and the inside shaped away from the cornea. This method is good for lenses with relatively thick edges.

ADJUSTING PERIPHERAL CURVES

Peripheral curves can be flattened, widened, or blended. The basic technique for flattening or widening the peripheral curves is to use a diamond-impregnated tool of the appropriate radius. The diamond tool should be soaked in water before use and kept wet during use. Silvo polish or other polishing compounds should not be used with such tools. The lens is held with a suction cup with its concave surface against the tool away from the center of rota-

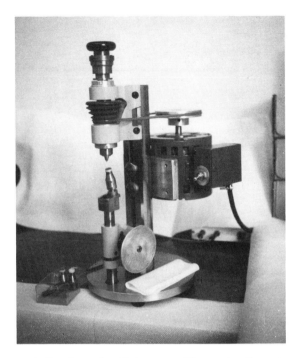

Fig. 13-11. Fenestration drill. There should be no visible cracks dispersing from the drill hole area because of stress caused by the drilling operation.

tion. The lens is rotated in a direction counter to the rotation of the tool. Once the desired peripheral curve is achieved, the lens should be polished with a felt-covered radius tool soaked with polishing solution.

FLATTENING THE BASE CURVE

Although infrequently done, flattening of the base curve of a lens can be done. The base curve of most rigid lenses can be flattened by about 0.50 diopter or 0.10 mm. The lens is with its convex side against the suction cup, and the concave side is placed against a tape-covered tool of the same radius of curvature as the lens. The lens is held directly on the center of the tool. Polishing solution should be added every 5 seconds to avoid burning and blurring of the optic figure. The base curve should be rechecked on the optic spherometer (Radiuscope) after every three of these 5-second applications on the tool.

The principle of this procedure is that the outer edge of the tool is rotating faster than the center and so a greater amount of material will be taken off at the periphery of the tool than at the center, resulting in a flatter lens.

IDENTIFYING THE LENS

If one specifies, most laboratories will put an identification mark on the right lens, such as a red dot, but again this can be done very simply by the fitter if the need arises. A toothpick shaved to produce a fine point or a similar thin-pointed object is dipped in lens identification ink, which is available from most lens manufacturers. After the toothpick is dipped into the ink, the tip should be touched to a piece of paper to remove any excess ink. The peripheral, convex surface of the lens should then be touched with the tip of the toothpick. After several minutes the lens should be rubbed with the fingers over the spot to remove any excess ink, and the lens should then be allowed to dry completely for 10 to 15 minutes before use.

Unfortunately ink or nail polish will wear off the lens with time. A small hole can be burred into the front surface of the lens with a dental burr or a small hand-held drill after which the hole is filled with nail polish. This type of identification never wears off; even though the nail polish may rub off, the red identification becomes a white dot because of the hole in the lens. This method is very good for office use. A small, inexpensive instrument may be purchased to burr the hole into the lens.

More elaborate instruments are available to mark "R" or any other letter on the lens.

FENESTRATING THE LENS

Putting a hole in a lens is not a way of allowing more oxygen to get to the cornea. Only 1 mm around the hole benefits from an added oxygen supply. Basically fenestration has the effect of loosening the fit of a lens. Holes can be applied to the center of a lens or at the outer periphery. Although this cannot be done with the modification unit, a small fenestration instrument can be purchased if necessary (Fig. 13-11). The fenestration unit contains drill bits, mounting arbor, dental wax to hold the lens in position, and a countersinking bit for removing burrs from the posterior surface of the lens. A fine oil is used to prepare the drill for cutting into the plastic lens without causing the heat to be absorbed by the lens itself. Fenestrating a lens affects the tear lens dynamics. The holes provide oxygen only in the area under the lens near the holes.

Comments. Although all the previously mentioned adjustments to lenses are possible, the ones most commonly done are blending transition zones, adding minus power, removing surface scratches, and dotting or redotting lenses for identification.

All modifications outlined in this chapter may be applied to any rigid lens that is not surface treated in some manner. Some helpful hints are as follows:

1. Use a fine polishing compound for all modifications to PMMA, CAB, and PMMA-silicone materials. When this is done, the same tools and pads may be used for adjusting any lens. Although the modification may take longer with the harder materials, it is not necessary for a total cleanup of the equipment after each adjustment.

2. Apply light pressure for short periods before checking the result. It is very easy to overadjust a lens.

3. Constantly add polishing solvent to avoid friction buildup, which will distort the lens.

Knowledge and expertise in making any of these adjustments increase the confidence of the fitter, which in turn is instilled in the patient.

Since many people lose at least one lens per year, it is advisable that a patient have a spare set of rigid lenses. This eliminates the problem of losing wearing time and the possible resulting overwear reaction that may occur if the patient tries to resume the same wearing schedule.

LENS SOLUTIONS FOR RIGID LENSES

WHAT IS WETTING?

A drop of liquid on a solid may behave in one of two ways. It may aggregate in droplets because of cohesion—the attraction of molecules in the liquid for each other—or it may spread over the surface of the solid because of adhesion—the attraction of molecules in the liquid to the molecules in the solid.

The relative values between the forces of adhesion and cohesion are expressed as the angle of contact—θ (theta) (Fig. 14-1). For water and glass, θ is 0 degrees, which is complete wetting of the solid by the liquid. Mercury on glass has a θ value greater than 90 degrees; it does not spread but gathers into spheric droplets. A hydrophilic solid has a contact angle of 0 degrees, since a liquid will spread over its surface. Polymethylmethacrylate is relatively hydrophobic; its contact angle with water is 60 degrees.

Wetting solution

A wetting solution serves to improve the wettability of the lens. This allows the tear film to uniformly spread over the surface of the lens rather than break up into droplets (Fig. 14-2). It also coats the lens and helps to prevent oils and debris from being transferred from the finger to the lens. During insertion it helps the lens adhere to the finger.

Tears will also wet polymethylmethacrylate, provided that the lens that is inserted into the eye is perfectly clean. There is a time lag, however, and the patient may experience discomfort until the tears coat the lens.

Saliva has been used by some patients as a wetting agent. Natural saliva is an excellent wetting agent because it contains a conjugated polysaccharide similar to that of the precorneal tear film. *Pseudomonas aeruginosa* is found as an indigenous oral flora in the saliva of 6.6% of the population. Besides this microbe, yeasts, fungi, protozoa, gram-positive and gram-negative cocci, and rods make up part of the host oral flora of saliva. Urine on the other hand is usually sterile. Neither is advocated, though the latter is the cleaner of the two.

Wetting solutions are composed of the following:

1. A preservative—benzalkonium chloride or thimerosal
2. A wetting agent—polyvinyl alcohol, poly-N-vinylpyrrolidone (PVP), or ethylenediaminetetraacetic acid (EDTA)

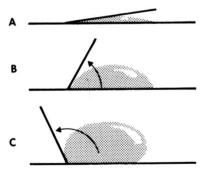

A

B

C

Fig. 14-1. The smaller the angle of contact (θ), the greater the spreading of a liquid over a solid. A rigid lens is hydrophobic and has a 60-degree angle of contact with water. **A,** Low-wetting angle; **B,** wetting angle of polymethylmethacrylate rigid lens; **C,** large wetting angle with droplet of mercury.

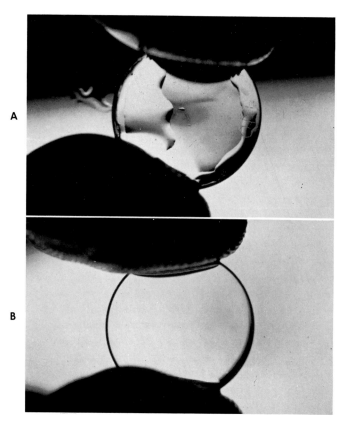

Fig. 14-2. A, Improperly cleaned and wetted lens. **B,** Lens properly wetted. (From Camp, R.N., Moore, C.D., and Soper, J.W.: Handling of the lens—insertion, removal, cleaning, and storage. In Girard, L.J., editor: Corneal contact lenses, St. Louis, 1970, The C.V. Mosby Co.)

3. A buffering system—the pH of the solution should be compatible with that of the precorneal film, 7.3 to 7.8
4. Methylcellulose—viscosity and cushioning effects
5. Sodium chloride—control of tonicity

Commercial solutions vary as to the concentrations of ingredients, buffering systems, and the substitution of act-alike compounds. No household product can be used as an effective substitute.

Improved wetting of a rigid lens has been aided by incorporating cross-linking agents that have an affinity for water and are part of the polymethylmethacrylate molecule. This new material, commercially sold under different trade names, is considered to be stable and easily fabricated and has a very low degree of water absorption. Improving surface wettability aids comfort and reduces lens awareness. Lenses of this material have a reduced surface

friction and resist the accumulation of mucus and other debris on the lens surface. A drawback of these lenses is that, over time, the lenses lose some of their wetting properties. The clinical significance of the slightly reduced wetting angles and the manufacturer's claims are controversial.

Storage solution

A storage solution primarily functions to eliminate or reduce to tolerable levels pathogens contaminating the surface of the lens. It also serves to clean the lens and keep it wet. Wetting of the lens should follow soaking to render the lens more hydrophilic (make the lens more wettable).

Soaking solutions should be changed daily. Some of the solutions evaporate, whereas in others inactivation of the preservative occurs by debris introduced into the solution by the lens or the patient's finger. The cost of a daily change of soaking solution is not great (approximately 10¢ per day), certainly within the means of any lens wearer.

The active disinfection ingredient in a soaking solution is the preservative. The common preservatives are benzalkonium chloride, chlorobutanol, and organic mercurials.

Benzalkonium chloride. Benzalkonium chloride is a quaternary ammonium compound. It is an effective germicide but in high concentrations (0.03% 1:2000) can cause superficial punctate keratitis, whereas in weak solutions it is not strong enough to provide a germicidal effect. Presently concentrations of 1.75, 0.0133% solutions are employed. Benzalkonium chloride is the best and most effective preservative against *Pseudomonas*. Benzalkonium chloride can reduce the surface wettability over time or certain silicone acrylates. In addition, adverse reactions such as corneal erosions have been reported.

Chlorobutanol. Chlorobutanol is a relatively slow bactericide and fungicide that possesses synergistic activit when combined with benzalkonium chloride. It is volatile, and conceivably its concentration can fall below useful levels. In recent years, some manufacturers have removed it from their products or have reduced the concentration by 50%.

Organic mercurials. Organic mercurials are largely bacteriostatic in activity and are not so effective as other preservatives against gram-negative organisms, especially *Pseudomonas*. However, in high-enough concentrations and when used with other agents, it can be an effective disinfectant. Thimerosal is the most commonly used mercurial. It can be irritating and sensitizing after repeated instillations.

WET OR DRY STORAGE

H.F. Allen has been largely responsible for the group that favors dry storage of rigid lenses. This group's criticism is that *Pseudomonas* has been cultured from lens solutions in liquid storage with a preservative.

The wet-storage faction argues that in these cases the concentration of benzalkonium chloride was too low—1:50,000—or that the preservative was leached out of the solution and deactivated by improper soaking cases containing sponge rubber. They also add that dry storage in ordinary atmospheric conditions results

in a moist lens that can still support bacterial growth. A rigid lens dehydrates in about 12 hours.

Clinical evidence favors wet storage. In dry storage the lens actually is quite moist when stored, supporting bacterial growth. Polymethylmethacrylate will also absorb approximately 0.2% of water by weight after 20 hours of immersion. Generally this hydration is not significant. If a dry, unsaturated lens is placed on the cornea, the affinity of the lens for water will result in water being absorbed from the tears. This causes a condensation of secretions on the surface of the lens. The storage solutions actually cut down the degree of bacterial contamination as opposed to a moist lens stored in a dry environment. The best adversary against contamination is to educate the patient to observe good hygiene with respect to the wearing of the lenses. Hands must be washed before handling, cases kept clean, soaking solutions changed daily, and lenses cleaned *when removed.*

Leaving the contamination issue aside, most fitters favor wet storage, since it makes the lens cleaner and more comfortable to insert and wear. Also a rigid lens tends to flatten with hydration, so that when the lens is stored dry its shape is constantly changing and only becomes stable after 24 to 48 hours of hydration. This is of particular importance when rigid gas-permeable lenses such as ones made of CAB are used because the water content is approximately 1.8%.

Ordinary tap water is sometimes used by patients for storage. This should be discouraged because the halogen component of tap water can be irritating and sensitizing to the tissues. Also tap water creates a hypotonic layer of water on the surface of the lens, which can be irritating when the lens is inserted.

COMBINATION SOLUTION

A combination solution is one with chemicals that permit cleaning, soaking, and wetting or just soaking and wetting. The major attractions of a combination solution are improved patient compliance, convenience, and some economy. The chemicals perform adequately together, but certainly not as well as when the individual solutions are used separately. For instance, the preservative is usually benzalkonium chloride

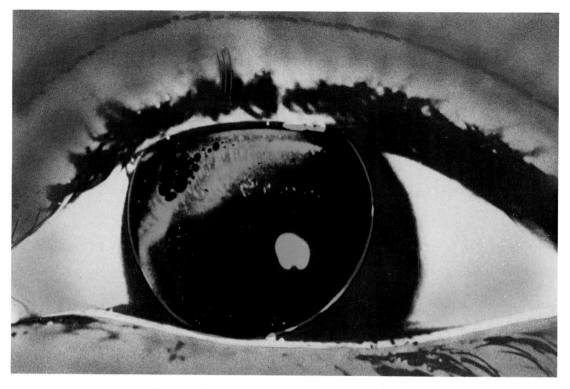

Fig. 14-3. Mascara deposit on the surface of the lens.

with ethylenediaminetetraacetic acid (EDTA) as a synergist. This preservative inhibits wetting so that a lens stored in a combined solution may cause discomfort upon insertion. In some combined solutions the preservative phenylmercuric nitrate 1:25,000 has been shown to be relatively ineffective against *Pseudomonas*. Thimerosal as a preservative has the same disadvantage. At the present time there is no all-purpose solution that is not a compromise.

CLEANING THE LENS

If a lens becomes smudged with dried mucus, oil, nail polish, nicotine, or a nonsoluble cosmetic (Fig. 14-3), it can be cleaned by the patient with a cleaner.

Some household cleaners, such as shampoo, may be used on PMMA lenses. However, some of this type of detergent may be harmful to gas-permeable materials or, if not properly rinsed off, may act as an ocular irritant.

Basic methods of cleaning

Basic methods of cleaning rigid lenses include friction rubbing, hydraulic cleansing, ultrasonic cleansing, and spray cleansing.

Friction rubbing. This is the application of a cleansing solution to the surface of the lens followed by rubbing of the lens between the thumb and forefinger. It is the least efficient method and over a period of time can lead to warpage of or scratches on the lens.

Cotton swab (Q-tip). With proper use, the Q-tip cotton swab is the most effective technique. One side of the cotton swab is saturated with the cleaner and gently rubbed over the surface of the lens. Then the other side of the lens is cleaned with the other side of the cotton swab. A new cotton swab is used for the second lens.

Hydraulic cleansing. In this method the lens is placed in a container that permits back-and-forth pumping action. Frequently this is accomplished by manual agitation of the entire unit. This is an adequate method.

Ultrasonic cleansing. In ultrasonic cleansing the lenses are placed in a cleansing solution through which ultrasonic waves are passed. Ultrasonic cleansing is efficient and excellent for the practitioner but too expensive for home use (Fig. 14-4).

Spray cleansing. The lens is placed in a per-

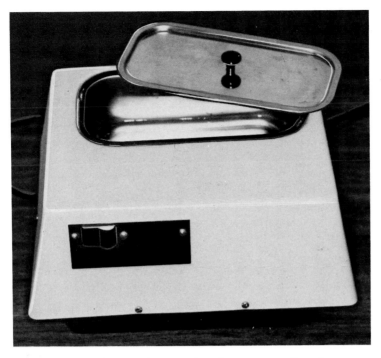

Fig. 14-4. Sonic cleaner for cleaning lenses. This device is excellent but too expensive for home use.

forated storage and cleansing kit (Swisher, Alcon/BP), which is then placed under a running faucet. Cleansing tablets such as Renex (Alcon/BP), a mild nonionic detergent, are added to the inner unit and dissolved to form a detergent solution. The running of the water provides the agitation and spray effect. This technique is theoretically sound if one can be sure that the tap water is sterile in the area and that the patient is conscientious about letting the tablet dissolve completely.

Routines employed by lens solution manufacturers

Barnes-Hind Pharmaceuticals, Inc. Lenses are cleaned by friction cleansing or hydraulic cleansing with the Hydra-Mat. With hydraulic cleansing a liquid cleanser is added to tap water and the lenses are put in a container that permits back-and-forth pumping action. The lenses are placed in a soaking container (Hydra-Kit) that is filled with soaking solution (Soquette [benzalkonium chloride 0.01%, chlorobutanol, EDTA]). The lenses are removed in the morning and wetting solution added. The storage unit (Aqua Cell/Mate, Fig. 14-8) has in-

ner and outer containers. The inner houses the lenses, and the outer contains tap water plus a cleansing agent. Manual agitation of the unit cleanses the lenses.

Alcon/BP. The lenses are soaked in Contique, which is really three solutions—wetting, soaking, and cleansing in one. The lenses are stored in a simple flip-top case that does allow safe rinsing of the lens in a separate storage compartment.

Allergan Pharmaceuticals, Inc. The lenses are placed in a receptacle that fits into a storage case (Clean-N-Soakit, Fig. 14-5). The container is filled with a combination cleansing and soaking solution (Clean-N-Soak). This solution has a cleansing agent and preservatives that include phenylmercuric nitrate 1:25,000.

Before removal the unit is shaken five or six times. The lenses are rinsed and a wetting solution applied before insertion. The wetting solution contains a wetting agent (polyvinyl alcohol with methylcellulose) and preservatives (EDTA and benzalkonium chloride 1:25,000).

Burton, Parsons & Co., Inc. The lenses are cleaned with friction rubbing with a cleansing solution (Clens), which contains the preservatives benzalkonium chloride 0.02% and EDTA 0.01%.

The lenses are then stored in Soaclens, a combined wetting and soaking solution, which contains thimerosal 0.004%, EDTA 0.1%, and polyvinyl alcohol as the wetting agent.

The combined solution is used for wetting before insertion.

Flow Pharmaceuticals, Inc. The lenses are spray cleaned in a combination cleansing and storage device (Porta-Flow, Fig. 14-6), employing the combination solution Hy-Flow, which has cleaning and storage functions.

The lenses are then transferred to a storage chamber and covered with the combination cleaning and storage solution duo-Flow. This solution contains benzalkonium chloride

1:7500, sodium EDTA 1:400, and polyoxyethylene-polyoxypropylene condensate.

Upon removal the lenses are rinsed with tap water and coated with Hy-Flow wetting solution before insertion.

Comment. Each approach to cleaning and storage has its faults, but each leaves the lens reasonably free of deposits. The greatest contamination comes from dirty lens cases, dirty fingers that carry the lens to the eye, and to some extent the eye itself, which harbors some pathogens on its surface. Wetting the lens with saliva will also negate any chemical decontamination attempts. The most important factor in lens cleanliness is still good patient hygiene.

If a patient does get an infection, it is important to do cultures and sensitivities of the lens case used and the conjunctiva as well.

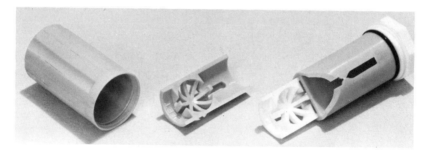

Fig. 14-5. Clean-N-Soakit. (From Dabezies, O.H., Jr.: Accessory contact lens solutions. In New Orleans Academy of Ophthalmology: Symposium on contact lenses, St. Louis, 1973, The C.V. Mosby Co.)

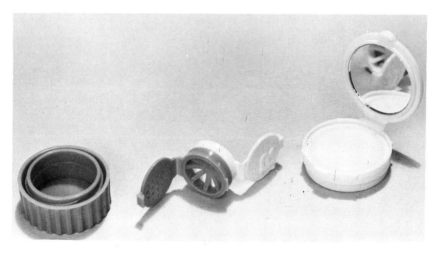

Fig. 14-6. Porta-Flow unit. (From Dabezies, O.H., Jr.: Accessory contact lens solutions. In New Orleans Academy of Ophthalmology: Symposium on contact lenses, St. Louis, 1973, The C.V. Mosby Co.)

LENS CASES (Figs. 14-7 to 14-10)

The design of the case is less important than the material from which it is produced. The lens-holding basket or compartment should be of a softer plastic than the contact lens so that the incidence of surface scratching is lessened. The patient should also be well instructed to avoid sliding the lens out of the case compartment. This will reduce scratching and the need for frequent lens polishing or replacement. The design of the case should be such as to allow a finger to be touched to the concave side of the lens, which will then stick to the finger when withdrawn.

A proper lens case can sidestep a number of problems. Ideally the lens case should fulfill the following requirements:

1. Should have a removable basket that will allow the lens to be rinsed without loss.
2. Should be stored loosely; patients tend to crack or bend lenses upon removal if they are fixed in a snap-on device
3. Should allow total immersion of the lens if it is going to be stored wet
4. Should be easy to clean; the snap-top variety is probably the easiest to contaminate
5. Should be made of plastic and should not contain any sponge rubber that can concentrate the chemicals of the soaking solution
6. Should be distinguished from mailing cases; the compartments of mailing cases are too shallow for germicidal solutions

GAS-PERMEABLE LENS CARE

Rigid gas-permeable lenses encompass a range of lens materials and material combinations broader than that of either soft or traditional rigid PMMA lenses. The care of a gas-permeable is simpler than that of a soft lens because cleaning is not so critical for the survival of the lens. Also heat sterilization is not used. Its care is a little more complicated than that for PMMA because deposits may form on the lens and should be removed.

Some common gas-permeable materials in use today are silicone-PMMA combinations, surface-treated silicones, CAB, and styrene. Although the advent of the gas-permeable material has been of great benefit to both fitter and patient, they have at the same time been accompanied by some characteristics not previously encountered.

Wetting and soaking

Most gas-permeable lenses tend to be somewhat hydrophobic. This is especially so in the case of silicone-PMMA materials such as the Boston and Polycon lenses. It is the silicone component that makes wetting more difficult. As in the case of any contact lens, poor wetting leads to complaints of blurred vision and discomfort. It is of importance that a compatible

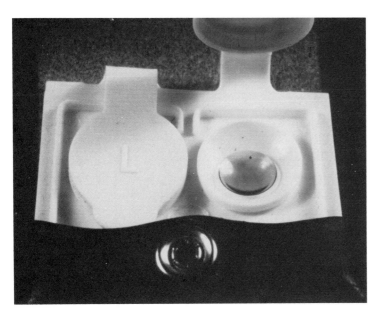

Fig. 14-7. Snap-top case is compact, inexpensive, and requires very little solution. The lens is easily exposed to contamination, it frequently is not immersed in soaking solution, and with time this case leaks. This case has limited use and is best for dry storage or as a mailing unit.

Fig. 14-8. Aqua Cell/Mate. The lens is held in place by a plastic holder. If the lens is not lifted out vertically, it may crack or bend. Improper sales of this type of case (if prong size too small) can result in the warpage of some large-diameter lenses.

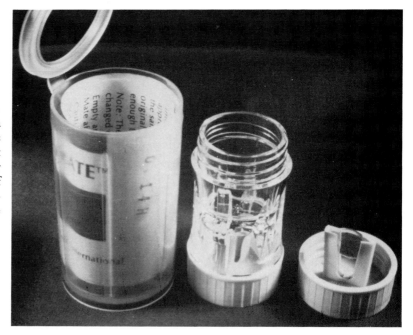

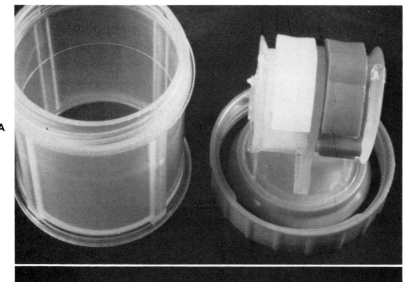

A

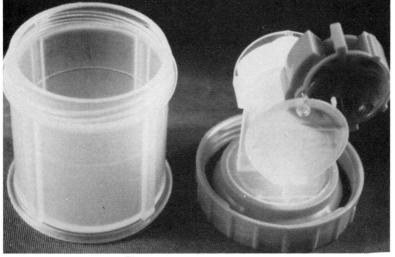

B

Fig. 14-9. A removable basket that prevents the lens from sticking to the case. This is an excellent case. **A,** Closed case. **B,** Open case. Patient must be certain lens is placed in center of drawer, with convex side down, or lens warpage can result.

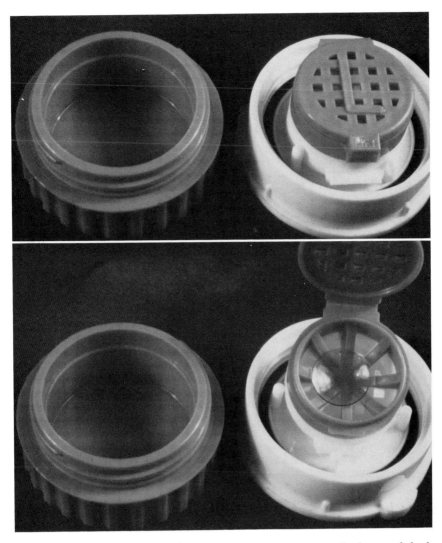

Fig. 14-10. It is difficult to contaminate this case, it is simple to remove the lens, and the lens can be rinsed without being removed. This case allows total immersion of the lens and is an excellent case. It is similar to the one shown in Fig. 14-6.

wetting agent be used with the gas-permeable lenses. Soaking in the same solution when the lenses are being stored is also recommended.

Most patients have the best wetting from wetting-soaking solutions that use EDTA as the primary agent. Polyvinyl alcohol, commonly used in rigid lens wetting solutions, does not seem to provide as good results as other agents. Some manufacturers, in an effort to obtain approval to market their lenses faster in the USA did so in conjunction with soft lens care systems. This method, however, is not acceptable from a practical standpoint, and soaking the lenses in a soft lens storage solution

does little more than keep them moist. There is little or no surface treatment or increased wettability achieved by these solutions.

Cleaning

The hydrophobic aspect of the gas-permeable lenses combined with their oxygen permeability can create a smearing such as that seen on a PMMA lens. However the coating is more of the proteinaceous and lipid type, which we would expect to see on a soft lens. The deposit, which is creamy to white, interferes with the comfort and clarity of the lens. One can best appreciate its presence by looking at the lens with the slitlamp after the lens has been rinsed and dried.

Because of the nature of the deposits, most soft lens surfactant cleaners do an adequate job of removal. In some 5% to 10% of patients wearing gas-permeable lenses, it is necessary to complement daily cleaning with weekly enzymatic cleaning to keep protein deposits in check.

Giant papillary conjunctivitis may occur around the protein deposits. It is usually found under the upper lid and has a cobblestone-like appearance. Each papilla usually has a blood vessel in the center in contrast to a follicle, which is virus induced and has a blood vessel on its surface. Also, virus-induced disorders frequently have a swollen preauricular node.

The tarsal side of the conjunctiva becomes heaped into large papules and produces even more protein, and so the circle of events goes faster. If the inflammation is giant papillary conjunctivitis, which can occur with hard or soft lenses, the reaction is usually seen on the center of the tarsus. With pure allergic reactions, the elevations are usually more at the edge of the tarsal plate.

Approximately 5% of PMMA lens wearers eventually get giant papillary conjunctivitis, whereas it can occur in some form in 20% of soft lens users. Oddly enough, its frequency is less with extended wear lenses.

People with this problem benefit with the weekly soft lens cleaner currently available. After one uses these proteolytic enzymes, the lenses should be rinsed with nonpreserved saline solution and conditioned with wetting solution before being used.

Tap water should not be used as a rinse for the lenses. Tap water in many cities may be contaminated with bacteria, including *Pseudomonas*. This is also true of distilled water taken off the pharmacist's shelf. In one survey we conducted on drugstore-purchased distilled water, some 50% of the samples were contaminated. The best rinse is physiologic saline solution. It is not contaminated when purchased but is not hypotonic like water.

Comment. Giant papillary conjunctivitis ensures a continuous supply of protein debris to the surface of the lens. Vigorous cleaning of the lens and the local application of steroids to shrink the papillas may not be sufficient to stop

the reaction permanently. Frequently the patient needs a new lens or a different type of lens. At times the patient has to resort to glasses for a while because a permanent solution does not seem to be present.

Cleaning devices

Some manufacturers advocate that patients clean their gas-permeable lenses with a velveteen cloth soaked in cleaner. This approach is not recommended because it may result in a distorted optic figure or unwanted treatment adjustments by the patient.

Patients who are extremely rough in handling their lenses may use a cleaning device, such as the Hydra-Mat II (Barnes-Hind Pharmaceuticals, Inc., Sunnyvale, Calif.), in which a dilute solution of cleaner is rinsed about the lenses. This type of cleaning, though not so effective as careful digital cleaning, may be best for the less careful individual.

Gas-permeable solutions for the Boston Lens

The Boston Lens has its own wetting and soaking solution, which has a hydrophilic component that binds to the surface of the contact lens, thereby enhancing its surface wettability. Other solutions are not recommended because of their ineffectiveness in wetting the surface of the Boston Lens.

The Boston Lens also has its own special cleaners, which are recommended. The method they advance is as follows. To clean the outside lens surface, attach a rigid suction lens holder to the concave surface and rub the outer surface in a circular motion over a taut piece of velveteen that has been saturated with the Boston Lens Practitioner Cleaner. To clean the inside surface, apply the lens holder to the outside surface of the lens. While rotating the lens, rub the velveteen soaked in the appropriate solution over the inside surface.

Although many patients dislike or will not use a device, great caution should be used in handling these lenses. Because of the silicone content, the lenses are more fragile, especially at the edges. Chipping is very easy to do. In a Boston Lens, the fragmentation is quite high because it does have a high silicone content for its high permeability and the ideal lens is fabricated with the edges in the order of 0.08 mm.

These lenses should be manipulated gently with no bending of the edges or rough handling.

Preservatives—a necessary troublemaker

Preservatives keep the solutions free of contamination while in storage and use. A solution without a preservative becomes contamined within 48 hours. *Pseudomonas*, which thrives in a wet environment, is the most serious pathogen. Preservatives also reduce surface contamination, especially by fungi, and act as a defense mechanism against the sloppy patient who will not change nonpreserved solutions regularly.

Commonly used preservatives in gas-permeable lens solutions are the following:

Benzalkonium chloride—primarily used as a preservative for rigid lenses; not used for soft lenses because it is absorbed into the lens itself. The absorption can reach toxic levels. It acts by a surface action in microbial organisms.

Chlorhexidine—used for soft lenses and has a tendency to bind protein to the lens.

Thimerosal—a mercurial that competes with the respiratory mechanism of microbial organisms by releasing mercury. It can be toxic to the tissues or act as a sensitizing agent.

EDTA (ethylenediaminetetraacetic acid)—deprives the organism of essential metal ions and disrupts the bacterial wall. EDTA is frequently found in soft lens solutions but is also present in some gas-permeable solutions. It tends to bind protein to the lens. If the concentration of the solution is reduced from 0.50 to 0.25, the binding effort is considerably reduced.

Chlorobutanol—another preservative commonly used. It is rarely used because of its volatility, and so it can become excessively concentrated in solution and reach toxic levels.

Some gas-permeable lens cleaners have preservatives that are especially troublesome, causing either toxic or allergic reactions. A toxic reaction is one that creates a harmful effect to tissues at the usual normal levels of concentration. It is caused by a direct insult to

cells in its metabolism. With toxic material, there is usually a history of progressive intolerance to the material used. An allergy is a reaction to an antigen, and the allergic inflammation is attributable to a specific antigen-antibody reaction. In the eye, the conjunctiva is the target organ of an allergy, whereas the cornea is the target organ in toxicity.

Chlorhexidine, though not directly toxic to the eye, binds proteins, fats, and mucus to the lens and renders it hydrophobic. The altered lens becomes an irritant to the eye and the eye becomes red. Most preservatives in full concentration are toxic to tissues. However, in many cases toxicity is not a problem because the preservatives of ocular solutions are immediately diluted by the tears.

Whereas chlorhexidine causes toxicity, thimerosal, a mercury-based preservative, is likely to cause an allergy. With an allergy, the patient is asymptomatic for a long time and suddenly a red eye occurs with contact of the allergen. The typical history is that a patient uses this agent 6 months or longer with no side effects and then suddenly develops an allergic inflammatory reaction. The eye simply becomes red and irritable with no change in the power or fitting characteristics of the lens. Although most preservatives can cause toxicity and allergic reactions, they are a necessary evil because they are needed to keep solutions free of contamination while the solutions are in the storage case.

There may be no clinical difference between an allergy, toxicity, and infection, except for the difference in history and the cytologic appearance, which would show a higher degree of eosinophils with an allergic case.

Comment. The weekly cleaners seem to be more toxic to the corneal conjunctival surface than the daily surfactant cleaners. When solution reaction is suspect, do an office cleaning, reassess the lens, and omit the weekly soft lens cleaners first. Also it is important to reassess the lenses once the offending solution is removed and the eyes have returned to normal (usually with the help of local steroids). The eyes may have become red because of tight-fitting lenses.

ASSESSMENT OF THE NEW RIGID LENS WEARER

General considerations

The eyelids

Tear film assessment

Tear deficiency—an analysis to consider before fitting

Role of blinking

Assessment of a new lens wearer

When to refit

Temporary glasses

GENERAL CONSIDERATIONS

Contact lens fitters tend to be cornea oriented. They look to the cornea for guidance in their base curve, optic zone, and diameter. In fact, they only look at a small segment of the cornea, that is the apical spheric portion called the "corneal cap." In the fitting with this type of approach the K measurements along with the refraction are sent to the laboratory, and a lens is made. And surprisingly it works a high percentage of the time. However, if a fitter wants better results and enjoys the pride of doing excellent work, there are a few other variables that must be considered—the eyelids, blinking patterns, and tear film.

The most neglected areas are the tear film and its layers and components. A poor or inadequate tear film will ruin the best of efforts. Blinking is also important, especially with a PMMA lens. The full blink response polishes the lens, provides tear exchange, and moves the lens to sustain centration.

THE EYELIDS

The lids have to be studied. If the lids are tight, a rotational force may be exerted on the lens or the lens may be drawn up to ride high. Also the lid configuration determines the size of the palpebral fissure opening, which in turn bears a direct influence on the size of the palpebral fissure. A small palpebral fissure may preclude the use of a large lens, which is especially significant with aphakic people. A retracted lid may cause lid impact, and a lid with

ptosis may not move the lens sufficiently to cause a tear exchange.

The inside tarsal surface has to be inspected. Any lens including rigid lenses can cause giant papillary conjunctivitis, the autoimmune inflammatory condition of the upper tarsal conjunctival surface. Some persons have this problem before they wear lenses, and the condition is aggravated by the lens. These persons may have vernal catarrhal or atopic allergies and may be poor candidates for contact lenses.

The lower lid may be important. If a truncated lens is employed, the lower lid cannot be too close to the margin of truncation because it will displace the lens upward or more commonly tip the lateral side of the lens in a clockwise rotational manner. The lower lid orientation, be it oblique, S shaped, low, or lax, is especially significant in the use of bifocal lenses.

TEAR FILM ASSESSMENT

The tear film is vital. Not only does it provide oxygen exchange as the lens is moved, but it also passes lysozyme, an antibacterial enzyme that inhibits bacterial proliferation.

Patients with a tear deficiency are more prone to infections and often cannot be fit comfortably with lenses. Ideally each patient should have the following:

1. Rose bengal test to stain areas of devitalized tissue.
2. A Schirmer test with and without a local anesthetic. Wetting of the paper strip 10

mm within 5 minutes is considered satisfactory.

3. BUT (tear film breakup time). Disruption of the tear film without blinking in less than 10 seconds is considered unsatisfactory.

4. Corneal assessment for erosions. If the dryness is severe enough to cause pitting of the corneal epithelium, rigid lenses should not be used. Not only is there a greater risk of infection but also a portal of entry is created. Associated findings that do not auger well include blepharitis for the contact lens patient and chronic conjunctivitis.

Serious problems can be anticipated. Suspect dry eye cases in menopausal women, women on birth-control pills, and patients with various forms of arthritis. Also normal tear production may be hampered by drugs taken orally such as antihistamines, belladona derivatives, and some tranquilizers.

Dry spots may be encountered in keratoconjunctivitis sicca or may be caused by inability of the epithelium to wet, as with old corneas scarred from trauma, herpes infection, and so on.

Contamination of the tear film may be patient induced by rubbing of the eyes with dirty fingers or be a consequence of high bacterial skin and conjunctival flora as found in acne rosacea.

Comment. Contact lenses, whether rigid or soft, by themselves do not cause an increase in the normal pathogens found in the eye. The contamination, if active, is usually external from dirty cases, dirty fingers, and so on. A higher conjunctival bacterial count may be encountered in acne rosacea, seborrhea, and ordinary acne. If such patients suffer from recurrent blepharoconjunctivitis or have recurrent hordeolum, they may be poor candidates for lenses.

TEAR DEFICIENCY—AN ANALYSIS TO CONSIDER BEFORE FITTING

The most common type of dry eye situation clinically found is keratoconjunctivitis sicca. In this condition there is a loss of the aqueous component of tears from the lacrimal gland.

Diseases commonly associated with tear deficiency include

Rheumatoid arthritis
Lupus erythematosus
Periarteritis nodosa
Sjögren's syndrome (keratoconjunctivitis sicca)—
dry eyes, dry mouth, and arthritis

Other causes include

Drugs such as belladonna derivatives
Menopause—hormonal changes

Normal tears are secreted at a low level—1 microliter per minute. The water-soluble components include proteins, inorganic salts, glucose, and oxygen. Aqueous tears form the *middle layer* of the tear film. This component is secreted by the lacrimal gland (Fig. 15-1).

The *top layer* is a *lipid film* over the aqueous layer. It is an oily layer secreted by the meibomian glands. Its function is to prevent evaporation of the tear film. Deficiencies in this section of the layer are rare.

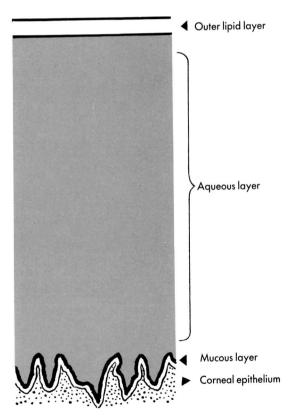

◀ Outer lipid layer

Aqueous layer

◀ Mucous layer
▶ Corneal epithelium

Fig. 15-1. Three-layer structure of the tear film. (From Stein, H.A., and Slatt, B.J.: The ophthalmic assistant, ed. 4, St. Louis, 1983, The C.V. Mosby Co.)

The *inner layer* is the *mucin film* obtained as a secretion of the goblet cells of the conjunctiva. Its purpose is to change the corneal epithelial hydrophobic surface to a hydrophilic surface upon which aqueous tears can spread. Mucin deficiency can be encountered in the following:

Stevens-Johnson disease
Ocular pemphigoid
Alkali burns

Signs of dry eyes:

Viscous mucous strands
Superficial epithelial erosions highlighted with rose bengal or fluorescein
Increased BUT (tear film breakup time), less than 10 seconds
Increased incidence of infection in terms of chronic conjunctivitis and blepharitis. These complications occur because of a loss of the normal antibacterial tear substances, lysozyme, β-lactam, and lactoferrin.
Positive Schirmer's test, wetting less than 5 mm after a piece of filter paper is placed into the lower conjunctival sac in a nonanesthetized eye for 5 minutes.

People with dry eyes or relatively dry eyes may make poor candidates for any contact lens. In a marginally dry eye a thin soft lens or a high water content soft lens with supplementary artificial tear drops can be used. Frequently a rigid lens works better in dry eye cases. This paradox occurs because the soft hydrated lens may cause an osmotic shift of fluid into the soft lens, making the tear film even dryer.

ROLE OF BLINKING

Poor blinking habits can make a well-fitted lens create as many symptoms as an ill-fitted one. The front surface of the lens becomes misty because of drying and lack of polishing by the lids, vision suffers, and in addition the lens does not move properly. The tear film under the lens becomes stagnant and corneal edema ensues. Such a situation can create mild symptoms of burning and photophobia or create such distress that continued wear of the lens is intolerable.

An equally disturbing event occurs when a patient does not have a full and upward Bell's response. In such a person, the eyes do not roll up and out. Instead, the eyes may not move or actually roll slightly downward. If the lids are not totally closed with sleep, the exposed corneas may show signs of dryness or desiccation. Such a person frequently wakes up in the morning with a grittiness in the eyes. Poor blinkers and people with a paradoxical Bell's response should not be wearing rigid lenses.

A normal blink is executed by the pretarsal fibers of the orbicular muscle. It is an automatic reflex movement. It should be distinguished from voluntary lid closure, which requires the action of the pretarsal, preseptal, and orbital segments of the orbicular muscle. The latter is a much stronger action and is accompanied by Bell's phenomenon. Patients with blinking problems are frequently instructed in voluntary lid-closure movements when it is the light pretarsal-mediated blink that must be restored to normal.

Comment. If blinking exercises are done, the second and third fingers should be placed just on the skin beyond the lateral canthus. Contraction of the underlying orbital segment of the orbicularis muscle should *not* be felt. With voluntary lid closure this muscle contraction can easily be felt.

The normal blink rate is quite variable. Approximately 15 to 18 blinks per minute is normal. Each blink lasts 0.3 seconds. The rate is higher for men than for women and is also increased with emotional outbursts or anxiety states. With a poor or tired blinker, the rate may go down as much as 60%. This occurs frequently with reading, driving, or watching computer screens during the full working day. Persons who have jobs that fatigue the normal blink response are best fitted with gas-permeable lenses, which do not depend heavily on blinking to relieve corneal hypoxia.

Types of blink activity with lens wearers

Partial blink. A partial blink is an incomplete blink in which the inferior half of the cornea remains exposed (Fig. 15-2).

Lid flutter. Lid flutter is a repressed blink. This typical habit appears in the apprehensive patient who tilts the head back, retracts the lids, and merely flutters the lids.

Normal blink. At first the lens is depressed by the descending lid. After full lid closure the lens rises as the lid elevates. Once the lid has achieved its full height the lens makes a slight gravitational movement downward.

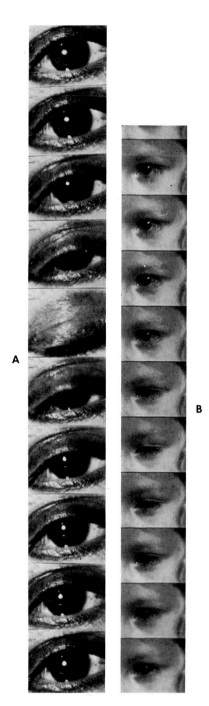

Fig. 15-2. A, Movement of the lens with blinking. The lens is initially depressed, is then elevated, and then gently drops to a central position. **B,** Incomplete blink. The lid is never fully depressed. It halts its downward progression at the margin of the lens. (From Girard, L.J., editor: Corneal contact lenses, St. Louis, 1970, The C.V. Mosby Co.)

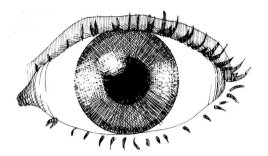

Fig. 15-3. Three and 9 o'clock staining resulting from inadequate blinking.

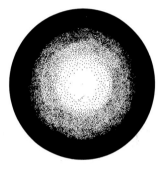

Fig. 15-4. Corneal edema with a poor blink response. There is tear stagnation and little lens movement.

Common findings with poor blink habits

The following are often found in persons with poor blink habits:

1. Low-riding lenses
2. Three and 9 o'clock staining (Fig. 15-3)
3. Corneal edema (Fig. 15-4)
4. Greasy or dry lenses with crystalline deposits

ASSESSMENT OF A NEW LENS WEARER
History

At the beginning, there will be many adaptive symptoms, such as flare, sensitivity to light, and tearing. These symptoms should be temporary and last no longer than 1 to 2 weeks.

Confusion should not be present between adaptive symptoms and those of a poor fit. Poor fittings will augment the normal conditioning to a rigid lens. If the patient complains of the lens falling out or being displaced on the sclera, the lenses are too loose. This problem will not get better with time. The patient may have difficulty removing the lenses. Aphakic persons do because their lids are often loose and floppy. New young patients may also have trouble because of normal anxiety and clumsiness in learning a new procedure. However the lenses may be tight. Adaptive symptoms must be separated from those of an ill-fitting lens. The former improves with time; the latter does not. If a patient is not making satisfactory progress, a reassessment is in order.

Visual acuity with lenses

Vision should be corrected for near distance since many persons with myopia, though content with their distance acuity, experience difficulty with reading. This is particularly true for myopic persons who are over 35 years of age.

The vertex distance must be considered in the refraction, especially with refractive errors greater than about 4 diopters. An over-refraction of the lens will usually show that more plus is needed for high hyperopic errors and less minus is required for high myopic refractive errors.

If this adjustment is not made, the hyperope will be undercorrected and the myope overcorrected, and significant problems with reading will occur in both.

If the vision is not adequate, the following difficulties may be present:

1. The lens may not be centered.
2. The sagittal vault of the lens may be too great, and so a plus lens effect is created. Excess pooling of fluorescein may be present.
3. Tearing may be excessive, and so the lens may slide around too much.
4. The lenses may be switched. In the early days of contact lens wear, anything could happen.

Manifest refraction over lenses

Frequently 0.50 D of myopia will be found and is an acceptable consequence of mild corneal edema. Greater changes should require reevaluation of fit. Residual astigmatism may be increased. Amounts of 0.50 D are very common and can be ignored. Excessive residual astigmatism may require a change in power equal to the spheric equivalent or an anterior toric lens.

Astigmatism of magnitude 1.00 to 5.00 diopters can now be fitted with large-diameter spheric gas-permeable lenses. This rule only applies if the cornea is the source of the astigmatism, that is, has toric curvatures in which the radius of curvature in one meridian is greater than in the other.

On the other hand, residual astigmatism, the astigmatism that is generated from the lens of the eye, should not be treated with a spheric lens. One can choose a front-surface toric soft lens (which we prefer) or a front-surface toric rigid lens.

An important cause of residual astigmatism is warping of the PMMA lens. Flexure of a lens may also contribute to residual astigmatism. This effect primarily occurs with thin small lenses and the softer gas-permeable lenses.

> If residual astigmatism is against the rule and the corneal toricity is with the rule, residual astigmatism is reduced.
> If the residual astigmatism is against the rule and the corneal toricity is also against the rule, the astigmatism is increased and a lens should not be used.

Lens position and movement

The lens should center over the apical zone of the cornea. The lens should move easily with a blink—first down, then upward as the lid is raised, and then gently downward as the lens drops by gravity to a central position. The lens movements should be fluid and smooth. A lens that drops quickly or moves upward in a jerky fashion does not fit properly. With ocular rotations the lens may lag 1 or 2 mm against the movement of the eye. The lag should not carry the lens over the limbus.

Slitlamp assessment (Fig. 15-5, *A*)

Sclerotic scatter (Fig. 15-5, *B*). Sclerotic scatter is the best way of detecting gross edema. The beam, directed at a wide angle at the periphery of the cornea, causes the area of corneal edema to stand out as a gray patch in relief at the center of the cornea.

Retroillumination. This is the best method of showing microcystic edema in the corneal epithelium (Fig. 15-6).

Focal illumination. Focal illumination with high magnification can reveal areas of corneal erosion or abrasion under the lens. It is also good for inspection of the lens to reveal scratches, edge chips, and so on.

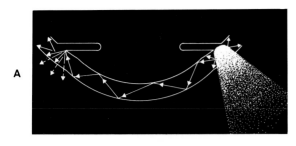

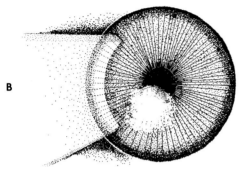

Fig. 15-5. A, Corneal edema can be detected grossly by angling the beam of the slitlamp 45 to 60 degrees at the limbus. **B,** Specular reflection. The internal reflection of light through the cornea makes the central edema stand out as a gray haze. The cornea is employed as a fiberoptic channel.

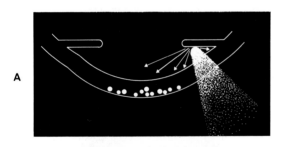

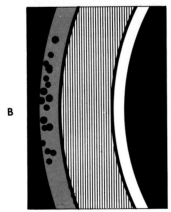

Fig. 15-6. A, Fine corneal edema. This is best appreciated through retroillumination. **B,** The corneal epithelium has a stippled appearance.

Fluorescein evaluation

Fluorescein evaluation using a Burton ultraviolet light or the cobalt blue filter of the slitlamp, employing a wide beam for an overview, and using a fine slitlamp beam and high magnification for detailed assessment of the tear film is a difficult assessment to make. The appearance of a normal fluorescein pattern depends on whether the lens is fitted on K or steeper than K, or whether a small, thin lens is employed versus a conventional or rigid lens, and so a normal pattern is a variable picture. For instance, a normal fluorescein pattern with a microthin lens can be considered steep with a conventional lens. The variability of "normal" fluorescein patterns is such that many fitters do not use it to assess fitting. Once the normal appearance becomes standardized for a given lens, the fluorescein test can yield interesting information on the corneal disorder and fit.

Serial keratometry

In serial keratometry (with the lens removed) K readings do not alter more than 0.50 D from well-fitting lenses. A cornea that varies from 42.50/42.75 to 43.50/43.75 D shows signs of steepening. This usually indicates corneal edema and is usually caused by a tight lens. During adaptation the horizontal meridian may increase appreciably, and the vertical meridian often decreases, sometimes staying the same, sometimes increasing, but usually increasing less than the horizontal. In the long-term wearer there is often a sharp reduction of the K reading in the horizontal meridian, meaning that it has become much flatter. There is usually a slight reduction in the K reading in the vertical meridian. There is seldom an increase (steepening) in this meridian.

In the new patient there is a change from K readings of 42.50 D × 180/42.75 D × 90 to 45.75/42.00 D (flatter in vertical). This is often a result of a lens decentered in vertical meridian.

A change on a mildly astigmatic cornea 42.50 D × 180/44.50 D × 90 to 42.75/43.75 D × 90 (if a spheric lens is being worn) would be considered normal and would be caused by a slight molding of the cornea by the lens.

WHEN TO REFIT

The patient who requires a refit should be treated as a new patient. The lenses should be removed, the tear film assessed, the K readings redone, and the spectacle correction reevaluated.

Most patients who require a refit have symptoms, that is, burning, poor vision, decreased tolerance for the lenses, increased awareness of the lenses, and so on. However, there are patients who are asymptomatic and require a refit. These patients tolerate poorly fitted rigid lenses. They may be indifferent to grossly ill-fitting lenses such as a lens that is too tight (the less the movement, the better they feel), too low (the blink rate is reduced to ameliorate lid impact), corneal edema or erosions (the sensation of the cornea is reduced), 3 and 9 o'clock staining (extensive marginal erosions with episcleritis may cause episcleral redness without pain), and decentered lenses that roll with each blink in a clockwise or counterclockwise manner.

These patients with quiet or minimal symptoms require a refit before an ill-fitted lens turns into a corneal complication. The general assessment should be the same. The problem in the past has been when to refit.

Ideally one should refit the cornea when the K readings are stable and the refraction unchanged. This may take a day, a week, or even months. Until the corneas become stable, the patient is not allowed to wear the lenses. Glasses must be purchased, a task that by itself takes time and leaves the person functionally blind until they are made. The arrival of glasses is hardly an event of joy in a lens wearer's life. Vision and its attendant distortions through thick spectacle lenses are intolerable to the pampered lens wearer. Moreover there is the added grief of change. The corneal curvature and the refraction change daily as the edema recedes, but the power of the spectacles remains the same. This solution is hardly ideal.

The most expedient line of attack is to fit the patient immediately with gas-permeable lenses or alternatively to use soft lenses until the cornea is stabilized. At least the patient can wear a contact lens while the corneas return to their original shape. Then changes in the lens can be made as changes in the contour of the cornea occur.

Many practitioners wait 48 hours while the corneas return to their original shape and then refit. The patient is asked to accept a weekend

of extremely poor vision that creates no inconvenience at work. The 48-hour rule of thumb has been shown to be useful but somewhat unrealistic.

These corneal and refractive changes move in the direction of flatter K readings in the primary meridian and less minus refractive error for a period of 3 to 4 days before these changes reverse or stabilize. Therefore any K readings taken 48 hours or later after lens removal will give values that are erroneous and certainly not so good as those taken immediately after lens removal.

The patient then should be progressively deadapted over a 5- or 6-day period or, better yet, given a hydrophilic lens.

It is wise to do a base refraction on a regular basis. Hartstein found large degrees of corneal astigmatism with the rule induced in 27 patients who, before wearing contact lenses, had no astigmatism or as little as 1.00 D of astigmatism.

Comment. Induced corneal toricity is quite unpredictable. It can last hours, days, or months or become permanent. At times the corneal astigmatism is irregular, and so spectacles will not suffice as a bridge before stability ensues. Soft lenses may not be adequate, especially if the sphere is a low power (-3 or less) and the corneal astigmatism is greater than 1.50 diopters. *The best solution is a gas-permeable lens.* Such lenses require no waiting time, yield the best acuity, and may be changed when the cornea regains its integrity.

TEMPORARY GLASSES

At times a person will want glasses to wear during some period of the day. Students studying at night are frequently happier to do prolonged reading with their glasses. Office workers are often relieved to remove their lenses at the end of the day to relax. The real message being relayed may be limited wearing time caused by a marginally fitted pair of lenses. Make sure the lenses are fitting properly.

Rigid lens patients who switch to spectacles are frequently miserable. The optic properties of spectacles are inferior, the visual fields are restricted, the distortions may be annoying, there are prismatic effects to overcome, the accommodative demands with spectacles are different, and there may be changing spectacle blur that makes a mockery of the fitter's attempt to arrive at a suitable power for the spectacle lenses.

If the person is unimpressed with the practitioner's arguments, the refraction should be done at the end of the day so that the prescription will more or less fit the time that the spectacles will be used.

A rest period during the day is advisable and beneficial. An hour break at supper may enable the person to read comfortably at night. It has been shown that patients who wear their lenses continuously are more likely to develop long-standing, toric corneal changes.

Comment. The major cause of intolerance to PMMA lenses after a workday is poor blinking, which in turn causes poor tear exchange. With fatigue or immobility of the eyes (looking at computer screens all day) the lenses move very little.

A gas-permeable lens has to be the best solution because the oxygenation of the epithelium is not so dependent on tear exchange.

CHAPTER 16

ADAPTIVE SYMPTOMS TO RIGID LENSES

Edges
Excessive movement
Lid impact
Excessive lens awareness
Flare
Optic-zone size
Decentration
Photophobia
Tearing
Difficulty with reading

There is no doubt that the symptoms initially labeled as adaptive were really limitations of the design and material of PMMA lenses. An adaptive symptom is usually manifested in an expression of the first few weeks of contact lens wear. Yet a soft lens can find harmony with the eye in a few minutes. So the duration and severity of these turbulent initial lens reactions are not attributable to the rejection of the device but the nature of the device itself.

Many early reactions to PMMA were hypoxic in nature. When the corneal thickness is measured on an eye in which a PMMA lens has been applied, with a −4.00 diopter model being used, the thickness can increase 10% or greater. Yet, when silicone is used, the increase in thickness of the cornea of the unadaptive eye is 4% or less.

Sudden shock to the cornea causes corneal edema and it symptoms of flare, sensitivity to light, tearing, inability to tolerate the lens, and the defense mechanisms of the lids, including abnormal blinking reactions. With time, corneal hypesthesia occurs, and these reactions may be reduced. Also, if blink posturing abates, proper tear exchange can reduce corneal edema to a tolerable 1% to 2%.

At times, the reactions of an early new rigid-lens wearer is simply the normal response to a bad or tolerable fit. For example, a small thin interpalpebral lens may be acceptable if the lens moves minimally. The reduced mass and thinness of the edges enable the lid to traverse the border of the lens without impact. The same fitting technique with a large-diameter lens would be intolerable, and clouding of the cornea would invariably result. Not only would there be corneal edema, but there would be blink inhibition to avoid contact with the heavy and thick edges.

Ideally, a rigid lens should be tolerable in a few days. There are modifications in design and oxygen permeability that permit faster physical and physiologic adaptation to the application of a lens.

In addition, patient selection is important. The fitting of a rigid lens on a high school student enjoying a summer vacation is a matter different from the application of an advanced student studying for a doctorate. If an eye is engaged in reading, the blinking rate is altered and may go down to as much as 75%. So the reader novice lens wearer may be faced with evaporation of tear film on the surface of the lens with resultant deposit formation, symptoms of a tight fit because of a lack of lens movement, and symptoms from a hypoxic cornea. The oxygen permeability of some widely used rigid lenses varies with the mode of measurement (Table 16-1), but it is apparent that PMMA has no permeability whatsoever.

The adaptation time to any rigid lens may be reduced significantly if gas-permeable lenses are used. Keep in mind that the permeability of any lens is a function of its thickness. In a +6.00 diopter lens the transmissibility at the center of the lens with a thickness of 0.3 to 0.4 mm may be virtually zero, with good transmissibility being enjoyed in the same kind of lens −4.00 diopters and 0.1 mm thick. Adaptability

Table 16-1. Oxygen permeability of rigid lenses

Material	DK (cm^2/sec)	Temperature
PMMA (polymethylmethacrylate)	0.2×10^{-11}	30° C
Silicone-acetate (Polycon, Boston Lens)	5.0×10^{-11}	30° C
CAB (cellulose acetate butyrate)	4.2×10^{-11}	21° C

is then a function of oxygen transmissibility of a lens, and that transmissibility in turn is governed by the thickness of the lens.

Initially displeasure and discomfort is a recognized feature of learning to cope with rigid lenses. The major causes of such reactions appear to be as follows:

1. Poorly contoured or thick edges
2. Excess movement
3. Lid pressure or impact
4. A lens that is stored dry
5. A lens that causes mechanical abrasion of the cornea.

EDGES

There is the possibility that the laboratory's quality control may be poor and must be checked with the optic spherometer (Radiuscope) and profile analyzer for evidence of careless manufacturing. However, the edge of the carrier of the peripheral flange may not be refined. For example, any aphakic lens should have a minus carrier to avoid the lid pushing a thick lens excessively low, instead of carrying the lens to its desirable up position with each blink. High minus lenses should have a plus carrier. Poor edges will make the process of adaptation much longer, if ever.

EXCESSIVE MOVEMENT

PMMA lenses need movement because tear exchange is the only vehicle for oxygen exchange. The movement of the lens causes lid impact and discomfort because the lens rides over a wide surface of the cornea.

The newer gas-permeable lenses offer more liberty in design. For instance, the Boston Lens permits a base curve 0.5 to 1.5 D steeper than K. This enables the lens to be fit tighter so that there will be less movement and initially less awareness of the lens. Ideally, the lens is fitted high under the upper lid so that there is less lid impact, and the comfort and period of adaptation are therefore shortened.

Another design feature is that these lenses can be made 9 mm or greater so that there is more stability. One drawback of the larger lens, however, is the problem of thick lens edges, which if not refined cause a lid gap and 3 to 9 o'clock staining. Lid gap occurs when there is a gap between the edge of the lens and the cornea sufficient to cause drying of the cornea at this site and subsequent desiccation.

LID IMPACT

Lid impact is more likely to occur when the lenses are small, movement is excessive, and the lenses are decentered inferiorly on the cornea as apposed to lenses covered superiorly by the margin of the lid.

A soft lens if made small enough to be an interpalpebral lens creates considerable interaction with the lid margin and is quite uncomfortable. So the initial discomfort of a lens can be decreased considerably by changes in its design. The lid should not engage the edge of the lens.

EXCESSIVE LENS AWARENESS

Lens awareness is caused by the conscious presence of a foreign body on the eye. However, like a new filling in a tooth, the feeling of "something there" should recede. Frequently patients who are very aware of their lenses and are anxious about their presence will demonstrate other features of their fear, such as not blinking, moving their eyes, especially upward, or tilting their head backward in an effort to reduce lens movement.

If the fit is good and the quality control of the lens is satisfactory, the use of a tear substitute or comfort drops may be sufficient to decrease the awareness of the lens.

FLARE

Seeing lights with a sunburst quality, especially at night, is a common initial symptom. There are two major reasons for flare, and they are related to the size of the optic zone and decentration of the lens.

OPTIC-ZONE SIZE

At times the optic zone may be adequate for the light-adapted eye but insufficient for the dark-adapted eye, in which the pupil dilates. Light streams in through the optic zone and around it because the optic zone is too small for the dilated pupil. Because of the movement of the lens, some flare may be acceptable, but it can be reduced when the optic zone and the lens diameter are enlarged.

A simple test to measure the adequacy of the optic zone is to have a patient simply observe in a dark room the quality of the square white blank image of your projector. If there is a great deal of streaming of lights, the lenses should be changed.

DECENTRATION

A decentered lens may be one that is off center and partially covering the pupil or a lens that is too flat and moving excessively. In both instances the remedy is either a larger or steeper lens. Obviously, if the optic zone is moving or not centered, flare will be excessive.

Initially some patients are extremely sensitive to light from oncoming cars when driving at night. If there are no faults in the fitting or lens movements, the flare with time recedes in intensity and usually is acceptable.

PHOTOPHOBIA

The pronounced sensitivity to light gradually recedes after the lenses have been worn 1 or 2 weeks, but in many cases it persists in a low-grade form. Some patients require sunglasses to go out on a cloudy day, whereas others are unable to work because of intolerance to fluorescent light. This is a more common symptom in blue-eyed individuals. If this does not abate after 2 or 3 weeks, it ceases to be an acceptable complaint and probably is indicative of persistent corneal edema.

The causes listed in Table 16-2 may be active in the production of photophobia.

Most of the time photophobia is the response to low-grade corneal edema. The solution is frequently a gas-permeable lens. Many people when outdoors have photophobia, which persists and requires the presence of deeply tinted sunglasses.

When photophobia occurs indoors, it is pathologic, especially if it persists. Such patients are really made into ocular invalids if they have to wear their sunglasses at night or indoors. Besides ruining contrast and resolution, the acuity that occurs with night driving is unacceptable.

How to cope with unacceptable photophobia:
1. Quality control on the lenses.
2. Consider gas-permeable lenses.
3. Check fit—if the lenses are too mobile, try slightly steeper fit.
4. Make sure the optic zone of the lens is sufficient for the size of the pupil.
5. Tinting the lens. If it is to be done, choose gray because it causes the least distortion of the color spectrum.

TEARING

Tearing usually stops after the patient becomes adjusted to the lenses. Sometimes the

Table 16-2. Causes of photophobia

Cause	Observe	Treatment
Corneal edema	Change in K readings or appearance of mires; pachometer change	If the lens fits, switch to gas-permeable lens
3 and 9 o'clock staining	Dry spots on cornea Deficiency of tears Lid gap because of thick edges	Tear film assessment and treat; modify lens edges
Large lens	Silicone-based lenses of high refractive error	Refined edges with good peripheral lens profiles May require switch to smaller PMMA lens or gas-permeable lens
	Blend and adequacy of peripheral curves	Modification of lens required

pooling of tears under and on the lens can create irritating reflections, and the patient complains of glare. A droplet of tears may dislodge the lens and create discomfort and variable vision because of the lens sliding around so much.

Dealing with tearing one has to look at several causes:

Inspect the edges—thick edges are uncomfortable and cause tearing.

Also check the lids. Lid impact can cause frothing because of the excessive liberation of sebaceous material. In addition, the lens develops a greasy film over its surface.

Inspect the periphery of the lens—even a new lens may have a poor edge profile.

Check the lens with a profile analyzer.

Look for signs of corneal edema that persists.

Change the fit, or change to a gas-permeable type.

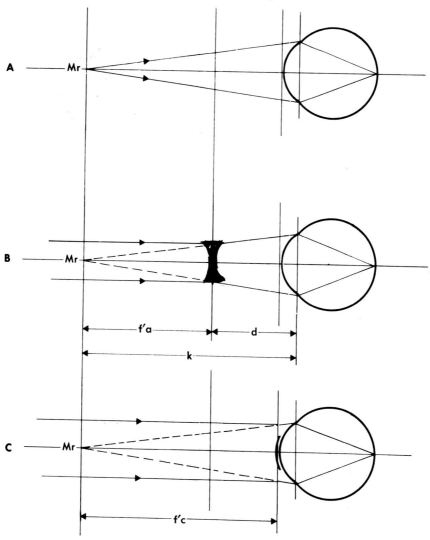

Fig. 16-1. A, Rays of light in the myopic eye in the uncorrected state diverge from a far point in front of the eye (Mr) and are focused on the retina, **B** and **C.** The focal length of the correcting spectacle lens (f'a) is less than the focal length of the correcting contact lens (f'c). Thus in myopia a weaker contact lens is needed as compared to a spectacle lens. It should also be noted that rays of light diverge after leaving a spectacle lens with the result that more accommodative effort is needed as compared to the accommodative demands of an eye corrected with contact lenses. A person with myopia who wears spectacle lenses and is developing presbyopia may find reading glasses a necessity when the switch is made to contact lenses.

DIFFICULTY WITH READING

More accommodation and convergence is required when a moderate to high myope exchanges his glasses for contact lenses (Fig. 16-1). There is an increase in accommodative demand and a loss of base in prism. With a young person these changes can be quickly overcome, but in a person 35 years or older with depleted accommodative reserves, reading becomes a difficult chore.

Added to these difficulties is the change in blink rate, which is often 75% less in a person doing concentrated work, and further problems may occur. The lens is not moved, and so tear exchange is poor. The eye may feel dry or gritty. Also evaporation occurs on the lens sur-

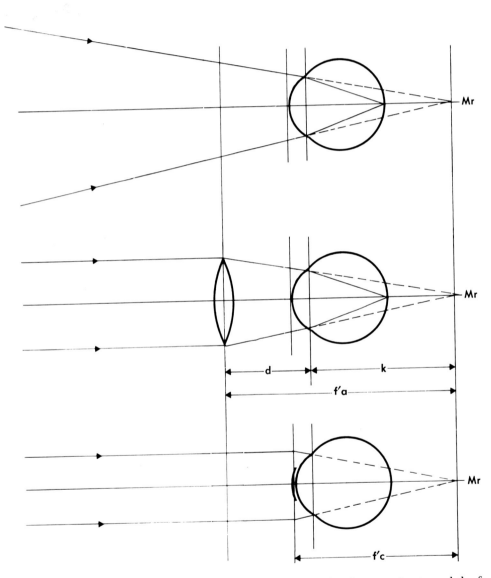

Fig. 16-2. Rays of light in the hyperopic eye that are uncorrected and converging toward the far point, which is behind the eye (Mr). The focal length of the spectacle lens (f'a) is greater than the corresponding focal length (f'c) of the contact lens. Thus in hyperopia a stronger contact lens is needed as compared to a spectacle lens. By the same token the hyperopic eye requires less accommodative effort when corrected with contact lenses. For the person with hyperopia who wears spectacle lenses and is developing presbyopia, this means that with contact lenses, reading glasses may not be required or may at least be postponed.

face and the visual acuity may become smoky. Dry spots may appear on the cornea just under the lens, and symptoms of burning and heat may result. These normal conversion symptoms can be ameliorated but not eliminated.

1. Do not prescribe rigid lenses for students in the intense part of their year of study.
2. Warn patients 35 years and up about the reading handicap.
3. Use of supplementary drops during periods of retarded blinking is helpful, as in driving, studying, and typing.
4. Consider gas-permeable lenses if the blink rate is normally infrequent or if the blink rate is retarded by the demands of the patient's occupation or hobbies.

Alterations in blink patterns may ensue. Changes in the blink rate, excursion, and style may occur if the rigid lens is perceived as

Table 16-3. Alterations in blink patterns

Blink pattern	Treatment
Lid retraction	A large lens, preferably gas permeable with the upper edge of the lens harbored under the upper lids
Lid flutter	Blinking exercises Good edges Normally tolerated lens movement
Incomplete blink	Blinking exercises and not voluntary forced lid closures
Infrequent blinking	Reschedule fitting if the patient needs his eyes for extensive reading or driving

something foreign to be avoided by the lids at all costs. The types of alterations that may be expected are shown in Table 16-3.

PRECAUTIONS

Precautions to minimize adaptive reactions to rigid lenses:

1. Do not fit PMMA lenses when the patient has recently become pregnant or has gone off or on birth-control pills or is becoming menopausal. Gas-permeable lenses are tolerated despite hormonal changes.
2. Try not to fit any patient under emotional distress.
3. Rigid lenses should be avoided in dry dusty working conditions, in arid places, like Arizona, and in polluted environments such as hair-dressing shops.
4. Do not prescribe rigid lenses in any myopic person who is edging into the presbyopic range because the lens may deplete his accommodative reserve (Fig. 16-2).
5. Do not use rigid lenses with patients with lid deformities, such as ptosis, retraction of lids, and active blepharitis.

Ideally there should not be any reaction to rigid lenses whether they are first applied or worn on an intermittent basis (though they should not be worn in this way). Adaptive symptoms are attributable to a combination of irritation and hypoxia, both of which can and should be minimized. Although an introductory period of rigid lens wear is commonly stormy, there is no reason to accept it as normal and not subject to improvement.

FITTING PROBLEMS AND THEIR SOLUTIONS

With the use of gas-permeable lenses, the problems have changed. The lenses are larger, override the superior limbus, create lid gap if the edges are not beveled, and create extensive 3 and 9 o'clock staining with greater frequency and severity than PMMA lenses. However, corneal edema is not a serious problem with gas-permeable lenses. Acute corneal hypoxia (the so called overwear syndrome) has been virtually eliminated (at least we have not seen a case). For this advantage alone these lenses have merit.

The variations from massive corneal edema with vertical striae on Descemet's membrane to epithelial microcysts have been effectively checked with the gas-permeable lens. But some of the PMMA complications were the result of chronic hypoxic changes in the cornea plus the added effect of molding, which produced an irregular corneal surface or a severe toric distortion in corneal shape. It is too early at this time to see whether these oxygen-permeable lenses will do the same because of molding alone, but we have been dealing with gas-permeable lenses over 5 years and permanent changes in the cornea contours have not been observed.

Also, fitting problems of a PMMA lens may be remedied with a gas-permeable lens. This is seen in any ill-fit PMMA lens that causes corneal hypoxia. In refitting the patient with corneal edema and distortion, one may use a gas-permeable lens right away without waiting for K readings to stabilize or the corneal surface to gain total regularity. This advantage represents considerable progress because these patients

were unable to wear this PMMA lens or see clearly with spectacles. The waiting period was often days. But commonly it was months before the corneas stabilized to prelens K readings. Because PMMA is still not a historic curio, we shall have to concern ourselves with its problems.

SYMPTOMS OF AN INADEQUATE FIT

Flare or streaming of lights. Frequently this is caused by a lens with a small optic zone that can be overshadowed by a large pupil. The typical story is that the person cannot stand driving at night because of the streaming around lights. When the pupil is dilated under dim illumination, there is a prismatic displacement of light coming in from the periphery of the lens. The same effect can occur from a lens that is decentered. In such a case the optic zone is displaced, and the pupil will not be fully covered. Flare is induced in aphakic patients who have had a sector iridectomy and are fitted with a lenticular lens fitted over a widely exposed coloboma. Corneal edema from any cause can create the same symptom. With the sensation of flare the zone of streaming of lights is always opposite in direction to the displacement of the lens. If the lens rides low the fringe of light will be above.

The detection of flare is quite simple. In the darkened examining room have the person look at the square visual acuity chart and report any distortions. If the flare is uniform, the optic zone of the lens is too small and it must be enlarged. If streaming occurs in only one direction attention must be directed toward center-

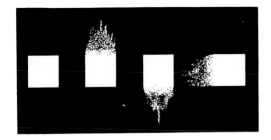

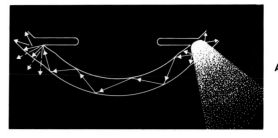

Fig. 17-1. Flare: The zone of streaming is always opposite to the displacement of the lens. Such a lens requires recentering. Uniform flare indicates that the optic zone of the lens is too small.

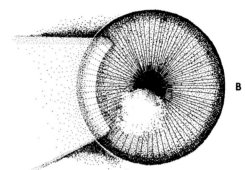

Fig. 17-2. A, Corneal edema can be detected grossly when the beam of the slitlamp is angled 45 to 60 degrees at the limbus. B, Specular reflection. The internal reflection of light through the cornea makes the central edema stand out as a gray haze. The cornea is employed as a fiberoptic channel.

ing the lens (Fig. 17-1). If the pupil is too large for the optic zone of the lens, constriction of the pupils by the application of light to one eye will abolish the flare. Flare around lights is rarely encountered at near range because of the synkinetic near reactions, which include pupillary constriction.

Large-diameter gas-permeable lens should be considered in anyone with huge pupils. This group is usually young, blue-eyed, and myopic people. Their pupils are 4 mm or greater and enlarge to 5 or 6 mm in dim illumination. The pupillary aperture is still smaller than the optic zone of a PMMA lens, but not when one considers the movement of that lens with blinking.

Gas-permeable lenses are effective because of the following:

1. The optic zone is normally large.
2. The movement of the large lens is less than that of a PMMA lens.
3. The lens is more likely to stay centered, especially with blinking.

Blurred vision. The most obvious cause of blurred vision is incorrect power of the lens and is simply handled by refracting over the lenses. If the manifest refraction brings the vision to normal by adding equal power to each eye but of the opposite sign, the lenses were probably switched.

At times the hazy vision may be caused by a grease smudge or coated lens. This becomes obvious the moment the retinoscope is used. An irregular reflex always ensues from the optically disordered front surface of lenses stained with a greasy deposit.

The most worrisome cause of hazy vision is corneal edema. Corneal edema always means a poorly fitting lens. When the edema is severe enough to create epithelial erosions that pick up fluorescein stain, it indicates severely decompensated corneal epithelium. For more subtle changes the slitlamp is used to best advantage.

Heavy edema accumulations in the cornea usually represent epithelial and stromal involvement. One can easily detect it by angling a broad slitlamp beam 45 to 60 degrees at the limbus (Fig. 17-2, *B*). By oscillating the beam, the specular reflection of light traveling throughout the cornea will make the central area of edema stand out in relief as a central, gray haze (Fig. 17-2, *A*). This device uses the cornea as a fiberoptic channel. Fine corneal edema and epithelial bedewing can also be demonstrated and are seen as a stippling of the epithelium. They are best seen in the shadow of retroillumination (Fig. 17-3).

The best antidote to corneal edema is a gas-permeable lens. This becomes most important with lenses with high refractive errors and thick centers (plus lenses), or thick edges (mi-

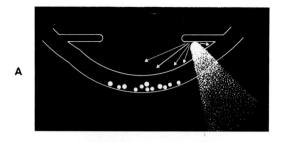

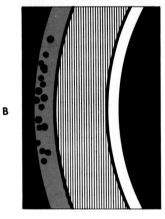

Fig. 17-3. A, Fine corneal edema. This is best appreciated through retroillumination. **B,** The corneal epithelium has a stippled appearance.

nus lenses), which are prone to cause corneal edema.

If a PMMA lens is used, the following points must be checked:

1. Is the lens warped? Check your Radiuscope findings.
2. Is the lens centered? Displacement can occur with blinking or eye movement. When this occurs, the lens, which normally rests on the central spheric portion of the cornea, is shifted to the flatter more ellipsoid section. The fit is then imperfect and molding of the cornea is a common complication.
3. Is the lens tight? Remember that small thin lenses are designed to be a little tight. A different lens may be needed.
4. Any change greater than 0.50 D in comparison with the amount found before a contact lens fitting is considered significant. Usually the K readings are steeper and may be blurred.

Burning. If burning occurs soon after the lenses have been inserted, it probably means that the lens is dirty or that the wetting agent used is irritating the eye. However, if the burning occurs after several hours of wear, it invariably suggests a poorly fitted lens or faulty blinking patterns. Burning is the symptom of equivalent of corneal edema and is a complaint to which one must pay attention.

Spectacle blur. This is such a common finding after wearing rigid lenses that it has been accepted as being a normal sequela of lens removal. However many authorities now believe that spectacle blur in excess of 0.50 D is symptomatic of a marginal fit. The thicker the lens, the greater will be the severity and duration of blur. Also, the larger the lens diameter, the more prominent spectacle blur is. It may be caused by corneal molding induced by the presence of a massive lens—certainly a microthin lens is less likely to cause spectacle blur of any consequence. The usual duration is variable. It may be present only a few minutes to half an hour, or it may persist for hours after the lenses have been removed.

Excessive spectacle blur of the type that lasts hours is usually caused by excessive corneal edema created by the presence of a poorly fitting lens (Fig. 17-4). Such a patient should be seen at the end of the day and examined for corneal edema, changes in the K readings, alterations in the refraction (the tendency is invariably toward being more myopic). Spectacle blur of this intensity should not be accepted as minor deviation of a normal lens event.

The tear exchange must be improved and appropriate alterations in the lens made depending on whether the lens is too flat, tight, and so on. Persistent flattening of the cornea by a poorly fitted lens can induce permanent changes in the corneal curvature. For those fitters whose sole interest is safely fitting corneal lenses this sequela should be regarded as a grave complication. The nuisance value of spectacle blur to the patient is one of the major drawbacks to rigid lens wear.

Corneal edema causes an increase in the radius of curvature of the cornea and produces a refractive change in the direction of myopia. It occurs most often with large-diameter PMMA lenses.

Spectacle blur from corneal edema can be resolved with the use of a gas-permeable lens. In some cases, the relief is dramatic. The wearer

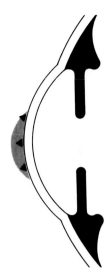

Fig. 17-4. Spectacle blur. With a rigid lens corneal edema is confined to the corneal cap, which results in a radical change of the corneal curvature. The location of the edema is central whether the lens is fitted steep or flat. Upon removal of a poorly fitted rigid lens there is often noticeable spectacle blur because of an increase in myopia.

can read or watch television within minutes of removing the lenses. This asset is one of the main features of a gas-permeable lens system.

Not all spectacle blur can be removed. In the higher grades of refractive errors, the aberration of spectacles in itself causes blurring of vision and discomfort. Nothing can be done about this type of spectacle blur. The person with a −8 D prescription will find the quality of vision poor regardless of the permeability of the lens or its fitting when the switch is made to glasses. That person will suffer chromatic aberration, spheric aberration, restriction of visual fields, image minification with myopic lenses, and parallax because the spectacle lens does not move with the eye. It is helpful to warn patients with large refractive errors of this spectacle-induced disturbance because they may harbor the notion that their prescription is incorrect.

With a PMMA lens, there are solutions to the problem of excessive spectacle blur.

To increase the tear exchange, a fitter can do the following:

1. Reduce the diameter of the lens
2. Blend the lenses
3. Flatten and extend the peripheral curve.
4. Switch to a microthin lens.

The easiest modification is to flatten the curvature of the peripheral curve.

Blending the junction between the optic zone and peripheral curve is effective, but this method reduces the size of the optic zone. Reducing the optical zone may cause flare if the

original lens was selected with the smallest optic zone.

The treatment of spectacle blur is important because it enables the patient to switch more comfortably from one system to the other. For the new patient, it is alarming that the new contact lenses have impaired visual acuity with spectacles.

Comment. The best solution to aggravating spectacle blur is a gas-permeable lens.

Mucus formation on lenses. This is a common complaint and has a variety of causes, none of which are too serious. Eyeliner, mascara, and lash thickeners, especially those that are water insoluble, can cake on the surface of the lens. Although the lens fitter is not supposed to be a beautician, it is helpful to warn female patients to keep their eyeliner behind the lash line, to confine the mascara to the outer half of the eyelashes, and to use water-soluble products. At times a poor edge of the lens can cause lid irritation and hypersecretion from the meibomian glands. Such a lens will appear greasy and coated, as though there is a film over it. Patients will usually complain of some discomfort and a lack of clarity. Frequently they will take their lenses out two or three times a day to try and clean them. With this kind of history the lens periphery must be suspect and the junction zones checked with the profile analyzer.

At times mucus secretions may be whipped into a froth by the fluttering action of the lids.

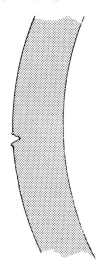

Fig. 17-5. A scratch consists of a ridge and a gutter. Only the ridge is removed with polishing.

This froth has the appearance of foamy, translucent bubbles and is seen around the lens edge.

A surface scratch, which consists of a ridge and a gutter (Fig. 17-5), can also irritate the lid. The lid is annoyed by the ridge, which can be eliminated with polishing. Too many gutters, however, require that a new lens be made because they fill up with debris and impair the transparency of the lens. It should be remembered that polymethylmethacrylate is more vulnerable to scratching than even the poorest grades of glass. However it is firmer than gaspermeable lenses are.

Imperfect lens edges account for more problems than any other defect. They can cause corneal abrasions, lid irritation, excessive meibomian gland secretion and dirty lenses, pronounced photophobia, and decreased lens tolerance (Figs. 17-6 and 17-7). The edges should be tapered so that they glide smoothly under the upper lid. The direction should be slightly posterior to prevent edge stand-off and displacement by the blinking lid. If the edge is too posterior (close to the corneal epithelium), tear exchange will be hampered.

Other complications with hard lenses

Toric or irregular cornea. Large amounts of astigmatism can be induced by a lens that is warped or fits poorly. Sometimes the astigmatism lasts for months and occasionally is per-

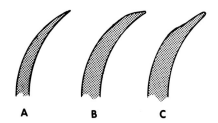

Fig. 17-6. Imperfect edges. **A,** Too sharp; **B,** too blunt; **C,** below center with lenticular ridge.

manent. The best treatment is prophylaxis. K readings of the cornea should be checked regularly, and quality control inspections of the contact lens for warpage should be done.

Persistent corneal edema. This is probably the most frequent complication and causes persistent redness around the limbus, flare, photophobia, haziness of vision as the day wears on, excessive and intolerable spectacle blur, and corneal erosion.

The presence of corneal edema is a sign of a poorly fitted lens, which must be corrected. Gross edema of the type that produces a gray blot on the apical zone of the cornea usually demands attention. Patients can tolerate corneas with microcystic edema indefinitely. They shorten their wearing time, take one or two breaks during the day, and glumly accept the murky vision of excessive spectacle blur. The fitter often tries to ignore such cases or treat them marginally. Such patients are told that the corneal edema will get better with time, are given a variety of drops ranging from vasoconstrictors to tear substitutes, or have their lenses fenestrated (the latter frequently works but does not deal directly with the cause). Any corneal edema causing a steepening of the K figures greater than 1.00 D requires reassessment.

Perhaps one of the most common forms of persistent corneal edema is 3 and 9 o'clock staining. These wedge-shaped corneal erosions at the nasal and temporal margins of the cornea may be indicative of a tightly fitted lens, inadequate blinking, or poor tears. It may occur when everything seems to be normal. Treatment is directed against the precise cause and, if no cause is found, consists in the use of tear substitutes. Some fitters ignore the problem because it may not disturb the patient or go on to ulcer proportions.

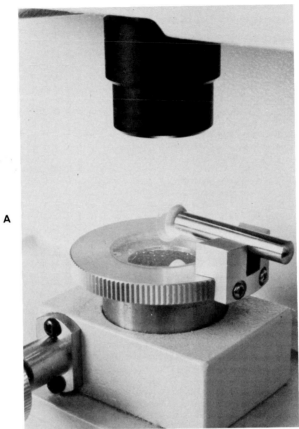

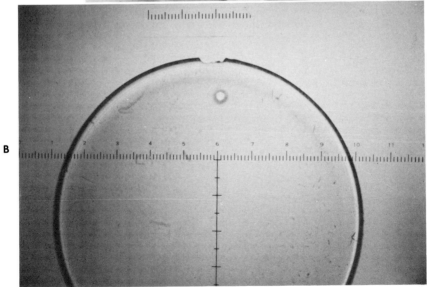

Fig. 17-7. A, Lens in position for inspection with shadowgraph. **B,** Chipped edge seen through shadowgraph.

Extremely rare complications. Some extremely rare complications that are frequently discussed because of their serious nature include the following:

Permanent loss of vision. This has been reported in only 14 eyes by Dixon. It is an extremely rare contingency with which most authorities will deny having any experience.

Keratoconus. It has not been proved that contact lenses cause keratoconus, but keratoconus can progress in a person who has the disease and who is wearing lenses.

Corneal ulcers. This is rare and usually unrelated to the lenses. The most common ulcer detected is a dendritic figure caused by the herpes simplex virus.

Endophthalmitis. Although we have never had a patient with this disease, it frightens us enough to demand strict hygiene from our patients and never to lose respect for possible serious contamination.

CHECKING THE OLD LENSES—A MUST!

It is important to check the old lenses. The profile analyzer is perhaps the most important piece of equipment for verification of the blend. Improper edges, though, are the most common cause of lens intolerance. The optic spherometer (Radiuscope) is useful to obtain the radius of curvature of the lens and to check for warpage. Warpage can be detected on the Radiuscope by noting that the line patterns do not come into focus at the same plane. Other parameters should also be checked, including the power, diameter, and thickness of the lens.

The next step is to check the fit of the lenses on the cornea. If the fit of the lens is grossly off, this will be obvious. At times, however, the fit is a little tight or a little loose and the fitter is not positive if anything is really wrong. It is helpful then to assess the patient only after the lenses have been worn for several hours. By that time there may be a little more corneal edema, and the situation may be easier to appraise. It is important to keep in mind that the adequacy of a lens-cornea relationship may be related to the movement of the lids. The blinking pattern should be analyzed. The symptoms of a tight lens that shows little movement may be caused by incomplete blinking motions.

Tight lens. A tight lens is a lens that hugs the cornea too tenaciously and shows little move-

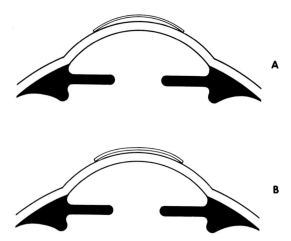

Fig. 17-8. A, Tight lens—base curve is too steep. **B,** Peripheral curves flattened—apical vault effect is decreased.

ment with blinking. The fluorescein pattern typically shows a dark band around or near the periphery of the lens with pooling in the center. A person wearing such a lens may be comfortable in the morning, but as the day progresses he or she develops hazy vision, burning sensations, and an inability to tolerate the lens during the day. When the lens is finally removed, it is frequently a struggle because the lens clings strongly to the cornea.

It is important to distinguish between a tight lens and a steep fit. The two are not always synonymous. A steep fit may be normal, as with microthin lenses, or may cause symptoms of a tight lens because either the peripheral or primary base curve impinges on the cornea.

Some causes of a tight lens include the following:

Steep base curve. When the base curve of the lens is much steeper than the corresponding radius of curvature of the corneal cap (Fig. 17-8), such a lens requires replacement with a flatter base curve. Because this solution is expensive and requires a new lens, many fitters prefer to make adjustments to the original lens. The peripheral curves are flattened and widened, and additional blending is often helpful. This technique works if the apical vault is great, since widening of the peripheral curves allows the lens to settle closer to the surface of the cornea (Fig. 17-9).

Reducing the diameter of the lens accom-

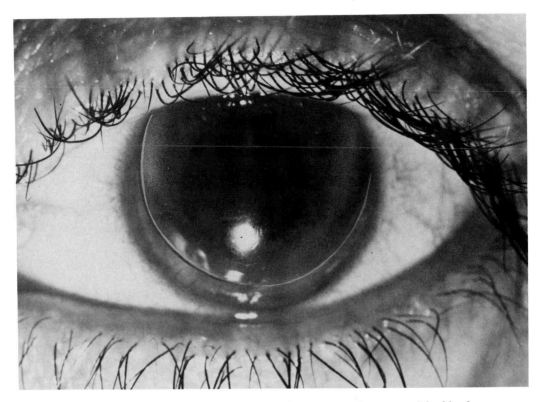

Fig. 17-9. Tight lens with compression of the cornea in the region of the blend.

plishes the same thing. Each time a lens is made smaller, one must add new peripheral curves to alleviate some of the stricture of a tight lens.

Steep peripheral curves. In this case there is minimal apical vault but tear exchange is hampered by steep peripheral curves (Fig. 17-10). The remedy is simple—the peripheral curves must be widened and flattened.

Decentered lens. When a lens is decentered, the optic zone of that lens is usually displaced to a flatter area of the cornea. The infringement of the steeper optic zone to a flatter corneal periphery results in a poor fit because of the trapping of tears under the center of the lens. A steep zone of the lens displaced to a flat area on the cornea is always noticeable; however, if the infringement is intermittent, the patient may tolerate it.

If a lens is decentered, it will cause tight-fitting symptoms. However tight symptoms can also occur when a lens that is too loose has been decentered. This can occur with a lens fitted too flat or displaced by a toric cornea.

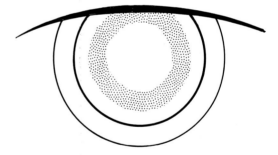

Fig. 17-10. Steep peripheral curve with absence of fluorescein staining in the periphery.

Too large a lens. An increase in the diameter of a lens increases the apical vaulting and makes the fit tighter. Reduction in lens diameter is a simple modification.

Infrequent and inadequate blinking movements. If blinking is incomplete or infrequent, the normal tear exchange and oxygenation of cornea will not take place. A lens normally moves with the action of a blinking lid. The upper lid pushes the lens down as the lid is lowered and then raises it up several millimeters

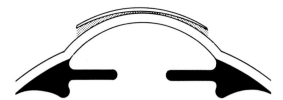

Fig. 17-11. Flat lens. Note concave meniscus of tears, edge stand-off, which allows for easy displacement by the lid, and minimal apical clearance.

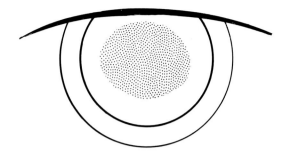

Fig. 17-12. Large central touch indicative of a flat lens.

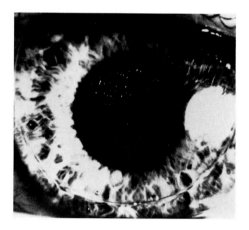

Fig. 17-13. Punctate staining of the cornea after flat-fitting lens is removed. (From Stein, H.A., and Slatt, B.J.: The ophthalmic assistant, ed. 4, St. Louis, 1983, The C.V. Mosby Co.)

as the lid is lifted. If the lid does not blink properly, the lens will not move sufficiently and there will be stagnation of tears. Such a lens, showing relatively little movement, will behave like a tight lens and give rise to tight symptoms. Blinking exercises are an even simpler remedy than office modifications of a lens in this situation.

Loose lens. A loose lens does not conform to the cornea because it is either too flat or too small in diameter and as a result moves too freely on the cornea.

Such a lens may be tolerated initially, but eventually the excessive movement or the apical corneal compression causes problems. Excessive lens movement leads to flare, intermittent hazy vision, and frustration from a lens frequently decentering or actually popping out of the eye. People with marginally flat lenses lose them with the slightest provocation (Fig. 17-11), including yawning, coughing, laughter, or a swift slap on the back by a well wisher. The weight of the lens bearing down on the corneal cap may cause a burning sensation after prolonged lens wear, foggy vision, and severe spectacle blur after the lenses have been removed (Figs. 17-12 and 17-13).

A lens may be loose because the peripheral and secondary curves are too wide or the optic zone is too wide. A lens made inordinately thick may also fit too loosely on the cornea. The primary base curve may be too flat, in which case a new lens is required.

Smaller diameter lenses can be worn with good movement patterns, but the lenses must be fitted steeper than normal to compensate.

The correction of a flat lens requires a new lens with steeper base curves and peripheral curves.

If the diameter of the lens is too small, it should be increased to improve stability and centration. A larger-diameter lens is more likely to be hidden by the upper lid so that it is less likely to be jarred out of position by the margin of the lid.

The symptoms of corneal edema, which occur with any poorly fitting lens whether flat or steep, are photophobia, burning, hazy vision, and excessive spectacle blur.

For a large-diameter lens of high refractive error that is too loose or too tight, a gas-permeable lens is the best solution. A gas-permeable lens can be fitted tighter because of its permeability. Its larger diameter leads to centration and retardation of lens movement, which checks the faults of a loose lens.

Low-riding lens. A low-riding lens may cause

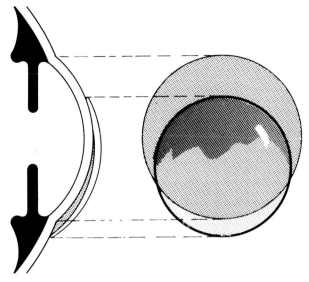

Fig. 17-14. Low-riding lens. Note vascular compression in the limbal region, corneal touch at the superior portion of the lens, and a wedge-shaped prism of tears with the base downward.

tight symptoms because of the inferior displacement of the optic zone if there is a lack of adequate movement, resulting in tear stagnation (Fig. 17-14). The lens can also irritate the lower lid by mechanically abutting against it with each successive blink. If the lens drops below the limbus at the 6 o'clock position, it can create vascular compression. Such a lens is uncomfortable to wear and is optically undesirable.

The most common cause of low-riding lenses is a thick, heavy, plus lens such as that prescribed for the ordinary aphakic patient. Not only is the lens weighted down by gravity, but also the convex anterior peripheral curve does not give the upper lid a proper edge to lift it. A low lens is frequently a lens that is flat or too small. Low lenses are common with patients with exophthalmos or just very prominent eyes. In such cases the lens diameter must be increased to permit more upper lid traction.

In large, flat, aphakic eyes the lens of choice is a lenticulus with a minus carrier. If the cornea is steeper than 45.00 D, a small-diameter, 7.8 mm, thin lens can be employed. For ordinary high-plus lenses, +3.00 D or greater, a microthin lens is frequently a satisfactory solution to the problem of a low-riding lens. Stronger powers can be added without making the lens heavy and bulky.

High-riding lens. Like all displaced lenses a high-riding lens suffers from a steep optic zone of a lens resting on a relatively flatter corneal periphery or even a limbal zone.

The most common cause of a high-riding lens is a high-minus lens that has a relatively prominent concave anterior surface. The periphery of the lens, which is similar to an hourglass, presents a ridge that is easily grasped by the upper lid.

Other causes include pronounced astigmatism with the rule and a high lower lid. A flat lens can be displaced upward, and a steep lens with a large optic zone may also ride high. The correction of this problem is not easy. The many solutions are indicative of the complexity of the situation and not of its simplicity.

Reducing the lens diameter seems to be the most direct route. Unfortunately this tactic often aggravates the condition and makes the lens ride even higher. This occurs because the lens is lighter and is more easily pulled up by the traction of the upper lid. Also the movement of a lens upward is basically stopped by the lens riding on a flatter peripheral area of the cornea or sclera. Therefore, if two lenses of different diameters have their upper most edge riding to the same point, it is apparent that the smaller-diameter lens will show a larger upward decentration than the larger lens will.

Incorporating a prism ballast, which makes the lens heavier, tends to bring it down. If this is combined with reducing the peripheral bevel on the periphery of a myopic lens, grasp of the upper lid is reduced. As a result gravitational effect of the lens is increased while the lifting power is minimized.

This is a good solution for high-riding minus lenses. A minus edge can be converted to a plus edge, that is, from a concave to a convex surface. This is called a plus-carrier lenticular lens.

If the cause is a pronounced astigmatism with the rule, a bitoric lens may be needed, though frequently a large-diameter spheric lens works as well but without the attendant troubles of a toric lens.

Patients with high lower lids usually have small palpebral apertures. A small, microthin lens is most helpful for this sort of problem.

It is important to recognize that a high-riding lens is not a single entity. At times trial and error must be used to correct the cause of it. For instance, reducing the diameter of the lens can make it better or, paradoxically, worse.

The high-riding lens is not a problem for the gas-permeable lens because it is designed to fit that way. The problem with these types of lens usually is a central or even low fitting position. When the lenses are low, 3 and 9 o'clock staining is intense and the lenses cause great discomfort. In such cases, the diameter may have to be reduced to allow the lids to lift the lens. Another solution is to fit the lens flatter to promote wider lens excursions so that the lens can be carried upward to the superior limbus.

Horizontally displaced lens. The most common cause of a nasal or temporal displacement of a lens is astigmatism against the rule (Fig. 17-15). If the astigmatism is 2.00 D or less, a spheric lens fitted steeper than K by 1.00 D is often enough to remedy the problem. For added stability and centration a large lens with a large optic zone should be employed.

Since there are no clear-cut numbers as to how much steeper than K is right for an individual patient or how large is large with respect to diameter, the simplest approach is to simply use trial spheric lenses. If a spheric lens will not become centered, a toric one must be employed. Again a gas-permeable lens is probably the best solution.

Edges—how to assess them. The treatment

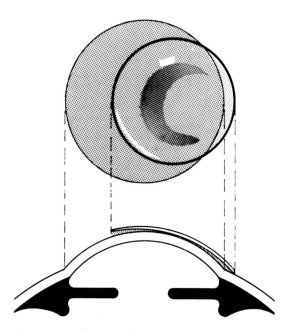

Fig. 17-15. A horizontally displaced lens caused by +2.25 D astigmatism against the rule. Note edge stand-off on the corneal side, limbal compression, and flat fit with paracentral corneal touch.

of the edge of the lens becomes more important with the use of gas-permeable lenses. These lenses are made large in diameter, 9.2 mm or greater, as opposed to a small microthin rigid lens, which may be 7.8 mm. Not only is there a 40% increase in the mass of the lens, but also the edges become very thick in the process.

A myopic profile on the anterior surface must be placed on lenses of a high-plus nature of plus five or over, to reduce the increased edge thickness.

Similarly a plus profile must be used to treat a high-minus lens, that is, −5 D or greater, so that again the edges are treated.

If the edges are not dealt with adequately, the following problems may occur:
1. Lid gap, which results in a very thin tear film at the meniscus of the lens edge.
2. Low-riding lens because of the lids pushing the lens down. This is especially true for high-plus lenses such as aphakic lenses.
3. Three and 9 o'clock staining.
4. Formation of dellen.
5. Discomfort because of lid impact. A blinking upper lid can create considerable pain if it engages a thick lens.

The edges should be checked with the profile analyzer and the shadowgraph with the lens being viewed in profile.

In the silicone-PMMA combinations, the edges are made too thin and they chip and fragment easily.

Good edging is difficult to fabricate because the problem of too little or too much is quite an easy trap to fall into.

Scratches on the lens. In times of frustration in dealing with a complaining patient many fitters will simply clean and polish the lenses and hope for the best. Unfortunately this device works only if there is accumulated mucus, grease, or salt crystals on the surface of the lens or actual scratches in the plastic. It is not a remedy for an ill-fitting lens.

If scratches are abundant, the furrow in the plastic will fill up with foreign debris, causing ocular irritation and hazy vision. A deeply scratched lens can be salvaged by removal of the disturbing ridges that line the furrows; however, if the scratches are very deep, removal of the ridges is not enough because the gutters will continue to collect dirt and foreign matter. In this case a new lens is needed.

Polymethylmethacrylate, the plastic of rigid lenses, is very soft and is more subject to scratching than even the poorest grade of glass. Because of this tendency to scratch, patients should be advised to be very careful with their lenses, especially regarding the following:

1. The lens should not be slid across a surface when one is picking it up.
2. Friction cleaning should be done gently, not vigorously, because this can cause scratches or warpage.

Gas-permeable lenses are even more prone to scratches because they are softer than PMMA.

Warpage of a lens. Warpage of a lens should be suspect in any patient who has been comfortably wearing lenses and then develops an intolerance to them. One can detect its presence by checking the lens curvature for cylinder with either an optic spherometer or a keratometer. Frequently the signs of warpage are gross and can be seen when one holds the naked lens with a smooth forceps in front of a good light source. If the plastic is internally fractured, the site of disruption in the lens looks frosted, like a series of crisscrossing translucent lines or a single, linear break. This dis-

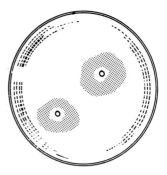

Fig. 17-16. Fenestrations only reduce corneal edema in a 1 to 2 mm zone around the aperture.

ruption of the plastic can be appreciated when one holds the lens under an incandescent light.

The most common cause of warpage is rough handling. Frequently an edge is internally cracked as it is pulled out of its container. Excessive pressure in the lens with cleaning can also cause ruptures in the plastic. Other causes include grasping a dropped lens between the thumb and index finger and excessive squinting with the lens in place. Occasionally a microthin lens can be reversed and then popped back. This not only disrupts the lens but also causes considerable warpage.

Lenses should be replaced if the warpage is creating residual astigmatism and visual difficulties or symptoms of corneal compression. If the warpage is excessive—greater than 0.50 D—lens replacement should be done to prevent induced corneal molding.

Warpage of a lens can mold a cornea to a toric shape. This can occur with large-diameter, thick lenses but is extremely unlikely with microthin lenses.

The other factor that causes induced toricity of the cornea is corneal edema. A soft cornea is more easily molded by a bulky ill-fitting lens.

Fenestrated lens. The prime purpose of fenestration in a lens is to make a marginal fit tolerable. It is particularly useful in a tight lens. The apertures serve to diminish the suction-cup effect created by a blinking lid pressing on a lens that is vaulting the cornea. It does not affect materially the presence of cornel edema. *In fact it only eliminates corneal edema in a 1 mm zone surrounding the hole* (Fig. 17-16).

Most commercial fenestrations are drilled on a finished lens. If they are not done properly, they can affect the optic properties of the lens. If the fenestrations are not finished, they can

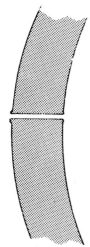

Fig. 17-17. An unfinished fenestration with a burr of plastic at the margin of the hole.

cause corneal abrasions resulting from irregular burs of plastic (Fig. 17-17).

The aperture should be straight, with a diameter not exceeding 0.4 mm, and should have a polished surface along its entire length. Apertures larger than 0.4 mm can cause visual blurring, whereas those much smaller tend to plug easily with mucus and debris.

Usually three apertures are adequate. Apertures can be easily drilled into the lens with a fenestration unit that contains drill bits, mounting arbor, dental wax to hold the lens safely, and a countersinking bit for removing burs from the posterior surface of the lens (Fig. 17-18). A fine oil is used to prepare the drill for cutting into the plastic lens without causing the heat to be absorbed by the lens itself. This operation has been popularized by Herschell H. Boyd and Paul Honan, who have been the major advocates of fenestrations. They fit only small, thin lenses and employ only one central fenestration. Four fenestrations is the usual limit. Fenestrations may also be useful in large, lenticular aphakic lenses.

Fenestrations have been receding in popularity as a cure for ill-fitting lenses. No one is really sure how the principle of fenestrations works. Although fenestrations may be helpful occasionally, they may be ruinous for both the patient and the lens if not done properly. We prefer to look for a precise cause for an ill-fitting lens and then treat it rather than drilling the lens full of holes.

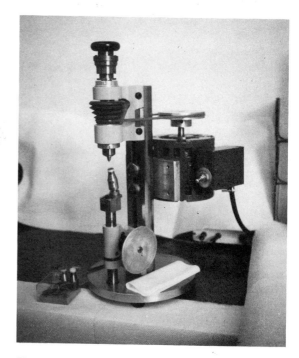

Fig. 17-18. Fenestration drill. There should be no visible cracks dispersing from the drill hole area because of stress caused by the drilling operation.

FITTING PROBLEMS RELATED TO THE CORNEA

The cornea should be assessed for corneal edema and its radius of curvatures checked with the keratometer. If there is corneal edema, the fit of the existing lens may be difficult to assess. An edematous cornea will exaggerate or even distort a preexisting marginally poor fit. For example, if the lens is tight, the edema will be confined to the apical cone of the cornea. When fluorescein is used to evaluate the fit, there will be corneal touch resulting from forward protrusion of the center of the cornea. Such a lens will appear to be fitting flat.

In cases of severe corneal edema the patient should be seen early in the day before the cornea becomes swollen and obscures the normal fitting pattern. The radius of curvature of the cornea should be evaluated in order to determine the presence of induced corneal astigmatism. These figures must be compared to previous K readings to determine the change in corneal curvature.

Corneal edema from an ill-fitting lens can be detected with the following:

1. Slitlamp—using indirect illumination
2. K readings
   a. Change in curvature
   b. Change in the quality of the mires—a muddy pattern with breaks and blurriness
   c. Distortion of the mires
3. Pachometer
4. Retinoscope—an irregular retinoscopy reflex
5. Placido's disc—distortion of the circles on the reflected image of the cornea.

Changes should be picked up when the corneal edema is present—large gray haze in the central area of the cornea, striae of Descemet's membrane, corneal erosions, large swing in the K readings, and pronounced changes in the refractive error to a more myopic correction.

ROLE OF BLINKING IN FITTING PROBLEMS

Patients with an unsatisfactory blink response frequently complain of intolerance to their lenses, especially PMMA lens wearers. The symptoms may be subtle or expressed as a total inability to wear their lenses. Some of the more common complaints include the following:

1. Failure to wear the lens for a full day. The patients can't wait to remove the lenses at 5 or 6 o'clock when they reach home.
2. Inability to wear the lenses for reading, studying, or driving.
3. Tight lens features.
   a. Spectacle blur that is excessive
   b. Burning of the eyes
   c. Grittiness of the eyes
   d. Poor vision
   e. Haloes and fringes around lights
   f. Discomfort and intolerance of the lens.
   g. Whitish strands on the lenses
4. A tendency to remove the lenses three or four times a day to clear them.
5. Excessive photophobia—tinted lenses are worn indoors and outdoors.
6. Discomfort symptoms—burning, irritation, pain with movement of the eyes, and so on.

Ocular signs of poor blinking

1. Erosions of the cornea inferiorly where the blink motion is arrested.
2. Deposits on the lens that is not polished by the action of the lids. With a rigid lens, a whitish film from deposited protein forms a band on the exposed inferior portion of the lens.
3. Features of a tight lens.
   a. Poor movement
   b. Lenses low and not rising properly with a blink motion
   c. Apical corneal edema
   d. Inferior corneal erosions
   e. 3 and 9 o'clock staining
4. Episcleritis and at times formation of dellen.
5. Features of corneal edema.
   a. Change in the quality of the mires of the keratometer
   b. Irregular astigmatism that one best appreciates by noting the distortion of the retinoscopy reflex or alteration of Placido's disc reflection
   c. Slitlamp findings of corneal edema usually best appreciated through indirect or retroillumination
   d. Change in pachometry readings, indicat-

ing corneal edema and increased corneal thickness

6. Dry spots on the corneal surface.

Purpose of blinking exercises

Blinking exercises, which in reality are a series of voluntary lid-closure movements, assist apprehensive patients who are excessively aware of their lenses. By consciously completing a blink patients soon learn to lose their fear of the lens. Also the lids get the feel of the lens and become accustomed to riding over the edge.

To avoid excessive contraction of the lids, the patient is asked to close the eyes slowly and naturally. The index fingers of both hands are placed just lateral to the outer canthi to become aware of any excessively forceful contractions. When the eyelids are closed, the patient is asked to pause for a moment. The eyes are then opened naturally, followed by another small pause before the exercise is resumed.

A series of 10 exercise blinks performed 10 times a day is usually adequate to correct faulty blink patterns. Most faulty blink patterns can be corrected within a week of earnest effort.

A change in the blink rate is not the only reason why many persons with myopia find it difficult to read when they first obtain lenses. Myopic spectacles offer the patient a base in prismatic effect, resulting in a decrease in the need to converge. The greater the refractive error, the greater the prismatic deviation of the spectacle lenses. A person with severe myopia changing to contact lenses frequently feels uncomfortable at first because of the need to converge. There is more accommodative demand from a contact lens compared to a spectacle lens of the same power. Rays of light are diverged by a minus spectacle lens before reaching the cornea, and so more accommodation is required. With contact lenses the convergence of light at the contact lens and the cornea are virtually the same. So a first-time myopic wearer of contact lenses requires more focusing power to read than previously was exerted with spectacle lenses.

If the person experiences hazy vision when reading is first attempted, this may indicate a loss of centration of the lens. When the eyes are lowered in the reading position, the lens may be displaced upward by the margin of the lower lid. This problem can be eliminated when the diameter of the lens is reduced.

Finally differentiation must be made between those patients who had poor blinking habits before wearing their lenses and those with faulty blinking induced by the wearing of lenses. Persons in the latter group are those whose poor blinking habits can be easily corrected by blinking exercises.

USE AND LIMITATIONS OF FLUORESCEIN IN ASSESSING FITTING PROBLEMS

The fluorescein pattern offers the clinician additional information regarding the fit of rigid lenses. A positive test is quite helpful in confirming or supporting a diagnosis of a tight or flat lens. However a normal fluorescein pattern is not necessarily evidence of an adequate tear exchange. It is possible that a patient, seen too early in the day and fit marginally, when first viewed, was shown to have a perfectly acceptable staining pattern. The time of examination may therefore be significant. The fluorescein paper acts as a Shirmer's test No. 1, which promotes reflex tearing in the unanesthetized eye. A flush of tears can certainly change the contact-cornea relationship, especially if the lens was initially slightly tight. There is no standard fluorescein test. A microthin lens is normally fitted much steeper than a conventional-sized or large lens, and so what is normal for one lens may be abnormal for another. In view of these drawbacks many authorities regard the presence of corneal edema detected by slitlamp examination as a better sign of poor tear exchange. It is undoubtedly more reliable, and there are still diagnostic clues provided by this simple, rapid test that cannot be determined in any other way.

A good method to apply fluorescein is to add a drop of anesthetic to the dry, sterile, fluorescein-impregnated paper and touch it to the upper sclera. This minimizes reflex tearing, and there is better control of the amount of fluorescein liberated. A single drop of fluorescein is adequate.

Take care to avoid dripping fluorescein on the patient's clothing because it stains vividly and is extremely difficult to remove.

Fluorescein in solution form is rarely used today because it has been shown to support the growth of *Pseudomonas aeruginosa*.

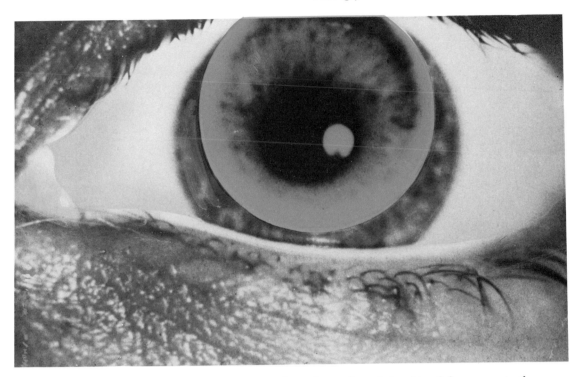

Fig. 17-19. Normal lens pattern. The pattern depends on the relationship of the cornea to the diameter and base curve.

The following are staining patterns associated with various lens characteristics:

Normal-lens-pattern lens with slight apical vault (Fig. 17-19). There is a slight vault over the apical zone of the cornea with slight central pooling with an absence of stain in the intermediate area. The peripheral portion of the lens should have a pooling of stain, indicating that the edge is standing off from the cornea.

Lens fitted too flat (Fig. 17-20). Typically with a flat lens there is apical touch with little fluorescein in the area of contact. The lens may also be decentered, a common finding with a flat lens. In this case the apical zone was too small. A large optic zone steepens a lens, whereas a smaller optic zone flattens it. This error was corrected by increasing the size of the optic zone from 6 to 7.3 mm. No other changes were made. There was apical staining of the cornea after the lens was removed.

Lens fitted too steep. The classic picture of a tight lens is central pooling with an intermediate or peripheral zone of touch (Fig. 17-21). In this case the lens is also decentered. A steep lens does not ensure centration; the centration was corrected by adjustment of the blend.

Astigmatic fit (Fig. 17-22). Characteristically there is a band-shaped area of touch on the flattest meridian. The degree of astigmatism was 6.00 D in this case, which is frequently too much for a spheric lens to vault. Over 3.00 D of astigmatism usually requires a toric lens.

Lens diameter too large (Fig. 17-23). The lens is in contact with both upper and lower lids with the eye in the primary position, and there is some central pooling. A large lens is effectively a steep lens and will present essentially the same fluorescein pattern. Note the frothing superiorly.

Lens diameter too small (Fig. 17-24). This lens is too small in diameter; as a result it is carried too high on the cornea by the action of the lid.

Foreign-body stain (Fig. 17-25). A false eyelash became trapped under the lens and created a typical abrasion.

Decentered lens (Fig. 17-26). The decentered lens overrides the flatter peripheral portion of the cornea and the limbus. This lens was too flat.

Ultrathin lens pattern (Fig. 17-27). The lens is fitted steeper than K, which is acceptable with

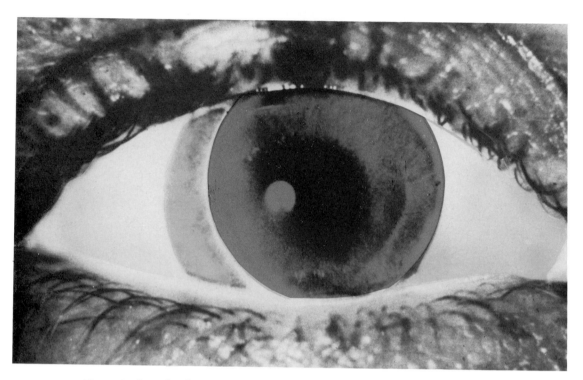

Fig. 17-20. Lens fitted too flat. This lens moves excessively and is easily displaced.

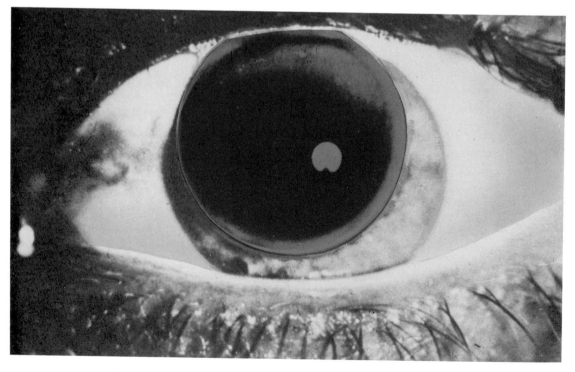

Fig. 17-21. Lens fitted too steep. Peripheral pooling, no apical stain.

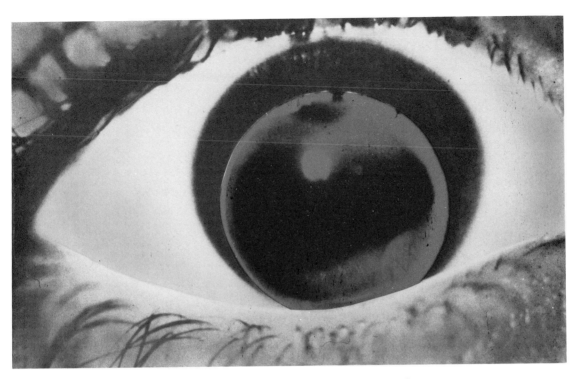

Fig. 17-22. Astigmatic fit. A band-shaped area of touch is characteristic.

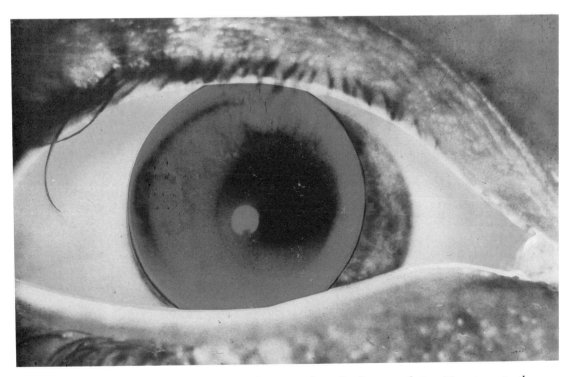

Fig. 17-23. Lens diameter too large. This lens is too large for the corneal size. More importantly, it is too large for the size of the palpebral fissures. The lens should not extend from lid to lid.

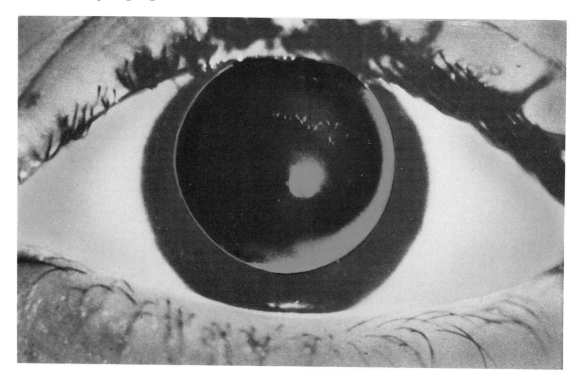

Fig. 17-24. Lens diameter too small. This lens showed too much movement. The looseness of the fit was improved by fitting with a larger diameter lens. The patient complained of streaming of lights because the size of the optic zone of the lens was too small to cover the pupil of the eye, which became semidilated in dim illumination.

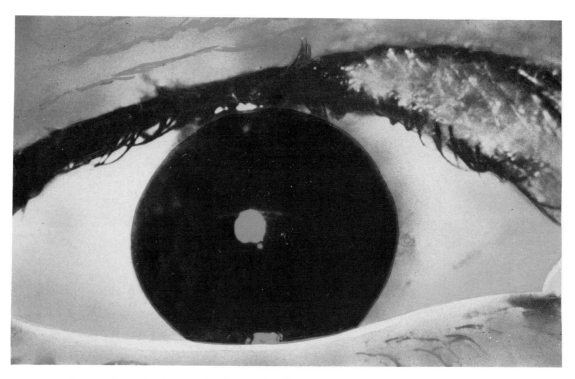

Fig. 17-25. Foreign body stain. An arc-like abrasion was caused by a small foreign body.

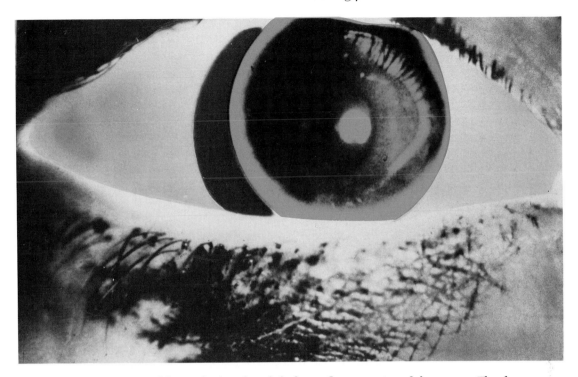

Fig. 17-26. Decentered lens. The lens has shifted to a flatter portion of the cornea. The decentered lens then acts as a tight-fitting lens. Flare is also a problem because the optic zone no longer covers the pupil.

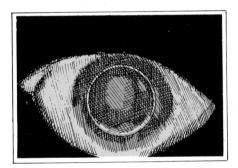

Fig. 17-27. Microthin lens fitted steeper than K. The ring of fluorescein around the lens is indicative of a very steep fit.

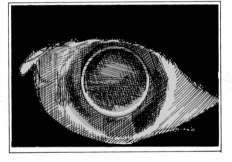

Fig. 17-28. The fluorescein pattern shows some central touch and pooling at the periphery of the lens because of the steep peripheral curves.

such a lens. The central pooling indicates a steep fit, which is present and, in this case, desirable.

Lens fitted on K (Fig. 17-28). A slight accumulation of fluorescein is present centrally. As with all microthin lenses a definite band of fluorescein is found at the position of the peripheral curve, which normally is fitted steep. This fitting pattern is also acceptable.

Abnormal staining patterns (Fig. 17-29)

Corneal edema from either a steep or flat lens is invariably central in location. It can create stippling, punctate staining, and central corneal hazing, which results from edema in the corneal cap.

Mechanical abrasions from foreign bodies create irregular superficial epithelial scratches. If the lens is fitted too flat, a central abrasion

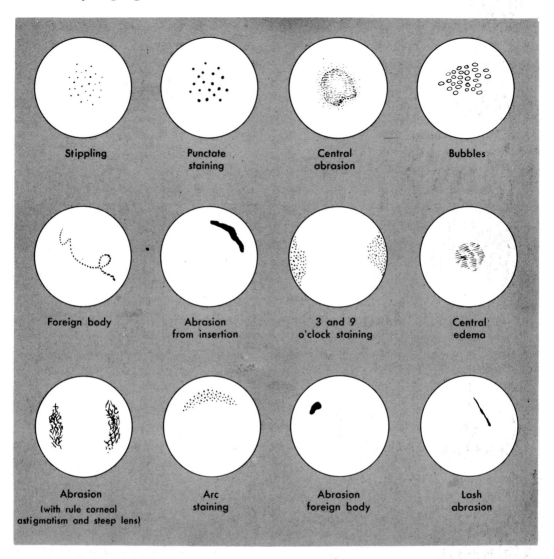

Fig. 17-29. Abnormal staining patterns. Notice that stippling, punctate staining, central edema, and central abrasion are largely apical and caused by an ill-fitting polymethylmethacrylate lens. (From Stein, H.A., and Slatt, B.J.: The ophthalmic assistant, ed. 4, St. Louis, 1983, The C.V. Mosby Co.)

will occur because the area of central clearance becomes converted to central touch, and compression of the cornea occurs. If the blend is too sharp or the peripheral curve too steep, the imprint of this poor fit leads to arcuate staining.

In 3 and 9 o'clock staining, a triangular wedge of corneal staining appears at the margins of the cornea.

There are several causes of the finding of 3 and 9 o'clock staining.

Lid gap. A lid gap occurs largely with large-diameter rigid lenses. It is particularly prone to

occur with gas-permeable lenses whose edges have not been reduced in size.

A gap occurs between the margin of the lens and the cornea. The meniscus of tears becomes very thin or absent at this border. It is a lens-induced dry spot.

The degree of staining is intense and often associated with episcleritis and even formation of dellen. It is particularly prone to occur with lenses that are low, that is, not brought up to a high position with a blink.

Low-riding lenses. Poor lid adherence may be a factor in causing a low-riding lens that results in 3 and 9 o'clock staining. If the lens is low, the lens should be made flatter, thinner at the edges, or smaller in diameter.

At times, the lens will rise with a blink and then suddenly drop to a low position. Such a lens requires a little alteration; flattening the blend and peripheral curves will frequently solve the problem.

Poor blinking. The incomplete blinker dehydrates the exposed position of the eye—the 3 and 9 o'clock portion. The lines of protein dehydration across the lens indicates its presence.

Treatment is blinking exercises.

Poor tear film. A poor tear film occurs with people with an insufficient tear film to support a large-diameter lens.

With these people, supplementary tears during the day and a bland ointment at night (such as Duratears) may be enough to remedy the problem.

The staining of the cornea is caused by desiccation of the corneal epithelium and not by corneal hypoxia.

CHAPTER 18

COMPLICATIONS OF RIGID LENSES

Keratoconus—a complication of contact lens wear?

Corneal edema

Corneal staining

Vascularization

Prolonged lens pressure

Loss of corneal sensitivity

Acute corneal crisis (overwear reaction)

Care-related problems

High-altitude risks

Inclusion blennorrhea

Birth control pill intolerance

There is no doubt that contact lens can cause complications despite the flippant way they are regarded by the media, some of the commercial optical shops, and the general public. Contact lens are advertised as a commodity, no different from shoes. It is no wonder that people are lax in their contact lens hygiene. They have no respect for the device.

Most serious ocular complications occur as a result of neglect. Failure to clean the cases in which the lens are stored can result in the growth of *Pseudomonas aeruginosa*, a virulent organism that can penetrate a small corneal ulcer and cause endophthalmitis. In 1 year, when rigid lens complications were surveyed, 14 eyes went blind and a few required enucleation because of total loss of ocular function and severe pain. This calamity was the result of infection from dirty cases and contaminated lenses. Dirty hands, dirty fingernails, dirty contact lens cases, dirty habits such as using saliva as a wetting agent, and failure to change soaking solutions on a regular basis are the most common causes of serious ocular infections.

Perhaps a warning message should be printed on each contact lens case stating that "contact lenses may be damaging to the eye if a strict hygienic procedure is not carried out."

KERATOCONUS—A COMPLICATION OF CONTACT LENS WEAR?

An area of controversy is whether keratoconus can be caused by a contact lens. Most contact lens fitters do not believe that it is possible. The increased incidence among contact lens wearers is probably attributable to the fact that the early symptoms of keratoconus may be progressive myopia. Both myopia and keratoconus begin in teen-agers. Most corneal edema in rigid-lens wearers is apical in location—on the corneal cap. Keratoconus usually is decentered, inferiorly and nasally, but not in the exact location where corneal edema is detected. Early keratoconus may be accelerated by the wearing of a contact lens, but in our opinion there is insufficient evidence to implicate rigid lenses as a cause of keratoconus.

CORNEAL EDEMA

Corneal edema is probably the most frequent complication and causes persistent redness around the limbus, flare, photophobia, haziness of vision as the day wears on, excessive and intolerable spectacle blur, and corneal erosion.

The presence of corneal edema is a sign of a poorly fitted lens, which must be corrected. Gross edema of the type that produces a gray blot on the apical zone of the cornea usually demands attention. Patients can tolerate corneas with microcystic edema indefinitely. They shorten their wearing time, take one or two breaks during the day, and glumly accept the murky vision of excessive spectacle blur. The fitter often tries to ignore such cases or treat them marginally. Such patients are told that the corneal edema will get better with time, are given a variety of drops ranging from vasoconstrictors to tear substitutes, or have their lenses fenestrated (the latter frequently works

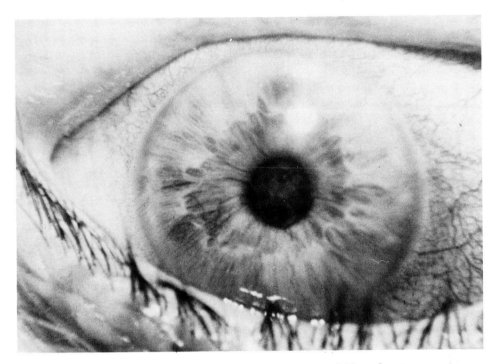

Fig. 18-1. Corneal edema centrally causing pain and blurred vision.

but does not deal directly with the cause). Any corneal edema causing a steepening of the K figures greater than 1.00 D requires reassessment. Corneal edema can assume a variety of forms and cause a variety of troubles for the contact lens wearer (Fig. 18-1).

CORNEAL STAINING

Stippling. Stippling or small dots may arise from lens defects in which there is inadequate tear exchange and so there is stagnation of tears resulting in anoxia to the cornea, heat retention, and inability to dissipate the end products of metabolism from the cornea. Changing the peripheral curve, blending the junctional zones, thinning and rounding the edges, or selecting a more appropriate diameter may correct this problem.

Punctate staining. Punctate staining in large areas may occur at the points of contact of either the edge of the lens, one of the curves of the lens, or the edge of the optic zone. It is a result of compression of the lens on the cornea. The lens may be too flat, have a sharp blend (which needs to be extended), have poor edges or edge profile, or be warped.

Arcuate staining. A poor edge that is not well rounded or one that is too sharp like a knife-edge can cause corneal insult of an arcuate nature. The junctional zones must be smooth and gently float over the peripheral cornea, or it may induce an arcuate staining defect. A lens that constantly decenters and positions itself eccentrically may cause arcuate staining.

3 and 9 o'clock staining. Three and 9 o'clock staining is sometimes referred to as peripheral corneal staining or nasal and temporal staining. It is usually light punctate staining found at the margins of the cornea but may coalesce to form a concentrated area of staining. Inadequate tear film, inadequate blinking, lid tension, and the relationship of the lens edge to the cornea are contributing factors. Redness is usually found adjacent to the area.

The presence of staining in the 3 and 9 o'clock positions of the cornea is regarded by most authorities as being attributable to a dehydration effect on the cornea occurring in this area. The 3 and 9 o'clock staining may be mild or cause a severe episcleritis or even marginal dellen of the cornea with ulcer formation. Physiologically, the mucoid layer from the goblet cells of the conjunctiva does not cover this area of the corneal epithelial cells and permit adequate wetting. It may lead to stromal thinning. This may occur with lacrimal insufficiency, a problem that has to be addressed.

Mild staining is not significant, but more advanced staining will often reduce the patient's wearing time considerably. The use of blinking exercises and artificial tears can lessen this considerably. Redesigning with thinner edges or making the lens large to bridge the defect in the case of gas-permeable lens will often help. With gas-permeable lenses this complication is common and is believed to be a complication of lid gap (drying of the tear film at the margin of a thick lens) and a low-riding lens, which impedes tear flow. To remedy this problem, one may also make the lens smaller with thinner and more polished edges. With gas-permeable lenses, one must thin the edges, that is, using a myopic profile on an aphakic lens, and the lenses must not be permitted to ride low.

VASCULARIZATION

Vascularization can occur because of a number of factors caused by a poor-fitting rigid lens. There may be chronic decentration of a rigid lens that continually rides on the limbus creating a vasogenic effect. This is more troublesome with thick lenses. There may be improper venting of the metabolic products such as lactic acid with its subsequent buildup behind the lens. Improper venting also leads to thermal buildup with a subsequent vascular response. Vascularization of the cornea is more likely to occur with soft lenses, which produce limbus-to-limbus corneal edema, whereas PMMA and gas-permeable lenses create corneal swelling in the corneal cap away from the limbal vasculature.

PROLONGED LENS PRESSURE

When a lens touches centrally on the cornea in any excessive amount, it causes a flattening effect of the apex resulting in a reduction of the myopic refractive error. Slight touching with graduated flattening of the curve of the lens and subsequent changes in the eye are the basis of orthokerotologic treatment. With regular lens fitting, flattening of the cornea is not desirable.

If the pressure area is excessive and the touch area becomes more than slight, there may be degradation in Bowman's membrane with resultant scar formation on a permanent basis. Because of this, moderate apical touch should be avoided with standard PMMA lenses. Slight touch may be valid in keratoconus. Soper-designed PMMA lenses with a deep central curvature permit maximal clearance at the apex. Gas-permeable lenses of the Soper design are one step better because if the cone does progress between visits, with prolonged pressure on the apex, the improved oxygenation of the cornea will prevent degradation of epithelium and Bowman's membrane and preserve corneal integrity.

Undue pressure or irregular corneal pressure on a normal healthy cornea may result in a change in corneal architecture in a manner that may result in astigmatism, not only of the regular type but also of the irregular type. Repeated keratometric monitoring is required for assessment of this phenomenon.

Comment. It seems that we are greatly overemphasizing the subject of induced toricity. In terms of frequency it is true. In terms of the magnitude of the complication on a healthy cornea, we are justified.

LOSS OF CORNEAL SENSITIVITY

The wearing of a rigid PMMA contact lens has been shown to decrease the corneal sensitivity. If a rigid lens is worn for 1 to 2 months, the corneal sensitivity is rapidly regained by overnight removal of the contact lenses. However, if the lenses have been worn for years, it may take several months for the corneas to regain their normal sensitivity. This is probably not a true atrophy of the corneal nerves but an adaptation effect to a constant foreign-body stimulus. Does this decrease in sensation put these patients at risk by eliminating a valuable warning sign of pain? Patients wearing PMMA lenses may have a corneal pathologic condition and not feel it. Included are the findings of 3 and 9 o'clock staining, corneal edema, and induced alteration of corneal topography.

Comment. One curious event of placing gas-permeable lenses on an eye with chronic corneal edema is the resumption of corneal sensation. Patients may initially find the new lenses are more difficult to wear because of an increase in that sensation.

Patience is vital if the lens fits. Otherwise your patient will not view your efforts charitably. If you have exchanged old comfortable PMMA lenses for uncomfortable gas-permeable lenses, the patient will believe that the device is worse than the disease. The patient should be forewarned about this contingency.

ACUTE CORNEAL CRISIS (OVERWEAR REACTION)

An acute corneal crisis is usually related to PMMA lens wear. It is strictly attributable to acute hypoxia of the corneal epithelium. Generally it occurs with a teen-ager who normally wears these lenses till 10 or 11 o'clock and then wears them to 2 or 3 o'clock because of a party or celebration. The normal wearing time is exceeded, and the corneal epithelium cannot tolerate the anoxia for such a length of time.

This condition always seems to begin in the early hours of the morning, several hours after the person has taken out his or her lenses the night before. Invariably there is an early morning phone call from a frightened mother that her child is totally blind and in excruciating pain.

A drop of local anesthetic goes a long way in reducing the patient's discomfort and furthermore in facilitating examination of the cornea. The typical clinical findings are central epithelial erosions, pronounced ciliary injection, swelling of the lids, and constricted pupils.

The cure is dramatic. With bilateral firm patching, an analgesic for pain, a hypnotic to allow the distressed patient to obtain some sleep, and a short-acting cycloplegic to relieve the ciliary spasm, the condition resolves in approximately 24 hours.

After such an occurrence the lens should not be worn for approximately 4 or 5 days until all signs of irritation and corneal edema are gone. A renewed, controlled wearing time is mandatory.

The patient should then be warned about overwearing the lenses. For any casualty of an overwear reaction, a 1-week rest period when renewed wear is established is advisable.

If there is no history of actually overwearing the lens, attention should be directed to reassessment of the fit of the lens. If the lens is slightly steep or flat, it may be tolerated, but not for a full day. This situation is not a true overwear reaction, though from the patient's point of view there is no difference in symptoms.

The best treatment is prophylaxis. The patient should trade these lenses in for oxygen-permeable lenses.

CARE-RELATED PROBLEMS

Scratches and cleaning. Feldman has pointed out that secretions of the meibomian glands will fill in the furrow of a scratched lens and will be difficult to remove because of the raised edge of the furrow. Polishing of these rigid lenses is required to permit adequate cleaning of lipoid material. Lester has suggested that edge buildup of material may be a causative factor in 3 and 9 o'clock staining.

Foreign body under lens. Any person who wears contacts may have a foreign body enter his eye. Because the tear exchange under a hard lens is about 50% to 80% with each blink, it is very easy for a conjunctival foreign body to enter and remain between the lens and cornea. In this position it will usually irritate and frequently scratch the corneal surface.

Of more particular concern is inadequate cleaning of a lens and leaving particulate matter on the inner surface of the contact lens. Not only may the matter act as a physical irritant to the cornea, but also chemicals remaining may cause toxicity to the underlying cornea. Careful washing of one's hands and using recommended care solutions are of utmost importance.

Fingernail scratches. Inadequate insertion technique with long fingernails is a frequent cause of corneal abrasions. This is usually noted by telltale markings on the inferior portion of the cornea. At least 6% of contact lens wearers experience corneal abrasion.

Improper care routines. The gas-permeable rigid lenses of the silicone-PMMA material do not wet well with standard rigid lens solutions. These standard rigid lens solutions will often impair the wetting surface of the newer gas-permeable lenses so that the person wearing these lenses will have blurred vision. One must follow recommended care systems.

Infection. The committee on Contact Lenses of the American Association of Ophthalmology reported in 1966 in the *Journal of the American Medical Association* on 14 eyes lost or blinded in patients wearing contact lenses from a population of almost 50,000 contact lens wearers. There were 157 other eyes permanently damaged in this series, attesting to the serious problems that can be accounted for with contact lenses. All the blinded persons were the result of a serious infectious process, a result of hand-to-eye contamination.

HIGH-ALTITUDE RISKS

People who live in high-altitude locations, such as Denver, Colorado, may experience great difficulty with hard lenses. In all probability the decreased tolerance is directly related to the decreased oxygen content found in high altitudes. Also the relative humidity at 5000 feet is lower than at sea level. The lowered humidity tends to increase the evaporation rate, and protein and salt deposits tend to crust on the surface of the hard lens. In addition to these problems the rare atmosphere allows more infrared and ultraviolet rays to pass through the lens with more intensity. The infrared rays create more heat and more evaporation. A polymethylmethacrylate lens acts as an insulation that raises the oxygen demands of the corneal epithelium. Coupled with the normal hypoxia of a lens covering the cornea, the added stress may be intolerable. The ultraviolet rays can create corneal epithelial irritation under the PMMA lens.

As one would expect, people who wear lenses in high-altitude locations frequently complain of photophobia, grittiness in the eyes, inability to tolerate their lenses for a full day, and burning sensations. Frequently they display superficial punctate staining of the epithelium, dry patches on the cornea, and 3 and 9 o'clock perilimbal congestion and keratopathy. These symptoms and signs frequently disappear when such a person either visits or moves to a low-altitude environment. Stewardesses frequently have trouble with their lenses while in flight. In the Boeing 747, for example, flying at 31,000 feet the cabin is pressurized to equal the pressure of about 5000 feet, whereas at 42,000 feet the cabin pressure is equivalent to an altitude of 7000 feet. Thus the atmospheric pressure is not at sea level. In addition, the air-conditioning system dehydrates the cabin, and so there are less tears to carry oxygen.

For permanent high-altitude dwellers who wear lenses, a reduction in wearing time to a range of 8 to 10 hours must be made. Other approaches include the use of multiple fenestrations, small microthin lenses, and the use of artificial tears during the day. Sometimes rigid lenses must be abandoned and, if the indications are present, soft lenses substituted, which usually are satisfactory.

Skiers do not seem to have any problems with their lenses and in fact enjoy them more while skiing. In all probability this comfort is caused by the increased tear production, stimulated by the cold and wind, and the cooler temperatures that prevent heat accumulation in the lenses. The hypoxia of high altitudes is compensated by the hypothermia, of a cooler environment.

Gas-permeable lens again are an excellent choice for the high-altitude dweller. Not only is the oxygen permeability better but also the thermal conductivity is enhanced. The temperature of the cornea is not raised by the presence of the lens. Regular PMMA acts as an insulator and consequently raises the oxygen demands of the cornea. With silicone-PMMA lenses, there is heat transfer through the lens and the oxygen needs of the cornea are reduced.

Comment. Ski goggles are still required for the protection of the corneas while contact lenses are worn.

INCLUSION BLENNORRHEA

An inclusion blennorrhea is a venereal disease that causes a subclinical infection resulting in follicular conjunctivitis, a few subepithelial infiltrates of the cornea, and a soft, palpable, preauricular node. This condition is tolerable until the patient tries to wear a lens and then suddenly develops symptoms that naturally are blamed on the presence of the lenses. These cases are best treated with sulfonamide drops until the punctate keratopathy and follicles disappear. The duration of the disease can seem to be endless, lasting from 6 weeks to 3 or 4 months, during which time lenses cannot be worn.

BIRTH CONTROL PILL INTOLERANCE

Women who begin wearing lenses and then begin taking birth control pills frequently find that they can no longer tolerate their lenses.

The vision becomes hazy, the wearing time is reduced, and the eyes are unusually sensitive to light. Some authorities believe that this results from a change in the tear film, whereas others who witness a haziness of the keratometer mires believe that there is an alteration to the shape or texture of the cornea itself. Women already on birth control pills usually do not suffer such reactions. Intolerance to the presence of rigid lenses has also been a problem during the early stages of pregnancy.

CHAPTER 19

HOW TO ASSURE YOUR RIGID LENSES ARE WHAT YOU ORDERED

G. PETER HALBERG*

Diameter
Surface quality and edges
Base curve
Power
Central thickness
Surface quality
Blend

If the lens received from the laboratory is faulty or does not conform to the design specifications ordered, the fit of the lens will be poor. No laboratory can mass-produce quality lenses all the time. Fitters must be able to verify the lens not only for their own satisfaction but also to keep the lens laboratory alerted to the fact that its work is being inspected. This helps to raise the standards for everyone concerned.

DIAMETER

The first parameter to be checked is the diameter of the lens. The diameter can be assessed, for rigid lenses, with a diameter gauge (Fig. 19-1). Care should be exercised not to use any force while inserting the lens into the gauge. The lens should fall into the proper position by its own weight. The lens should check in at least two meridians for roundness. It should also be dry, as a wet lens will have a water collar at the edge and will appear larger. The tolerance for diameter should be ±0.05 mm. The diameter of rigid lenses can also be assessed with a measuring loupe, which serves the dual purpose of measuring the diameter and the width of the peripheral and optic zones. In addition the hand loupe serves to assess the surface quality of the lens (Fig. 19-2).

SURFACE QUALITY AND EDGES

A more elaborate and precise check of the surface quality and diameter of the lens can be

*M.D., F.A.C.S., Chairman, International Contact Lens Council of Ophthalmologists; Professor of Clinical Ophthalmology, New York Medical College, New York, New York.

performed with the various projector type of inspection devices available. Typical of these projection devices is the Wesley-Jessen Inspectocon (Figs. 19-3 and 19-4).

Comment. It is important to check the edges, since an imperfect edge is probably the greatest source of discomfort from wearing rigid lenses.

BASE CURVE

The curvature of the lens can be assessed by the Bausch & Lomb keratometer or the CLC Ophthalmometer of the American Optical Corporation (Figs. 19-5 to 19-7). A holder is attached to the keratometer that has a receptacle for the lens and a concave test plate. The lens is held in the well of the holder with an adhesive substance such as clay or cream. An excellent type of holder (called Con-Ta-Check) is one that allows the lens surface to be placed horizontally while the keratometer remains in its normal position. A front-surface mirror placed at a 45-degree angle to the optic axis of the keratometer reflects light from the mires to the lens. For optic purposes it is the same as if the lens were placed in front of the keratometer. By allowing the lens to lie flat, no adhesive substance is needed; this eliminates annoying distortions. The lens is placed so that its convex surface is in contact with the fluid, which can be glycerin, water, or wetting solution. Because the refractive index of the fluid approximates the index of the lens, the convex surface is neutralized and the posterior lens surface is measured.

More reliable inspection and measuring of

Text continued on p. 222.

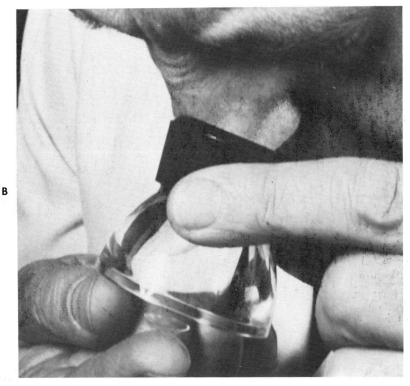

Fig. 19-1. Diameter gauge for rigid lenses.

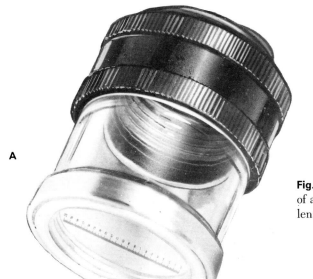

A

Fig. 19-2. **A,** Measuring hand magnifier. **B,** The use of a hand magnifier to inspect a rigid or soft contact lens.

B

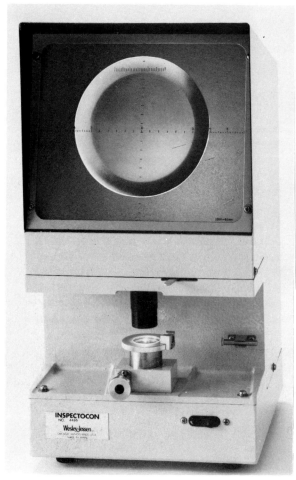

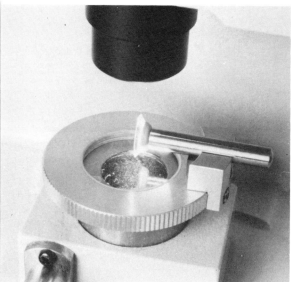

Fig. 19-3. A, Inspectocon projector device. (Courtesy Wesley-Jessen, Chicago.) **B,** Close-up of a lens attached to a suction cup for inspection by Inspectocon projector.

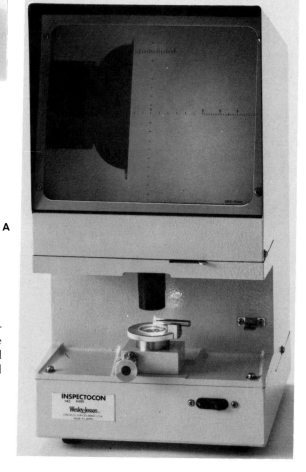

Fig. 19-4. A, Inspectocon projection device has provision for examination of the lens edge in a profile view. **B,** Close-up of the finished edge of a rigid lens. **C,** Shadowgraph projection of a thick blunted rigid lens edge.

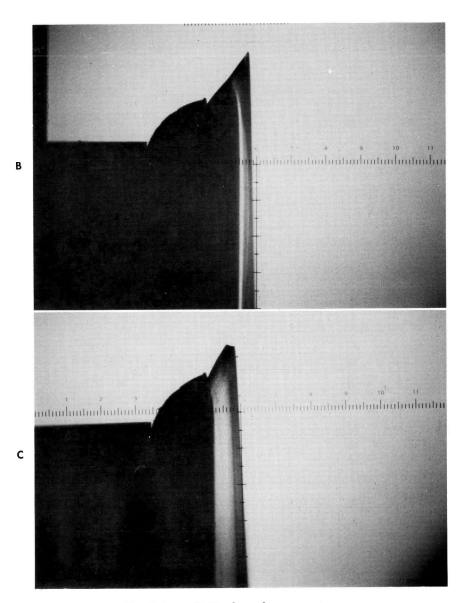

Fig. 19-4, cont'd. For legend see opposite page.

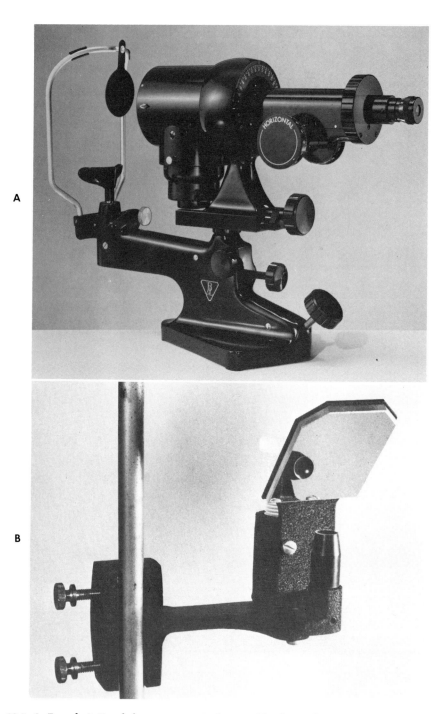

Fig. 19-5. A, Bausch & Lomb keratometer. **B,** Con-Ta-Check attachment for keratometer. (Courtesy Wesley-Jessen, Chicago.)

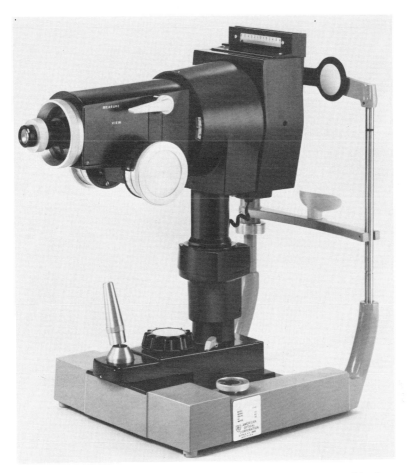

Fig. 19-6. CLC Ophthalmometer. (Courtesy American Optical Corp., Southbridge, Mass.)

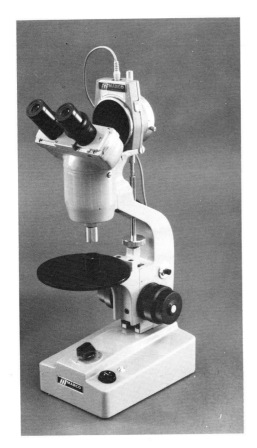

Fig. 19-7. Binocular Digital Radiusgauge optic spherometer for measuring the dioptric power of a contact lens. Note the digital readout. (Courtesy Marco Medical Products, Jacksonville, Fla.)

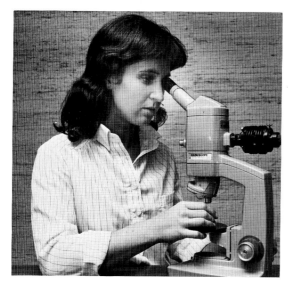

Fig. 19-8. Measuring curvature of a contact lens with the optic spherometer (Radiuscope). (From Stein, H.A., and Slatt, B.J.: The ophthalmic assistant, ed. 4, St. Louis, 1983, The C.V. Mosby Co.)

the lens curvature can be performed with the Radiuscope (American Optical Corporation), Figs. 19-8 and 19-9.

The Contacto Gauge (Fig. 19-10, *A*) works on the same principle as the optic spherometer (Radiuscope, Fig. 19-8) but is lower in price and has the added advantage of a built-in thickness gauge.

Besides being a part of the routine verification of a lens, evaluation of the base curve is the best method for determining warpage. Contented lens wearers who suddenly develop hazy vision, intolerance to their lenses, or astigmatism must be suspected of having a warped lens. The base curve should be accurate to within 0.025 mm of specifications (Fig. 19-10, *B*).

The optic spherometer is specifically designed to measure the optic-zone radius. It is more accurate than the keratometer, is simple to use, and yields rapid results. It is an excellent instrument for determining the base curve or the presence of warpage. Its major disadvantage is its cost.

The technique is straightforward. The concave surface of the lens is used as a concave

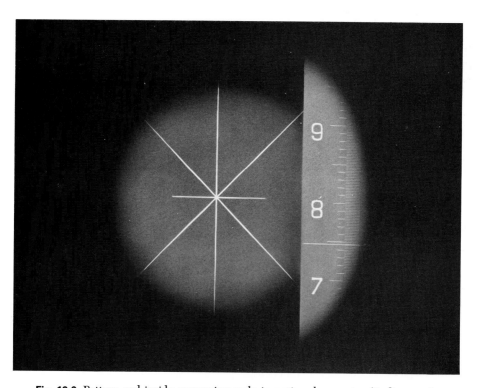

Fig. 19-9. Pattern and inside measuring scale in optic spherometer (Radiuscope).

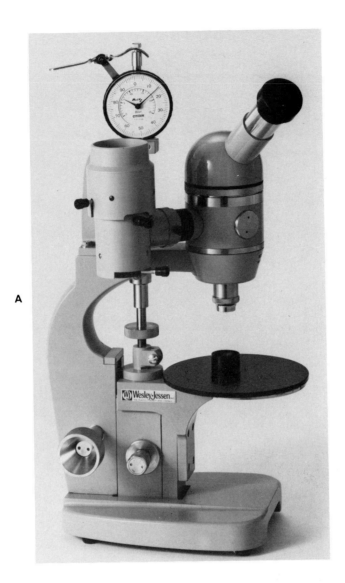

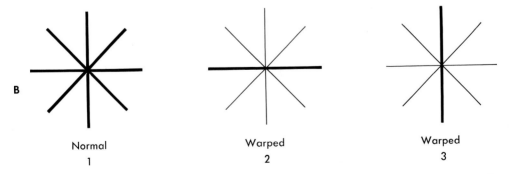

Normal
1

Warped
2

Warped
3

Fig. 19-10. A, Wesley-Jessen Contacto Gauge with built-in thickness gauge. **B,** Warpage is indicated if the mires are not in focus in all principal meridians as indicated in *2* and *3*.

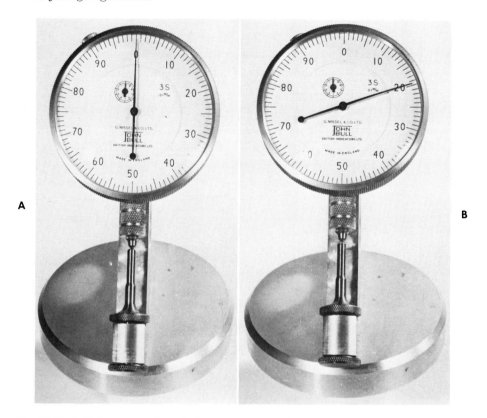

Fig. 19-11. A, Before measuring, thickness gauge must be set to zero. **B,** Thickness gauge.

mirror. The convex surface is neutralized by a drop of glycerin placed under the lens. The image is reflected from the posterior surface of the lens and is viewed on the lens and at the radius of the mirror. The focusing device is adjusted to its lowest position until the bottom image comes into sharp view. This image should be adjusted for zero. The barrel is moved upward until the first image is seen. The radius of curvature is read in hundredths of a millimeter.

POWER

The dioptric power of a rigid lens is determined with the lensometer. Since most lensometers are designed for large, flat posterior curvatures of spectacle lenses, they cannot be completely converted to measure the power of a highly curved, corneal lens. An error in power is introduced that is equal to the sagittal depth at the back of the lens and the plane of the aperture. This error can be reduced with an accessory conic choke, which reduces the aperture size. The convex side faces away from

the eyepiece, that is, against the lensometer stop when the power at the front-vertex surface is measured. However, most laboratories measure the back-vertex power; that is, the concave surface is placed away from the examiner and toward the lensometer stop. This is done because refractors, corrected trial lenses, and spectacle lenses are all specified this way. This is the back-vertex or corneal-plane–vertex power of a lens, the most reliable one to use. This difference in approach can yield different results. The practitioner should make sure that he or she and the laboratory are doing the same thing. Plus lenses show less plus for front-vertex powers than for back-vertex powers. The lens power should be exact within ± 0.25 D of power ordered and less than ± 0.12 D of uncalled-for astigmatism.

CENTRAL THICKNESS

A thickness gauge is the most useful device for measuring central thickness. The most reliable measurement is calibrated in tenths of a millimeter, but some lathe-cut machines

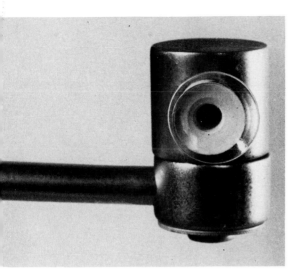

Fig. 19-12. Holder for lens in slitlamp inspection.

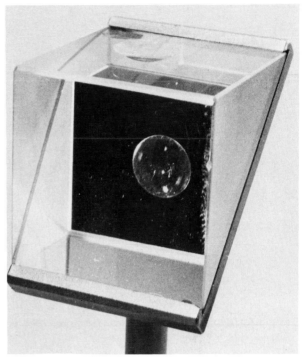

Fig. 19-13. Zeiss prismatic lens inspection device for the slitlamp.

(Wesley-Jesson) for fabricating lenses are set for thousandths of an inch, and so one must make a conversion, for example, 0.001 inch = 0.02 mm.

The most common instrument used is the dial gauge. The lens is placed convex side down on its base. A spring-plunger tip is released until it touches the lens. The amount by which the plunger is separated from the base indicates the thickness of the lens (Fig. 19-11).

All gauges have arrangements for zero setting. Before measuring, the gauge must be set meticulously to the zero point.

SURFACE QUALITY

Surface quality of the rigid lens can also be assessed by use of attachments for the slitlamp, which then permit detailed inspection in diffuse or slit illumination, or both. If necessary, one can use monochromatic light, switching in the various filters available on the slitlamp. Fig. 19-12 shows a simple device readily available for slitlamp inspection of lenses. The holder rotates the slitlamp, and the lens is held in place by a standard rubber suction cup.

A more elaborate slitlamp inspection device is the Zeiss prismatic lens holder, which will fit on the Zeiss photographic slitlamp and with some ingenuity can be easily attached to other slitlamps. We use it on the 900 Haag-Streit slitlamp by inserting the metal rod of the prismatic device into the Hruby lens holder socket (Fig. 19-13).

BLEND

The transition zones of the rigid lens in our view should be thoroughly blended. Instantaneous assessment of the transition zones can be achieved with the profile analyzer, a product of Gulf Coast Contact Lens, Inc., of New Orleans (Fig. 19-14). This instrument gives an optic projection of the inner (concave) surface of a narrow section of the lens diameter, vividly displaying any defect that may be present in the blending. One look at a poorly finished transition zone in the profile analyzer will make it instantly clear to the fitter why the patient cannot tolerate the otherwise well-fitting lens. In our view this is an essential quality-control instrument in medical lens practice (Fig. 19-15).

A sharp junction at the blend is a major source of rigid lens defects, but a faulty edge creates more problems. If a profile analyzer is not available, Honan and Garland have described the following technique to examine the peripheral curves and blend of a rigid contact lens.

The fluorescent tube should be in front of and higher than the examiner. The examiner should position himself so that the bare fluores-

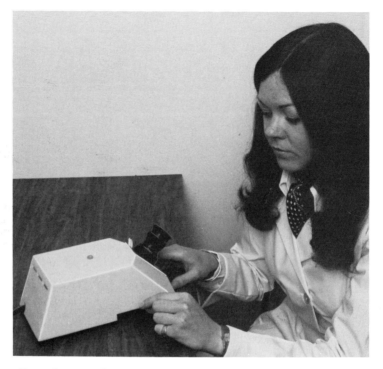

Fig. 19-14. Profile analyzer used to evaluate the blend of the peripheral curves of a lens. (From Stein, H.A., and Slatt, B.J.: The ophthalmic assistant, ed. 4, St. Louis, 1983, The C.V. Mosby Co.)

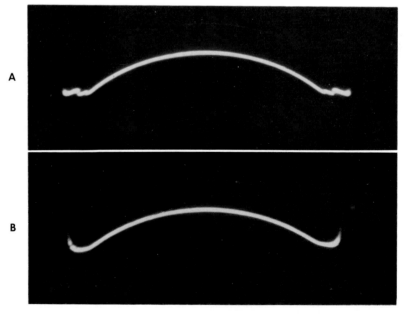

Fig. 19-15. A, Poorly finished transition zone as determined by the profile analyzer. **B,** Perfect transition zone with ski contour at its periphery.

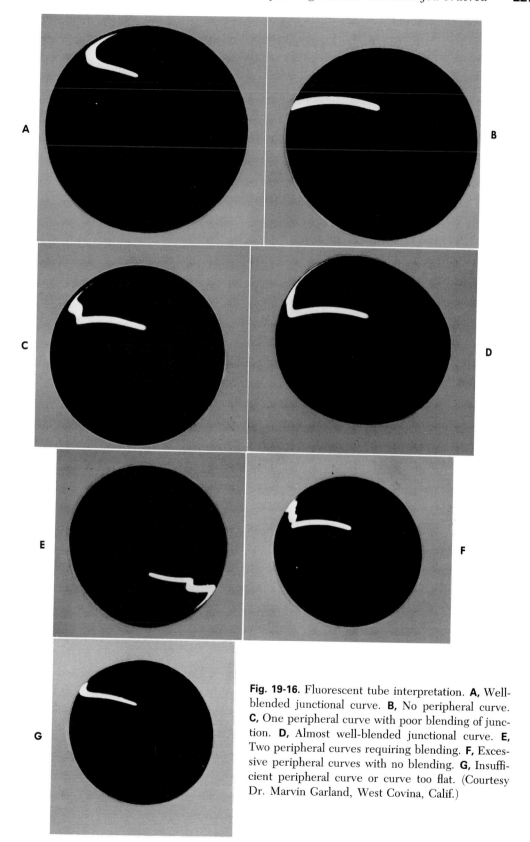

Fig. 19-16. Fluorescent tube interpretation. **A,** Well-blended junctional curve. **B,** No peripheral curve. **C,** One peripheral curve with poor blending of junction. **D,** Almost well-blended junctional curve. **E,** Two peripheral curves requiring blending. **F,** Excessive peripheral curves with no blending. **G,** Insufficient peripheral curve or curve too flat. (Courtesy Dr. Marvin Garland, West Covina, Calif.)

cent tube is *directly* in front of and parallel to the examiner's shoulder. One should be situated slightly back from the fluorescent tube so that the reflection is thinner and easier to interpret. The lens must be held so that the reflection of the light on the posterior surface of the lens falls on the inferior portion of the lens, approximately 65% to 75% of the distance from the top to the bottom of the lens. The lens must be tilted and positioned slightly to the side so that the reflection is continuous to the edge of the lens. The positioning of the lens under the fluorescent tube is the most difficult part to perform. Wearing a loupe or using a hand magnifier helps one to see details better.

An ideal blend in peripheral curve should show a J-shaped or ski pattern in a nice smooth curve. The J is horizontal and curves inferiorly at the edge (Fig. 19-16, *A*). If there is no peripheral curve present, the reflection of the fluorescent tube continues to the edge in a straight or upward pattern (Fig. 19-16, *B*).

If there are peripheral curves, the area where the reflection starts to curve inferiorly is a junction of the optic zone and peripheral curve. If the peripheral curve is poorly blended, the reflection appears as in Fig. 19-16, *C*. An almost well-blended curve is shown in Fig. 19-16, *D*. If there are two peripheral curves requiring blending, this pattern appears as in Fig. 19-16, *E*. If there are excessive curves, the pattern looks like a Z as shown in Fig. 19-16, *F*. Appropriate blending will convert this pattern to the ideal J or ski pattern. If there is an insufficient peripheral curve or the peripheral curve is too flat, this deficiency is shown in Fig. 19-16, *G*.

Comment. Quality control of contact lenses starts with the manufacturing phase. However, the practitioner should have sufficient equipment to determine that the specifications conform to what was requested. the edges are smooth and carefully lathed, and a proper blend is constructed between curves. Without these assurances, one cannot adequately analyze improper fitting and proceed to rectify the problem.

Section three

Gas-permeable lenses

CELLULOSE ACETATE BUTYRATE (CAB) LENSES

The gas-permeable CAB lens is made of a unique plastic (cellulose acetate butyrate, a cellulose derivative) that has the ability to permit oxygen to diffuse into and carbon dioxide to diffuse out of the lens. This gas-permeable plastic, which is made from natural substances, was developed by Eastman Kodak for photographic purposes. Cellulose is derived from wood and cotton, acetic acid from vinegar, and butyric acid from natural gas. Although the plastic has been available since 1938, it was not utilized as contact lens material until 1974. It was the first of the gas-permeable lenses.

The material's prime attraction appeared to be that it was not flammable. This plastic dissipates heat much better and wets much easier than that of ordinary hard lenses and thus permits tears to flow better under it. Kodak is still the prime manufacturer of this material.

ADVANTAGES

The gas-permeable lens has the following advantages:

1. Increased comfort.
2. Longer wearing time.
3. Reduction of corneal edema, spectacle blur, and overwear syndrome.
4. Elimination of edge glare seen with smaller lenses because lenses can be fitted larger.
5. Increased capillary attraction resulting from its greater flexibility.
6. Rapid adaptation to spectacles after lenses removed.
7. Permeability to oxygen 40 times greater than that of soft lenses but not so much as the pure silicone lenses or the silicone-PMMA varieties.
8. Better sport lenses because they can be fitted tighter than the rigid lenses; consequently less chance of loss.
9. Larger optic zone; consequently increased visual field and less flare.
10. Better heat conductivity.
11. Very tough and difficult to break.

The CAB lens has a smaller contact angle than the PMMA lens, making it more wettable than the PMMA lens. This advantage is particularly helpful in patients with moderately dry eyes. The surface tension is 35 degrees lower and the wetting angle 18.5 degrees less than those of PMMA. Although the major advantage of this plastic is its permeability to oxygen and carbon dioxide, the newer rigid lenses, including the silicones, the silicone resins, and the silicone-PMMA combinations are much better in terms of their DK values and permeability factors.

DISADVANTAGES

These lenses have the following disadvantages:

1. Visual acuity may be reduced because of poor surface optic patterns. This was a problem of poor quality control observed in some early lenses.
2. Some lens awareness because of thickness at the center and the edges.
3. Susceptibility to scratches and chips.
4. Center and edge thickness is much greater (approximately one third) when compared to silicone-based lenses. These

lenses have been improved and made thinner recently.

5. Unavailability of toric lenses and prism ballasts, color, and other special designs.

6. Lack of stability. Lenses frequently change after hydration and occasionally steepen after several weeks. Also the lenses can warp after 1 year of wearing time. Lens warpage, however, is not too much of a problem if the lens is not manufactured too thin.

7. Verification of the base curve requires rapid measurement after drying of the soaked lens since the properties of the same lens differ depending on whether it is wet or dry.

The primary disadvantage of CAB is its low module of elasticity or poor shape retention. The material does not retain its contours when flexed or distorted. Clinically, this leads to warpage of the lens from handling during cleaning procedures. The material tends to be distorted by a lathing bit, and during manufacturing the material may require special hardeners to keep it compact. One method to retain hardness is boiling the buttons in silicone oil. Unless excellent quality controls in the fabrication are present, the softness and heat sensitivity of the materials can result in unsatisfactory peripheral curves and edges. Finishing procedures require care. Special compounds must be used in its fabrication. The polishing compounds should be cool or cold and water-based. Ammonia-based compounds like Silvo hydrolyze and the lens material can turn it yellow. Alcohol and petroleum products also cause opacification of this material. The plastic must be bathed at 98° F (39° C) for hours after finishing.

The finished lens is relatively thick in contrast to the thin PMMA or hydrogel lenses. The recommended minimal central thickness is approximately 16 mm. These lenses are fit steeper initially, since the material tends to flatten because of its inherent softness or perhaps its molding to the corneal surface. As with any gas-permeable lens, the permeability feature allows for larger diameters, which in turn allow one to have a larger optic zone than a smaller-sized PMMA lens would have. The large lenses about 9 mm in diameter also afford stability and centration. The steeper base curves are permitted because of the ancillary

feature of diffusion of oxygen. There is less movement to a good fit, and hence there is more comfort. In the aphakic lens, the added thickness of the lens makes warpage less of a problem. However, the thicker lenses also significantly reduce oxygen permeability, and such a reduction makes extended wear unsatisfactory or marginal.

Comment. Excessive lens flexure may cause unwanted astigmatism with CAB lenses.

FITTING THE CAB LENS

Any size, curvature, or thickness similar to regular rigid lenses can be ordered. A good fit is one that is positioned somewhat high with minimal movement but with complete corneal clearance. One should fit either from a trial set or from K and refractive error measurements. There is a high index of refraction to this plastic; consequently about 0.50 D more plus than the normal refractive power is required.

The CAB lens is made of a tough, gristle-like material that may have microscopic waves. Verification of the base curve on the optic spherometer may show errors as a result of the very small segment measured. The keratometer, which measures a larger area, will show the true base curve.

Fitting from K

The first step in fitting is to determine the base curve:

1. If the two ophthalmometric readings are alike (spheric cornea), a base curve that is 0.25 D flatter than the readings should be adopted.

2. If the person has corneal astigmatism with the rule:
   a. When the difference between the two meridians is not over 0.75 D, the lowest reading (fitting on K) should be adopted as the base curve of the lens.
   b. When the difference between the two readings is between 0.75 and 1.50 D, a base curve 0.25 D steeper than the lowest reading should be adopted.
   c. When the difference is greater than 1.50 D, a base curve 0.50 D steeper than the lowest reading is needed.

3. If the corneal astigmatism is against the rule, the base curve should be made 0.25 D steeper than the above indications.

The curvature of the cornea is a better indication of the diameter of the lens because of the amount of surface area involved. The following scale has been computed on this basis and is a good guide to follow, at least tentatively, until more experience is gained.

Base curve (D)	Recommended diameter (mm)
52.00	8.4
50.00	8.5
48.00	8.7
46.00	8.8
45.00	8.9
44.00	9.0
43.00	9.1
42.00	9.2
40.00	9.3
39.00	9.4

If the lenses are to be made smaller or larger than shown on this scale, the base curve should be steepened for smaller lenses and flattened for larger lenses at an approximate ratio of 0.50 D for each 0.5 mm of change.

Diagnostic fitting set for CAB lenses

A diagnostic fitting set of 10 to 12 lens is recommended for fitting.

1. Select the initial lens based on the base curve.
   a. Base-curve selection. Slightly steeper than the flattest corneal meridian, that is:

   $$43.00 \times 44.50 \text{ diopters}$$

   Base-curve initial selection 43.50
   b. Diameter. Selection is related to base curve. The flatter the cornea, the larger the lens.

	Use
40.00 to 43.00 D	9.4 mm
43.25 to 45.00 D	9.2 mm
Greater than 45.25 D	9.0 mm

2. Insert the lens and allow to settle for 20 minutes.
3. With good centration, over-refraction can be done.
   a. Optical power. Power of sphere plus the degree of additional minus power to account for steepening of the base curve, that is:

   −2.00 sphere plus (−0.50) for K variation
   Total power = −2.50 D

   b. Alterations must be made for a vertex distance of more than 4.00 D.
4. If centration and movement are not adequate, select another lens 0.5 D steeper or flatter as the need demands.

The lens is shipped in vials in the wet stage so that it is readily compatible with the eye. It is stored wet in Soaclens solution and then rinsed with water, and a drop of Soaclens is added. The lens should be worn 2 hours the first day and then increased 1 hour or more each additional day. Adaptation is rapid, and comfort is usually achieved by the end of the first week.

Patients should clean their lenses immediately after removal and rinse and store them in fresh soaking solution.

Comment. Because of the oxygen transmission of the CAB material, this lens may be fitted somewhat tighter than normal. However for best results, fit the lens according to its best position and comfort. Do not worry if the base curve is a little steep or flat.

REFITTING THE PMMA LENS WEARER WITH CAB LENSES

If a patient has 20/20 visual acuity in each eye with PMMA contact lenses, but has corneal edema and spectacles, the following steps should be followed in refitting with CAB lenses.

1. Do not immediately discontinue wearing of the PMMA lenses, unless there is corneal scarring, severe induced corneal toricity or other major problems.
2. Reduce daily PMMA lens wear by 3 hours per day so that the cornea is clear within 5 days.
3. Obtain original K readings. If possible, obtain original K readings before the patient wore contact lenses. Match the fit of the PMMA lens with the CAB lens, but not necessarily the lens specifications.
4. If the PMMA lens is under 9 mm in diameter, fit CAB lens 0.5 D flatter and 0.6 mm larger in diameter.

   Example: PMMA = 7.80, −2.00, 8.4
   CAB   = 7.90, −1.50, 9.0

Always verify with a diagnostic lens.
5. If PMMA lens is over 9.2 mm in diameter, match exactly for every 0.4 mm dif-

ference in the optic zone. Make CAB base curve 0.25 D flatter than the PMMA optic zone.

> Example: PMMA = 7.90, −3.00, 9.4, 7.6
> Standard CAB lenses have 0.7 mm width in the center of the lens
> CAB = 7.94, −2.75, 9.4, 8.0

TWO TYPICAL REFITTING CASES
Case 1

Best refraction:	−1.75 −1.50 × 20 and
	−2.00 −1.50 × 160
Original K:	45.50/46.50 and 45.50/46.75
Original prescription:	−3.75 −0.25 × 5 and
	−2.75 −0.75 × 175
New K's:	43.25/45.00 and 43.75/46.00
Old PMMA lenses:	7.60 −2.75 8.4 7.5
	7.58 −2.50 8.4 7.5
CAB lenses prescribed:	7.67 −2.37 9.2
	7.67 −2.00 9.2

New lenses are larger and flatter. Fitting was done by use of diagnostic lenses because K readings and refraction are *unreliable* after

PMMA lens have been removed. The duration of induced change may last for weeks or even months.

Case 2

Original K:	42.00/42.50 OU
New K:	40.75/42.50 and 40.00/43.00
Old PMMA lenses:	8.04 +17.00 10.1
	7.94 +15.50 10.2
CAB lenses designed:	7.98 +16.00 9.8
	7.98 +15.50 9.8

The corneas have been flattened by the old lenses. These large-diameter lenses were best treated with CAB lenses of smaller diameter. The rules are merely guides. Flexibility in fitting is vital.

Comment. The CAB lens never achieved widespread popularity because of its dimensional instability. Although improvements in design and structure have been made, the silicone-acrylate lens is still the most popular rigid gas-permeable lens.

CHAPTER 21

SILICONE-ACRYLATE LENSES

Gas-permeable lenses have added a new dimension to the fitting of rigid lenses. Because of the ability to transmit oxygen, they have significantly reduced the complications of rigid PMMA lenses that are attributed to anoxic changes in the cornea. Also, because of the ability to design larger rigid lenses than before, one can overcome the optic disadvantages of the PMMA lenses. With this technologic improvement to the time-honored PMMA lens, the silicone-acrylate (sometimes referred to as siloxanyl-acrylate) lenses promise to replace PMMA lenses as the rigid lens of choice. Other gas-permeable lenses, such as the styrene lens of Wesley-Jessen (Chicago) and the rigid fluorocarbon lens of 3M (St. Paul, Minnesota) may someday be a threat to the dominance of the silicone-acrylates in the market place.

The principal silicone-acrylate lenses are known clinically as Polycon I or II (Syntex Ophthalmics, Phoenix, Ariz.), Boston lenses I & II (Polymer Technology Corporation, Wilmington, Mass.), lenses derived from the GT buttons giving rise to a number of trade names, and Menicon O_2 (Toyo Contact Lens Company, Tokyo, Japan). In addition, Optocryl 60, Paraperm, and B&L Gas Perm are three new entries into the field. These lenses should be differentiated from cellulose acetate butyrate

(CAB), basically a wood product that is also gas permeable but thicker and less stable, being subject to warpage. Rigid lenses of 100% silicone (silicone resin, Dow Corning Ophthalmics, Conforma Labs, Norfolk, Va.) are even more permeable than the polymer combinations and are discussed in Chapter 22.

THE LENS
Material considerations

The essential component of this group of gas-permeable lenses is silicone.

After oxygen, silicon is the second most abundant element in the earth's crust. From its position below carbon in the periodic table, one would expect silicon chemical behavior to be similar to that of carbon, but it is not. During the past several decades, there has been a burgeoning synthesis industry so that today thousands of organosilicones are known.

The preparation of silicones starts with the isolation of pure silicon or silicon carbide. For contact lens usage, most polymers stem from silicon oxide and carbon groups—R_2SiO—and various polymers are added. Organosilicone polymers are polyacrylates and have radicals attached to make the material more functional.

Methyl groups contribute to flexibility.
Phenyl groups contribute to stiffness.

Increasing the length of the organic group attached to silicone increases its softness and water repellency. As the ratio of organic groups to silicone decreases, the polymer becomes less fluid, less soluble, and harder to produce (that is, goes from a rubbery to a glassy state).

The oxygen bond of the silicone contributes to high heat resistance, oxidation resistance, and permeability toward gases.

Pure silicone polymers are soft and nonwettable (hydrophobic). In combination with polymethylmethacrylate (PMMA), the hardness and stability of the silicone are enhanced. To ensure sufficient wettability, there is a polymerization of the silicone with additional hydrophilic monomers. When this is done, no surface treatment or special solutions are thus required to attain good surface wettability. Different additives such as dimethacrylate may be used to enhance tensile strength and resistance to deformation.

In the marriage of silicone with PMMA, normally the addition of silicone decreases the wettability, stability, and strength. This has been overcome by some manufacturers of silicone-acrylate lenses: the wettability, stability, and strength of the hybrid material has been maintained when the two components are mixed usually in the ratio of about 65% PMMA and 35% silicone.

Table 21-1 reflects the technical comparisons of the numerous available lenses. Silicone polymers fall between PMMA and CAB (cellulose acetate butyrate) in terms of hardness on the Shore D scale.

PMMA	88.5
Silicone-PMMA	84.0
CAB	77.5

In terms of wettability, silicone-based gas-permeable lenses are close to PMMA and CAB—between 23 and 25 degrees.

Fabrication

The fabrication of silicone-based lenses is similar to that of PMMA lenses. However, the silicone polymer is somewhat more sensitive to heat and pressure. Thus the diamond-tipped cutting tool must always be sharp; *carbon-tipped tools are not satisfactory. Compressed air cooling of the diamond tip is advisable.

Wax or pitch polishing is strongly recommended especially for outside surfaces. Pillow pads may be used for base curves. White Nissel wax is ideal for polishing base curves. Conventional nonammoniated polishes may be used for edge finishing and generating peripheral curves. However, polishing compounds with a particle size less than 0.4 µm should be used for polishing both surfaces. If done properly, the optic quality of these lenses should match that of PMMA.

Aliphatic (saturated) hydrocarbons solvents are best for the removal of wax, pitch, and tape adhesive. Alcohols, esters, ketones, and aromatic hydrocarbons will damage the plastic and *should be avoided.*

Because these lenses may be less resistant to breakage than PMMA lenses are, they are frequently made slightly thicker than a regular rigid lens.

The following are common problems in quality control.

Lens warpage. The presence of warpage usually indicates that excessive heat was applied during the blocking or lathing procedures or excessive force was applied as the lens was removed from the blocking pitch or wax. If this problem persists after you confirm the alignment and sharpness of the diamond tool, reduce the depth and speed of each cut and check the results of increasing the turning speed of the lathes.

Poor surface optic properties. If this problem is present, increase the polishing time using a polishing compound. Also, the alignment or sharpness of the cutting by the diamond tool may be unsatisfactory.

Comment. Silicone polymers that are made with PMMA can be made as thin as regular rigid lenses. The only problem with these hybrid lenses is they are slightly more brittle and tend to chip easily at the edges.

Thermal conductivity

PMMA acts as a thermal insulator. Not only does it create corneal hypoxia, but by insulating the cornea it also raises the basal metabolic rate and increases the oxygen demand of the epithelium of the cornea. However, silicones, either in the pure form or mixed with PMMA, are thermal conductors, which take the heat of metabolism away from the corneal surface and thereby decrease oxygen requirements.

Thermal conductivity: 10,000 cal/sec/m^2/°C/cm
ASTM test   C 177
CAB   6.4
PMMA   5.0
Silicone   12.6

Optic and surface properties

These silicone polymers transmit most of the light in the range of the visible spectrum, that is, 400 to 750 nm. Commercially available contact lenses have a refractive index in the range of 1.35 to 1.45.

For the investigation of the wettability of polymers, most reports deal with angle measurements. However, these measurements are not absolute because the figures change drastically when lenses are worn. For example, the addition of protein or lipid to the surface of a lens effectively reduces its wettability and permeability. As one might expect, surface coatings reduce vision and comfort.

UNDERSTANDING GAS PERMEABILITY

The permeability of a contact lens is largely related to the following:
1. Permeability of the polymer, or D_1
2. Solubility coefficient or partition coefficient, or K_1
3. Thickness of the lens

Permeability can be enhanced by increasing DK or reducing the thickness of the lens.

The permeability coefficients of contact lens materials to oxygen are usually expressed at a constant relative humidity (water-vapor activity) and at a constant temperature, preferably at 34° C (Table 21-1).

Silicone groups offer high oxygen permeability, whereas an ordinary PMMA lens has no oxygen permeability. Also, pure silicone polymers are chemically stable and transparent. Unfortunately, in the pure form they are not very wettable and they can warp. The incorporation of moderate amounts of silicone monomers by copolymerization with PMMA increases the permeability of oxygen through these lenses without losing the dimensional stability of the lens.

True gas-permeable rigid lenses range from 2 to 14 in terms of their DK values. It should

be noted that a cosmetic HEMA lens of 38.6% water content and 0.15 mm center thickness allows no physiologically significant oxygen to reach the cornea. All rigid and most conventional soft lenses present a barrier to oxygen diffusing directly to the cornea. After wearing a nonpermeable test lens, the cornea develops an increased demand for oxygen. With PMMA, for example, with the lens being −4.00 D, the application of such a lens to the cornea can increase its thickness by 10% or greater because of hypoxia.

If a goggle is placed over the eye with different percentages of oxygen until that oxygen degree producing the same corneal demands as the test lens is found, it it said that that value represents the equivalent oxygen performance of the lens. Without proper oxygen, the cornea becomes hypoxic. A silicone lens that is gas permeable creates only a 4% increase in corneal thickness when first applied to the eye.

Edema results if the available oxygen falls below the level of 1.5% to 2.5%. This can be measured with the pachometer as an increase in corneal thickness. Glycogen (glucose-storage level) begins to dissipate if there is less than 5% oxygen available.

The amount of equivalent oxygen in air is 20% with the eyes open. With the eye closed as when sleeping and no lens applied to the eye, the amount of oxygen drops to 7% equivalent of oxygen to the corneal surface. It is therefore desirable that any gas-permeable day-wear lenses allow between 7% to 10% oxygen to the cornea. Normally the present-day gas-permeable silicone-acrylate lenses provide about 7% equivalent oxygen performance (EOP). However, with adequate blinking the tears introduce more oxygen, and so the EOP in the blinking state is over 8% (Fig. 21-1). Permeability of one manufacturer's lens from another will vary considerably (Tables 21-2 and 21-3). As technology improves, each manufacturer tries to leapfrog over the other in the production of a better material.

TEAR-LAYER OXYGEN

Oxygen at the corneal site under a gas-permeable contact lens reaches the cornea through tear exchange and by diffusion through the lens itself. Diffusion is controlled by the

Table 21-1. Available specifications of some gas-permeable rigid lenses*

Rigid oxygen-permeable lenses	Manufacturer	Index	Hardness		Permeability ($DK \times 10^{-11}$)	Wetting angle
			Shore D	Rockwell		
		(1.490)	(95H)	(94H)	(0)	(25°P, 46°H, 50°A, 20°)
(Polymethylmethacrylate for comparison)						
Polycon I	Syntex Ophthalmics	1.479	86	71H	5.0; 5.82 ± 0.9132‡	22°P, 43°H, 56°A, 30.4°R
Polycon II	Syntex Ophthalmics	1.479	N/A	N/A	10.0	50°A, 15°R
Boston Lens I	Polymer Technology	1.471	116 79H	85	116 79H; 10.66 ± 0.7590‡	22°P, 47°H, 29° others
Boston Lens II	Polymer Technology	1.471	N/A	N/A	12.6	24°
CABCurve	Hydrocurve	1.475			4.2†	56°S, 24°B
Modified CAB	Hydrocurve	1.475	76		4.2	20°S, 13.5°B
Meso	Danker-Wohlk	N/A		116	11.5†	21°, 23°P
AquaCAB	Union	1.47		110	6.64	21°
W/J Airlens	Wessley-Jesson	1.533	86		12.2	54°B
Sil-O₂-Flex	Fused Contacts	1.47	89		7.7 5.2†; 8.2 Hill	25.4°P
Menicon O₂	Toyo Contact Lens	1.481	N/A	N/A	7.5 10.5†; 9.1 others	16° to 23°
ParaCAB	Paragon	1.47		110	5.0; 8.86 ± 1.3712§	20°
Opticryl 60	Capital	N/A	N/A	N/A	12.4	N/A
Persecon	Titmus-Eurocon	N/A	N/A	N/A	N/A	N/A
Oxyflow	Hirst	1.47		31	32.01 22.0†	42.3°H
Alberta (SM38 and XL30)	Calgary Contacts	1.469	88		8.73 ± 1.0872§	24.8° to 30°, 30.4°P
Calgary (XL20)	Calgary Contacts	N/A	N/A	98H	4.05° 1.8246§	28°, 46°H
Oxyflex	Cantor & Silver	1.47	N/A	N/A	13.0 7.2 others	23°P
Experimental (Hyperm?)	Hydron	N/A	N/A		22.45 ± 1.4380§	
Hartflex	Wohlk	N/A	N/A	N/A	11.15†	21°, 23°P

*Data tabulated and supplied by Dr. Josh Josephson, Toronto.
†Morris: RM (rotation of mirror) = 21° to 25°; eye = 35°.
‡Morris, 1981.
§Morris, 1982.
N/A, Not applicable.
A, Advanced; B, bubble; H, Hirst; P, poster; R, receded; S, sessile drop.

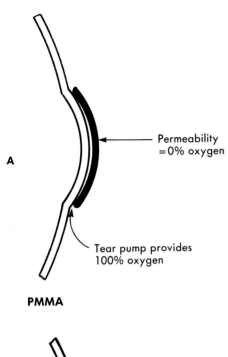

A

Permeability
=0% oxygen

Tear pump provides
100% oxygen

PMMA

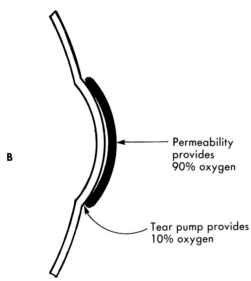

B

Permeability
provides
90% oxygen

Tear pump provides
10% oxygen

Gas permeable

Fig. 21-1. A, Normally with a polymethylmethacry-late lens, 100% of the oxygen must be provided by tear pump. **B,** With the gas-permeable lens, 90% of the oxygen diffuses through the contact lens, and so only 10% is required through the tear pump.

Table 21-2. Oxygen permeability (DK)

Silicone	Highest permeability
Boston Lens	
Alberta	
Polycon	graded in ml O_2–cm^2/sec ×
CAB	mm Hg at room temperature
HEMA	
PMMA	Lowest permeability

Table 21-3. Relationship between center thickness and equivalent oxygen performance for gas-permeable contact lens materials*

Center thickness (mm)	Equivalent oxygen performance (%)
HEMA (hydroxyethyl methacrylate) (35% water)	
<0.05	6.0-3.0
0.05-0.10	3.0-2.0
0.10-0.20	2.0-1.0
>0.20	<1.0
CAB (cellulose acetate butyrate)	
<0.05	7.5-6.5
0.05-0.10	6.5-3.5
0.10-0.15	3.5-2.0
0.15-0.20	2.0-1.0
>0.20	1.0
Silicone-organic copolymer	
<0.10	12.0-9.0
0.10-0.20	9.0-7.5
>0.20	7.5-6.0
Polycon	
<0.10	10.0-7.8
0.10-0.20	7.8-4.5
>0.20	4.5-2.5
Hard silicone	
<0.10	17.5-12.0
0.10-0.20	12.0-8.5
>0.20	8.5-7.0
Permalens	
<0.10	19.0-15.0
0.10-0.20	15.0-10.0
>0.20	10.5-8.5
Silicone	
<0.10	21.0-20.0
0.10-0.20	20.0-19.0
>0.20	19.0-18.5

*From Goldberg, J.: Int. Contact Lens Clin. 6(6): 64, 1979.

difference between external and internal oxygen tension. The factors that control the available oxygen supply are quite variable, as in the following:

1. Different eyes may have different oxygen needs. The difference may be in the integrity of the corneal epithelium and the nature of the tear film. For example, a cornea with a previous epithelial nebula from trauma or with dry spots will have oxygen needs different from those of a totally normal corneal epithelium.

2. Time during the day in which the oxygen supply is measured is important. With fatigue or reading or any activity in which the blink rate is down, the oxygen supplied through tear exchange will be depressed.

3. The external oxygen tension is a variable that is partially dependent on altitude and weather conditions. Oxygen tension decreases when the altitude is increased. The oxygen pressure at sea level is 155 mm Hg; whereas in Mexico City it is only 126 mm Hg. At the top of Mount Everest it is between 20 and 30 mm Hg. Under a contact lens it varies from 0 to 30 mm Hg. An oxygen tension greater than 20 mm Hg is required to supply the cornea's adequate oxygen needs.

Comment. Certainly the use of gas-permeable lenses must be appreciated in high-altitude places like Aspen where the oxygen pressure is considerably lower than it is at sea level.

ADVANTAGES OF A GAS-PERMEABLE LENS

1. *More comfort.* The high-riding lens with minimal movement is a very comfortable lens. It is much more comfortable than a small 8 mm ultrathin interpalpebral lens.

2. *Rapid adaptation.* The gas-permeable lens can frequently be worn for full-time day wear within a week.

3. *Spectacle blur.* Blur that is largely caused by corneal hypoxia is reduced. It is not eliminated because some spectacle blur is attributable to the aberrations of conventional spectacle lenses and is not related to corneal edema, or induced myopia, or molding of the cornea.

4. *Corneal distortion.* Corneal distortion from an ill-fitting PMMA lens will usually disappear with gas-permeable lenses. The distortion is best appreciated when one notes the irregular mire pattern of the keratometer by observing the irregular reflex from a retinoscopy light or the muddy reflex from the reflection of a Placido disc. Good refractions with stable corneas are frequently found 4 to 12 weeks after a gas-permeable lens is worn. Of great importance is that an oxygen-starved cornea can be immediately covered with a gas-permeable lens and the repair can occur under the lens. With rigid lenses a period of days to weeks, even months, may be required before K readings and mires are stabilized. During this time, the patient is incapacitated in visual needs.

5. *Larger lens permitting better centration.* Better centration makes the lens more stable and less irritating because of smaller excursions, and a large lens can cover astigmatism of the cornea up to 5 diopters.

6. *Greater safety.* The incidence of an acute hypoxic syndrome, better known as an "overwear reaction" is minimal. We have not seen a single case in over 1000 cases fitted. Long-term hypoxic changes, which include corneal molding, corneal hypesthesia, and irregular astigmatism, do not occur as with PMMA lenses.

7. *Less flare.* There is less flare because the optic zone is usually large enough to accommodate a young, blue-colored pupil dilating in dim illumination. With a lens 9.5 mm in diameter the optic zone is 8.4 mm, larger than the entire diameter of many PMMA lenses.

8. *Coverage of astigmatism.* Gas-permeable lenses in a spheric form can cover large amounts of astigmatism. The large lens offers stability and centration. Up to 5 diopters of astigmatism can be attempted with a regular lens. With corneal astigmatism of 1.00 D the base curve should be 0.20 to 0.30 flatter than the flattest K. With corneal toricity of 4.00 D or greater, the selected base curve should be on K.

    Rule. As the corneal astigmatism increases, so should the steepness of the base curves and center thickness increase (see Harrison-Stein nomogram).

9. *Sucked-on lens syndrome.* Reported with pure silicone lenses greater than 12 mm in diameter, the sucked-on lens syndrome is

more likely if the patient has a marginal tear film. It has not been reported with the silicone-acrylate lens.

In this syndrome the lens adherence to the epithelium becomes advanced toward the end of the day when the blink rate is decreasing and the tear film has shown some evaporation, with the visible formation of dry spots. Also, these lenses, which are usually silicone, are fitted a little steep to allow for perfect nonfluctuating acuity.

Clinically what occurs is that the lens movement ceases and the eye suddenly becomes inflamed. There is circumcorneal injection, corneal edema with striae of Descemet's membrane, iritis, and so on. The patient is in severe pain and has pronounced photophobic and extremely blurred vision.

Comment. This complication can result in the tearing of the epithelium when the lens is removed. The lens is best removed with an eye cup with saline solution so that pulling off of the entire epithelium is avoided. This type of response is to be anticipated in pure silicone lenses of high elastic content that are fitted steeper than the flattest corneal meridian. The steep fit can be recognized early because it may cause pressure at the 6 to 12 o'clock meridian causing lens buckling at the horizontal meridian. This creates against-the-rule astigmatism.

DISADVANTAGES OF A GAS-PERMEABLE LENS

1. *Quality control.* Quality control must be excellent because the large diameter can create edge and peripheral curve problems. Check edges and peripheral curve profile with the profile analyzer. If the edges are thick, as one might find with a high myope, lid impact will be excessive and the lenses uncomfortable. Also, lid gap becomes a problem. The frequency and severity become common and severe. Many patients develop exposure episcleritis and formation of dellen. The edge thickness for a regular myopic lens should be no greater than 0.09 mm.

2. *Increased fragility of lens.* More care is required in the cleaning of these lenses because breakage can occur.

3. *Waxlike deposits.* Because silicone is lipophilic, lipid deposits may form on the lens.

After 12 months of wear, creamy deposits are best identified when the rinsed and dried lenses are examined with the slitlamp. Appropriate cleaners can be used to clean the lens.

4. *Protein deposits.* If protein deposits are excessive, they may not come off manually. The lens is cleaned with a soft-lens cleaner, or some of the specific cleaning agents for gas-permeable lenses. Avoid rigid-lens cleaners because cleaners with polyvinyl alcohol can degrade the wettability of the lens.

    For professional cleaning the lens is held with a suction cup, and the outer surface is rubbed in a circular motion with velveteen saturated with the appropriate cleaner. One cleans the inside surface by applying the suction cup to the outside surface and applying the cloth impregnated with cleaning solution gently. This procedure must be stressed because the lens edge may fragment and chip with excessive manual application.

5. *Early scratched surfaces.* Gas-permeable lenses are softer than PMMA ones and tend to scratch easier.

    Comment. It is advisable to select your patients with the softness of the plastic in mind. Teen-agers who are rough with their lenses and may be a little careless with handling of them are often better off with PMMA lenses, which are hard and resistent to breakage.

6. *Initial transfer irritability.* Patients who are being refit to gas-permeable lenses for induced toricity, corneal edema, or irregular astigmatism, or excessive spectacle blur, may on initial exposure be unhappy with the comfort of a gas-permeable lens even if the lens is perfectly fit.

    This paradox occurs because the corneal sensation frequently improves when a gas-permeable lens is worn. The same patient who will tolerate corneal edema, corneal erosions, or infiltrates of the epithelium, may be quite irritable with new lenses that are gas permeable. Usually the "symptoms of increased corneal sensation" lasts 2 to 4 weeks. Unless the practitioner is aware of this change in corneal sensation, he or she will make endless modifications of a lens that may be fitting perfectly for a patient who seemingly can never be satisfied.

PATIENT SELECTION FOR GAS-PERMEABLE LENSES

We are of the opinion that if gas-permeable lenses were available throughout the world PMMA rigid lenses would become obsolete. However, because of the availability and delays in receiving properly ground silicone-PMMA lenses, one may be initially called on to select candidates for this type and pick and choose (see the chart in the next column).

Our experiences, dating back to 1976 when gas-permeable lenses became available to us in limited quantities, was to select patients who would benefit the most from the features of gas-permeable lenses. These candidates are as follows:

1. PMMA wearers who develop corneal edema caused by chronic hypoxic changes; also those patients who end up in the emergency room of a hospital because of acute hypoxia or "overwear syndrome."
2. Patients who have persistent spectacle blur after removing their glasses. This is caused by corneal edema producing an increase in myopia.
3. PMMA rigid lens wearers who cannot achieve satisfactory wearing time.
4. Patients with high degrees of corneal toricity that may be more simply remedied by a rigid lens than a soft toric lens.
5. Patients who develop flare with standard PMMA lenses. The gas-permeable lenses may be made larger with a larger optic zone.
6. Patients who have developed warped corneas with PMMA lenses. It has been traditional to advise these patients with corneal warpage to discontinue use of their lenses until their eyes are stable; that is, the K readings are normal, mires undistorted, and the refractions back to baseline findings. Unfortunately such advice may make a visual cripple of the person. The induced astigmatism may last for months. Refitting these people with gas-permeable lenses of the same measurements as that of their rigid contact lenses will in most cases permit the cornea to regain its normal undistorted mires.
7. Patients whose corneas developed vascularization from hypoxia at the limbus.
8. Keratoconus patients with thinning or scarring of the cornea.

Indications for a gas-permeable lens

Giant papillary conjunctivitis
History of soft lens damage
Keratoconus or irregular cornea
Cornea astigmatism up to 5 diopters of astigmatism
Epithelial infiltrates with soft lenses
Rotational instability with toric soft lenses
Rigid lens dropout
    Poor comfort
    Corneal edema
    Flare and glare

Comment. Over 97% of our patients fitted with a rigid lens for astigmatism over 1.25% could be fitted with a gas-permeable spheric lens, whereas less than 3% required a toric gas-permeable lens.

The least successful candidate for this lens has the following:

1. A large corneal diameter.
2. Lids that barely cover the upper limbus.
3. Inadequate blink responses—incomplete blink, infrequent blinking, and so on.
4. A low centration despite modifications in the lens.

FITTING GAS-PERMEABLE LENSES

Obviously there will be differences from one company to the next and from one expert to another according to preferences and clinical experience. We shall attempt to deal with general principles and be specific on occasion to present a broad picture.

Which lens to choose

There is obviously, even now, a large selection of gas-permeable lenses. One might assume that the higher the permeability of a lens, the more desirable the lens. We did a study on two lenses. At that time only the Boston and Polycon lenses were available. The Boston Lens had a DK value greater than 10, whereas the DK value of the Polycon lens was 5.5. Thus one lens had almost twice as much oxygen permeability as the other. The following considerations were made.

Corneal edema. There was no difference in the function of the two lenses.

Corneal complications. There were more problems with the Boston lenses. These early lenses had thick edges with all the attendant problems.

Durability. The Polycon lens was better. It was less fragile.

Wetting angle. The Polycon lens was lower.

Care. They were about the same.

Conclusions. The design characteristics of the lens is as important as its permeability. A lens with good quality control should be chosen over a lens with sloppy manufacturing techniques. Note the following points:

1. The laboratory that can produce reproducible high quality control lenses.
2. A lens laboratory that customizes a lens if needed.
3. A lens that uses a variety of cleaners so that availability is not a problem.
4. Any lens that will effectively eliminate corneal edema.
5. A thin lens with thin edges that do not break.

Positioning the lenses

The ideal fit for any gas-permeable lens is one in which the lens position is high, even when the lens overlaps the superior limbus (Fig. 21-2). The upper lid should cover a position of the lens during the full cycle of each blink. The purpose of the high-riding lens is to tuck the edge of the lens under the lid to avoid lid impact. This "full-sweep" blink also enhances lens surface wetting. The engagement of the upper lid margin with the edge of the lens is a major cause of discomfort. Even a soft hydrogel lens will be uncomfortable if it is made small and interpalpebral.

At times, the ideal may not be achieved (Fig. 21-3). The position of the upper lid may be too high to cover the upper position of the lens or there may be excessive astigmatism, which because of the corneal topography resists the upper motion of the lens. In these cases, the central position may be accepted, provided that the patient accepts this type of fit or modifications can be made. The lens diameter may be reduced to increase the lid lift, or a flatter base curve can be chosen. A central fit on the cornea is adequate, but a low-riding lens is unsatisfactory. When the lens is low, the blink rate is frequently suppressed to a minimum or the blink itself is incomplete. Also, a low lens is frequently a source of lid gap, which causes 3 and 9 o'clock staining of the cornea. The margin of the upper lid slides over the low lens, and it bridges the nasal and temporal cornea between the edge of the lens and limbus. Lid

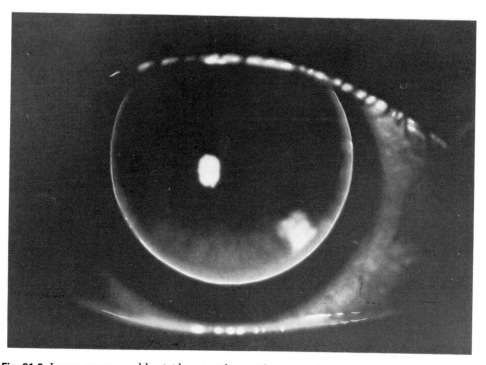

Fig. 21-2. Large gas-permeable rigid contact lens with upper edge under upper lid. Normal fit.

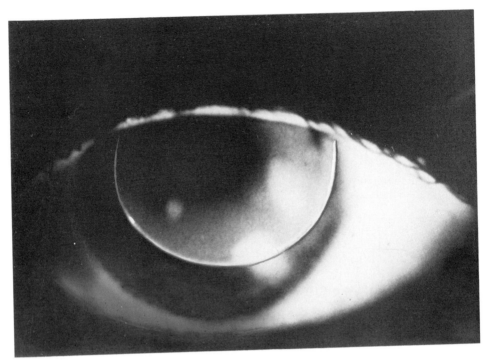

Fig. 21-3. A flat-fitting lens riding too high.

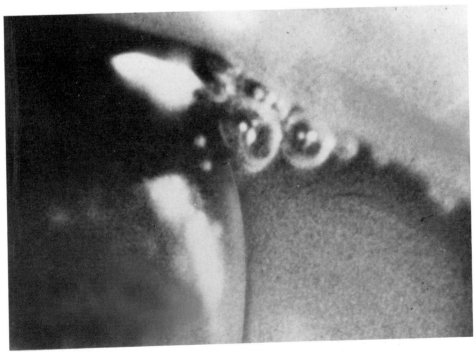

Fig. 21-4. The gap at the edge of the eyelid and contact lens may lead to corneal desiccation if the lens is thick.

gap is especially common with highly myopic refractive corrective lenses because the edges of the lens are prone to be thicker than usual and the trough between the edge of the lens and the margin of the cornea is likely to be deep (Fig. 21-4). Because these lenses are usually of large diameter, the proper edge treatment is essential (Fig. 21-6). A plus edge or configuration for myopic lenses with power greater than −4.00 D and a minus edge for lenses +4.00 D or greater.

SYSTEMS FOR FITTING
Diagnostic lenses

For trial purposes, gas-permeable lenses can be fashioned from PMMA material. As a result, it is quite acceptable and even preferable to use PMMA trial lenses. They should be made up in PMMA material for practicality of maintaining a firm surface and wetting characteristic without use of conditioners. It is best to use large-diameter trial lenses. For example, for the Boston lenses, a trial lens of 8.5 mm diameter is chosen. The base curve should be 0.5 to 1.5 steeper than the flattest K. If the lens is high or just overriding the limbus, the lens power is determined by an over-refraction. If the lens rides excessively high, a larger diameter is chosen sufficient to cover the pupil in dim illumination. *As the diameter of the lens increases to 9 mm or greater, the lens base curve should be made flatter*—to the flattest corneal meridian. This rule applies to all gas-permeable lenses.

For those who wish to work with diagnostic sets we have identified the most commonly used lenses in our practice to serve us as a diagnostic set (Table 21-4).

Comment. Polycon uses three standard diameters for myopes, 8.0, 9.0, and 9.5 mm. The initial 9.0 mm lens is usually chosen flatter than the flattest K, but the final lens is not chosen in terms of the base curve but from the *positioning of the lens* and *its comfort.* At times, the lens rides high after a blink and then drops. The after-blink position should be maintained in the high-riding position. If it is not, a flatter lens should be chosen.

If the lens rides low, increase the diameter and make the base curve flatter. Ideally the apex of the lens should not slide below the center of the cornea between blinks. Lenticular

Table 21-4. Diagnostic set for gas-permeable lenses

Base curve (D)	Diameter (mm)	Power	Peripheral curve width (mm)
40.00	9.6	−3.00 −6.00	0.6
41.00	9.4		0.6
42.00	9.2		0.5
43.00	9.0		0.5
44.00	8.8		0.5
45.00	8.6		0.4
46.00	8.4		0.4
40.00	9.8	+14.00	0.6
41.00	9.6		0.6
42.00	9.4		0.5
43.00	9.2		0.5
44.00	9.0		0.5
45.00	8.8		0.4
46.00	8.4		0.4

Diagnostic set
  14 minus lenses
  7 plus lenses

lenses should have a minus carrier. If the lenticular lens is low, choose the smallest single-cut lens with a base curve steeper than K.

Inventory fitting

There is a belief among some fitters that lens design and manufacturing is of primary importance and that soft lens systems may be applied to the gas-permeable lens. In effect, one manufacturer (Syntex Ophthalmics) believes that three diameters of lenses, 8.5, 9.0, and 9.5 mm, for myopia will satisfy almost all requirements for patients, and they recommend 9.5 and 10.0 for aphakia. If adequate base curves are available, these lenses will simplify fitting.

For myopic patients, the larger 9.5 mm diameter is recommended for levels of high astigmatism and also for flatter corneas.

Comment. Inventory fitting by lenses with preselected diameter simplifies fitting because one has fewer variables to deal with. In addition, one can rely on the quality control in providing lenses and controlled edge designs by one manufacturer.

Lid sensation is directly dependent on the edge finishing. It must not be left thick but thinned out to minimize lid sensation and the

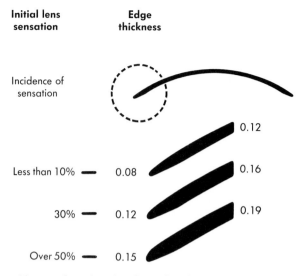

Fig. 21-5. Sensation of lens is directly related to edge thickness. Lens edges must be made thin to reduce lens sensation. Over 50% of patients with a lens edge 0.15 mm as noted in the lower lens will complain of sensation because of lens-lid impact. (Courtesy Syntex Ophthalmics, Inc., Phoenix, Ariz.)

uncomfortable fitting of a lens that lies under the upper lid (Fig. 21-5). A good reliable laboratory is most important.

Polycon, in an effort to maintain as high a permeability as possible, manufactures all minus lenses to a center thickness of 0.08 to 0.1 mm. This may not allow for lens flexure on high astigmatics. Custom lenses of greater center thickness may be better for these cases because the thicker lens marks the corneal toricity.

Harrison-Stein nomogram method of fitting

The ideal method of fitting silicone-acrylate lenses is from a trial set where the lens is placed on the eye. There are a number of low-volume fitters and occasional fitters who do not wish to have and maintain a standard fitting trial set. We have developed, over the past few years, a nomogram that is designed to be a guide for the best possible starting point in lens selection (Table 21-5). With a nomogram, one may order the lens directly by referring to the nomogram for the initial lens factor.

The nomogram takes into account the progressive increase in diameter required for flatter corneas and the decrease in diameter for the steeper corneas. The second factor takes into account the increased thickness required for the soft silicone-acrylate lenses to avoid

flexure on the cornea. The base curve is selected according to the corneal toricity. If the corneal cylinder is 0.75 D or less, we select the flattest K. If the corneal cylinder is between 1 and 2 D, we add one fourth of the difference of the two K's to the flattest K reading. If the corneal cylinder is over 2 D, we add one third of the difference to the flattest K.

Example. If the flattest curve of the cornea was 42.0 D and the cylinder axis was less than 75°, we would select a lens 9.2 mm in diameter and provide the lab with the details of the peripheral curves.

In developing this nomogram, we have reviewed almost 1000 eyes. We found that 75% could be fitted on a first-fit basis using this nomogram and most of the remainder fitted with less than two subsequent lenses.

WEARING SCHEDULE

A simple safe conservative wearing schedule can be applied to most patients.

Day	Hours
1	4
2	5
3	6
4	7
5	8
6	9
7	10
8	11
9	12

Table 21-5. Harrison-Stein nomogram: initial lens selection

If corneal cylinder < 0.75:   select flattest K.
      1.00 to 2.00 D: add ¼ of difference of 2 K's to flattest K.
      > 2 D: add ⅓ of the difference of 2 K's to flattest K.
      (All plus prescriptions over +2.00 D should be in lenticular form.)

Base curve (D)	Diameter (mm) Minus power	Diameter (mm) Plus power	Peripheral curves (mm/D)
40.00 and 40.25	9.6	9.8	0.2/36.00 0.2/31.00 0.2/27.50
40.50 and 40.75	9.5	9.7	
41.00 and 41.25	9.4	9.6	0.2/36.00 0.2/31.00 0.2/27.50
41.50 and 41.75	9.3	9.5	
42.00 and 42.25	9.2	9.4	0.3/32.00 0.2/27.50
42.50 and 42.75	9.1	9.3	
43.00 and 43.25	9.0	9.2	0.3/33.00 0.2/27.50
43.50 and 43.75	8.9	9.1	
44.00 and 44.25	8.8	9.0	0.3/34.00 0.2/29.00
44.50 and 44.75	8.7	8.9	
45.00 and 45.25	8.6	8.8	0.2/36.00 0.2/29.00
45.50 and 45.75	8.5	8.7	
46.00 and 46.25	8.4	8.6	0.2/36.00 0.2/30.00
46.50 and 46.75	8.3	8.5	

Additional hours may be added until the person is wearing gas-permeable lenses full time. Despite their permeability, we do not now recommend wearing of these lenses on an extended basis overnight.

In many cases an accelerated schedule can be used.

Day	Hours
1	2 hours morning, afternoon, and night
2	same
3	3 hours morning, afternoon, and night
4	same
5	4 hours morning, afternoon, and night
6	same
7	full-time wear

Most adaptation is of a physical nature (lid-lens) rather than physiologic nature (cornea-lens).

CARE OF GAS-PERMEABLE LENSES

Giant papillary conjunctivitis, which is an autoimmune papillitis of the upper tarsal conjunctiva, occurs with gas-permeable lenses but not with the same frequency as with hydrogel lenses. It is important to keep these lenses clean. Daily nonsensitizing cleaners such as Pliagel assist in reducing the incidence of papillary conjunctivitis. After cleaning, a saline solution, preferably without preservatives, should be used to rinse the lens. At times, reactions can occur to the saline solution and the cleaners. Usually, it is the preservative thimerosal that is the sensitizing agent. In such cases, nonpreserved saline solution made fresh daily or dispensed from an airtight container should be used. Weekly or bimonthly cleaning may be necessary. Soft-lens weekly cleaners can be best employed for the more thorough cleaning. How does a patient know the lenses are dirty? After cleaning, the lenses should be clear and transparent. If the lens is exposed to a light source, the dirty deposits will become visible instantly.

Special solutions are required for silicone-acrylate lenses. The wetting and soaking solutions used at least 15 minutes before insertion conditions the lens and improves its wetting angle. They also remove any accumulation of surface deposits.

Comment. It has been our experience that wetting agents composed primarily of polyvinyl alcohol do not wet silicone-PMMA lenses as well as EDTA does.

APHAKIC GAS-PERMEABLE LENSES

The large lenticular contact lens is recommended in aphakia. The trial lens should have a large diameter and myopic edge (minus carrier) design. The base curve should show minimal clearance. If the lens rides low, use a double lenticular design. If this lens is not successful, attempt to fit a steeper single-cut lens.

Comment. With the thickness required for an aphakic lens, the permeability of the lens at its center is drastically reduced. For example, the Boston Lens with outer lens thickness of 0.1 has a DK value of 10, whereas at a thickness of 0.30 to 0.40, the usual range of an aphakic lens, the DK value drops to 5. CAB at a center thickness of 0.1 has a DK value of 4, whereas at 0.3 to 0.4 mm thickness the DK value drops to less than 2. For extended-wear purposes, the equivalent oxygen performance should be 7% or greater. The lack of permeability to support the oxygen requirements of the cornea and during sleep makes the gas-permeable lens a questionable choice for extended wear. For this reason, a gas-permeable lens is not so important to the aphakic person. Central permeability is lowered, but it is still higher than that of PMMA, yet PMMA may be chosen because it is sturdier and less likely to fracture peripherally during handling.

If higher peripheral permeability is required, a lenticular lens with a wide flange of plano or plus design may be manufactured.

SPECIAL PROBLEM SOLVING WITH GAS-PERMEABLE SILICONE-ACRYLATE LENSES

Many of the major and disabling complications of PMMA lenses have been eliminated by the use of the new generation of gas-permeable lenses. There are still, however, a number of lens-regulated problems of the gas-permeable lenses that need to be addressed. By an understanding of these problems and solutions, practitioners are able to direct their attention to achieving happiness and success in a lens wearer.

Three and 9 o'clock staining

There are several causes of the finding of 3 and 9 o'clock staining.

Lid gap. A lid gap occurs largely with large-diameter rigid lenses. It is particularly prone to occur with gas-permeable lenses whose edges have not been properly thinned.

A gap occurs between the margin of the lens and the cornea. The meniscus of tears becomes very thin or absent at this border. It creates a lens-induced dry spot. The degree of staining is intense, often associated with episcleritis and formation of dellen. The staining of the cornea is attributable to desiccation of the corneal epithelium and not to corneal hypoxia. It is particularly prone to occur with lenses that ride low, that is, not brought up to a high position with a blink. Poor lid adherence is another cause of a low-riding lens.

The treatment is to make the lens flatter, thinner at the edges or smaller in diameter.

At times, the lens will rise with a blink and then suddenly drop to a low position. Such a lens requires a little alteration; flattening the blend and peripheral curves will frequently solve the problem and permit tear flow.

Poor blinking. The incomplete blinker dehydrates the exposed position of the eye at the 3 and 9 o'clock portions. Lines of protein accumulation caused by dehydration across the lens indicates its presence.

Poor tear film. Some people have an insufficient tear film to support a large-diameter lens. With these people, supplementary tears during the day and a bland ointment at night (such as Duratears) may be enough to remedy the problem.

Comment. Three and 9 o'clock staining is more common with large gas-permeable rigid lenses. Despite the intensity of the corneal erosions and episcleritis, patients do not seem to have much pain. Some fitters do not treat it because it may be an asymptomatic condition. This is an error. Breaks in the epithelial integrity should not be tolerated. More often than not, these patients primarily complain of the redness of their eyes.

Lens-flexure problems

The softer silicone component that is added to the silicone-acrylate mixture combined with the thin-designed lenses permits the lens to flex with each blink because of the pressure effect of the eyelid on the lens, which may rock on a toric cornea. This phenomenon results in blurring of vision, along with a residual astigmatism that is not corrected by the tear film.

Against-the-rule corneas create even more lens flexure as the lid sweeps over the lens. Steeper fitting of the lens also will create more opportunity for lens flexures. Smaller lenses may produce even more flexure than the larger-diameter lenses, which have a greater stabilizing force.

These problems of lens flexure are problems that are presenting themselves because the new generation of lenses are being used to correct astigmatism. These problems were apparent with soft HEMA lenses in the early years. Their use for corneal toricity was minimal because one soon learned that the soft HEMA lenses draped entirely over the cornea since they did not have any hard component. These lenses did not significantly correct large measures of corneal astigmatism.

To remedy this problem, one needs to increase the thickness of the lens. This will vary with the degree of corneal cylinder present. As a general rule, one should increase the thickness by 20% to 30% for larger lenses and 40% to 60% for the smaller lenses because the smaller lenses are more subject to flexure.

The lens should also be fitted high under the upper lid because doing so minimizes flexure, which may occur with an interpalpebral lens.

Comment. Because of lens flexure with the silicone-acrylate lenses, one of use (B.S.) uses a trial set made from the material to be dispensed. One of us (H.S.) believes, however, that this factor can be estimated quite reasonably and that PMMA lenses used in trial sets are preferable because they maximize the durability of the trial set and minimize the care required in conditioning the wetting angle of the lens.

Lens breakage

Gas-permeable lenses, because of their soft component, are liable to breakage. Patients must be taught the same careful care and cleaning routine that one has learned to establish for soft lenses.

Fabrication more difficult

The manufacture of these lenses does require more sophisticated care or the breakage rate in fabrication can be very high, particularly if they are made thin. A good manufacturing facility is important. This additional manufacturing capability may be reflected in a higher cost than that of PMMA lenses.

More deposit formation and greater drying

The new generation of lenses have a greater propensity to pick up proteins and lipids onto their surface than PMMA lenses have. They are not quite so vulnerable as the soft lenses. The lenses also dry easily between blinks. If one watches the patient carefully with the slit-lamp, one can readily see the evaporation of the tear film and a drying of the lens surface.

A number of good cleaners specifically designed for gas-permeable lenses are available for these lenses. Conditioners are also important to maintain the proper wetting angle of the contact lens.

CLINICAL PEARLS ON THE GAS-PERMEABLE LENS

1. In regard to thickness, not all gas-permeable lenses are the same. The CAB lenses tend to be thicker than the PMMA-silicone lenses. CAB usually has a center thickness of 0.19 mm compared to 0.10 mm for Polycon (silicone-acrylate). However, some of the recently developed CAB lenses (Rynco) are very slim. Edge thickness of CAB is often 0.18 mm, whereas edge treatment of silicone-acrylate can be refined to 0.08 mm. Thinner lenses mean better permeability, but thinner edges also mean greater breakage.
2. Large refractive errors require special attention to lens edges so that irritation is minimized (Fig. 21-6).
    Comment. For every 1 to 2 D of corneal cylinder we order the lenses 0.04 mm thicker to reduce lens flexure.
3. PMMA-silicone is not a homogeneous mixture when manufactured into buttons. Therefore permeability may vary slightly from one lens (of the same material and manufacturer) to another.
4. PMAA-silicone lenses must be well finished, as with blended edges. Despite their forgiving properties, quality in manufacturing is still all important.
5. The reduction in spectacle blur with a well-fitted gas-permeable lens is impres-

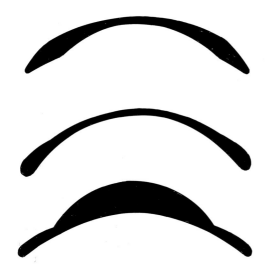

Fig. 21-6. For large refractive errors, the edge treatment is essential.

sive. Close to 90% of rigid lens patients sampled were vastly improved when the switch to a gas-permeable lens was made. Of course, the smaller the refractive error, the better the result because the distortions, minification, and aberration of a thick-lensed glass system still cannot compare to the visual accuracy obtained by use of any contact lens.

6. Frequently a lens will ride high just after a blink and then drop. When lens drop occurs, it usually means either a flatter lens is required or the blink is incomplete. If the latter is the case, the patient requires blinking exercises.

7. Gas-permeable lenses are best fitted steeper and larger than comparable PMMA lenses are.

8. Signs of corneal disaster under a PMMA lens include the following:
   a. The retinoscopy reflex on the naked cornea is irregular.
   b. There is irregularity from the reflection of a Placido disc.
   c. The mire reflection from the keratometer is distorted.
   d. Corneal edema is present with changes also in the corneal thickness. This change is apparent when one measures the central corneal thickness through the pachometer.
   e. Corneal hypesthesia occurs.
   f. These are corneal pitting and erosions of the epithelium.
   g. There is a change in the refractive error because of greater astigmatism, greater hyperopia attributable to flattening of the cornea, greater myopia in a mature adult, or suspicion of diabetes.

   Comment. When one is removing a PMMA lens, if the keratometer mires are distorted, refraction is difficult to refine and visual acuity is reduced. The contact lens should be checked for warpage with the Radiuscope. What to do? Refit with gas-permeable lenses preferably when the keratometer reading and refraction are stable. If vision is too poor with spectacles, it is permissible to refit immediately with gas-permeable lenses.

9. Gas-permeable lenses should be considered in any area where the temperature is generally warm or hot. Lenses such as the gas-permeable lens have a 25% greater thermal conductivity than PMMA lenses do, permitting a greater dissipation of heat. A PMMA lens acts as an insulator, increasing the metabolic activity of the epithelium and increasing the oxygen demand. So, if you live in Arizona or Texas, a gas-permeable lens should be on top of the list.

10. Flexure may result in astigmatism, which is aggravated if the lens is very thin, the fit is steep, or there is against-the-rule astigmatism (Fig. 21-7).

11. The major flaws of these lenses are improper edges. Because these lenses are frequently large in diameter, the edges tend to be thicker. There should be a plus-carrier lenticular lens for high-minus lenses. A minus-carrier lenticular lens should be used for low-minus lenses. A minus-carrier lenticular lens should be used for high-plus lenses. Any projection device will illuminate the edge profile. The integrity of the edge design is easily checked with the profile analyzer or the soft-lens analyzer.

12. Blinking may cause an epithelial defect at the 6 o'clock position (Fig. 21-8). This is particularly true if the edges are thick or the lens is steep. It will also occur if there is against-the-rule astigmatism with the

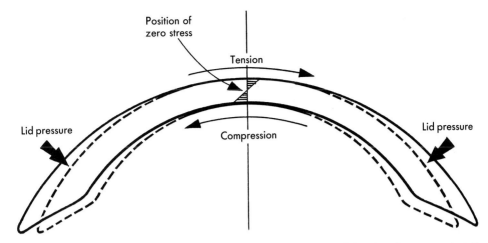

Fig. 21-7. Flexure-induced residual astigmatism. This is aggravated by thin lenses, against-the-rule toric corneas, steep fits, interpalpebral designs, hydrogel lenses, and silicone-acrylate lenses.

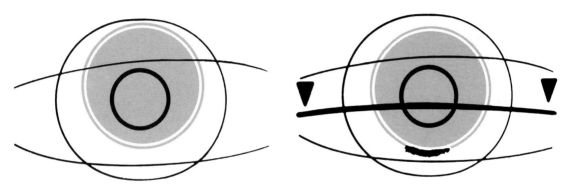

Fig. 21-8. Blinking may cause arcuate epithelial defect if edges are thick.

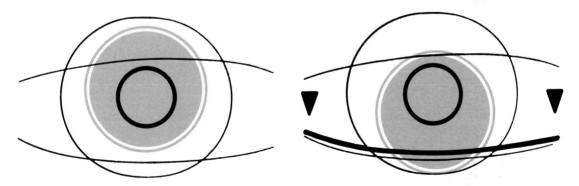

Fig. 21-9. Blinking may cause the lens to ride low.

flatter meridian vertically (see Fig. 24-6, *B*, on p. 302).

13. Blinking may also predispose to the lens riding low (Fig. 21-9). This may also occur if there is a moderate amount of with-the-rule astigmatism with the flatter meridian

placed horizontally. It may also occur if the lens is heavy or the edges are thick.

14. Lid gap or a thick lens may result in a gap of mucin tear film at the corneal surface adjacent to the contact lens. This may result in drying of the cornea, corneal ero-

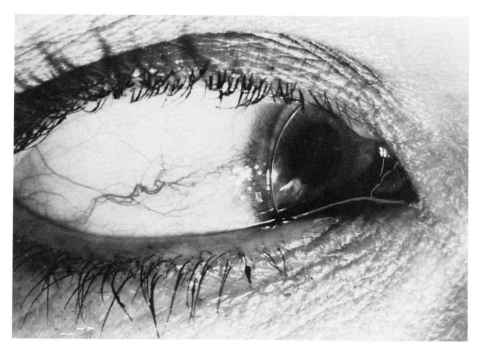

Fig. 21-10. Three to 9 o'clock staining and neovascularization caused by edge thickness with drying of the cornea at the edge of the lens.

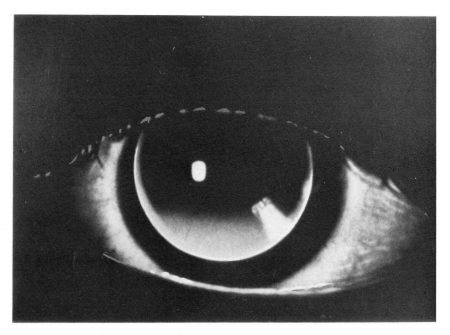

Fig. 21-11. A gas-permeable rigid lens fitted on a cornea with 4 diopters of astigmatism. Note the dark horizontal flat band.

sion, and eventually vascularization (Fig. 21-10). This usually occurs at 3 and 9 o'clock.

Summary of advantages. It would seem that gas-permeable lenses have a few more virtues than a PMMA lens does.

They are more comfortable.

They are safer.

They are better for use in warm climates or areas of low oxygen tension because they are a thermal conductor.

They are easier to adapt initially, and the adaptation time is reduced by 50%.

Some of these lenses are more wettable than other types in this classification.

They can hide up to 5 D of corneal astigmatism without going to a toric lens design (Fig. 21-11).

They are useful in keratoconus and in post-graft cases with irregular astigmatism and are better tolerated in children.

They give more satisfactory results in cases of piggyback fitting.

They cause less flare, glare, and photophobia because they have a large optic zone, and they relieve hypoxia created by an ill-fitting rigid lens.

They rarely require fenestration.

They are fitted with rigid-lens trial sets. Inventory is not generally required.

Why don't all wearers abandon PMMA and use gas-permeable lenses? They are. PMMA lens sales are dropping 10% to 15% per year. Eventually they will be an anachronism.

One benefit for PMMA lenses is that they are durable and may find use in teen-agers who are rough with their lenses.

FITTING SILICONE CONTACT LENSES

John F. Morgan*

Silicone resin contact lenses
Silicone elastomer (rubber)
contact lenses

The search for a contact lens material that was highly gas permeable has been pursued since the late 1950s. The use of silicone as a contact lens material dates to 1958, when Walter Becker of Pittsburgh working with the Mellon Institute and Dow Corning Ophthalmics, Inc. fabricated a relatively crude contact lens from silicone rubber (Fig. 22-1).

Contact lenses containing silicone are beginning to dominate the rigid contact lens market. Rigid contact lenses that contain silicone and other compounds are referred to as "silicone-acrylates." Rigid contact lenses made from silicone alone are silicone resin lenses. The rubberlike lenses made from silicone alone are called silicone elastomers.

The rigid contact lenses marketed by Dow Corning Ophthalmics, Inc. (Norfolk, Va.) are trade-named "Silcon" (Fig. 22-2) from a material termed "silafilcon A." Rubberlike contact lenses manufactured by Dow Corning Ophthalmics are trade-named "Silsoft" (Fig. 22-3) from a material named "elastofilcon A." These silicone contact lenses are the ones that are discussed in this chapter. They are the lenses that will be most readily available in the North American market. Silicone elastomer lenses have been manufactured by other companies in Europe and Japan. The availability of these lenses in North American is very likely to be limited.

*M.D., F.R.C.S.(C), Professor, Department of Ophthalmology, Queen's University, Kingston, Ontario, Canada.

SILICONE RESIN CONTACT LENSES

The silicone resin lens is a rigid lens. The information that pertains to the fitting of rigid lenses made from polymethylmethacrylate (PMMA) applies, in general, to the fitting of the silicone resin lenses. However there are very important exceptions relating to the physiologic tolerance of the eye for the silicone resin lens compared to the polymethylmethacrylate lens.

The physical parameters of the silicone resin lens, trade-named "Silcon" (silafilcon A), manufactured by Dow Corning Ophthalmics, are as follows (Fig. 22-4):

Specific gravity, 1.15 ± 0.2
Refractive index, 1.52 ± 0.005
Light transmission measures greater than 90% when dry
Surface character, wettable (hydrophilic)
Water absorption, 0.02% for 24 hours
Oxygen permeability (polarographic determination) in DK values, 8.3×10^{-11} at 21° C, and 16.3×10^{-11} at 35° C

The finished lens is treated to make the surface wettable (hydrophilic). This is not a surface addition but a treatment of the surface of the silicone resin material. To maintain this surface as wettable as required, one should always store the lenses in one of the solutions that are recommended for it. If a lens is allowed to dry, the wettability of the surface of the lens will be considerably reduced.

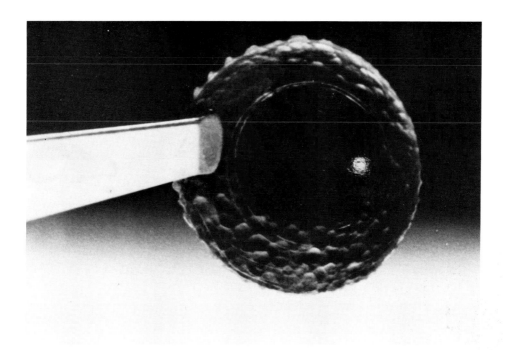

Fig. 22-1. Original silicone elastomer lens fabricated by W. Becker in 1958.

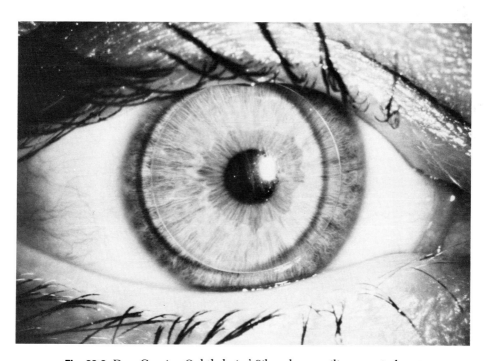

Fig. 22-2. Dow Corning Ophthalmics' Silcon lens, a silicone resin lens.

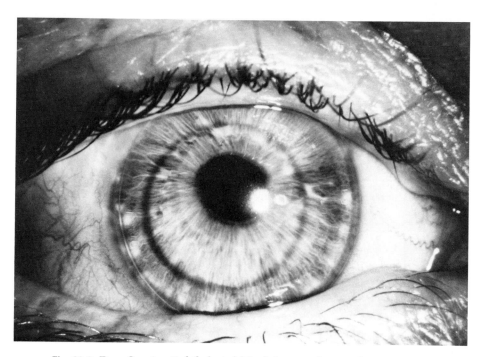

Fig. 22-3. Dow Corning Ophthalmics' Silsoft lens, a silicone elastomer lens.

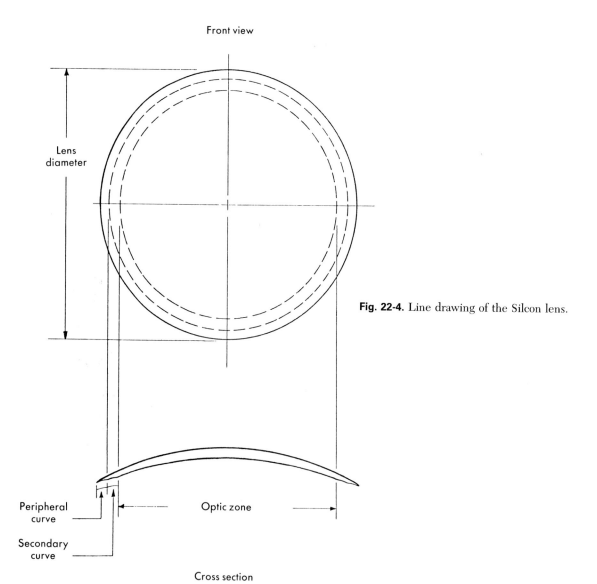

Front view

Lens
diameter

Fig. 22-4. Line drawing of the Silcon lens.

Peripheral
curve

Secondary
curve

Optic zone

Cross section

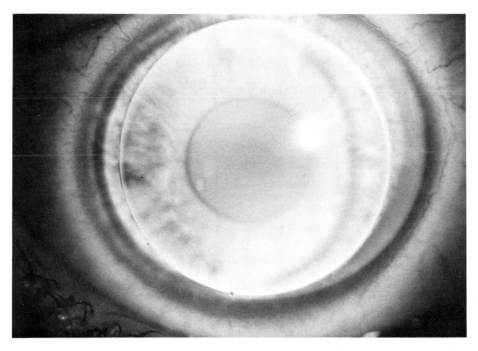

Fig. 22-5. An apical-fitting rigid contact lens with apical clearance from the steeper-than-K fit.

Available parameters

The Silcon lens can be obtained as an inventory lens or as a lens designed to the specifications of the fitter.

The inventory lenses have the following characteristics

Diameter, 8.8 mm
Optic zone, 7.6 mm
Power range (minus powers only), from −1.00 to −6.00 diopters
Base curves, 7.25 to 8.23 in 0.25-diopter steps
Lens center thickness, 0.12 mm nominal at −3.00 diopters

Method of fitting inventory Silcon lenses

The very important but basically common-sense indications for the selection of patients for the wearing of contact lenses of course apply. A detailed examination of the eye is mandatory, as for all patients being fit with any type of contact lens. The fundamental information obtained by ophthalmometry and refraction must be recorded.

The inventory lens being discussed has a relatively small diameter at 8.8 mm. This diameter means that the lens will be essentially an apical fitting lens (Fig. 22-5). This means that the lens will not be a high-riding lens sitting well up toward the superior limbus, beneath the upper lid. The lens, by virtue of its diameter of 8.8 mm, will tend to sit apically between the lids in the palpebral-fissure area of the cornea. The method of fitting then has to be steeper than K, with very few exceptions.

Ideally the fitting of the lens should be done with assessment lenses. It is *not* necessary to have the assessment lenses made from the silicone material. In fact, it is preferable in many respects to have the assessment lenses manufactured from polymethylmethacrylate. Polymethylmethacrylate will not changes its surface wettability significantly if it is stored dry. In an office setting, it is preferable to have lenses that can be stored dry without concern that their surface wettability will be significantly changed. Polymethylmethacrylate lenses are less expensive to have fabricated for an assessment set. The concerns of initial expenditure and breakage are less. It is, however, very important that the polymethylmethacrylate lenses have very similar parameters to the Silcon inventory lens that will be prescribed. A useful assessment set would consist of the following, made in polymethylmethacrylate:

Base curve, 7.25 to 8.23 in 0.50-diopter steps with 12 lenses involved.
Lens diameter, 8.8 mm
Optic zone, 7.6 mm
  Peripheral curve, 0.3 mm. in width
  Intermediate curve, 0.3 mm in width
Power, −3.00 diopters
Center thickness, 0.12 mm

With this set of lenses, one should be able to assess the adequacy of the diameter 8.8 mm for a given patient. The rules of thumb for the initial selection of lenses are based on the relationship of lens curvature to the patient's K (K, the longer radius meridian or flatter curve of the cornea). If the patient has less than a 1-diopter difference between the meridians of the cornea, a lens with a base curve that is 0.25 to 0.5 diopter steeper should be selected. If a patient has a difference in corneal meridians of 1 to 2 diopters, the lens selected should be between 0.5 and 1 diopter steeper than K.

The assessment lens that most closely approximates the desired corneal curvature to base-curve configuration is tried on the patient's eye. I do not recommend the use of a topical anesthetic in the trial of rigid lenses. I believe that the anomalies this introduces are far greater than any particular value it may present. With any rigid contact lens there will be a period of at least 20 minutes before one can assess the lens on the patient's eye. This period of 20 minutes must be allowed for. The initial tear response must be reduced to allow the fitter to accurately obtain the details of the lens-corneal relationship.

The adequacy of fit of the assessment lens can be determined by its centering and movement characteristics. The lens should be centered so that the optic pathway of the lens is properly encompassing the visual axis of the eye. The lens should move at least 1 mm with a full blink. The lens should not consistently lag low after blinking.

The adequacy of the fit can be further assessed by the use of fluorescein. The ideal fitting pattern should show minimal apical clearance with moderate edge lift. Noticeable pooling of fluorescein in the apical region indicates that the lens is potentially too steep. Evidence of lack of fluorescein in the apical area would indicate the lens is too flat.

Once the adequacy of fit has been assessed and considered to be functionally good, an over-refraction of the lens for power can be carried out.

If an adequate fit can be obtained with the 8.8 mm diameter lens available from inventory and the patient's power requirements fall within the currently available powers in inventory, a lens can be ordered for the patient.

Custom fitting of Silcon contact lenses

If the practitioner finds that the 8.8 mm diameter is not a diameter that gives satisfactory results, the Silcon lens can be fabricated with any set of parameters that the practitioner feels will be functionally good.

Many practitioners, with several years of experience with rigid gas-permeable contact lenses, have come to the conclusion that the larger diameters are functionally much better. They are better primarily because of the comfort that they provide. The advantages of relatively large rigid contact lenses have been known since rigid contact lenses were first found to be practical. Diameters in the range of 9.2 to 10 mm were found to be more comfortable, with the added advantage of allowing for a large optic zone.

It is recommended that a diameter for a myopic patient be 9.2 ± 0.2 mm. An assessment contact lens set is very necessary for the fitting of these lenses. An assessment set that could be useful should contain lenses as follows:

Diameter, 9.2 mm
Base curves, 7.25 to 8.23 mm in 0.5-diopter steps (12 lenses)
Optic zone, 8 mm (intermediate curve, 0.3 mm wide; peripheral curve, 0.3 mm wide; recommended that the intermediate curve be 1 mm longer than the base curve; recommended that the peripheral curve be approximately 3.5 mm longer than the base curve)
Center thickness, 0.12 mm
Power, −3.00 diopters

This assessment lens set is used in the same manner as described for the 8.8 mm assessment set.

Because the lens is slightly larger in diameter, 9.2 mm compared to 8.8 mm, a close to, if not on K, fitting may be used for patients with no significant difference in the corneal curvature of the two meridians. If, however, there is more than 1 diopter difference in the two me-

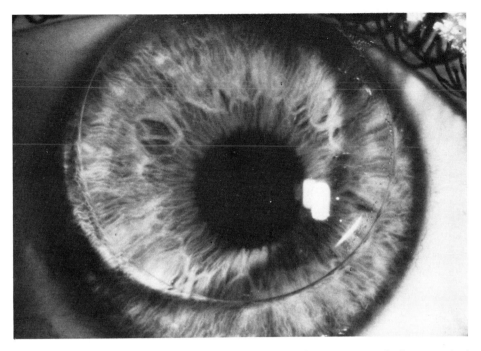

Fig. 22-6. A moderately large diameter rigid gas-permeable lens, 9.4 mm, which centers high.

ridians as measured by the ophthalmometer, it is considered advisable that the fitting be at least 0.5 diopter steeper than the flattest meridian (K).

The appropriate assessment lens is selected, the lens is placed on the patient's eye without topical anesthetic, and the lens is allowed to settle for 20 minutes. One then assesses the fit of the lens by observing the way the lens centers and moves. The large-diameter lenses of 9.2 mm or greater will or should center high. The upper edge of the lens should be beneath the upper lid near the limbus (Fig. 22-6). The movement pattern of the lens should indicate a degree of downward movement, but not the wide excursion that is seen with lenses of the 8.6 ± 0.2 mm diameter range. The lens will be venting with the blink, rather than having a wide excursion of movement when the upper lid moves down.

The fluorescein pattern should show apical clearance with a thin band of fluorescein present beneath the surface of the lens. A large pool of fluorescein in the apical area indicates that a lens will be too snug with inadequate movement. A very thin to nonexistent pool of fluorescein in the apical zone indicates that a

lens may have an apical touch. This will produce discomfort.

Once a lens that meets these criteria has been found in the assessment set, the over-refraction is then carried out. The final lens can be ordered to these parameters.

The occasional patient will be found for whom a lens of diameter 9.2 mm does not give an adequate fit. It is possible to extrapolate from the fitting characteristics of a 9.2 mm lens up to a lens of 9.4 mm or down to a lens of 9.0 mm. However, it is somewhat risky to extrapolate to diameters larger or smaller than those mentioned. Depending on the type and size of the practitioner's practice, it may be wise to have an assessment lens set of a larger diameter. A diameter of 9.8 mm would allow the practitioner a range of 9.6 to 10 mm when ordering a lens for a given patient. The lenses required in a 9.8 diameter and made from polymethylmethacrylate, as emphasized before, should be of the same base-curve selection as quoted previously.

Nonassessment lens method of fitting

If the practitioner does not have assessment lenses to utilize in the fitting of the Silcon lens as just described, one can fit the patient using rules of thumb.

This technique is not recommended because in essence what is being done is to produce a customized assessment lens for that particular patient. If this technique is used, the practitioner should be prepared to change the specifications of the lens. If the practitioner is going to utilize this particular technique, the only practical way of ordering the lens is on a per case plan.

The rules of thumb that should be followed are basically the same as those outlined for the selection of the assessment lenses. The diameter should be 9.2 mm. The selection of the base curve will be dependent on the ophthalmometer readings. If there is less than a 1-diopter difference in the corneal meridians, the base curve of the lens should be 0.50 diopter steeper than the flattest meridian (K). If the difference between the corneal meridians is between 1 and 2 diopters, the base curve of the lens ordered should be 0.75 diopter steeper than the flattest meridian (K). If the difference between the meridians is greater than 2 diopters, the base curve of the lenses ordered should be the radius of curvature of the flattest meridian of the cornea plus one half the difference of the two meridians. An intermediate curve of 0.3 mm in width that is 1 mm longer than the base curve is recommended combined with a peripheral curve that is 0.3 mm in width, approximately 4 mm longer than the ordered base curve. Maximum blending of the point of change between the curves is suggested.

The power of the ordered lens would be arrived at when one uses the rules for vertex distance based on the power that the patient requires with glasses and compensating for the plus tear lens that would be formed by the apical clearance of the contact lens on the cornea. For example, if the patient required a −3.50-diopter power in the glasses, vertex distance could be ignored. If the apical clearance of the lens is 0.50 diopter, a −0.50-diopter power must be added to the lens to compensate for the +0.50-diopter tear lens that should be present. The resultant power of this particular lens would be −4.00 diopters.

This method is reasonably successful provided that the cornea is symmetric between its meridians. As more corneal astigmatism is encountered, this technique is less likely to produce an acceptable fit.

When this lens is received from the manufacturer, it is used as a customized assessment lens. If changes in the lens must be made to achieve a better fit or better visual acuity, one would order a second lens incorporating the changes found to be required.

Lens handling and care

The silicone resin lenses are rigid lenses. The methods of insertion and removal that are appropriate to other rigid lenses are utilized with this lens. Illustrations and details of lens handling can be found in other sections of this book.

I must emphasize that the silicone resin lenses will wet poorly if they are left out of their fluid medium. Lenses that are allowed to dry for any period of time will be found to wet poorly. Each new Silcon contact lens will be shipped in a sterile sealed glass vial filled with purified water (Fig. 22-7).

Silicone-derived lenses, both the silicone resins and the silicone-acrylates, in clinical practice have a tendency to be coated more rapidly than polymethylmethacrylate lenses are. Regular cleaning of the lenses on their removal each day must be strongly recommended to the patients. In addition, it has been found most helpful to have the patients use the papaine-based enzymatic cleaning tablets every 10 to 14 days.

The lens may be cared for by use of either a heat decontaminating system or a chemical decontaminating system.

With a heat decontaminating system, it is recommended at this time that one use Soft Mate (Barnes-Hind, Sunnyvale, Calif.) to clean the lens by placing two drops on the lens surfaces and rubbing very gently between the thumb and index finger or between the palm of one hand and a fingertip of the other hand. After the lens is cleaned, it should be rinsed in preserved saline solution. The lens is then placed in the heater unit filled with preserved saline. It is wise to avoid saline preserved by thimerosal.

The chemical care system can employ wetting-storage solutions that are clearly marked for gas-permeable lenses. Dow Corning Oph-

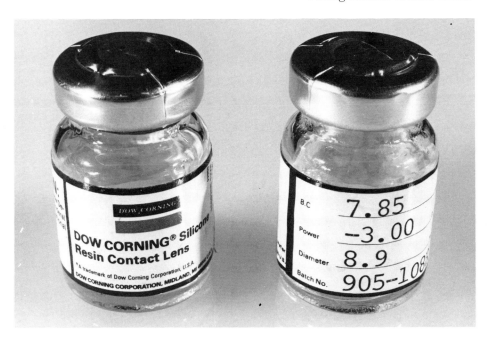

Fig. 22-7. Vials for shipping the Silcon lens by Dow Corning Ophthalmics.

thalmics currently recommends, based on the approved materials for lens care at the time of the clinical studies, that one use Normol* to rinse the lens after cleaning with Preflex. The lens is stored in Flexsol.* The other chemical care is based on Flex-Care,* which is used both to rinse the lenses and to store them overnight.

If the patient warps the lens, either by rough handling or by squeezing it in the case, the curve of the lens may be restored by heating of the lens. The silicone resin material has an excellent shape retention, and if the lens is heated in distilled water or normal saline solution, the original curvature of the lens will be restored. The method that we use in our office is to place the lens in its vial and to heat it in the units designed to care for soft (hydrophilic) contact lenses. If the patients are using a chemical care technique in the decontamination of their lenses, it may be necessary for them to bring their warped lenses to your office to have this procedure carried out. If however, the patients are using a thermal care technique, they can return the lens to its prewarped curvature by passing the lens through two or three heat cycles.

*Alcon/BP, Ft. Worth, Texas.

Custom lenses

Dow Corning Ophthalmics will supply lenses to any prescription that the practitioner wishes. They can provide any power, plus or minus, and any base curve. They will produce a lens of any diameter, with any optic zone or center thickness or secondary or bevel curves. They will also manufacture special designs including toric curves and bifocals, but facilities for this may be limited and the practitioner is wise to check with Dow Corning to find out what special lens configuration can be fabricated.

To avail oneself of this complete range of lens parameters, the practitioner should use the assessment-lens approach to fitting his patients. The emphasis thus far has been in fitting the myopic patient. The hyperopic patient and the aphakic patient can be fit with the Silcon lens.

Fitting the hyperopic patient

The patient should be fit with the appropriate assessment lenses manufactured from polymethylmethacrylate. It is not considered advisable to use lenses other than those of similar configuration of the final ordered lenses. A minus lens, even a very low power, will have significantly different fitting characteristics from those of a hyperopic lens. The fitting set that is recommended for hyperopes would have the following characteristics:

Base curves, diameter, 9.4 mm
Base curves, 7.25 to 8.23 mm in 0.50-diopter steps
Method of manufacture, single cut
Optic zone, 8.2 mm in diameter (intermediate curve, 0.3 mm in width; peripheral curve, 0.3 mm in width)
Power plus four

The principles of fitting the assessment lens are the same as those described for the myopic patient. Corneas that have no significant difference between their meridians on the ophthalmometer reading can be fit 0.25 to 0.50 diopter steeper than the flattest meridian. The large diameter of the lens will produce a large sagital depth, and an on K fitting may be the best choice depending on the fluorescein appearance. If the assessment lens that is 0.25 to 0.50 diopter steeper shows a significant apical pool with very little fluorescein evident in the midperipheral zone, an assessment lens that is on K, that is, a lens whose base curve has the same radius of curvature as the flattest curve of the cornea, may be a better fit. A cornea that has a difference in its meridians of 1 to 2 diopters should be tried with an assessment lens that is 0.75 to 1 diopter steeper than the flattest meridian. If the difference in the corneal meridians is greater than 2 diopters, the initial assessment lens should have a base curve that is equal to the flattest meridian plus one half the difference between the two meridians.

If the practitioner does not have an assessment lens set of these parameters, the per case method of ordering may be used with the initial lens based on the previously stated rules of thumb.

Fitting the aphakic patient

The aphakic lens is, of necessity, relatively heavy. To minimize the tendency of the lens to drop low and override the inferior limbus, the weight of the lens is reduced by lenticularizing the lens. An optical zone of 8 mm should be aimed for. To achieve this, one often requires a large-diameter lens. The assessment-lens set for the aphakic would consist of lenses that have the following specifications:

Diameter, 9.8 mm
Base curves, 7.25 to 8.23 mm in 0.50-diopter steps (12 lenses)

Method of manufacture, plano carrier lenticulus with an optic zone as close to 8 mm as possible (intermediate curve, 0.3 mm in width; peripheral curve, 0.3 mm in width)
Power, +14.00 diopters

The lens selected from this assessment set for a given patient should have a base curve that is 0.75 diopter steeper than the flattest meridian (K) if the difference between the meridians is less than 1 diopter. If the difference between the meridians is between 1 and 2 diopters, a lens that has a base curve of 1.00 to 1.25 diopters steeper than the flattest meridian should be selected. If the difference in the corneal meridians is greater than 2 diopters, the assessment lens selected should have a base curve that is equal to the flattest meridian's radius of curvature plus one half the difference between the radius of curvatures of the two meridians.

The aphakic assessment lens should become centered with its optic zone well over the visual axis of the eye. The lens should not override the inferior limbus. The visual acuity with the lens, after the initial period of 20 minutes to allow the tearing to subside, should be stable with the over-refraction.

The final power of the lens that is to be ordered will be dependent on the over-correction that is required in the case of both the hyperope and aphakic patient.

If the lenses are being ordered without an assessment lens being utilized, the power of the lens will be a result of the vertex rules applied to the power of the patient's glasses with compensation for the plus tear lens that is formed by the contact lens on the cornea. As the power requirements of a given patient increase, the chances for error in ordering power increase. The power requirements of an aphakic patient are less likely to be arrived at accurately by the rules-of-thumb method than they are by over-refraction of a well-fit assessment contact lens.

Wearing schedule

In theory, with the gas permeability of the silicone resin lens, the patient should be able to put the lens on and wear it all waking hours from the first day. Although this may be true in theory, it is not a practice that is carried out for a variety of reasons.

I still recommend to the patients that they

build their wearing time up over a period of time. I suggest that the patient wear the lens 3 hours the first day and, if he or she is comfortable at the end of that time, add 2 hours a day to the wearing schedule until all-day comfortable wearing is achieved. If a patient is free of discomfort, he or she should be able to achieve all waking hour wearing times within a week, following this schedule. However, patients are strongly advised that if an eye is uncomfortable when the lens is taken out at the end of any one particular time period the patients should not exceed that time period the following day. For example, if the patient finds that the eyes are uncomfortable after wearing the lenses for 7 hours, he or she should not exceed 7 hours the following day. If the eyes are still uncomfortable the following day, the lenses should not be inserted and the patient should be assessed in the office.

The reason for continuing to follow a relatively slow buildup of lens-wearing time, in the face of good gas permeability, is based upon the following clinically observed facts. The first is that more patients fail with contact lenses because of poor blinking patterns than any other single factor. Although a patient may have a "normal" blinking pattern without a lens in, the presence of a foreign body on the cornea may significantly suppress the patient's desire and ability to blink. A reestablishment of a "normal" blink rate and excursion may take some time in many patients. If the patient were allowed to wear the lens all the waking hours, the decreased blinking rate and excursion would lead to dry eyes with redness and discomfort. I have found that some patients cannot tolerate their lenses beyond 6 hours. Almost invariably when such a patient is assessed with the lenses in after 3 to 4 hours, one will find that the blink rate has been decreased significantly in frequency. In addition, the patient may have a pseudoblink. The excursion in a pseudoblink is not full. The lid contacts the upper edge of the lens and does not fully sweep the palpebral area of the eye.

Having the patients wear their lenses over gradually increasing periods of time also provides a safety factor for those who cannot handle their lenses adeptly in the first few weeks. If the cornea is slightly traumatized during insertion or removal, this minor problem may be turned into a major one should the patient attempt to wear the lens for prolonged periods of time during the waking hours.

Despite extensive checking in the office to ensure that the lenses have met specifications with good blends of the curves and a good edge finish, borderline inadequate lenses may still be placed on patients' eyes. By limiting the amount of wearing in the initial period, patients may avoid significant problems caused by poor blends and edge finish.

SILICONE ELASTOMER (RUBBER) CONTACT LENSES

Contact lenses made from the silicone elastomer (rubber) are the only lenses that are flexible under all conditions. This presents problems in their manufacture. Silicone elastomer lenses made by Dow Corning Ophthalmics and trade-named "Silsoft" (elastofilcon A) are manufactured by precision molding under high temperature and pressure. The lenses are then laser-marked with their individual power, base curve, and lot number. The fact that the material is flexible under all conditions makes edging a difficult technical feat.

The lens design of the Silsoft contact lenses includes a tricurve posterior surface and a lenticular anterior surface in the hyperopic configuration (Fig. 22-8). The myopic configuration does not have a lenticular anterior surface. The lenses are available in a diameter of 11.3 mm in the minus series. They are available in 11.3 and 12.5 mm in the plus series.

Diameter selection has been a significant point of interest. Numerous semiscleral designs (13 to 14 mm diameter) were tried. These lenses were undoubtedly much more comfortable than the smaller diameters currently being marketed. However, loss of lens motion was a common occurrence with the large-diameter lenses.

The silicone elastomer lenses produced by Dow Corning Ophthalmics, trade-named "Silsoft," have a hydrophilic surface. This surface is not a coating or an additional level of a different substance. The normally hydrophobic characteristic of the silicone material has been changed by a patented process to allow the surface of the lens to be wettable. The technique involves producing hydroxyl (OH) groups on the surface of the lens. These hydroxyl groups on the lens surface provide the hydrophilic (wettable) characteristic needed for a contact lens.

Front view

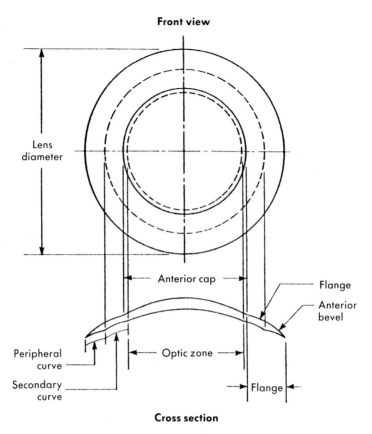

Lens
diameter

Anterior cap

Flange

Anterior
bevel

Peripheral
curve

Secondary
curve

Optic zone

Flange

Cross section

Fig. 22-8. Line drawing of the Silsoft lens for the correction of high hyperopia (aphakia). (From Morgan, J.F.: In Hartstein, J., editor: Extended wear contact lenses for aphakia and myopia, St. Louis, 1982, The C.V. Mosby Co.)

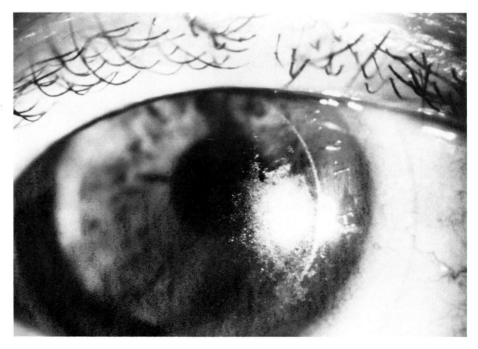

Fig. 22-9. Poor wetting of the surface of a Silsoft lens after it had been lost from the eye for 24 hours.

This hydrophilic surface of the lens maintains itself as long as it remains in a water environment "most of the time." The natural tears maintain the wettable lens surface as do the cleaning, disinfecting, and storage solutions used with the lenses.

However, it is very important to remember that any prolonged period of drying of the lens may drive off sufficiently large numbers of the hydroxyl groups on the lens surface so that it loses some or all of its wettability. In practical clinical terms, this means that the lenses must always be stored wet in the office. Patients must be warned that if the lens is lost from the eye and not found for several hours, it is quite probable that it will not be functional because the surface will not be adequately wettable (Fig. 22-9).

Lens parameters

The Silsoft contact lenses are currently available with the following parameters

Base curves, 7.3, 7.5, 7.7, 7.9, 8.1, and 8.3 mm radius of curvature
Diameter, 11.3 mm in the minus series; 11.3 and 12.5 mm in the plus series
Power, -0.75 to -5.00 inclusive in 0.25-diopter steps in the minus series; $+7$ to $+20$ inclusive in 0.5-diopter steps in the high-plus (aphakic) series
Index of refraction, 1.44 ± 0.02

Center thickness, 0.10 mm nominal in the minus series; 0.35 mm at $+14$ diopters in the high-plus series
Optic transmission, greater than 85% when dry
Oxygen permeability (DK), 34×10^{-11} at 21° C

Prolonged (extended) wear

The remarkably high oxygen-permeability coefficient of the silicone elastomer material makes it the best candidate for prolonged-wear lenses among all the materials that are currently being used for contact lenses. For practical purposes, the oxygen equivalent that is available to the eye while wearing a silicone elastomer lens is essentially the same as that available in the atmosphere. Thickness does not significantly change the amount of oxygen that is available. This is in contrast to the silicone resin lenses or silicone-acrylate lenses, the rigid materials, in which the oxygen transmission decreases as the lens thickness increases. For example, a silicone elastomer lens with a center thickness of 0.1 mm has an equivalent oxygen performance of over 20%. Even when the thickness of this lens is increased to 0.4 mm the equivalent oxygen performance is above 19%. In contrast the silicone resin lens at a center thickness of 0.1 mm has an equivalent oxygen performance of approximately 12%, and at a center thickness of 0.4 mm it has an equivalent oxygen performance of approximately 7% (Fig. 22-10).

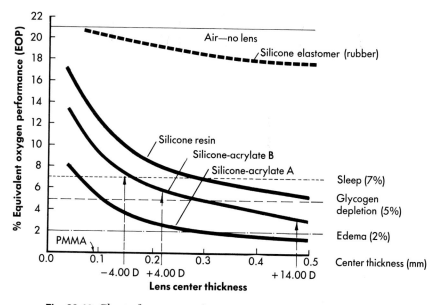

Fig. 22-10. Chart of oxygen performance versus lens center thickness.

Fitting the silicone elastomer contact lenses (Dow Corning Ophthalmics Silsoft Lens)

Minus series. A set of assessment lenses is mandatory for the fitting of the elastomer lens. No rules of thumb for ordering a lens based on measurements that can be done in the office are really practical. The assessment lens set for the minus series should consist of one of each of the available base curves (7.5 to 8.3 mm in 0.2 mm steps) in a power of −3.00 diopters.

The necessary prerequisite examination must of course be carried out. The contraindications for the utilization of contact lenses must be reviewed. With these fundamental steps having been done, the initial lens that is selected from the assessment set should be one that is on K. This means that the base curve of the assessment lens should have the same radius of curvature as the flattest meridian of the cornea. Because only one diameter, 11.3 mm, is available in the minus series, there is no difficulty in selecting which particular diameter should be considered.

It is always wise to start with the lens that parallels the flattest K. If there is a significant degree of difference between the two meridians of the cornea, that is, a significant degree of corneal astigmatism, it is probable that the visual acuity achieved with the silicone elastomer (Silsoft) contact lens will not be adequate. The Silsoft lens will mask or compensate for more astigmatism than a thin hydrophilic (HEMA) contact lens will but not significantly more. If good visual acuity cannot be achieved with the silicone elastomer contact lens, it is probably not indicated. A lens that is significantly steeper than the flattest meridian of the cornea may mask a degree of astigmatism and may initially feel quite comfortable. However, this lens almost invariably will lose movement. When movement is lost, there is no tear exchange beneath the lens and the lens may lock on. The locking-on of a silicone elastomer lens is discussed in more detail later.

After selection of a silicone elastomer lens in the minus series that has a base curve approximately the same as the flattest meridian of the cornea, it is placed upon the patient's eye and allowed to remain there for at least 30 to 40 minutes. A word of caution, a well-fitted silicone elastomer lens in the minus series is quite

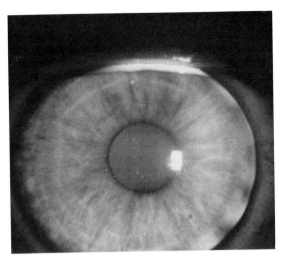

Fig. 22-11. "Fluting" of the edge of a Silsoft lens.

uncomfortable compared to a well-fitted hydrophilic (HEMA) contact lens. Associated with the discomfort will, of course, be the reflex tearing. Adequate time must be given for allowance of this reflex tearing to decrease toward the normal base-line level.

After waiting at least 30 minutes, the patient is assessed for fit. The ideal fit is one that shows slight apical clearance, slight intermediate zone bearing, and peripheral clearance. Fluorescein may be used with these lenses because they will not absorb this material. The lens should move at least 1 to 2 mm with each blink. The lens should maintain a degree of stable centering to permit stable visual acuity. The practitioner may note that there is a degree of what has been termed "fluting" or "scalloping" of the lens edge on the cornea (Fig. 22-11). This particular appearance was more evident when the 12.5 mm diameter lens for the minus series was available for clinical trials. The presence of this change is in itself not an indicator that the lens is a poor fit. In fact, just the opposite was the case in the clinical trials. The presence of fluting indicated that there was a high probability that the lens would not lose movement over the wearing time of the patient.

Once one has established that the lens becomes centered, has movement, and has minimal apical clearance, one carries out an overrefraction to arrive at the power that would be required for the patient with the particular base curve of the lens on the eye. If the lens is moving excessively and will not stay centered, the practitioner has one of two options. He may elect to wait another half hour and reassess the lens because the excess movement may be the result of increased tearing related to relative lens discomfort. He may elect to go to a lens with a steeper base curve.

It is probably wise to wait another half hour provided that the lens is not decentering to the degree where it will not maintain itself on the cornea for most of the time under observation. If it is constantly getting displaced off the cornea, selection of a steeper base curve is indicated.

These lenses do tend to lose movement with time. It is for this reason that waiting a further half hour, with what appears to be a borderline fit of the lens, is advised. If, after one waits a further half hour and the lens appears to be more stable with a more stable vision, this may be the base curve of choice for the lens.

If the practitioner elects to go to a steeper base curve, he should not progress beyond more than 0.2 mm "steeper" than the patient's cornea; that is, the radius of curvature of the base curve of the lens selected should not be more than 0.2 mm less than the radius of curvature of the flattest meridian of the cornea. If the steeper curve lens will provide the criteria that have been set out for a well-fitted lens, it may be the lens of choice. It is mandatory that this lens have movement. When the lens lacks movement in the initial fitting procedure, the patient may note that it is significantly more comfortable than the lens that does have movement. However, the practitioner must beware of the lens with minimal movement during the fitting procedure. Almost invariably this lens will lose movement over a period of time measured in days, and a locked-on lens may ensue.

If the initially selected lens that was on K appears to be a good fit and satisfies the criteria noted above, the practitioner should then move to the next flattest lens. The object of the fitting exercise is to fit the cornea with the flattest lens that will maintain centering and provide stable visual acuity. When one reaches a lens that is flatter than K that will not stay centered and provide stable visual acuity, the lens that was steeper by one step should be the lens

of choice, provided that it did have adequate movement.

Having gone through this exercise, the practitioner should then observe the patient, with the lens that the practitioner believes is the best choice on the eye for a period of not less than 3 hours. If the lens is maintaining movement at the end of three hours, it would be the assessment lens whose base curve would be that of the final lens chosen for the patient.

Fitting the aphakic patient. The same basic directions discussed previously in the fitting of the minus series apply to the high-plus (aphakic) series of elastomer lenses manufactured by Dow Corning Ophthalmics (Silsoft).

Fitting the aphakic person cannot be achieved without a set of assessment lenses. A lens in each of the base curves that are available, 7.5, 7.7, 7.9, 8.1, and 8.3 mm, in each of the diameters 11.3 and 12.5 mm, with a power of +14.00 diopters would be required in the assessment lens set.

From this assessment lens set one selects a lens the base curve of which has the same or approximately the same radius of curvature as the flattest meridian of the cornea (on K fitting). The smallest diameter of the two available, 11.3 mm, should be used. This on K fitting lens in the smaller diameter is then placed on the patient's cornea and allowed to remain there at least 30 minutes. The hyperopic series of lenses, interestingly enough, are more comfortable initially than the minus series lenses are. However, they are less comfortable than a well-fitted hydrophilic (HEMA) aphakic contact lens. They are more comfortable than a rigid contact lens for an aphakic. Because of the decreased sensitivity of the average aphakic patient's cornea, an aphake has less awareness of the lens than a myopic patient has.

After waiting 30 minutes, one assesses the lens. The criteria for fitting are the same as the minus series. One hopes to have minimal apical clearance, mild intermediate zone bearing, and peripheral clearance. This can be determined by the use of fluorescein (Fig. 22-12). The lens should have 1 to 2 mm of movement with the full blink. The lens should become centered so that its optic zone is over the visual axis of the patient. The lens should not become decentered dramatically off the cornea. Decentering off the cornea, even with what turns out

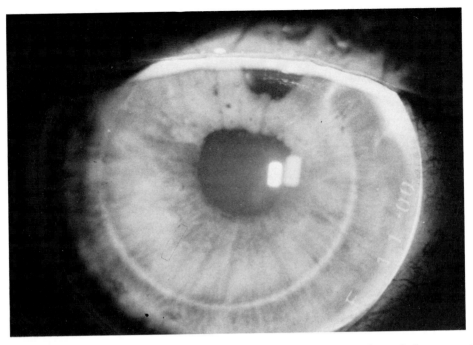

Fig. 22-12. Fluorescein pattern of a well-fitted Silsoft lens showing minimal apical clearance with intermediate bearing and peripheral clearance.

to be a functionally good fitting lens, is not uncommon in the aphakic patient. If the patient is closely watched, it will be found that rather than blinking in a normal manner, the aphakic patient is squeezing his lids closed. As he releases the blepharospastic lids, the lens is often displaced off the cornea by the snug upper lid. If this appears to be the reason for the lens getting displaced, reassurance is given to the patient and a further 30 minutes of wait is deemed necessary. If the lens is displacing off the cornea despite the appearance of a normal blinking pattern, the larger-diameter lens, 12.5 mm, should be tried on this patient. This larger-diameter lens for the patient should have the same base curve as the 11.3 mm lens that was being displaced.

When the practitioner is satisfied that the reflex tearing has become significantly reduced and the patient's blinking pattern is normal, the lens fit should be assessed. If the criteria have been met, that is, movement of 1 to 2 mm with a normal blink and a minimal apical clearance with light intermediate bearing and peripheral lift, an over-refraction can be carried out to determine the power of the lens re-

quired for the individual patient with that particular base curve.

The configuration of the silicone elastomer lens for the aphake entails a relatively thick center portion of the lens where the optics are. This thicker central area, compared to the relatively thin central area of a minus configuration lens, permits the lens to compensate for moderate degrees of astigmatism. It is not uncommon to see 1.5 to 2 diopters of corneal astigmatism compensated for by the high plus series of silicone elastomer lenses produced by Dow Corning Ophthalmics. In those patients in whom there is residual corneal astigmatism present, an over-correction of the appropriate amount of astigmatism can be given to the patients in their glasses. The aphake often wears glasses with his contact lenses for reading. If these are made in the form of bifocals, the incorporation of a correction for astigmatism is not a difficult thing to achieve and is functionally quite satisfactory from the patient's standpoint.

After the practitioner has obtained a good fit, he should then try an 11.3 mm diameter lens in the next flattest base curve. The aim in fit-

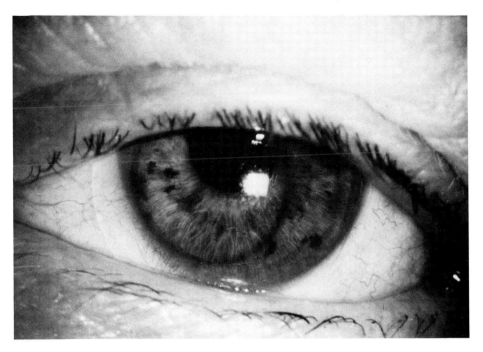

Fig. 22-13. Decentering Silsoft lens.

ting is to find the lens with the flattest base curve and the smallest diameter that will stay centered on the cornea to permit stable vision. He should never really be satisfied that he has achieved this until he has placed a Silsoft lens on the eye that will not maintain a centered position with stable visual acuity (Fig. 22-13).

Having found a lens of base curve and diameter that promises to be clinically satisfactory, the practitioner should then observe this lens on the patient's eyes after the patient has worn it for a minimum period of 3 hours. I must emphasize that these lenses lose movement with time. In the clinical studies, the recurring theme associated with problems was the selection of a lens whose base curve was steeper than what was required. The lenses that were steeper appeared initially to be good fits and were certainly initially comfortable. The passage of time with the lenses that did not initially show adequate movement produced, in a number of cases, a tendency for the lenses to lock on. When the figures were studied for the lenses that did lock on, almost invariably they were steeper than the flattest meridian of the cornea.

With the presently available parameters of the Silsoft high plus series of lenses, the practitioner should not be too upset when he finds a patient he canot fit. Data from the studies indicated that there were 5% of patients who could not be fit with the parameters available. Hopefully, with the passage of time, a greater range of parameters will be available so that this small percentage of patients can be fit with the Silsoft lens.

"Locking-on" syndrome

Reference has been made several times to a tendency for lenses to lock on. The Silsoft contact lens is not the only lens available that will lock on to a cornea. Hydrophilic lenses were seen to lock on corneas. The reasons for a hydrophilic lens "locking on" a cornea vary. One type of hydrophilic lens has demonstrated a change in its physical characteristics with a change in pH of the tears during sleep. The reasons for the locking on of a silicone elastomer contact lens are somewhat different. Two probable mechanisms can be presented. The first of these is the fact that the silicone elastomer material is no more a barrier to water va-

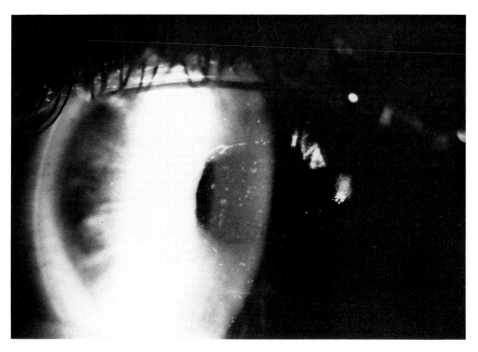

Fig. 22-14. Ring of trapped debris beneath a Silsoft lens that has lost movement.

por than it is to oxygen. Water vapor will flow freely through the material. This means that the tear pool will have a tendency to vaporize through the lens to the atmosphere and be significantly reduced in volume. The second factor is the elastic properties of the silicone elastomer material. This material is very rubberlike because it is elastic. With the blink the lens is pressed against the cornea and the tears tend to be expressed from beneath the lens. As the lid comes up off the cornea, the peripheral portion of the lens exerts its elastic characteristics and may contract against the corneal periphery and stop the inflow of tears.

This "one-way valving system" is more likely to be present with the minus series of lenses. In the minus configuration, the thickest part of the lens is at its periphery. Consequently, greater elasticity is present at the periphery of the lens. With the high-plus (aphakic) series the lens is thinnest at the periphery, and this elastic phenomenon is less likely to occur.

The basic finding for a lens that may lock on is its loss of movement with a blink. If a lens is observed not to move with a blink, it is a potentially dangerous lens. If the practitioner believes that the range of movement of the lens

is borderline in its adequacy, he should closely observe the character of the tears beneath the lens. If these tears contain a ring of debris, he can be certain that this lens is not moving adequately (Fig. 22-14). The presence of a trapped ring of debris beneath the lens is a certain sign that this lens is losing its ability to move and that locking on of the lens will take place shortly.

The effect on the corneal epithelium of a lens that loses movement can be profound. The trapping of the desquamated epithelial cells in the stagnant residual minimal tear layer beneath the lens leads to toxic effects (Fig. 22-15). The desquamated epithelial cells, as they break down, release potent destructive enzymes. In addition, the accumulation of the products of metabolism of the epithelium contribute to the toxic changes that may take place. The reader may recall that we noted the fact that the hydrophilic surface of the lens maintains itself *as long as it remains in a water environment*. With the loss of tears beneath the lens, the water environment is significantly reduced. The back surface of the lens now tends to become hydrophobic. The anterior surface of the cornea is relatively deprived of

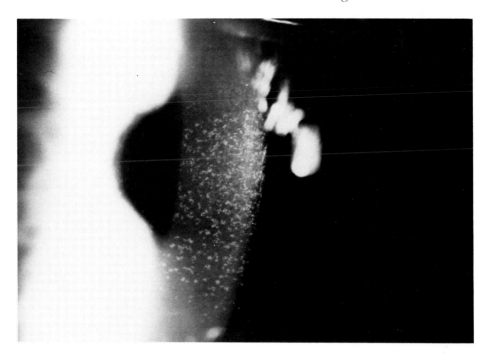

Fig. 22-15. Central corneal punctate keratitis present when the lens shown in Fig. 22-14 was removed.

its layer of mucin, and so it too tends to become hydrophobic. One now has two hydrophobic surfaces approximated to each other and they stick.

It is thus of fundamental importance that the initial fitting of the silicone elastomer lenses ensures a lens with movement. It is fundamentally important that the patient be followed closely over the first 3 months and be continually monitored for movement of the lens.

Comment. A lock-on lens causes an acute form of red eye and may be accompanied by adherent corneal epithelium when the lens is removed.

Handling and care

The Silsoft contact lens can be inserted and removed by use of the same techniques that are employed for rigid contact lenses. The lenses are stiff enough that the "blink-out" method of removal can be successful. Patients that have utilized hydrophilic lenses and are used to the "pull-down pinch-out" method of removal can often employ this same technique with the silicone elastomer lenses.

The lenses can be cared for by use of either a heat or chemical care technique.

The thermal or heat method of care involves cleaning of the lens with an appropriate surface cleaner such as the Barnes-Hind Soft Mate, followed by rinsing of the lens with a preserved saline solution, preferably non–thimerosal preserved, and placing the lens in its case filled with the preserved saline for heating in the heater unit. The papaine-based enzyme tablets should be used every 10 to 14 days to minimize deposit formation.

The chemical care material that has been approved for use with the silicone elastomer lenses produced by Dow Corning Ophthalmics (Silsoft) are those that were utilized in the study and consist of Preflex as a cleaning solution; Normol as a rinsing solution; Flexsol as a soaking, disinfecting, and storage solution; the papain enzyme tablets for cleaning; and Adapettes for intermittent lubrication of the lens while in the eye.

Wearing schedule

The silicone elastomer lenses are extended or prolonged wear lenses as well as daily wear lenses.

The minus configuration lens is not likely to be the first choice of a lens for a myopic patient. The comfort factor of the minus configuration lens does not compare well to a well-fitted hydrophilic lens or to a well-fitted large (9.2 mm or greater diameter) gas-permeable rigid lens. The comfort factor of the minus lens, at this point in time, is such that only a few selected patients are likely to be able to accept the lens. For those patients that have shown a degree of vessel invasion of the cornea and who wish to continue wearing contact lenses, the minus-configuration silicone elastomer lens may be their only option. It is probable that the peripheral edge design, the diameter, or other configuration characteristic of the minus series of lenses may be changed in the future to provide greater patient comfort. When greater patient comfort is achieved with the minus-configuration lens, it may then become the lens of choice for those myopes for whom it gives adequate visual acuity.

The high-plus (aphakic) configuration lens is a relatively comfortable lens. The patients must be told, particularly if they have worn soft lenses before, that this lens will be initially more uncomfortable than the hydrophilic lens that they were accustomed to. However, in our practice invariably the comfort factor of the silicone elastomer (Silsoft) aphakic lens has been significantly better after the patient has achieved all-day or prolonged wear of the lens. It may be necessary to reassure the patient that as the wearing time progresses the comfort increases. The silicone elastomer Silsoft lens is currently my first choice for prolonged wear in aphakic patients.

It is my personal philosophy that all patients entering prolonged wear of any contact lens have a period of daily wear of the lens. I follow this because I believe that it is mandatory that the patient or relative or nearby friend have the ability to insert and remove the lenses with confidence. One can best achieve this by having the patient wear the lens on a daily basis for at least a week, preferably 2 weeks.

The wearing time with the lenses is built up over approximately 5 days. The patient is requested to wear the lenses for 3 hours on the first day and add 2 hours per day provided that the eye was comfortable at the wearing time of the preceding day.

When the patient has achieved comfortable all-day wearing and demonstrated his ability to handle the lens or the practitioner has become assured that a relative or friend can and will handle the lenses, the patient then proceeds to prolonged wear of the lenses.

The patient is seen after the first 24 hours of prolonged wear of the lens. If the lenses are maintaining movement, the patient is comfortable, the cornea is clear, and the visual acuity is stable, the patient then continues to wear the lens on a prolonged basis.

The patients are always strongly advised to remove immediately a lens that is uncomfortable. The patient is then seen 1 week after he has been wearing the lenses on a prolonged or extended basis. If everything is satisfactory at that time, he is then seen in 2 weeks. If conditions continue to be satisfactory, he will be seen in 1 month, 2 months, 3 months, and then at 6-month intervals.

When a patient is wearing the lenses on a prolonged basis, the intervals between removal will depend entirely on the comfort factor of the lens and the clarity of the visual acuity. As debris begins to build up on the surface of the lens, the comfort will decrease and the visual acuity will be less satisfactory. This time interval will vary from patient to patient. There are some patients who find they must remove the lenses at least every week. There are others who find that they can wear them 3 months or longer without problems. The practitioner will be able to assess the probable time between removals during the initial 3 months of follow-up when he is seeing the patient at relatively frequent intervals.

Helpful hints

The silicone elastomer (Silsoft) lens is often well tolerated by patients with borderline tear production. Unlike the hydrophilic lenses, the silicone elastomer lens will not dry in the eye. If adequate movement can be achieved with the patient with borderline tear production, the lens will probably function well.

If the lens should lock on, flooding the eye with normal saline or Balanced Salt Solution may significantly assist in the removal of the lens from the eye. Locking on of the silicone elastomer lens has not been the major problem with the Silsoft lens that it was with the European and Japanese lenses. There, a combination of a different type of lens surface, which

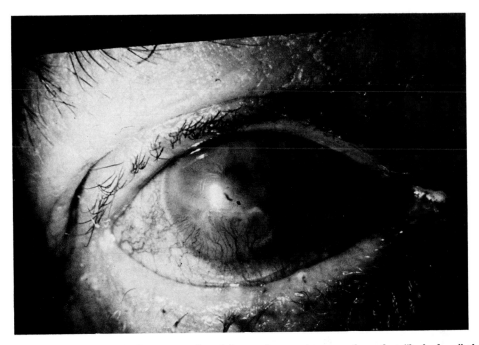

Fig. 22-16. Severe corneal changes produced by a silicone elastomer lens that "locked on" the cornea. The silicone elastomer lens that produced this problem was manufactured by a German lens company. (Courtesy Dr. Hans Roth, Ulm, West Germany.)

tended to be more hydrophobic under stress, and a lack of good instruction of practitioners to be aware of this problem led to very significant problems (Fig. 22-16).

No difficulties have been encountered when topical medications are used with the silicone elastomer contact lenses.

If a patient has persistent discomfort with a silicone elastomer (Silsoft) lens that cannot readily be explained by either corneal changes or the fitting characteristics of the lenses, be suspicious that you have a lens with a poor blend or a poor edge. As I noted before, the silicone elastomer is the only material that remains soft under all conditions. Consequently edging and placing good blends on the lens is technically difficult. Researchers at Dow Corning Ophthalmics have done a commendable job in this area and are constantly improving it.

However I have experienced on several occasions a lens that is persistently uncomfortable. Replacing the lens with a new one of the same parameters has lead to significantly improved comfort. I can only attribute this improvement to having obtained a lens with a better peripheral finish.

The silicone elastomer lens in the high-plus (aphakic) configuration is a tough entity. It will withstand handling. This makes the lens a good daily wear lens if the patient should so wish. It may be the only lens that an eye will tolerate.

If, on follow-up, you note a lens that wets poorly, be sure to ask the patient if on any occasion the lens was lost from the eye. I must emphasize that the silicone elastomer and for that matter the silicone resin lenses must be maintained in an aqueous medium or they will lose their hydrophilic surface characteristics.

PART III

FITTING GUIDE FOR MORE ADVANCED FITTERS

KERATOCONUS

Treatment with contact lenses
Single-cut rigid lenses
Soper keratoconus diagnostic
  fitting set
Dura-T lenses
Hydrophilic lenses
Piggyback lenses
Gas-permeable lenses: types and
  application

Keratoconus is a bilateral, progressive, conic deformity of the central or more commonly paracentral cornea. The apex of the cone is invariably located downward and nasally from the visual axis and may protrude 10 to 15 D or an additional 2 mm in relation to the normal height of the cornea, which is 2.5 mm (Figs. 23-1 and 23-2). The area of ectasia is generally limited to 3 to 6 mm in diameter; this characteristically is the zone of greatest thinning of the cornea.

The condition begins in adolescence, frequently in one eye, and then undergoes remissions and relapses until the ages of 40 to 45 years, when it seems to stop. With repeated attacks of corneal breakdown the apex of the cornea becomes thin and scarred and loses the regularity of its front-surface optic properties. The diagnosis is simply made with a Placido disc, a flat disc on which has been painted alternating black and white rings that encircle a small, central, round aperture. The cornea is

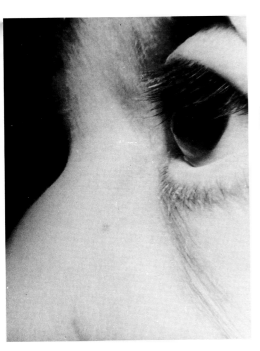

Fig. 23-1. Keratoconus. (From Hartstein, J.: Questions and answers on contact lens practice, ed. 2, St. Louis, 1973, The C.V. Mosby Co.)

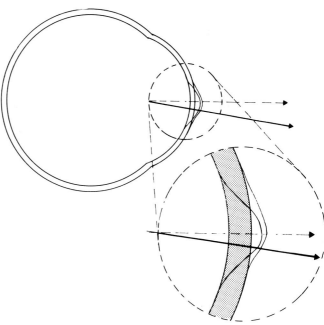

Fig. 23-2. The apex of the cone and the visual axis are not in alignment. The cone is usually displaced downward and nasally.

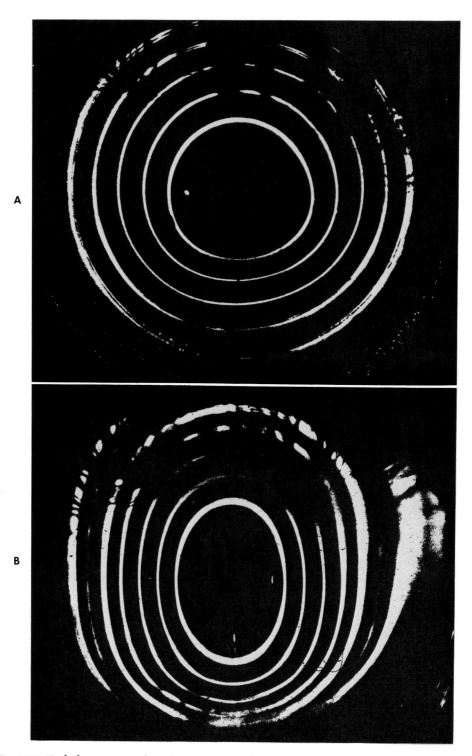

Fig. 23-3. Early keratoconus, less than 48.00 D, which shows, **A,** some distortion but within the variation of an astigmatic cornea. **B,** Moderate keratoconus, 52.00 D, which shows considerable distortion.

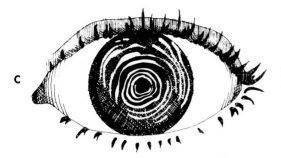

C

Fig. 23-3, cont'd. C, Severe keratoconus with many distortions and breaks in the concentric circles.

Table 23-1. Classification of keratoconus

	Mild	*Moderate*	*Advanced*	*Severe*
K reading	<45.00 D	>45.00 D	>52.00 D	>60.00 D

used as a front-surface convex mirror that reflects from the normal cornea a series of perfectly uniform, concentric circles. In a cone-shaped cornea the reflected target is distorted and the concentric circles are uneven, frequently broken and without symmetry (Fig. 23-3).

The limitation of this instrument in the diagnosis of early keratoconus should be appreciated. If the Placido disc on the keratoscope (an electric Placido disc) is tilted, the reflected circles may also be ellipsoid in a normal cornea, simulating early keratoconus.

A slitlamp diagnosis is difficult to make in the early phase, whereas in the late stages the diagnosis becomes obvious with apical thinning, Fleischer keratoconus ring, increased endothelial reflex, increased visibility of the nerve fibers, scarring of Bowman's membrane, and so on.

Keratometry is very helpful in the early phase of this disease since the mire images appear distorted and irregular. The two principal meridians are not at right angles to each other, and the dioptric value of the readings is quite high—48 D or higher.

Perhaps the best instrument for diagnosis of keratoconus in the early stages is the retinoscope, which reflects irregular light reflexes from the surface of the cornea.

The diagnosis of keratoconus in the early stages is often elusive. It depends on the following:

1. The keratometry reading indicating high cylinder axes or irregular mires
2. Changing astigmatic refractive errors
3. Vision that is not correctable by spectacles to 20/20
4. Scissor movement on retinoscopy
5. Placido-disc reflection
6. Slitlamp findings including Fleischer's ring and evidence of corneal ruptures with scarring
7. Pachometric findings to indicate a thinning of the cornea

Keratoconus may be classified according to the degree of conicity of the apex of the cone. Classification is noted in Table 23-1. An example of an advanced keratoconus is indicated in Fig. 23-4.

Distinction should be made between two clinical types of advanced keratoconus. There is the round or nipple-shaped cone that lies most commonly in the lower nasal quadrant. It is the most common type and is limited in diameter.

The other type is oval or sagging, is longer, and sags in the inferotemporal quadrant. It is most prone to corneal hydrops. It is steeper than the round cone, having an average keratometric reading of 68 D. The round cone is rarely greater than 65 D.

The round cone has the best prognosis in terms of contact lens fitting. Fortunately, it is the most common type.

Comment. There is some controversy whether rigid contact lenses cause keratoconus. Most authorities do not support this hypothesis because if it is true the incidence of keratoconus should be much higher than it is in the general population. The starting age of a contact lens patient and the age of a keratoconus patient are similar. Also, in the early phases of

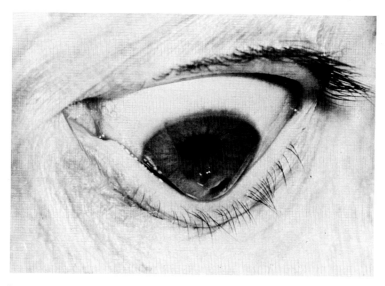

Fig. 23-4. Advanced case of keratoconus. (Courtesy Dr. Dean Butcher, Australia; in Stein, H.A., and Slatt, B.J.: The ophthalmic assistant, ed. 4. St. Louis, 1983, The C.V. Mosby Co.)

keratoconus the person may be merely myopic, and so it is quite natural to assume that one causes the other. There are however some who believe that a rigid lens may accelerate the development of early forms of keratoconus.

TREATMENT WITH CONTACT LENSES

The purpose of a lens is to cover the irregular astigmatism and the disordered anterior surface optic properties of an ectatic cornea by providing a regular, spheric optic surface before the eye. The lens does not retard the progression of the disease, which by itself may have long periods of natural remission. Spectacles are only satisfactory in early mild cases.

Several approaches using contact lenses may be used:

1. Single-cut small, steep PMMA or gaspermeable lenses
2. Soper two-curved method of vaulting
3. Thin lenses
4. Scleral lenses (these are virtually obsolete now)
5. Soft lenses
6. Piggyback soft and rigid lenses

The first three approaches can be used with either PMMA or gas-permeable lenses.

SINGLE-CUT RIGID LENSES

Ideally corrective rigid lenses should touch the apical cone lightly and rest on the peripheral cornea where there is little or no thinning

(Fig. 23-5, *A*). Lenses fitted excessively flat eventually cause corneal abrasions (Fig. 23-5, *B*). Minimal apical clearance of the cone has been advocated, but this point of view represents a minority opinion. Attempting to obtain central clearance in even moderate cone cases will necessarily result in considerable pooling of tears around the periphery of the cone because of increased elevation of the conical area (Fig. 23-5, *C*). This pooling frequently leads to hazing, bubble formation in the vaulted area, and discomfort.

Trial lens fitting (Table 23-2)

In the early phases of keratoconus, K readings are a guide to selecting a lens. As the condition develops, the mire image becomes irregular and the cone becomes steeper than 50.00 D so that the radius of curvature cannot be determined by ordinary keratometry. The only alternative is to fit the patient by trial and error.

The range of the keratometer can be extended to 61.00 D with an auxiliary +1.25 D lens (Table 23-3 and Fig. 23-6). However, because of the disordered mires, problems in fixation, and optic defects in the system, the results merely serve as a guide to trial lens selection. Fixation can be improved when one employs the viewing light of the topogometer.

A good fit should have a central touch of 2 to 3 mm centrally with a thin band of touch at the lens periphery, as determined by the fluores-

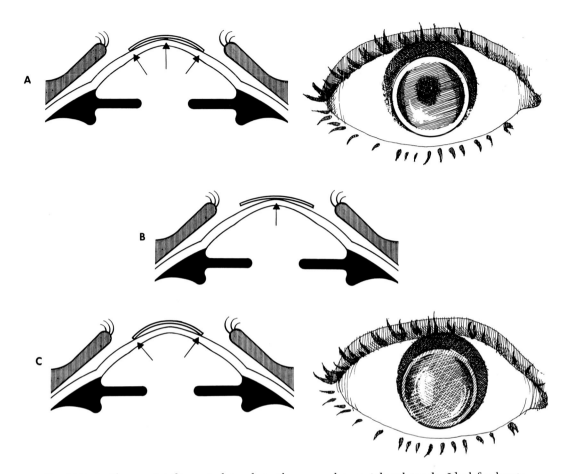

Fig. 23-5. A, Three-point fit—apical touch to the cone plus peripheral touch. Ideal for keratoconus because of the distribution of weight of the lens. **B,** Flat fit—apical touch but poor centration because of rocking on the corneal cap and edge stand-off. **C,** Steep fit—two-point touch with an air bubble between the lens and the cone. The apical cone is cleared.

Table 23-2. Specifications of 10-lens keratoconus trial set

Scribed lens (D)	Radius (mm)	Diameter (mm)	Second curve (mm)	Power (D)
42.25	8.0	9.2	0.3 (12.25)	+1.25
43.50	7.75	9.2	0.3 (12.25)	+0.25
45.00	7.5	9.2	0.3 (12.25)	−2.00
46.50	7.25	9.2	0.3 (12.25)	−3.50
48.25	7.0	9.4	0.4 (12.25)	−5.25
50.00	6.75	9.4	0.4 (12.25)	−7.25
51.87	6.5	9.4	0.4 (12.25)	−9.25
54.00	6.25	9.6	0.2 (9.50), 0.3 (12.25)	−11.25
56.25	6.0	9.6	0.2 (9.50), 0.3 (12.25)	−13.50
58.75	5.75	9.6	0.2 (9.50), 0.3 (12.25)	−17.00

Courtesy Plastic Contact Lens Company, Toronto, Canada.

Table 23-3. Dioptric curves for extended range of keratometer

High power (with +1.25 D lens over aperture)		Low power (with −1.00 D lens over aperture)		High power (with +1.25 D lens over aperture)		Low power (with −1.00 D lens over aperture)	
Drum reading (D)	True dioptric curvature (D)	Drum reading (d)	True dioptric curvature (D)	Drum reading (D)	True dioptric curvature (D)	Drum reading (D)	True dioptric curvature (D)
52.00	61.00	42.00	36.00	47.37	56.37	37.50	31.50
51.87	60.87	41.87	35.87	47.25	56.25	37.37	31.37
51.75	60.75	41.75	35.75	47.12	56.12	37.25	31.25
51.62	60.62	41.62	35.62	47.00	56.00	37.12	31.12
51.50	60.50	41.50	35.50	46.87	55.87	37.00	31.00
51.37	60.37	41.37	35.37	46.75	55.75	36.87	30.87
51.25	60.25	41.25	35.25	46.62	55.62	36.75	30.75
51.12	60.12	41.12	35.12	46.50	55.50	36.62	30.62
51.00	60.00	41.00	35.00	46.37	55.37	36.50	30.50
50.87	59.87	40.87	34.87	46.25	55.25	36.37	30.37
50.75	59.75	40.75	34.75	46.12	55.12	36.25	30.25
50.62	59.62	40.62	34.62	46.00	55.00	36.12	30.12
50.50	59.50	40.50	34.50	45.87	54.87	36.00	30.00
50.37	59.37	40.37	34.37	45.75	54.75		
50.25	59.25	40.25	34.25	45.62	54.62		
50.12	59.12	40.12	34.12	45.50	54.50		
50.00	59.00	40.00	34.00	45.37	54.37		
49.87	58.87	39.87	33.87	45.25	54.25		
49.75	58.75	39.75	33.75	45.12	54.12		
49.62	58.62	39.62	33.62	45.00	54.00		
49.50	58.50	39.50	33.50	44.87	53.87		
49.37	58.37	39.37	33.37	44.75	53.75		
40.25	58.25	39.25	33.25	44.62	53.62		
49.12	58.12	39.12	33.12	44.50	53.50		
49.00	58.00	39.00	33.00	44.37	53.37		
48.75	57.75	38.87	32.87	44.25	53.25		
48.62	57.62	38.75	32.75	44.12	53.12		
48.50	57.50	38.62	32.62	44.00	53.00		
48.37	57.37	38.50	32.50	43.87	52.87		
48.25	57.25	38.37	32.37	43.75	52.75		
48.12	57.12	38.25	32.25	43.62	52.62		
48.00	57.00	38.12	32.12	43.50	52.50		
47.87	56.87	38.00	32.00	43.37	52.37		
47.75	56.75	37.87	31.87	43.25	52.25		
47.62	56.62	37.75	31.75	43.12	52.12		
47.50	56.50	37.62	31.62	43.00	52.00		

Courtesy Baush & Lomb, Inc.

cein test. The three-point touch adds to the stability of the lens on the cornea and distributes the weight of the lens not only over the apex but over other bearing areas as well. The peripheral touch area corresponds to the zone of the intermediate curve. The initial lens selected, with the K readings serving as a guide, should have a base curve flatter than K. Then, with use of the fluorescein test, the lens is exchanged until one is found that results in slight apical touch of 2 to 3 mm or from 1 to 4 mm flatter than K. A light, apical touch is desirable so that the lens can function as a pressure bandage on the thin, central corneal apex.

It is important to follow the keratoconus patient closely on a weekly basis because of progressive flattening of the cone by the initial lens. As the area of touch increases and the cone flattens, a new lens with a flatter base curve can be tried. Lens changes should be made until changes in the shape of the cornea are stabilized. With flattening of the cone it is

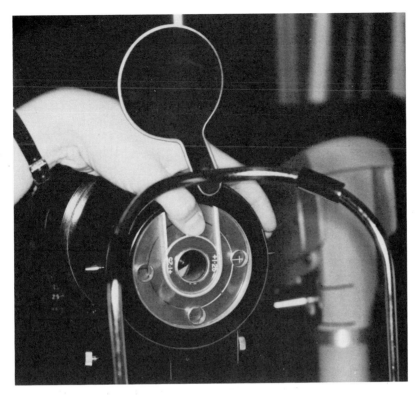

Fig. 23-6. INNS extension disc to extend range of keratometer.

not unusual to find that over a period of time as much as 4.00 to 6.00 D of plus power over the original lenses will be needed. Flattening may occur without a change in power if there has been a compensatory change in the lacrimal lens.

A guide to lens selection

Diameter. Large lenses with a diameter of 9 to 10 mm are generally used to provide stability and support whereas small lenses with diameters of 8 to 8.5 mm have been employed successfully for milder forms of keratoconus, that is, less than 52.00 D. A smaller lens may be used if it does not show excessive movement (Fig. 23-7). Basically small lenses are made quite steep and are employed when the cone is truly central. Small-sized lenses are lighter; so they can be fitted flatter. On the other hand this same merit can lead to loss of stability. Small lenses for keratoconus are usually bicurve with a narrow peripheral curve that rests on the apex of the cone end near its limiting border.

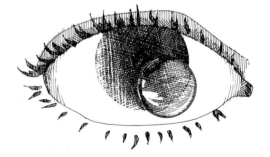

Fig. 23-7. Smaller lenses are used only for central cones, which are rare. If smaller lenses are fitted on an eccentric cone, they frequently slide off the cornea.

Comment. Small lenses were used only with early keratoconus when PMMA was the only material available. With gas-permeable lenses, it is preferable to use larger lens for centration, comfort, and stability with blinking. Also a large-diameter lens invariably has a large optic zone.

Optic zone. The size is usually determined by trial and error with fluorescein. The size will depend on the site, protrusion of the conic deformity, and the amount of corneal touch. The optic zone should be larger than the pupil size in average illumination and should allow for the amount of decentration of the apex of the cone, which frequently is 1 mm nasally and 1 mm inferiorly. With a 5 mm pupil the average optic zone is approximately 7 mm.

Peripheral curves. Peripheral curves can be tricurve or even pentacurve in advanced cases. The intermediate curve should be 1 or 2 mm flatter than the base curve. The peripheral curve is approximately 4 mm flatter than the intermediate curve.

In advanced cases additional peripheral curves are needed to avoid sharp blends. The difference in radius of curvature between the primary base curve and the peripheral curve is frequently considerable, as from 45.00 to 60.00 D to 35.00 to 40.00 D. These additional curves prevent abrupt changes in the radius of curvature as the lens undergoes radical flattening from the apex to its periphery.

Power. One can best determine the power by refracting the patient wearing trial lenses. A contact lens provides the cornea with a smooth and regular anterior surface so that light is evenly refracted. With spectacles, compensation cannot be made for the irregular astigmatism and distortion that accompanies keratoconus. The refraction through a contact lens can yield remarkable results with acuity improving from 20/200 to 20/30 or 20/25. The lens power usually has a range between −5.00 and −15.00 D. Sometimes a local anesthetic must be used for a trial-set refraction to reduce irritation and tearing during the examination.

Evaluating lens fit

1. A large bubble indicates the lens is too steep. Also vision is poor.
   Treatment. Try on a flatter lens. Gaspermeable acrylate lenses permit a flatter fit without compromising the epithelium.
2. Apical touch is indicated by the absence of fluorescein-stained tears at the apex of the cornea and indicates that the lens is touching the cornea at that area.
   Treatment. Try a steeper lens.
   Comment. Slight apical touch is acceptable.
3. The presence of fluorescein-stained tears under the central area but not under the peripheral curves near the edge of the lens in-

dicates that the lens may be close to the desired central posterior curve, but too steep in the periphery.
   Treatment. The same-diameter lens could be ordered and wider, flatter posterior peripheral curves used. Over-refraction will reveal the lens power needed.
4. Refraction over the trial lens may provide only poor vision. A small pupil test (accomplished by flashing a light in the opposite eye to create a small pupil by the consensual reflex) may improve vision. If so, the optic zone is too small.
   Treatment. Try to order a larger-diameter lens. A larger lens is invariably tight, and so a flatter fit may be required.
5. A new lens may provide good vision and may have apical clearance, but be too tight at the periphery as indicated by the absence of fluorescein-stained tears under the lens edge. A small bubble may be trapped under the lens.
   Treatment. It is best to modify the lens. Use diamond radius tools (such as 11.50, 9, or 8 mm down to 1 mm flatter than the central posterior curve) to widen the posterior peripheral curves. Reapply to cornea and reevaluate fluorescein patterns.
6. The lens may fit well, but vision may be improved with additional cylindric over-refraction.
   Treatment. If the cylinder addition is large, incorporate the added cylinder in a spectacle. Some people wear a soft lens and a rigid lens and spectacles. It is a little too much of a hassle for the average patient.

SOPER KERATOCONUS DIAGNOSTIC FITTING SET

The Soper lens (Fig. 23-8) is our fitting set of choice because we have had excellent results both in moderate and advanced cases of keratoconus. By concentrating on increasing or decreasing sagittal depth and by choosing an appropriate base curve or size one can fit most keratoconus patients with a minimal number of trial lenses (Table 23-4). Over-refraction is used to arrive at the best visual correction.

Progression of the cone can be detected by observation of an increase in apical staining and the presence of large abrasions. When this occurs, it indicates that the cone has moved for-

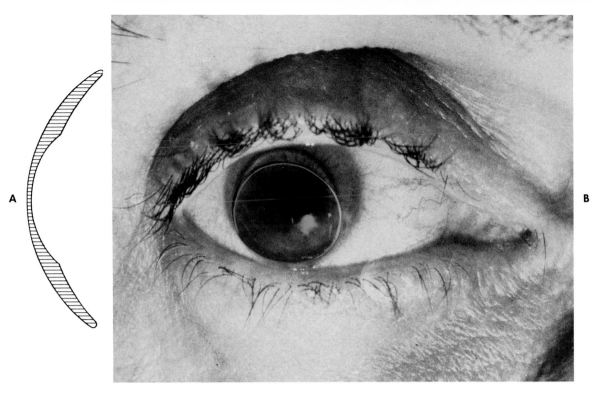

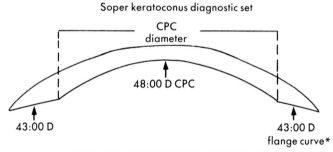

Fig. 23-8. A, Soper cone lens for keratoconus. There is a steep central posterior curve and a much flatter flange surrounding it. **B,** Soper cone lens over a moderate keratoconus deformity.

Table 23-4. Soper keratoconus diagnostic fitting set

Soper keratoconus diagnostic set

CPC diameter

48:00 D CPC

43:00 D

43:00 D flange curve*

Cone	Try first	Sagittal depth (mm)	Central posterior curve (D)	Power (D)	Lens diameter (mm)	Thickness (mm)	Central posterior curve diameter (optic zone mm)
Moderate	A	0.68	48.00/43.00	−4.50	7.5	0.10	6.0
	B	0.73	52.00/45.00	−8.50	7.5	0.10	6.0
	C	0.80	56.00/45.00	−12.50	7.5	0.10	6.0
	D†	0.87	60.00/45.00	−16.50	7.5	0.10	6.0
Advanced	E	1.00	52.00/45.00	−8.50	8.5	0.10	7.0
	F	1.12	56.00/45.00	−12.50	8.5	0.10	7.0
	G	1.22	60.00/45.00	−16.50	8.5	0.10	7.0
Severe	H†	1.37	52.00/45.00	−8.50	9.5	0.10	8.0
	I	1.52	56.00/45.00	−12.50	9.5	0.10	8.0
	J	1.67	60.00/45.00	−16.50	9.5	0.10	8.0

*There must be at least a 5-diopter difference between the central posterior curve (CPC) and the flange curvature for the lens to be effective.
†The sagittal value (vaulting effect) of lens H (a 52.00 D lens) is *much* greater than lens D (a 60.00 D lens), which is attributable to the *much* larger diameter (9.5 mm) of the H lens.

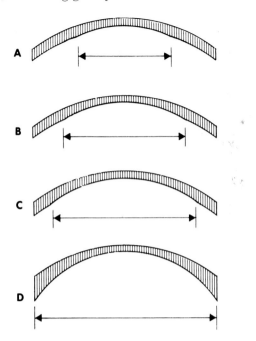

Fig. 23-9. The Soper lens. An increase in the sagittal depth can be made by an increase in the diameter of the lens. The base curves of **A** to **D** are the same.

ward, touching the lens. In such cases a new lens must be ordered with greater apical vaulting.

The Soper lens has been designed with a very steep, central posterior curve to accommodate the cone of the cornea and a much flatter flange surrounding it to rest on the more normal, surrounding cornea. The cornea is fitted from a trial set of lenses with base curves ranging from 48.00 to 60.00 D and lens diameters ranging from 7.5 to 9.5 mm. By varying the base curve and the size of the lens the axial depth can be increased or decreased. As the size of the lens is increased and the base curve held constant, the vaulting effect is enhanced (Fig. 23-9). One of these two variables can be altered to obtain clearance. A good fit results when the lens has a slight touch or slight vaulting at the apex and a touch all around the periphery as detected by fluorescein. A central air bubble indicates that the lens is vaulting too much. A large central touch indicates that the lens is vaulting too little over the cone.

Soper fitting procedure

If the patient to be fitted is wearing contact lenses, it is *absolutely imperative* that the lenses be discontinued at least 48 hours before

refitting is started. Fitting these lenses takes only the time needed to try on several lenses and locate the lens that meets the criteria of a well-fitted lens. The first lens from the set tried is one that relates to the degree of conic progression. If the cone is moderate, the lenses A to D are tried first; if it is advanced, the lenses E to G are tried; if severe, H to J are used first. If this lens has excessive apical vaulting, air will be trapped over the cone. In that case the lens with the next smaller sagittal values is tried, and if necessary, additional lenses, until the bubble is no longer observed. If, however, apical touch is observed, this indicates a need for a lens with a greater sagittal value and thus a need for a lens with a greater sagittal value, and therefore the lens from the trial set with the next greater sagittal value is tried and the process is continued until the apical touch is alleviated.

The criteria for a well-fitted cone lens are as follows:

1. Apical clearance with circulation of tears between the lens and the apex of the cone and some lens movement. Apical touch should not exceed 1 mm.
2. Centration and no displacement.
3. Movement of the lens with blinking.

Interpolating the best fit

In some few cases the best fit may fall between two trial lenses; that is, the lens with the greater sagittal values demonstrates a small bubble whereas the lens with the lesser sagittal value shows a slight apical touch. In that instance the fitter must interpolate.

Example:
  A 48/43 lens gives a slight touch.
  B 52/45 lens produces a small bubble over the apex of the cone.
  Interpolated lens to order: 50/45

Comment. Whenever it is possible, the lens central posterior curve (CPC) and diameter ordered for the patient should be the same as the diagnostic lens. The lens made for the patient will fit exactly as the diagnostic lens. When interpolation between two lenses is done, some degree of guesswork is involved.

Calculation of patient lens power

One can determine lens power *only* by refracting over a trial lens. The lens used for this purpose should not have an air bubble over the visual axis.

Example:

Trial lens CPC	52/45	
Trial lens power		−4.50
Over-refraction		−2.00
		−6.50
Lens to order:	52/45	−6.50

If the central posterior curve to be fitted is 54:00 (by interpolation as previously discussed) and the trial lens and over-refraction are as above, the central posterior curve to be fitted will be 2.00 diopters steeper than the trial lens; therefore an additional −2.00 must be added to the power of the lens to be ordered. In this case the lens ordered would be 54/45 −8.50.

DURA-T LENSES

The use of Dura-T lenses has been advocated by Gasset. The major point in this technique is that the lenses are made thinner. The central thickness of these keratoconus lenses are only 0.08 mm thick.

The thinness of the lens reduces the weight of the lens by 30% approximately. The reduced mass assists patient tolerance and centration. It is especially useful with large inferiorly placed cones.

Fitting procedure

These lens are fit from inventory. There are 30 lenses in a set, with a power range of −2.00 diopters in 0.5-diopter increments to −23.00 diopters and base curves from 47 to 60 diopters.

A −10.00-diopter soft lens is used as a base on the patient's eye. Select the proper K readings with this lens.

Comment. The soft lens is employed to extend the readings of the keratometer. The power (−10.00 D) must be added to the final reading.

Power is obtained by over-refraction.

This method is very simple. Only the base curve and power changes need to be considered. The other parameters, such as the size of the optic zone, peripheral curves, and blend, are all standardized.

The initial lens should have a base curve halfway between the flattest and steepest meridian; for example, if 52 and 58 are the K readings, select 55 as the initial base curve.

The fit should be assessed by fluorescein. A three-point touch is important—central and midperipheral touch with peripheral clearance. If the lens does not conform to this pattern, go flatter or steeper as the fitter sees fit.

The refraction should be expressed in minus cylinders. Use the sphere and drop the cylinder. The over-refraction should then follow.

Example:
−12.00 +5.00 × 90
Minus cylinder form, −7.00 −5.00 × 180
Power of the lens, −7.00 plus
Over-refraction required, −4.00
Total power, −11.00 D

The inventory method makes sense if a fitter has a large volume of patients with keratoconus. Besides being simple to calculate and evaluate, this method allows one to fit a large number of patients and to give them their lenses the same day.

HYDROPHILIC LENSES

Empirically it has been found that hydrophilic lenses are useful in the treatment of keratoconus. Although such a lens normally does not mask astigmatism, it has been shown to reduce by three to four times the amount of astigmatism present in keratoconus, making overcorrection with spectacles a simple task.

These lenses are comfortable and extremely useful for the patient who cannot tolerate a hard lens. Discomfort from hard keratoconus lenses is quite common; keratoconus patients rarely tolerate their lenses as well as persons with myopia. The base-curve selection is usuallly flat, 8.1 to 8.4 mm, and the diameter large, 13 to 14 mm, to provide lens stability.

A good fit is a lens that centers well with a minimum of movement. If the lens does not center, the diameter can be increased or the base curve made steeper. If there is an air bubble over the apical cone, a flatter lens must be used.

Fitting procedure

1. The diameter of the lens should be 2 mm larger than the corneal diameter.
2. Select a lens with a steep base curve as a starter lens. If it is too steep, an air bubble will be captured under the lens, there will be no movement, and the eye will be red because of compression and banking of the conjunctival blood vessels.

Reduce the steepness of the lens until the fit is satisfactory.

3. Allow a few moments for the redness and tearing to subside. Wash the lens with non-preserved saline solution before insertion.

4. A properly fitted lens should have 1 mm of lens motion and no drag with lateral motion. The lens must be centered.

The reason why a soft lens works in keratoconus is poorly understood. However, it has been shown that a soft lens is able to reduce the amount of required cylinder up to 5 diopters.

Another way to employ a soft lens is to allow it to become the base for a rigid lens—piggyback style.

PIGGYBACK LENSES

To avoid the use of auxiliary spectacles, spheric, curved rigid lenses placed over the soft lens, piggyback style, work surprisingly well (Fig. 23-10). (See also Fig. 26-1.)

This approach was introduced by Baldone. A soft lens forms the base lens and assures the patient of comfort. A soft lens with an 8.4 mm base curve and 14 mm diameter will fit most corneas. The power range is between −5 and 15 diopters.

Over the soft lens a rigid lens may be either placed to ride freely or placed into a depression to insert into the plastic that has been designed to hold a rigid lens. Usually, an 8.5 to 9.5 mm rigid lens is the best diameter to ensure centration and stability. Evaluation of the fit is standard.

Refraction over the trial rigid lens will give the power of the lens to be used.

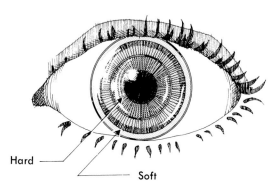

Fig. 23-10. A rigid lens riding piggyback over a soft lens.

If centration is a problem, an aphakic high-plus lenticular soft lens should be tried. The anterior lenticular bulge provides a convex surface, more appropriate to the fitting of a rigid lens.

Comment. This method should not be the first one tried. It requires double handling and double care systems—one for a rigid or gas-permeable lens and one for soft lenses.

An ultrathin permeable soft lens base with a gas-permeable rigid rider lens provides the best combination.

GAS-PERMEABLE LENSES: TYPES AND APPLICATION

These lenses, which include silicone and silicone resin lenses, CAB (cellulose acetate butyrate), the silicone-PMMA combinations (silicone-acrylates), and styrene, have been used with great success for fitting the patient with keratoconus. These lenses, which are fundamentally a rigid lens, can be made 9.2 mm or greater and still eliminate hypoxic changes because of their oxygen permeability. Most patients with keratoconus have a corneal cylinder of 5.00 D or more. Most gas-permeable lenses can cover 5 D of astigmatism when spheric lenses are used. The large-diameter lens 9.2 mm or greater with an optic zone of 6.5 mm or greater permits this type of fitting without sacrificing centration and stability.

The fitting of such a lens requires a small fitting set with minimal selections available. Gas-permeable lenses can be fabricated to the Soper lens or any other lens chosen for keratoconus. The only problem with pure silicone is its brittle qualities and loss of dimensional stability. For best results, the composite lens with PMMA and silicone, the silicone-acrylate lenses, are best employed.

We recently reviewed our management of patients with keratoconus who have contact lenses. We found that 55% of patients with keratoconus could be fitted with standard rigid gas-permeable lenses whereas 40% of the more advanced cases required a Soper-style gas-permeable lens and 5% required a piggyback lens.

Spectacles may work in mild cases of the *forme fruste* of keratoconus that does not progress. Contact lenses may be the only treatment necessary for most patients with keratoconus, and they should be the first and preferred remedy. However despite the presence of contact lenses many corneas continue to deteriorate. Keratoconus below 55.00 D generally lends itself to correction with lenses. Once the keratoconus exceeds 60.00 D, the use of lenses becomes difficult.

Keratoplasty should probably not be considered until there is pronounced corneal scarring reducing best corrected visual acuity in the better eye to 20/50 or less, acute corneal hydrops, conic thinning in the range of 0.3 mm where perforation is a distinct possibility, and a large eccentric cone greater than 5 mm in diameter. If a patient cannot tolerate a lens for at least 10 to 11 hours, keratoplasty may be the best alternative.

Comment. Fitting the patient with keratoconus requires patience and expertise. These persons afflicted with this disease have fears about losing their sight every time they need a change or modification of their contact lenses. Success in fitting these persons requires the fitter to be optimistic, reassuring, and calm because the patient will be tense, agitated, and worried.

CHAPTER 24

THE CORRECTION OF ASTIGMATISM

Soft lens correction

Ridid contact lenses for astigmatism

Correcting astigmatism with a PMMA bitoric lens

Use of gas-permeable rigid lenses

Astigmatism, the result of a variation in the shape of the cornea, may be caused by a difference in the radius of curvature of the principal meridians of the cornea. It may also be the result of a different meridional refracting surface posterior to the front surface of the cornea. This form of astigmatism is called "residual astigmatism" because it persists despite the correct fitting of a lens to the cornea. It may be caused by a partially dislocated lens, a posterior toric corneal surface, or a toric crystalline lens. It is important to distinguish between these two entities because the remedy for each is quite different (Fig. 24-1).

Residual astigmatism is that amount of astigmatism that remains after a lens has been fitted to the cornea. The most common source is lenticular astigmatism. In a previous lens wearer the appearance of a new astigmatic error invariably indicates warpage of the lens. A poorly fitted lens, especially one that is decentered, may also demonstrate residual astigmatism be-

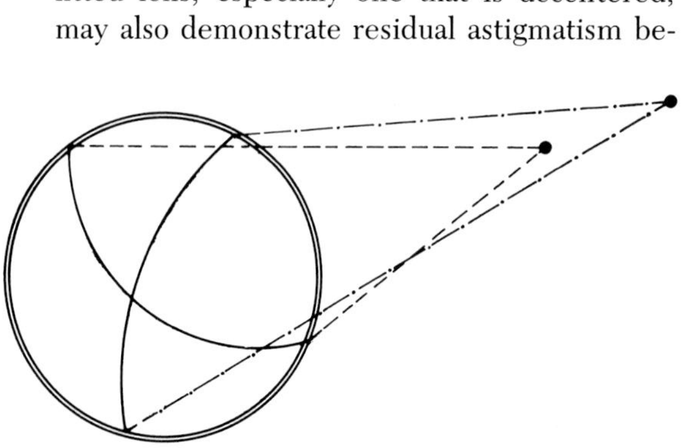

Fig. 24-1. A toric cornea. The two curvatures have different focal points.

cause of oblique incidence of light. At times a hard lens may mold the cornea, but such induced astigmatism is usually masked by the tear layer.

Most residual astigmatism is against the rule; that is, the meridian of greatest power lies nearest the horizontal meridian or the correcting plus cylinder is at 180 degrees. Actually it is quite common—approximately 30% to 40% of patients will demonstrate some low order of an astigmatic defect of 0.50 D. However the vision of most of these patients is normal, perhaps not optimal, but does not require any special attention. It is only when the visual acuity declines to 20/30 or 20/40 with lenses or the patient suffers from visual distress that attention should be directed toward correcting the defect.

Over 25% of all patients interested in contact lenses demonstrated astigmatism over 1.25 diopters according to Holden (Table 24-1).

There are a number of options open to the fitter in correcting astigmatism; one may use a soft lens, either a spheric soft lens or a toric soft lens, or a rigid lens, either spheric or toric.

A gas-permeable lens, because it is larger than a PMMA lens, is more stable on a toric cornea and can correct up to 5 diopters of cylinder with a spheric lens design. The soft hydrogel toric lens can also correct a similar amount of astigmatism on those lenses in which the cylinder is ground on the anterior surface. Besides, the hydrogel lens, even in a toric configuration, has unsurpassed comfort. However, each system has its flaws, and these are reviewed as well as their advantages.

Table 24-1. Distribution of astigmatism in prospective contact lens patients

0.25 D or more	0.50 D or more	0.75 D or more	1.00 D or more	1.25 D or more
76.5%	61.5%	45.4%	34.8%	24.8%
1.50 D or more	1.75 D or more	2.25 D or more	2.75 D or more	3.00 D or more
19.2%	15.8%	10.0%	6.0%	3.4%

From Holden, B.: Aust. J. Optom. **58:**279-299, Aug. 1975.

SOFT LENS CORRECTION
Spheric soft lenses

Spheric soft lenses can mask anywhere from 20% to 70% of corneal astigmatism. The astigmatism is not truly masked, but merely tolerated. The higher the spheric refractive error, the more this can be tolerated. If the total astigmatism is +1.25 D and the overall refraction is −6.00 D, that degree of astigmatism may be tolerated. However, if the degree of spheric refraction is −2.50 D or less and the total amount of astigmatism is +1.25 D, in all likelihood that amount of astigmatism will not be tolerated. Thus the ability of the eye to tolerate the lack of any astigmatic correction depends primarily on its absolute value and secondarily on its relative value in relationship to the total refractive error. As a rule, if the astigmatism represents one third or greater of the total refractive error, that degree of astigmatism needs to be corrected by means other than spheric soft lenses.

Comment. In higher refractive errors, less astigmatism may be tolerated; for example, −8.00 sphere may tolerate a +2.00 D astigmatic correction. The maximum tolerable astigmatic error however should be about 1.50 cylinder, regardless of the refractive error.

Standard-thickness lenses should be used where possible for toric corneas. The use of ultrathin lenses will leave a considerable amount of cylinder uncorrected. If there is still defective vision because of uncorrected cylinder, one may have to switch to a toric soft lens or a gas-permeable lens.

Toric soft lenses

The following are indications for astigmatism correction by toric soft lenses:

1. Corneal astigmatism.
2. Lenticular astigmatism.
3. Combinations of 1 and 2.

The following are contraindications for fitting:

1. Irregular corneal astigmatism, as in a cornea scarred by previous herpes simplex infection.
2. Abnormal lid closure, as in partial Bell's palsy.
3. Any conditions that contraindicate the wearing of a contact lens in general.

Candidates for a soft toric lens include the following:

1. Rigid lens dropouts for any reason, such as induced toricity, discomfort, and corneal edema.
2. Soft lens dropouts, who were fitted with spheric lenses with poor visual results because the astigmatism component was not dealt with.
3. Patients with residual astigmatism. The front surface soft lens toric is ideal for the candidate whose astigmatism is largely lens induced.
4. Large degrees of astigmatism, between 3 and 5 diopters.

The problems of fitting toric soft lenses are similar to those of any soft lens, with the added difficulty of sustaining lens stability. It is this balance between a proper fit and alignment of lens axis to corneal toricity or to the zone of residual astigmatism that provides the challenge.

The major mechanisms for stabilizing the soft toric lens in either lenticular or corneal astigmatism and incorporating a toric surface include the following:

1. Prism ballast, 1 D or 1.5 D.
2. Truncation, either single or double.
3. Dynamic stabilization, the use of inferior and superior thin zones on the lens.
4. Aspheric back surfaces. This design sets up a drag phenomenon through a surface-tension zone between the lens periphery and the corneal periphery.
5. Posterior toric lenses.
6. An eccentrically placed lens that is weighted inferiorly, not being a prism but

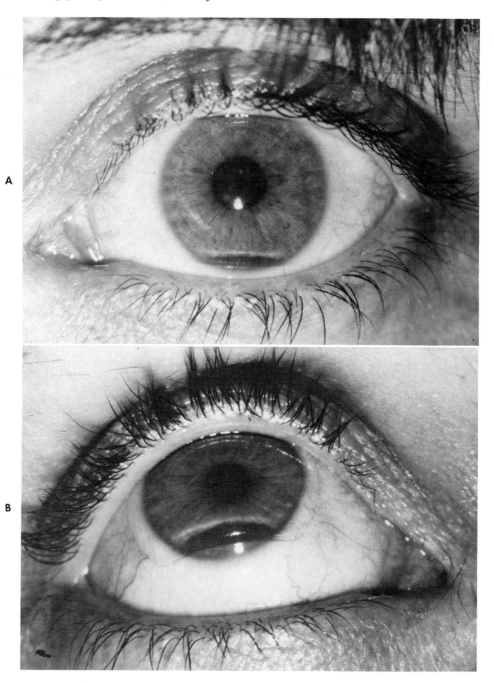

Fig. 24-2. A, Soft toric contact lens: a truncated-prism ballast lens in normal position. **B,** Looking up. The lens should stay in place with eye movement and yet be loose enough to move with a blink.

having a thicker inferior edge called a "bioflange."

7. Combination of the preceding; that is, the Hydron lens uses an aspheric back surface with a central base curve with an eccentricity of 0.7 D, a prism ballast, and truncation.

Stabilization techniques

Prism ballast. The amount of prism ballast varies between 1 and 1.50 diopters. The heavier prism ballast is required for eyes with tight lids, flat corneas, and an oblique axis of astigmatism. The prism factor adds weight to the lower portion of the lens, and its thickness precludes any significant oxygen permeability in the inferior zone of the cornea. Hypoxic disturbances and arcuate staining of the cornea are occasionally encountered in the region of the prism. Manufacturers such as Bausch and Lomb and Hydrocurve, presently provide lenses with pure prism.

Truncation (Fig. 24-2). The contact lens is sectioned off 0.50 to 1.5 mm on the lower edge and occasionally on the upper edge as well. Smaller-diameter lenses of 13.5 mm use 1 mm of truncation, whereas the larger diameters of 14.0 or 14.5 mm employ 1.5 mm of truncation. A good truncated lens will be beveled so that edge compression of the cornea will not occur. Truncation tends to loosen a toric lens, which some manufacturers fix by making these lenses slightly steeper.

Truncation on the inferior edge permits the lens to rotate so that the lower flat edge comes to lie adjacent to the lower eyelid margin and thus stabilizes it. The lid configuration, which frequently varies from person to person, will affect the rotation of the truncated lens. A truncated lens may also be rotated if one edge, especially the lateral one, hits the lower lid before the other. A sloping lid that is higher laterally usually causes this to happen.

Truncation provides stability but is not a guide to the axis of the correcting cylinder. The 0- to 180-degree axis must be made with the slitlamp. The bottom of the truncated lens may not be parallel with the orientation of the lower lid, which frequently is sloping.

Often truncation is combined with prism ballast, so that the heavier dependent and thicker part is cut off. This also aids in reducing the overall lens weight of the contact lens. In addition, palpebral fissures that have sclera exposed inferiorly may require larger soft toric truncated lenses to permit the lower truncated edge to be in juxtaposition to the lower eyelid. These types of lenses are typified by the toric lens made by Hydron (Woodbury, N.Y.) called the "Hydron T" and by Wesley-Jessen (Chicago) called the "Durasoft TT."

Truncation adds discomfort to the toric system. If the lower lid is in proximity to the truncated edge, lid impact occurs. Also there is displacement of the lens upward as the eyes are lowered to the reading position. Variable vision with reading results when upward decentration of the lens occurs.

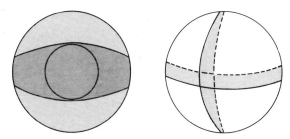

Fig. 24-3. Double slab-off soft lens used to correct astigmatism. The lens is made thinner superiorly and inferiorly so that the thinner portions tend to rotate and come to rest under the upper and lower eyelids.

Thick-thin zones (double slab-off lens, dynamic stabilization). This lens system is perhaps the best for comfort because there is no lid impact on the inferior surface, but it does not offer lens stability as well as the truncated or posterior toric devices. The central body of the lens that lies in the palpebral fissure is thick, but the superior and inferior edges of the lens are thin (Fig. 24-3). When this lens is placed on the eye, the thinner zones come to lie under the upper and lower eyelids.

Many lenses, rigid and soft, rotate with blinking. However, such rotation is unacceptable with a toric lens system. Thus corrective cylinders are usually ground into this lens on the front surface, so that the lens will stop rotating on the eye. Weicon (West Germany), CIBA-Geigy (Summit, N.J.), and Dominion Contact Lens Company (Toronto) produce this type of thick-thin lens. These double slab-off lenses may also be combined with prism ballast to prevent displacement of the axis and rotation with blinking.

The thin-zone lens is best when the axis of astigmatism is in the major lines of power, that is, 180 or 90 degrees. Also it functions best when the drag between lids and lens is not excessive. The thin-zone lens is usually marked with etchings on the 0- to 180-degree axis, which provide easy orientation to the axis of the cylinder.

Posterior toric lenses. Posterior toric lenses are perfect for patients with an imperfect corneal toricity because the axis of the lens can be aligned with the axis of the cornea that requires correction. This type of lens is stabilized by the toric correction being placed on the posterior side of the lens. It is valid for astigmatism that

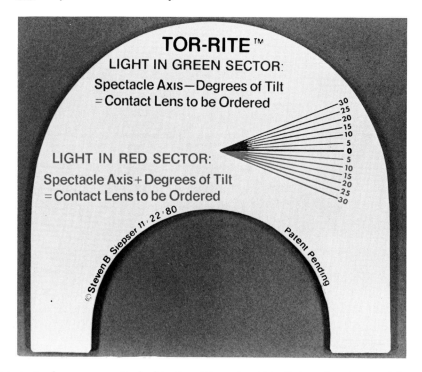

Fig. 24-4. A simple accessory attached to the slitlamp to aid in fitting of toric contact lenses. The slit is projected on the device, focused, and read.

is largely generated by a toric corneal surface. Hydrocurve utilizes this principle in the fabrication of their lenses.

The limitation of the system is that Hydrocurve toric lenses are available in only two power choices and work best with major meridional astigmatism. Also this system is not ideal for residual astigmatism, which does better with a spheric or aspheric lens and an anterior toric surface.

Aspheric lens surface. An aspheric lens surface aids in lens-axis stabilization by adding drag to the motion of the lens. It is not used as the primary force in lens stability but rather as an adjunct. Usually prisms or truncations are added to the system. Unfortunately such a lens becomes very tight with time, and so it is made flatter in the fitting, a shape that reduces lens stability.

Identifying marks. Soft toric lenses may be identified by either etch marks or laser marks on the 3 and 9 o'clock areas of the lens, or at the 6 o'clock area. This will vary with the manufacturer. Dr. Steven B. Siepser of Paoli, Pennsylvania, has developed a toric soft contact lens fitting aid that attaches to the slitlamp and

is an accessory aid in fitting toric lenses on astigmatic patients. The device, called Tor-Rite, is placed on the chin set of the slitlamp and the slit-beam focusing on the guide provides an accurate means for estimation of the cylinder axis and an increase in the reliability of toric soft contact lens selection (Fig. 24-4).

Quality control. A toric soft lens design is an efficient correcting modality for astigmatism greater than 1.50 D. It is essential that the truncation is properly aligned with respect to the base of the prism.

To do this control, one uses a projection vertometer. The lens is mounted so that the truncation is positioned parallel to and adjacent to the observer doing the inspection. When observing the screen, the optic center of the mires should be in line with the central vertical line inscribed on the projection screen (90-degree axis); that is, the truncation is perpendicular to the axis of the prism. If the center of the mires is not in line with the central vertical line of the projection screen (assuming the lens has been centered) the cylinder axis will be off.

If this axis is not aligned correctly at this position of the lens, the lens should be rejected and remade. *Lens verification is critical for success when one fits the astigmatic patient with toric hydrogel lenses.*

One can check the power of the lens with a lensometer by blotting the lens dry with a piece of lint-free tissue paper and aligning the lens of 0- to 180-degree markings horizontally with the lens properly centered. The power can be read as one would for a spherocylinder spectacle prescription.

Lens fitting. The toric lens has so many variables that trial-set fitting is used for best results. Only 60% of first fits can be achieved with a trial set of spheric lenses. With toric lenses results are better by 10%.

The fitting varies with the manufacturer and is dependent on the device employed for lens stability. For lenses stabilized by prism and truncation, the following method may be employed:

1. *Lens diameter selection.* Add 2 to 2.5 mm to the visible iris diameter.
2. *Selection of base curve.* The arithmetic mean of the K readings is taken and converted to millimeters of radius. For example, if the K readings are 40.25 × 180° and 42.50 × 90°, the mean radius would be 41.38 D. When this is converted to millimeters, the selected lens is 8.15 mm.

   A flatter base curve is selected and this is achieved when one adds on 0.7 mm to the mean radius, which in this case would make the initial lens 8.75 mm.
3. *Over-refract in minus cylinders.*
4. *Record the vision of the back vertex distance.* One arrives at the cylindric component by doing a conventional over-refraction. The base curve of the final truncated prism-ballasted lens is compensated by the laboratory for the reduced vertical diameter that results from truncation.
5. The movement of the lens should be 1 to 2 mm with each blink. Check on the fit. The mires should be sharp and the retinoscopy reflex crisp.

To fit a double slab-off lens, we employed as an example of this technique the Dominion Contact Lens, a Canadian lens. This is a lathe-cut double-slab-off lens made from the Toyo material. The lens has a front-surface toric design; the back surface is spheric and consists of two curves, a base curve and a peripheral curve, which varies with the base-curve radius. The meridional orientation of the lens is stabilized by a superior and inferior slab-off off the front surface and has 1.25 to 1.50 D prism ballast within the optic zone. The spheric power selection is unlimited up to −20.00 to +20.00 D, whereas the cylinder correction is limited to 0.50 to 3.50 D.

The recommended fitting set has 10 lenses that vary from 30.00 to 42.50 D in 0.50 D steps. The diameter is 14.5 mm for lenses 40.50 D and flatter and 14 mm for lenses 41.00 D or steeper.

The following method is employed for double slab-off lenses:

1. The base curve is selected on the basis of a lens 4.00 D flatter than the flattest K.
2. Evaluate the lens on a cornea relationship to position, movement, and quality of the K.
3. Over-refract and include the minus cylinders and the vertex distance.

The best candidates for selection are those with cylinders ranging from 1.00 to 2.00 D and those with regular astigmatism. Oblique cylinders between 30 and 60 degrees are difficult to orientate. Patients with tight lids and small palpebral fissures are screened out because of previous poor results with such patients.

Note that this particular lens, as opposed to others that employ the same type of slab-off inferiorly and superiorly, has a toric zone only in the optic area of the lens. The lens has engraving at the 9 and 3 o'clock positions, and it is stabilized below as indicated by the presence of a blue dot.

Comment. Thin-zone lenses are the least stable but most comfortable. Also the permeability of these lenses to oxygen is much greater than similar lenses stabilized by prisms.

Assessing the fit. Once the lens has "settled" on the eye, always note the final lens orientation relative to the true 180-degree axis. At least 15 minutes is required for lens settling. If the lens orientation and stabilization is not achieved, a different stabilizing technique should be used.

Correcting the axis. Axis corrections can be defined with etch marks, or laser beams, on all lenses at 0 to 180 degrees, a blue dot at the 6 o'clock position, or a vertical line. These marks are reference points to the orientation of the toric axis. A spectacle trial frame with axis lines is employed. The lens is then rotated until the axis lines are in alignment with the prism base marked on the contact lens. The amount of rotation is directly read from the scale. The marks are usually in 5-degree intervals. For example, a lens at 5 o'clock will be rotated 15 degrees.

The 0- to 90-degree zone of the lens is regarded as the *subtractive inclination*. If the axis of the correcting cylinder toric lens is wrong, subtract the inclination in that zone. For example, if the minus cylinder axis is 20 degrees (which is in the 0- to 90-degree quadrant) and the over-refraction yields 15 degrees of axis correction, the final cylinder axis would be 5 degrees, that is, 20 degrees − 15 degrees.

The *additive quadrant* is between 90 and 180 degrees. So, if the axis is 140 degrees and the correct axis is 10 degrees, the final axis is 140 degrees + 10 degrees = 150 degrees.

Posterior toric lenses are always gauged for lens orientation on the measurement of exact corneal toricity determined by cylinder scales.

Visual results. The degree of visual acuity is not absolute. Some patients with high degrees of astigmatism are content to have 20/25 vision, whereas others with low degrees of astigmatism are not content with this level of performance. However, as with all soft lenses, there are people with 20/20 vision who still complain of poor vision. Technically they are not rejects. In absolute terms 70% of our patients received 20/20 visual acuity with toric corrections, 80% of patients get visual acuity equal to or greater than the spectacle visual acuity, and 20% of cases required a second fitting to yield good visual results.

The results of soft toric lens fitting is directly proportional to the enthusiasm of the fitter. At best, 70% of patients are easy and require only one fitting. After a year an additional 20% may require refitting.

Protein on the lens can change the comfort of the lens, alter the lens contour, and interfere with visibility through the lens.

Problems in soft toric lens fitting. The causes of rejection of the toric lens are (1) discomfort, which can be created by foreign-body sensation of the lens, excessive movement of the lens, and awareness of the lens because of the abut-

ment of the lens against the lower lid; and (2) poor vision, which can be attributable largely to rotation of the axis of the lens, which cannot be stabilized. This is particularly true with astigmatism of oblique axis 20 to 80 degrees and 110 to 160 degrees. Axis mislocation is a significant problem that was substantially reduced by the use of a truncated prism-ballast trial set. In some cases, the poor vision is related to variable vision symptoms of a tight or a flat fit and other visual defects that can confront any hydrogel lens wearer. There are cases in which poor vision is directly attributable to some diffuse corneal edema and the incorporation of fine subepithelial precipitates.

Signs of inadequate fit
1. Corneal edema or diffuse corneal stippling, especially under the thicker prismatic portion of the lens.
2. Inability to stabilize the lens axis.
3. Too much edge lift causing the lens to slip out of position.
4. Decentered lens or an inability to make the lens system flat enough to ensure adequate movement.
5. Discontinued lens wear because of limbal compression with engorgement of the limbal capillaries, which could eventually lead to corneal vascularization.

Factors that favor a good fit
1. Corneal astigmatism at the 90- and 180-degree meridians. If the astigmatism is oblique, say, at 60 degrees, the lids will create a rotational force on the lens with each blink. This movement is largely caused by the lens thickness not being the same on each side of the lens. As the lid moves down, it creates a greater drag or rotational force on the thicker side than on the thinner side.
2. Normal lid motion with small and tight palpebral fissures. Narrow palpebral tissues and tight lids create excessive movement of the lens and upset the toric alignment.
3. A lower lid that does not abut the truncated edge of a toric lens.
4. Astigmatism greater than 1.00 diopter. Small amounts of astigmatism should be ignored.
5. Use of a toric-lens trial set to evaluate correction and rotational characteristics

of the lens on the eye. The trial lenses have prism ballast, truncation, and toric surfaces.

6. Cylinders of about 2 diopters are ideal. The more cylinder that is found in the treatment, the greater the difficulty in centration and the heavier the lens.

7. A minimally flat fit. If too loose, a lens will cause variable vision. A tight lens adds to stability but causes other undesirable signs and symptoms.

8. Lid configuration and lid tensions are important considerations. The closure of the eyes on blinking, particularly if there is increased tension, or downward or upward sloping lateral canthi, will effect the performance and stabilization of toric lenses.

9. The double slab-off design is best for comfort.

10. Prism ballast plus beveled truncation is best for lens stability and precise axis correction.

11. Posterior toric lenses are best for a correction of moderate to high corneal toricity.

12. Aspheric lens design is a helpful adjunct to any lens system.

13. Large diameters, such as 14.5 mm, assist in centering the lens. One must compensate for the added tightness that a large-diameter lens confers by fitting the lens flatter.

14. Higher water content and thinner lenses aid comfort and oxygen permeability. Because lens thickness is usually measured at the optical center of a lens, the extra dimension of the prism in these lenses may not be included.

Comment. The fitting of a soft toric lens is not easy. One has to stay within the small zone of fitting too tight or too loose to ensure lens stability without adding complications.

Also, the frequency of lens replacements is higher than that of a spheric lens. With time, axis mislocation may occur because of protein debris in the lens, which can alter the fitting characteristics of the lens.

Unless the fitting criteria are present for a favorable hydrogel toric lens fit, a gas-permeable lens may be a better choice.

If residual astigmatism is present, we have found soft toric lenses better than rigid lenses because the larger diameter permitted with soft lenses permits better stabilization. Also the extra power required can easily be ground on the front surface of the lens.

RIGID CONTACT LENSES FOR ASTIGMATISM

Today, the emphasis in the types of rigid lenses is on the gas-permeable lenses. We will however include discussion of PMMA lenses because there are still fitters who prefer these lenses because of their greater durability. Also the gas-permeable lenses may not be readily available in every country.

Spheric rigid lenses

A spheric rigid lens should first be tried with any cornea of 3.00 D or less of corneal astigmatism. It is the lens of choice for toric corneas of small magnitude simply because a spheric lens is the easiest to fit, modify, and duplicate. A spheric lens is our choice of diagnostic lens to be used first, regardless of the degree of astigmatism.

It may be employed in the following manner:

1. An ultrathin lens may be used to correct low levels of residual astigmatism of 1.00 D or less. Such a lens will normally flex with blinking and will tend to nullify residual astigmatism against the rule. It is a good lens for residual astigmatism.

2. A conventional spheric lens may be used. One method is simply to "split K" so that the radius of curvature of the lens is *halfway* between that of the steeper and flatter meridians. Another approach is simply to ignore any astigmatism of 2.00 D or less. For each 0.50 D over 2.00 D of corneal astigmatism, fit 0.25 D steeper than K.

3. A large diameter lens of *9.5 to 10.5 mm fitted on K may be used.* A large spheric lens provides stability on a toric cornea and is the lens of choice when a regular-sized lens fails to achieve adequate centration. Large lenses have also been used with success in some cases with astigmatism of 3.00 to 5.00 D. Only gas-permeable lenses should be used with large degrees of astigmatism where large diameters are required to ensure centration and stability.

Comment. We have found that spheric rigid lenses account for over 90% of our rigid lenses used for correcting astigmatism whereas only 4% required a custom-ordered toric rigid lens.

Thin, spheric lens. A microthin lens with 0.12 mm or less central thickness will flex on a toric cornea with astigmatism with the rule and will reduce an astigmatism against the rule. However if the residual astigmatism is against the rule and the corneal surface has astigmatism against the rule, a thin lens will only augment the residual astigmatism.

Spheric equivalent. In patients with residual astigmatism of 1.00 D or less, the simple device of increasing the power of the spheric lens by an amount equal to the spheric equivalent of the remaining refractive error can be employed very effectively. For example, if the residual refractive error is -1.00 D cylinder axis 180 degrees, the spheric equivalent to be added to the spheric correction would be 0.50 D.

Toric rigid PMMA lenses

For historic reasons we should consider toric PMMA lens. As noted previously this accounts for only a minimal number of fittings to correct astigmatism today.

Prism-ballast lens. This lens has a spheric back surface, a prism base down of 1.5 prism D, and a toric front surface that provides the necessary correcting cylinder. Prisms greater than 2.00 D have such a heavy edge that they are seldom tolerated. For weaker power, -5.00 D or less, 0.75 prism D is frequently satisfactory. The bottom of the lens may be truncated to add stability and proper orientation. Truncation may produce problems however. It can weight down the lens so that it overrides the lower limbus and can also irritate the lower lid by bumping it. Moreover a truncated lens is difficult to fit for residual astigmatism against the rule because there is conflict between the gravitational movement of the lens downward and the need to contour the lens against a steep, horizontal meridian. Many fitters prefer a circular prism-ballast lens since it is easier to center and manufacture. One should use a trial lens for the refraction and determine the lens orientation by marking it with a grease pencil. This indicates the axis of the front-surface cylinder.

If one eye is fitted with a prism-ballast lens it is frequently necessary to fit the other eye in a similar fashion to avoid creating an intolerable vertical phoria. A prism-ballast lens should not be ordered unless absolutely necessary. What is gained by correcting residual astigmatism may be lost by the reduced optic quality of the lens imposed by the prism.

CORRECTING ASTIGMATISM WITH A PMMA BITORIC LENS (Table 24-2)

A bitoric lens is employed to fit a toric cornea when a spheric lens has been tried and found inadequate. It is usually required in any cornea if the toricity exceeds 4.00 D of astigmatism with the rule or 2.00 D of astigmatism against the rule. The spheric lens may center poorly and rock or cause poor acuity. For example, if the astigmatism is against the rule, the lens will rotate along the vertical meridian and slide either temporally or nasally. Such a lens will irritate the eye and will not be tolerated for full-time wear. A toric arc of touch is characteristic of the fluorescein pattern. Its prime purpose is to correct a physical disturbance in the cornea and not to remedy a refractive error.

A bitoric lens has cylinder correction on the front and back surface. The back-surface cylinder is in relation to the toric shape of the cornea. The front-surface cylinder is used to correct the residual refractive error or the added astigmatism induced by the posterior cylindric correction. A toric, peripheral curve lens may provide the stability and centration for a spheric lens and should be considered before one uses back-surface toric lenses.

Occasionally a bitoric lens is needed when a prism-ballast, front-surface, cylindric lens is tried to correct residual astigmatism and the lens fails to center.

Fitting a bitoric lens

Base curve. The lens is usually fitted flatter than K in either principal meridian. The flattest meridian is made flatter by 0.25 D and the steeper one flatter by 0.50 D.

Diameter. These lenses are generally not made larger than 8.5 mm to avoid flare. The optic zone is generally 1 mm less in dimension. Some leeway in diameter size can be considered on the basis of normal factors such as cor-

Table 24-2. Dioptric values for light passing through the two primary meridians of an inside toric lens and cornea

Vertical meridian	V1	V2	V3
	r = 8.036 mm	r = 7.542 mm	r = 7.336 mm
Dioptric values immediately after light passes through the surface	+60.98 D	+40.76 D	+40.76 D

Interface n' − n	*Anterior lens and air*	*Posterior lens and tears*	*Posterior tears and anterior cornea*
	1.49 − 1.00 = 0.49	1.3375 − 1.49 = −0.1525	1.3375 − 1.3375 = 0

Horizontal meridian	H1	H2	H3
	r = 8.036 mm	r = 8.036 mm	r = 8.036 mm
Dioptric values immediately after light passes through the surface	+60.98 D	+42.00 D	+42.00 D

Formula: $\dfrac{n' - n}{r}$

$$V1: \quad \frac{0.49 \text{ mm}}{8.036 \text{ mm}} = +60.98 \text{ D}$$

$$V2: \quad \frac{-0.1525 \text{ mm}}{7.542 \text{ mm}} = -20.22 \text{ D}$$

$$V3: \quad \frac{0}{7.336 \text{ mm}} = 0$$

$$V1 - V2 = +40.76 \text{ D}$$

$$H1: \quad \frac{0.49 \text{ mm}}{8.036 \text{ mm}} = +60.98 \text{ D}$$

$$H2: \quad \frac{-0.1525 \text{ mm}}{8.036 \text{ mm}} = -18.98 \text{ D}$$

$$H3: \quad \frac{0}{8.036 \text{ mm}} = 0$$

$$H1 - H2 = +42.00 \text{ D}$$

$$V1 - V2 - V3 = +40.76 \text{ D}$$

$$H1 - H2 - H3 = +42.00 \text{ D}$$

$$V - H = 40.76 - 42.00 = -1.24 \text{ D} \times 180$$

Assumptions

Lens (anterior)	V1: 8.036 mm (42.00 'K' D)	H1: 8.036 mm (42.00 'K' D)
Lens (posterior)	V2: 7.542 mm (44.75 'K' D)	H2: 8.036 mm (42.00 'K' D)
Cornea (anterior)	V3: 7.336 mm (46.00 'K' D)	H3: 8.036 mm (42.00 'K' D)

Assumptions
1. Index of cornea and tears both same as keratometer calibration—1.3375 mm
2. Infinitely thin thickness of lens and tears
3. Incident light is parallel

Thus light entering the eye (past the anterior corneal surface), after passing through this lens system, shows a (residual) astigmatism of −1.24 D × 180 that has to be corrected without an outside cylinder of +1.24 D × 180.

Courtesy Dr. Stanley Gordon, Rochester, N.Y.

A.

	Example 1	*Example 2*
Spectacle prescription	Plano -4.00 D $\times$ 180	Plano -4.00 D $\times$ 180
Keratometer cylinder	-3.00 D $\times$ 180	-5.00 D $\times$ 180
Predicted residual (or determined by over-refraction)	-1.00 D $\times$ 180 (correcting cylinder)	$+1.00$ D $\times$ 180

B.

Determine *induced* cylinder = 45% of inside cylinder prescribed expressed in K diopters; prescribed for both 3.00 D $\times$ 45% = -1.35 D induced (requiring correction with a $+1.35$ D correcting cylinder).

B − A

Induced cylinder	-1.35 D $\times$ 180	-1.35 D $\times$ 180
Predicted residual	-1.00 D $\times$ 180	$+1.00$ D $\times$ 180
Total anticipated residual	-0.35 D $\times$ 180	-2.35 D $\times$ 180
Required correction by this outside cylinder	$+0.35$ D $\times$ 180	

neal diameter, palpebral fissure size, and K readings.

Power. The power of a toric surface in plastic is considerably higher than an identical amount of toricity of the cornea because of the higher index of refraction of plastic. The power, measured in air, of a lens cylinder is approximately 1.45 times the cylindric power of a cornea of the same toricity.

Example

℞ -2.00 D -4.00 D $\times$ 180 = 41.00 D $\times$ 180/ 45.00 D $\times$ 90. If the full 4.00 D of cylinder were generated in a back toric lens, its power would be -5.81 in air at 180 degrees, which is -1.810 D of excessive cylinder. This requires a correction with a $+1.181$ D outside cylinder $\times$ 180.

The induced cylinder is independent of the corneal cylinder and is related to the outside toricity of the lens only.

$$n' - n: \frac{\text{Plastic} - \text{Air}}{\text{Tears} - \text{Air}} = \frac{1.49 - 1.00}{1.3375 - 1.00} = \frac{0.49}{0.3375} = 1.4519$$

The induced cylinder is therefore 45% of the inside cylinder, when the inside cylinder is expressed in K diopters as usual (if the inside cylinder is expressed in millimeters the induced cylinder is 31%).

A simple method to arrive at the correct power is to trial-fit the patient with toric base curve, spheric, front-surface lenses. An over-refraction is done, and the added cylinder is simply put on the front surface of the lens.

The determination of the outside cylinder required (or, for that matter, whether an inside toric or bitoric is required) should be left to a competent laboratory to calculate because most practitioners do not have the understanding of the optics involved. The way it may be done is as follows:

Determine the predicted residual astigmatism or, for even greater accuracy, have the practitioner refract over a *rigid*, well-centered, spheric lens. (See top of page.)

It should be evident that for the special case where the outside cylinder used is equal to and corrects all of the induced cylinder the power of the cylinder in air of this lens is equal to the K dioptric power of the inside cylinder. To illustrate, take the 4.00 D inside toric lens, which has a cylinder power in air of -5.81 D $\times$ 180. By placement of a $+1.81$ D front-surface cylinder on this lens D the power in air now becomes -4.00 D cylinder $\times$ 180, and all of the induced cylinder is corrected.

A bitoric lens is difficult to manufacture accurately. Office modifications require great skill to avoid removing the peripheral toricity. The cost of these lenses is high, and they are difficult to reproduce for replacement. Frequently there is a power difference between the two toric surfaces, causing residual astigmatism. Move with caution and be sure that both you and the laboratory are capable of handling a bitoric lens before suggesting one.

Sampson and Feldman have popularized the

Table 24-3. Use of negative toric (back cylinder) contact lenses for high corneal toricity and residual astigmatism*

Cornea	Lens	Cornea	Lens
Cylinder of inside lens surface (D)	Refractive cylinder values in air (D)	Cylinder of inside lens surface (D)	Refractive cylinder values in air (D)
−0.25	−0.36	−4.25	−6.17
−0.50	−0.73	−4.50	−6.53
−0.75	−1.09	−4.75	−6.90
−1.00	−1.45	−5.00	−7.26
−1.25	−1.82	−5.25	−7.62
−1.50	−2.18	−5.50	−7.99
−1.75	−2.54	−5.75	−8.35
−2.00	−2.90	−6.00	−8.71
−2.25	−3.27	−6.25	−9.08
−2.50	−3.63	−6.50	−9.44
−2.75	−3.99	−6.75	−9.80
−3.00	−4.36	−7.00	−10.16
−3.25	−4.72	−7.25	−10.53
−3.50	−5.08	−7.50	−10.89
−3.75	−5.45	−7.75	−11.25
−4.00	−5.81	−8.00	−11.62

Courtesy Dr. Stanley Gordon, Rochester, N.Y..
*Corneal values based on refractive index = 1.3375; lens values based on refractive index = 1.490.

use of posterior toric lenses as a better alternative to bitoric lenses. These lenses are easily fabricated, have a spheric front surface that can be polished, rarely required any truncation or prism ballast for proper meridional orientation on the cornea, and will handle over 90% of all cases requiring toric lens design, residual astigmatism, or both.

In terms of corneal dioptric toricity, the total amount that may be generated on the posterior surface of a lens is about two thirds of the corneal toricity, which is given more accurately in Table 24-3.

To calculate such a lens consider the following example:

K = 42.00 D × 46.00 D × 90
Refraction −1.00 D with −2.50 D × 180
From Table 24-3, 1.75 D of corneal toricity is equal to 2.50 D of plastic toricity.
CPC = 42.00 D × 43.75 D
Lens = −1.00 D with −2.50 D × 180
or
CPC = 43.00 D × 44.75 D
Lens = −2.00 D with −2.50 D × 180

Comment. The PMMA lens in the correction of significant astigmatism has given way to gas-permeable lenses and hydrogel lenses. The family of gas-permeable lenses offers the benefits of an oxygen-permeable system and a large-diameter lens between 9 and 10 mm, which ensures axis stability. Also, these lenses can be fitted with a spheric lens up to 5 diopters of cylinder, which adds to the ease of fitting.

The soft lens is still the most comfortable lens, being flaccid, thin, and hydrated. It is more complicated than a gas-permeable spheric lens in that the fitter must contend with a system that requires a toric lens. The rigid gas-permeable lens offers better crispness of vision if the toricity is great or is found in an oblique axis. The best part of it is that a spheric lens can be used to handle most astigmatic corrections. *When dealing with astigmatism that has to be corrected with a contact lens,* the fitter should think first of a *good gas-permeable lens,* then of a *soft lens,* and finally of a *PMMA lens.*

USE OF GAS-PERMEABLE RIGID LENSES

Gas-permeable rigid lenses include cellulose acetate butryate, silicone-acrylate, silicone resins, and styrene. There has been a dramatic increase in the use of gas-permeable lenses. They have superseded PMMA as a rigid lens. With their use has come increased safety for the cornea, comfort, and better visual performance for the wearer. This has been discussed previously. Newer types of polymers with higher gas permeability than before have entered the field. This change has dramatically resulted in a wider use of the gas-permeable rigid lenses for correcting astigmatism.

Of more importance has been the increased size, which can be tolerated. This has enabled the fitter to utilize these lenses for the correction of astigmatism. The average diameter for nontoric spheric lenses should be 9.2 mm ± 0.2 mm. These lenses can be used in much greater diameter for larger corneal toricity. Even a 10, 11, or 12 mm gas-permeable lens may be required for corneal toricity greater than 5 diopters. They are particularly useful for aphakic corneas and for distorted corneas with irregular astigmatism. The larger lenses permit better centration and vaulting over the corneal

toricity. In addition to an increase in size, the gas-permeable lenses can be fitted flatter than PMMA lenses can without induction of corneal hypoxia.

Tips on fitting gas-permeable lenses for astigmatism

1. A spheric trial set is needed for assessment of the fitting characteristics of the lens. These sets should be made up in PMMA material because they not only are more durable but also do not require any conditioning effect by solutions as some gas-permeable materials do, such as the Boston Lens.

2. Because these gas-permeable lenses have a large diameter and the refractive power or cylinder correction may be large, attention must be given to the edges of the lens to ensure comfort. A high-minus lens should have a

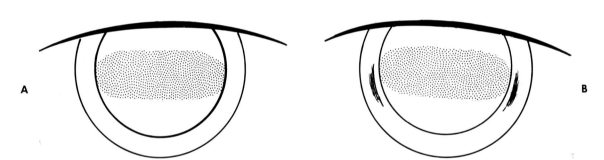

Fig. 24-5. A, With-the-rule astigmatism, which creates a flatter horizontal meridian in which the lens may decenter vertically. **B,** During blinking the lens may cause compression on the flatter horizontal meridian and may result in epithelial erosion at the 3 and 9 o'clock position.

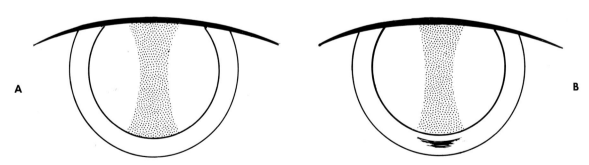

Fig. 24-6. A, Against-the-rule astigmatism, which creates a flatter vertical meridian in which the contact lens may decenter side to side. **B,** During blinking the lens may cause compression on the flatter vertical meridian and may result in epithelial erosion at the 6 o'clock position.

plus profile and a high-plus lens a myopic profile.

3. Fit first with spheric gas-permeable lenses. Our studies indicate that over 90% of cylinder may be corrected with a spheric rigid lens, which is the simplest type of lens to fit.

4. With high cylinders, one should have some thickness increase to the lens to prevent flexure on the steepest corneal meridian. Our rule of thumb is to add 0.01 mm extra thickness for every 1 to 2 diopters of cylinder to be corrected.

5. If centering is a problem with the trial lens, one should go to a larger-diameter lens as first choice.

6. In with-the-rule astigmatism, one may develop vertical decentration because the lens rocks on the flatter meridian (Fig. 24-5, *A*). The rocking may cause corneal epithelial erosion at the 3 and 9 o'clock positions (Fig. 24-5, *B*). This problem may require a larger lens, and the lens must have perfect blend and thin edges.

7. Against-the-rule astigmatism may cause side-to-side decentration because of rocking on the vertical flatter meridian (Fig. 24-6). Also, with each blink there may develop corneal erosions at the 6 o'clock position because the edge of the lens indents on the flatter part of the cornea inferiorly. This problem may require a larger lens or a steeper lens.

8. One should use a toric trial set if standard spheric lenses cannot be fitted. One is often surprised that a lesser degree of toricity is required than would be expected. One may have 5 diopters of corneal astigmatism as determined by K readings but only require a 3-diopter toric lens.

9. A gas-permeable lens does not function optimally unless it rides high. Low-lying lenses create discomfort because of lid impact, cause 3 to 9 o'clock staining with marginal episcleritis, and create variable vision. Because the diameters of these lenses must be large, the high-rising interblink position can only be achieved when one fits these lenses somewhat flatter and pays special attention to the edges of the lens and to the thickness so that the lids will lift the lens as opposed to pushing it down.

10. The gas-permeable lenses of larger refractive power and large diameter may ride low because the lenses are likely to be heavy. This means that the lenses may not function optimally, as in (9).

One manufacturer (Syntex) has simplified gas-permeable lens into three diameters, along with applying soft lens design systems. By selecting one of the three diameters in appropriate base curves, one not only can achieve a remarkably high first-fit lens but also can retain a smaller inventory of gas-permeable lenses for immediate fitting.

Comments. In a retrospective analysis of correcting astigmatic errors over 1.25 D, we used the percentage of lenses as shown in the following:

Retrospective fitting analysis of cylinder > 1.25 D (869 eyes)

Soft lenses	
Spheric	30%
Toric	19%
Rigid lenses	
Spheric	48%
Toric	3%

In most cases a spheric gas-permeable rigid lens will work to correct astigmatism and only rarely do we have to utilize a front or back surface toric lens.

Gas-permeable rigid lenses are preferred for clarity of vision and ease of fitting for toric corneas. They are preferred for large errors of cylinder over 4 diopters. Soft toric lenses, on the other hand, may be utilized for comfort and for residual astigmatism.

It is uncommon now for us to use a rigid PMMA lens.

PRESBYOPE BIFOCAL LENSES: RIGID AND SOFT

There is a huge untapped market of presbyopic people. It is a condition that sooner or later affects 100% of people. Not all will want to wear contact lenses, but a considerable number will want them when they are perfected.

One of the main reasons that few presbyopic spectacle wearers wear contact lenses seems to be lack of interest. It has been shown repeatedly that the major reason that young persons with myopia want lenses is for cosmetic purposes, a factor of lesser importance to middle-aged persons. Bifocal lenses are difficult to fabricate, modify, and fit precisely. These lenses do not center well and may require either truncation or prisms for stability. They are thicker than normal and, with the optic weighting at the bottom of the lens, their movement with blinking is restricted and the vision through the near segment is fair at the J_3 to J_5 level.

The trick of prescribing so that one eye sees well for distance while the other is employed for near work is only a compromise solution until a better one is found. The aspheric lens with its variable-focus features seems to be the most promising. It is basically a single-vision lens with no prism or segment. As such, patients are not bothered with image jump, flare, or bifocal segments that ride too high or slip too low. The lens is more comfortable because it can be prescribed with standard thickness. It is also quite new in application, which means that the list of its disadvantages is not yet finished. The aspheric lenses show promise, but our initial experience with them was disappointing. Once we acquired some expertise, our clinical results improved.

Approximately 65% of patients achieve adequate near vision, but we have been unable to predict in advance those most likely to succeed. We have enjoyed our best success by overplussing the nondominant eye using single-vision lenses. A mixed technique is also effective: bifocal lenses with slight overplussing in the nondominant eye.

The arrival of a reliable, effective rigid bifocal contact lens has not yet materialized. The newer gas-permeable lens may be of help in fabricating an adequate bifocal rigid lens. These lenses will have a larger optic zone for distance and near vision, so that the shift in vision will be more readily accomplished. Also the permeability features may allow stabilizing devices such as prisms to be more readily tolerated. Motivation should be present to yield a higher success rate among those patients who are fitted with rigid bifocal lenses to provide the stimulus for a better solution. A strong desire to wear contact lenses is especially important for the patient who is a first-time lens wearer.

The soft bifocal lens has also made its way on the scene. Its debut is appreciated. Although not perfect, it eliminates one problem for the middle-aged novice presbyopic patient, that is, discomfort. It is important to appreciate that from a clinical point of view the fitting of a bifocal lens may be an exercise in futility. Some fitters do better than others with bifocal lenses largely because of expertise and motivation. Expertise can be acquired.

Without adding fresh cases, we know that there are in everyone's practice people who have worn rigid contact lenses for 20 years or more and who have become presbyopic. These people require a contact lens for general vision and are not happy utilizing a pair of reading glasses. So despite the imperfections in the systems available for total contact lens application for distance and near vision, it is necessary to deal with the subject, like it or not.

So it behooves the fitter to learn bifocal techniques, even to become a little excited about them.

Comment. Our results are similar for rigid and hydrogel lens wearers. One major problem is quality control. Often the bifocal reading areas in both lenses is too weak in power or one lens is correct in power and the other does not appear to have any bifocal addition.

BIFOCAL RIGID LENSES
Annular bifocal lens

This lens is designed with the distance power ground into the center and the near power into the periphery of the lens. The power of the lens may be incorporated into the front or back surface. Vision may be simultaneous with the eye seeing clearly at distance and out of focus at near range or alternating with the lens designed to shift its position if sight is directed from distance to near range (Fig. 25-1).

This lens is not popular. Using the principle of simultaneous vision, the patient always experiences one out-of-focus image. With this method of using the bifocal lens there is difficulty in producing a lens that moves up adequately for clear near viewing.

Prism-ballast bifocal lens

This bifocal lens is stabilized in one of two ways: (1) it is made so that the lower portion is heavier and wider than the upper or (2) the bifocal segment is made in the form of a prism by fusion of an insert on the distance lens or by grinding of the segment on the front surface of the lens.

The segment may be fused into an insert on the distance lens. The added power is derived from the fused segment having a higher index of refraction than the upper portion of the lens.

Fused bifocal (Camp) lens. The fused bifocal (Camp) lens (Fig. 25-2) is thinner with a sharp division between distance and near vision and

---

Specifications for annular bifocal lens

Front surface
   Diameter: 9 mm
Bifocal addition
   Base curve: fit on K to allow movement
   Optic zone: 3.5 mm—relative to pupillary size for distance power only
Back surface
   Diameter: 8.5 to 10.5 mm
Bifocal addition (de Carle)
   Base curve: tight fit—0.50 D steeper than K
   Optic zone: smaller than pupillary zone; approximately 3 mm in size

---

Specifications for fused bifocal (Camp) lens

Bifocal segment: 6.5 mm
Diameter: 8.5 to 9.5 mm
Prism ballast: 1.5Δ
Segment height: fitted 1 mm higher than the pupillary margin for plus lenses and 1 mm lower for minus lenses
Truncation: 0.4 to 0.5 mm

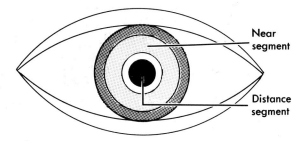

Fig. 25-1. Annular bifocal lens. The near segment is pushed up by the lower lid.

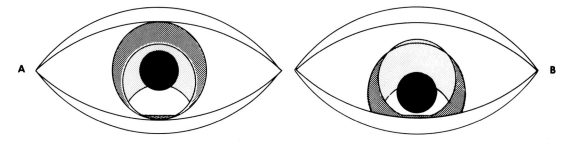

Fig. 25-2. **A,** Camp bifocal lens. The bifocal segment is pushed up, **B,** for reading.

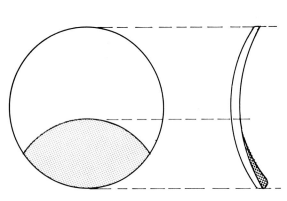

Fig. 25-3. Camp fused bifocal lens.

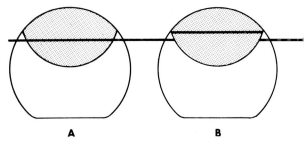

Fig. 25-4. Monocentric bifocal lens. Each lens is calculated so that no image jump occurs along the segment line. It is a one-piece lens, truncated at the bottom. If a bifocal lens is not monocentric, a line seen through the lens will be displaced as in **B.**

with a front surface free for a cylinder correction. The area of the fused segment is frequently of poor quality and becomes an area of optic distortion (Fig. 25-3).

The one-piece monocentric bifocal lens, in which the segment has been ground on the front surface of the lens, has the advantage of a segment selection and no image jump (Fig. 25-4). The bifocal addition can be shaped to suit any purpose.

One-piece bifocal lenses

Crescent bifocal (Black) lens (Fig. 25-5). The crescent bifocal (Black) lens is a crescent-shaped bifocal lens with the flat surface on the top. This lens offers minimal image jump as compared to the round-top bifocal lens. It is necessary to fit the segment so that it is in the lower pupillary border, since it induces diplopia if it is above or below it.

Monocentric bifocal (Mandell) lens (Fig. 25-6). The monocentric design of this lens eliminates image jump because the distance and near vision sections lie in the same focal plane. The top of the bifocal segment should be

slightly higher than the lower margin of the pupil.

Comment. The monocentric bifocal lens does not have a prism on the lens blank. It is ground on the front surface. The absence of a prism in the basic segment eliminates such visual problems as monocular diplopia and ghost images. Its concave shape affords a wider range for near viewing (Fig. 25-7). It is superior to the fused bifocal lens because of its better optic properties and wider field of near vision.

Truncation. Truncation serves to provide a flat edge for better contact with the lid and reduces overall lens weight (Fig. 25-8).

The truncation should be flat with rounded corners and tapered evenly on both surfaces. The bevel is usually 0.4 to 0.5 mm in diameter. The truncated edge should remain on the lower lid as the eyes shift down. With the lenses on the lower lid the upper pole of the lens should not override the upper limbus. Adding truncation has the same effect as adding more prism ballast. It adds stability to the lens and stops rotation.

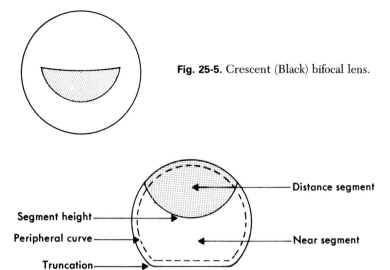

Fig. 25-5. Crescent (Black) bifocal lens.

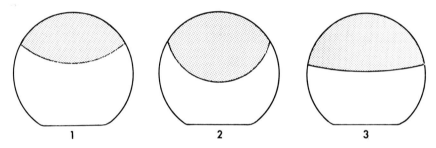

Fig. 25-6. Monocentric (Mandell) bifocal lens. The advantage of this lens design is that the entire pupil is covered by the bifocal segment as the lower lid pushes the lens upward during the act of reading.

Fig. 25-7. Variations in design of one-piece bifocal lens. *1*, Standard lens design; *2*, concave lens design—this lens affords greater side-to-side viewing for a near object; *3*, flat lens design—this lens affords a wider sweep for distance vision.

Difficulties with near vision with prism-ballast lenses. If the lens is too tight, it may not shift upward in the reading position. With the patient looking straight ahead, the lens should be picked up 1 to 2 mm in the blink and then dropped back to a lower position. A lens that fits too tightly may be improved if one flattens the peripheral curve, reduces the diameter, or flattens the base curve.

If the lens drops too low (Fig. 25-9), one may solve this problem by broadening the truncation area, increasing the flat surface of the lens, or decreasing the prism by 0.50 D.

If the vertical diameter is too great, the lens will not be able to move up with reading (Fig. 25-10). The solution for this problem is to reduce the lens diameter.

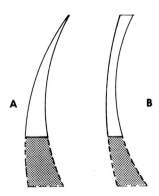

Fig. 25-8. Truncation provides lens support, reduction in lens weight, and a wide edge of contact to engage the lid. The effect of truncation depends on the refractive error. It adds ballast on a plus lens, **A,** and reduces ballast on a minus lens, **B.**

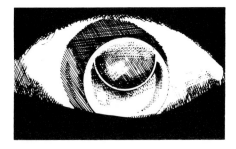

Fig. 25-9. Bifocal lens is decentered. The lens is too small.

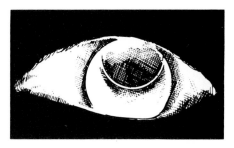

Fig. 25-10. Bifocal lens. The diameter of this lens is too large—the lens touches the upper lid.

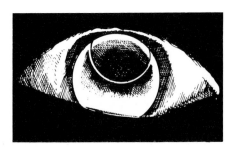

Fig. 25-11. Bifocal segment too high.

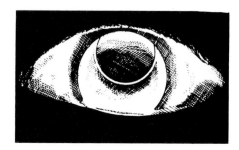

Fig. 25-12. Bifocal segment correct height.

Specifications for monocentric bifocal (Mandell) lens

Monocentric diameter: 9 to 10.5 mm
Optic zone: 1.2 mm less than diameter
Prism ballast: 1.5Δ
Truncation: 0.4 to 0.5 mm

Insufficient height of the reading segment to cover the pupil for all positions of gaze inferiorly can be solved when the height of the segment is increased.

If the distance vision is impaired, this problem may indicate that the bifocal segment height is too high (Figs. 25-11 and 25-12). It can be solved in two ways: one can prescribe a new lens with a lower segment height or reduce the diameter of the lens, especially at the truncated edge. It may also indicate that the lens is too tight and is not positioning low enough. Reducing the diameter of the lens, flattening the peripheral curve, or adding 0.50 D more prism will solve this problem.

Multifocal lens

The multifocal rigid lens is an aspheric, variable-focus, corneal lens that provides clear distance and near vision (Fig. 25-13). It has no segments or prisms. The power of the lens increases from the central area of the lens to the periphery. This produces an increase in plus power toward the edge of the lens. The central rays from a distant object are focused on the retina, whereas the paraxial rays are focused in front of the retina (Fig. 25-14). To achieve a +2.00 D effect for reading, the posterior aspheric base must flatten approximately 6.00 D within the pupillary area.

Spheric aberration is greatly increased by the shorter focal length toward the periphery provided by an aspherically based multifocal lens. This increase in spheric aberration reduces the effective aperture and increases the depth of focus of the lens. The base curve is aspheric but should be fitted steeper than the flattest corneal curvature by 0.35 mm. The front surface is spheric.

This lens can be fitted using diagnostic lenses or the photokeratoscope.

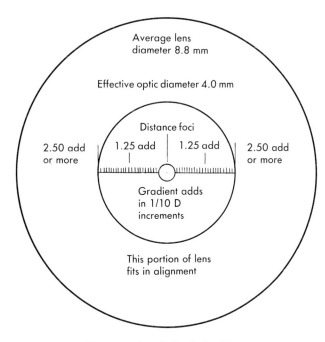

Fig. 25-13. Presbiflex bifocal lens.

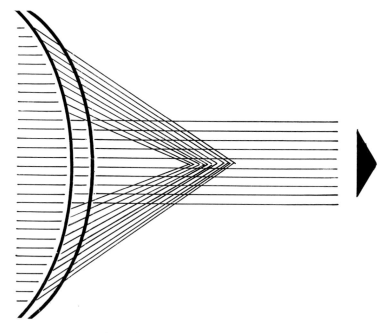

Fig. 25-14. Presbiflex lens of $+2.50$ D has between 35 and 40 foci.

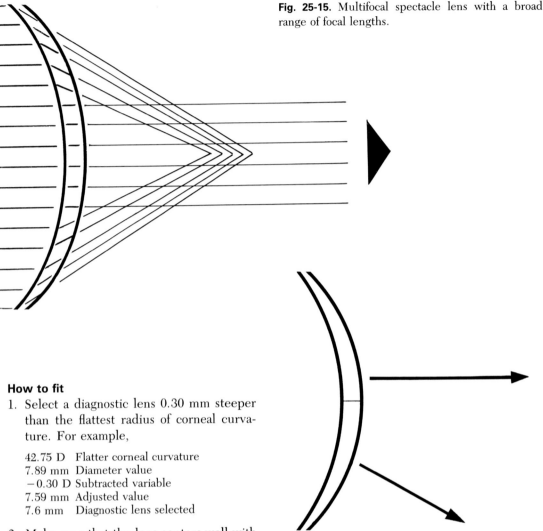

Fig. 25-15. Multifocal spectacle lens with a broad range of focal lengths.

Fig. 25-16. Traditional bifocal lens with distance and near focal lengths.

How to fit

1. Select a diagnostic lens 0.30 mm steeper than the flattest radius of corneal curvature. For example,

   42.75 D   Flatter corneal curvature
   7.89 mm Diameter value
   −0.30 D Subtracted variable
   7.59 mm Adjusted value
   7.6 mm   Diagnostic lens selected

2. Make sure that the lens centers well with a minimum of movement—1 to 2 mm.

3. Over-refract through the trial lens to obtain the best distance correction. Initially the patient may report that the vision is blurry and that a short rest period is frequently needed to adapt to the lenses.

4. Instruct the patient to look at a near-vision card. Add 0.25 D at a time until the print J$_2$ can be read. Do not overplus the patient because doing so can be quite easy. The best guard against this problem is to have the patient look alternately at the distance chart to ensure that vision at 20 feet still remains clear.

   The final power should be
   −4.50 D—distance refraction
   +0.75 D—near over-refraction
   −3.75 D—for total lens

5. If vision is blurred at near range, check the centration in the reading position. If the lens is displaced by the lid so that the patient is looking through the peripheral portions of the lens while reading, the acuity will be poor and variable. One can verify this displacement by determining whether the vision clears when the reading card is held at eye level. In such a case a steeper or larger lens might be employed.

   Base curve. Because 55% of the lens rests on a paracentral position of the cornea, the degree

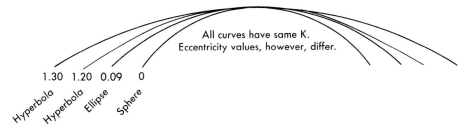

All curves have same K.
Eccentricity values, however, differ.

1.30   1.20   0.09   0

Hyperbola   Hyperbola   Ellipse   Sphere

Fig. 25-17. Each curve has the same base curve. They differ only in the rate of flattening. An aspheric curve is determined by its central curvature and its E value, that is, peripheral curvature. Represented are a sphere, ellipse, and hyperbola.

of flattening of the cornea should be known. Because each cornea has a different topography and is even different from temporal to nasal sides, only an approximation value can be assigned to the peripheral contours of the cornea.

K reading	Curve values of paracentral cornea (diopters flatter than K)
7.20 to 7.50	5.00 to 8.00 D
7.60 to 7.90	4.00 to 7.00 D
8.00 to 8.40	3.00 to 6.00 D

The optic section is generally 3 to 4 diopters steeper than K. To give an adequate range of reading, add 2.50 diopters or more. With an aspheric lens, the rest of the lens is in alignment to the paracentral cornea even though the optic zone is 4.00 diopters steeper.

Diameter. Most lenses are fitted with a diameter that averages 8.8 mm.

Power. The spheric power of the refraction is the base power. But an equal amount of minus must be added to the base reading to neutralize the amount of steepness over the flattest K.

Example. The base curve is −4.00 D steeper than K; add −4.00 D to the spheric power. If corneal astigmatism is present, one half of the corneal cylinder over 1.00 D should be added to K for better alignment.

Optic zone. There is a *Catch-22* situation with the optic zone. If the optic zone is too small to engulf the pupil in dim illumination, the patient will suffer from flare and glare, that is, ghost images, stars around lights, and so on. However, if the optic zone is made too large, it rests on the flatter paracentral cornea and tight symptoms are produced, since this problem causes corneal edema. With an aspheric lens, there is no junction between the optic

zone and the peripheral segment of the lens. Flare is not a problem, and so an 8.8 mm lens is sufficient size to cover a 6 mm pupil, which is considered large.

The lens. The anterior surface is spheric. The posterior surface is both spheric in the range of the corneal cap and aspheric in the periphery. The geometric center of the lens houses the distance correction. As the lens begins to flatten (Figs. 25-15 and 25-16), 0.10 D extra power is added in a gradual fashion in 0.10 D gradients. The aspheric optic section has an individual focal zone. The gradual increase in power toward the periphery creates a smooth transition of power without image jumps. This effect can be measured in terms of eccentricity values.

Eccentricity values. This value of eccentricity is determined by the measurement of the rate of flattening of the curve in the distance. The value is measured with an optic spherometer (Radiuscope) coupled with an attachment called the eccentroscope (Fig. 25-17). The following formula is applied:

$$\text{Eccentricity} = \frac{1 - \dfrac{TR}{MR}}{\sin \theta}$$

TR is the transmeridian radius.
MR is the meridian radius.
The angle theta (θ) is the tilt of the lens on the off-center reading.
This is measured on the Radiuscope-eccentroscope.

Measurements required for ordering a lens include K reading including the axis, spectacle prescription, spectacle addition, diameter of cornea, diameter of the pupil in dim illumination, and palpebral fissure.

Patient selection. Those patients least likely to succeed with bifocal contact lenses:

1. Flat spheric corneas
2. Astigmatism greater than 2.00 D
3. New lens patients and previous contact lens failures
4. Low distance refractive errors ± 1.00 D

The best candidates for bifocal contact lenses:

1. Those who were successful single-vision lens wearers
2. Those who are highly motivated and have a highly motivated fitter
3. Those who have an occupational need for bifocal contact lenses, such as waiters and people in the media (including films)

Comment. The results of this lens system is not apparent at the first fitting. A vision of 20/30 to 20/40 may improve to 20/20 in 4 to 5 days. Changes in refraction and lens changes should not be made until refraction is stable over two visits. Patience is a must.

Special problems in fitting relevant to the aspheric bifocal lens. *Decentration* of the lens will cause blurred vision. This error can be fixed in routine ways. The lens base curve must get tighter as the diameter of the lens is increased.

Poor vision at near range is usually caused by a lack of tear pooling. The central vault must be 3 to 4 diopters steeper than K. Optimum results are obtained in a lens with 2 to 4 mm of central pooling and a thin tear bearing area peripherally. The tear film is best appreciated through a fluorescein test. A narrow bright-green pool at the very edge should be present to reveal a meniscus tear accumulation at the bevel.

With *variable vision,* the movement of the lens should be fast, not slow. A distance of 0.5 to 1.5 mm is ideal. With the soft lens only 1 mm of lens motion should be tolerated. Excessive movement is often caused by tear pooling. This is most evident on insertion of the lens. The lens must settle before it is assessed.

Comment. The VF-II Silicon lens has proved to be a reasonably good presbyopic lens for most of our patients. (VF means 'variable focus.')

Monocular over-correction of plus power

The gambit of over-correction is often successful, especially in previous rigid lens wearers who become presbyopic. Despite a difference of 1.50 to 2.00 D between the lenses there is sufficient vision in both areas to maintain binocularity. One eye sees well in the distance, whereas the other functions primarily in the near range. It is a simple method to apply, but about 20% of patients complain of headaches, disorientation, and lack of clarity for precise vision.

Because of the great simplicity of fitting, this lens is our starting method for fitting all persons with presbyopia. One can use trial lenses, which are not really practical for bifocal lens wearers. It is wise to choose the least myopic or the more hyperopic eye for the near correction. If the refraction is the same in both eyes the overplussing should be done on the nondominant eye.

Comment. Baldone refers to this type of vision as "Omni vision." He selects the overplussed eye by holding a + 1.50 D lens in front of alternate eyes and observes the patient's reaction as to which eye is more comfortable with the lens rather than select the nondominant eye arbitrarily. For the target shooter or Olympic shooter who is presbyopic it is important that the dominant eye be overplussed so that the front sight of the rifle is in sharp focus while the target is blurred.

Patient selection for bifocal lens

1. Patients who are difficult to fit should be avoided if possible. This includes people with lax or low lids because of the lack of support of the heavier bifocal segment, those who are poorly motivated, and those with severe or residual astigmatism.
2. Persons with hyperopia do better than those with myopia. Hyperopic patients need less bifocal addition than persons with myopia of equal power. A minus lens requires more prism ballast than a plus lens does.
3. Patients who require bifocals for both distance and near range are preferred over patients who primarily need reading glasses. A previous single-vision lens wearer is also a good candidate.

BIFOCAL SOFT LENSES
Patient selection

Of prime consideration are the refraction present and the type of work required to be done by the patient. *Ideally:*

1. The addition required should be between +1.00 and +1.75 D.
2. The spheric-equivalent addition should be between −4.00 and +2.00 D with the minus cylinder deleted, not being greater than 1 D.
3. The patient should understand the limitation of the bifocal system and still be motivated to want them, because for very small print and reading in poor lighting a reading glass may still be required. To eliminate "readers" entirely, overplus one eye perhaps up to +0.75 D.

Fitting procedure

One obtains the distance correction by using the spheric equivalent and adding −0.50 D to this power; for example, a −3.00 D lens would require a −3.50 D lens as the initial selection of power. An over-refraction is done to achieve the best vision.

Near vision is estimated with the appropriate lens, that is, −2.50 D. In other words, using the above example, choose the addition that requires the smallest prescription commensurate with normal reading requirements. If this lens does not satisfy the near needs of the patient, additional plus power is added. The maximum amount of plus power to be added is the power that does not affect the distance vision. If the vision is barely adequate, +0.75 D can be added to the nondominant eye. This technique borrows from the monovision device to achieve satisfactory vision.

Problems in fitting

Decentration of the central zone will usually cause fluctuating vision or ghosting. The lenses can be made larger or tighter if this occurs. One can stabilize lathe-cut lenses by adding truncation and prism. Spin-cast lenses are stabilized with an aspheric posterior surface.

Fluctuating vision can be attributable to excess lens movements. These lenses should not move more than 0.5 to 1.5 mm.

Hyperopes require less power addition than myopes to achieve the same results. Also patients will not tolerate more than 0.50 D of uncorrected cylinder at near range. These restraints of optic correction should be appreciated before one fits such a lens.

Patients with low lower lids do poorly on those lenses with truncation and require the lower lids to push up the lenses with reading.

The spin-cast bifocal lens is designed so that there is a gradual increase in power of the lens. But both the distance and reading portions lie within the pupillary diameter permanently. This position produces two images all the time, one from each part of the lens. The patient soon learns to disregard the more out-of-focus lens. This lens requires minimal movement and so has to fit relatively tightly. The simultaneous-vision lens requires maximum correction to achieve adequate power. Simultaneous-vision lenses function best on patients with large pupils. Elderly patients and glaucomatous patients on miotic drugs do poorly.

For the Olympic-style shooter who is a presbyope it is imperative that the dominant eye be overplussed and not for distance because it is the front site of the gun that must be in sharp focus whereas the larger target can be somewhat blurred.

Comment. The best candidates for these lenses are people who have worn soft lenses for distance in the past. Persons with occupations that require sharp acuity, such as architects, may not have sufficient clarity through soft bifocal lenses.

Our best success is using the soft bifocal lens along with overplussing the more hyperopic eye, or the nondominant eye. With good patient selection, successful results were obtained in approximately 65% of cases. By success, we mean that the patients were satisfied with their vision through these lenses. It does not imply 20/20 vision in each eye for both distance and near range. Also we took our sample 1 year after the bifocal lens was worn.

In our series of 100 cases, only previous lens wearers were selected, with 100 eyes having soft lenses, and 100 eyes having rigid lenses. The results were about the same.

The use of the lathe-cut bifocal lens is hampered by the prism, which can cause the lens to be quite thick at the base. This design can create discomfort. Also, if the line of truncation is not contoured to the lower lid, rotation of the lens will occur when the eyes look down.

Up to now our best results have been with the variable-focus design in which there is a power change from the lens center to the lens periphery. The optic principle is that the pupil changes its position relative to the lens center on down gaze into a greater plus zone.

Finally, required additions of $+2.00$ D or greater in myopic patients do not have a good success-performance ratio. It is better to exclude these people from consideration.

Comment. Better results are obtained with gas-permeable lens than with PMMA. The size of the optic zone for distance and near range can be made larger. With soft lenses, durability is often a problem because these lenses become more quickly coated than a lens on an eye that is 20 years younger. In all probability the increased incidence of deposit formation in the middle-aged person is related to increased viscosity of the tear film.

CHAPTER 26

SPECIAL USES FOR RIGID AND SOFT LENSES

X-CHROM lens
Piggyback contact lens system
Lenses for sports
Nystagmus
Colored soft lenses
Contact lenses for children
Orthokeratology

X-CHROM LENS

Persons with normal color vision can see all ranges in the spectrum of white light in wavelengths from 380 to 760 nm and can differentiate a wide range of hues of color ranging from red to blue. However 8% to 10% of males and 0.5% of females have some impairment in color vision ranging from mild to almost complete impairment. This failure of differentiation is for the most part in the red-green area and to a much lesser extent in the blue-yellow area.

An X-CHROM corneal lens, which transmits light in the red zone from 590 to 700 nm has recently been introduced. This lens can improve color discrimination for the individual who is partially blind in the red-green area. A red lens is fitted to the nondominant eye of a person with red-green partially defective vision. The other eye remains uncovered. The uncovered eye will perceive a red or green object as usual, but the eye with the red lens will perceive the red wavelengths of light and will absorb the green wavelengths. The brain now receives two different intensities; by a rapid self-learning process the patient can identify both colors properly.

The manufacturer claims that the person wearing a single X-CHROM lens can read the numbers in Ishihara's test and can identify traffic signals and color-coded wires and that the rapid self-learning process with the single red lens permits the individual to perceive the world more vividly than ever before.

The American Committee on Optics and Visual Physiology has offered the following statement on the use of the X-CHROM lens.

A red tinted contact lens worn over one eye may help color defectives to discriminate colors by changing the relative intensities of red and green objects viewed through the filter. Examiners should measure color vision of each eye separately as well as together and compare the color test scores achieved with and without the use of the lens. In evaluating color vision qualifications, particular attention should be given to the ambient light levels under which the activity is carried out and the level of color recognition required by the task. Consideration must also be given to the detrimental effects of wearing such a lens on space localization of moving objects and other aspects of binocular vision. Persons operating moving vehicles wearing a tinted lens over one eye may experience hazardous distortions of the positions of perceived objects and may, therefore, be dangerous drivers in certain circumstances. Conservative judgments are justified until the extent of these hazards is better understood.

How to fit

The lens must be thin to permit adequate vision, must be large to avoid edge awareness (8.5 to 9.3 mm), and must center well. The lens should be fitted steeper than usual to achieve reduction in movement.

Comment. Although we have had limited experience with this lens, it seems that the motivation to correct the color defect must be extremely high to overcome the cosmetic disadvantage of the person's appearance while a single red lens is worn. On the other hand, parents of children with color-defective vision should be made aware that congenitally inherited color defects of vision can be altered. If the child's vocational or avocational direction is toward a field requiring good color discrimination, such as marine navigation or aviation, this type of lens is available. We have fitted a few art-college students with this lens, which aids them with art work. Although it does not correct the color defect, it does permit them to make a discriminatory judgment of color.

PIGGYBACK CONTACT LENS SYSTEM

The piggyback lens is basically the wearing of a soft lens against the cornea to provide comfort and a rigid lens over the soft one to attain useful vision (Fig. 26-1). A standard soft lens is applied to make the new anterior surface of the lens-cornea combination have a smooth anterior spheric surface.

On the surface of the soft lens is placed a cone lens, which has a steep central posterior curvature surrounded by a much flatter peripheral zone. The steep zone is stabilized over the corneal cap and the flatter zone rests on the periphery of the lens.

In corneal grafts, the steep zone vaults over the astigmatic graft. A set of cone lenses is required to see which lens provides optimum

clearance, centration, and movement. After the lens has been fit, a manifest refraction is done over the selected diagnostic lens to determine the final power.

A lenticular soft lens with its high-plus power is used for the base lens whether the eye is aphakic or not. This provides compensation for the myopia induced by the steep-fitting cone lens and provides a better base for fitting.

In patient selection these lenses can be used for the following conditions:
1. Postoperative corneal keratoplasty
2. Aphakia
3. Keratoconus
4. Traumatic induced irregular astigmatism

Problems with the system are as follows:
1. Inability to center the rigid lens
2. Inability to handle the combination of lenses
3. Confusion over rigid and soft cleaning and soaking solutions.

Two separate systems are required. The time and cost of two separate lenses may be a burden. Also the handling of two lens systems

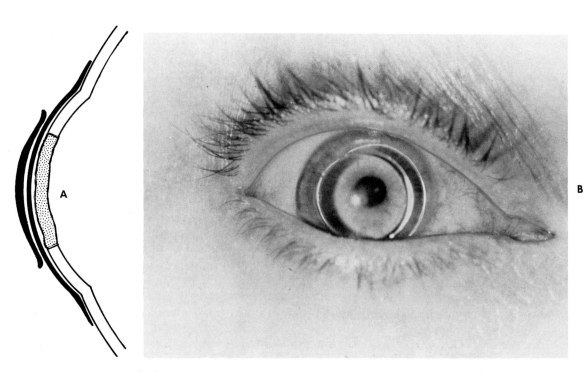

Fig. 26-1. A, Piggyback system of soft contact lens riding on a corneal transplant with a surface rigid lens to provide optical correction. **B,** Piggyback contact lens system with a gas-permeable lens resting on a larger soft lens.

must be taught, and so patient compliance must be exceptional.

Some laboratories will create an anterior depression in the soft lens in order for the rigid lens to fit. This feature permits better centration because the rigid lens fits into the shallow depression of the soft lens.

Comment. This system, first introduced by Dr. Joe Baldone of New Orleans, is the last device to be used. It is applied to those patients who have been failures in the wearing of rigid PMMA, soft, and gas-permeable lenses.

Although the results are good in the majority of problem cases reported, the system is too cumbersome and expensive for routine use except for complicated cases. One really ends up with a mixture of soft and hard lens problems, plus the difficulty of having one lens ride over the other.

LENSES FOR SPORTS

Generally a soft lens is preferred for any contact athletics because of the danger of a lens being jolted out of the eye. So frequently has this happened that the National Basketball Association has passed a ruling that games cannot be stopped to look for a lens that accidentally popped out of a team member's eye.

Athletes, like everyone else, have astigmatism and frequently need a rigid lens. A hockey player, such as a goalie, who is trying to follow a puck traveling 50 miles per hour needs the best vision attainable.

There are two ways to handle the problem. The rigid lens may be fitted steeper than K by 1.00 to 1.50 D. If a microthin lens is used, such a lens will apply itself tenaciously to the cornea. This lens cannot be tolerated for full-time use because tight symptoms frequently develop after 4 or 5 hours of wear. Alternately the lens may be increased in diameter over its regular size by 2 mm. Additional peripheral curves must be added to reduce the apical vaulting produced by the larger-diameter size. An aspheric lens is a perfect choice for this situation. Its elliptic design ensures a good peripheral contour, and it comes in rather larger sizes—up to 10 mm.

Comment. If there is a high-degree of astigmatism, that is, 7 rather than 3 D, a gas-permeable lens of large diameter 9.2 mm or more is the lens of choice. Dynamic visual acu-

ity, the ability to see clearly a moving target, is enhanced in comparison to a soft lens.

Which lens to choose for sports

The rigid PMMA lens has been rendered virtually obsolete by the gas-permeable lenses and the soft lenses for sports.

Gas-permeable lenses offer the following advantages:

1. They are larger than PMMA lens and so center better and are not easily displaced.
2. They are more comfortable.
3. They do not need special design for most sports.
4. They are less likely to cause photophobia because they move less and have a larger optic zone than PMMA lenses do.
5. They are better tolerated with fatigue.
6. They are more likely to be worn on a regular basis. If a contact lens is worn intermittently for sports, the player will always have to adjust to a size difference, which will affect his eye-hand co-ordination.
7. The optic characteristics of the lens are as good as those of the PMMA lens.

Soft lenses have other features:

1. They are best for body-contact sports because they move the least and are almost impossible to knock out.
2. They create the least photophobia.
3. They are the most comfortable lens and can be worn full time.
4. They are always centered with eye movement. Their displacement is rarely more than 2 mm with a blink.
5. They are best in situations in which there is irritation to the eyes because of dust, wind, and sun because they cover the entire cornea and a few millimeters of the sclera. This feature makes it the lens of choice for soccer, football, tennis, rugby, cricket, lacrosse, and polo.

The major disadvantage of a soft lens is that the contrast sensitivity is not so good as that for PMMA or gas-permeable lenses.

Tennis

For tennis, a soft lens is preferred. In the service shot, the head and eyes go up to watch the ball. A soft lens has very little drag and drop. So centration and stability are maintained in the up position. With a rigid lens, the lens frequently drops as the eyes move up.

Also, a rigid lens is more likely to cause photophobia and glare. This problem is especially true on outdoor courts under a sunny sky. These effects can be ameliorated with sunglasses. However, tinted lenses reduce contrast, which in a moving game is essential. Dynamic visual acuity is largely predicated on contrast. Note that the professionals rarely use sunglasses during play even during day matches.

Squash and racquetball

It is important to remember that a contact lens does not provide any special safety over the naked eye. Eye protection is mandatory because the incidence of eye injuries is high, especially for the creation of a hyphema with severe damage. With the use of high-speed photography ball speeds in racquetball have been reported at 78 mph for the novice and 127 mph for the A-level player. Professional squash and racquetball players move the racquet at speeds of 108 to 125 mph.

A lens 3 mm thick or a polycarbonate plano lens are best over the contact lens.

Again a soft lens is preferred because of the dynamics of the serve and the high illumination from direct and reflected light (Fig. 26-2).

Skiing

Most skiers tolerate any lens because the cold weather depresses the basal metabolic rate of the corneal epithelium. Thus the oxygen demands are reduced. This advantage is partially reduced by the decrease in oxygen tension that prevails at high altitudes.

Tinted rigid lens do not offer protection against ultraviolet rays because the central surface of the cornea is not protected. Gas-permeable lenses are better than PMMA lenses and can now be tinted. Soft lenses are comfortable and can be tinted.

Actually, all these lenses are tolerated well. The soft lens is preferred because there is less photophobia, more protection against the wind, and good oxygen permeability if a thin lens is used. Goggles that are polarized and tinted are still recommended regardless of the lens type employed for better protection against direct and reflected ultraviolet rays.

The gas-permeable lens is an excellent alternative for those people with astigmatism. The lens is large and not likely to be displaced by

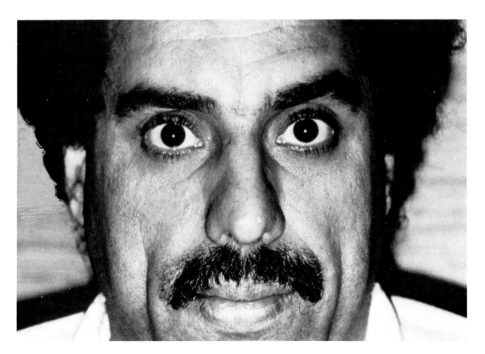

Fig. 26-2. Sharif Khan, world-famous squash player, who wears soft contact lenses that permit him to excel in squash.

tearing. Also the permeability features make the tolerance of this lens excellent. The optic characteristics are better than those of a soft lens especially in the area of contrast sensitivity. When a large size is used, 9.2 mm or greater, the chance of a lens being lost in a fall is negligible. A properly fitted gas-permeable lens should fit under the upper lid margin. In a spill, the upper lid should retain the lens.

Football, hockey, and basketball

Obviously in these rough sports dislodgment by bodily contact is the major issue. The most desirable lens must be the soft lens; it will not be popped out by a hard body check into the boards or with an aggressive tackle or by a basketball giant pushing another player to the side. Besides, a soft lens can be worn intermittently because many professionals only want lenses for sports.

We must emphasize that a contact lens of any type offers no protection from trauma to the eye. With children playing hockey or football, *eye protection still must be worn.* On the other hand, the wearing of a contact lens does not add any special liability to the eye.

Swimming and soft contact lenses*

Soft lens manufacturers place limitations on their lenses when it comes to swimming. This area of sporting activity makes visual cripples of those wearing high corrective lenses.

Information from a number of patients who wore soft lenses while swimming led us to undertake this study to determine whether soft lenses are safe for swimming and if so under what conditions and what safeguards should be taken. Our study was based on four factors:

1. Is there a high risk of losing the lenses in the water?
2. Are the lenses damaged by the various swimming conditions?
3. Is there a significant loss of vision or damage to the eye?
4. Most important, are the lenses safe for the wearer while swimming and what precautions should be taken?

Experiments were conducted in chlorinated pool water and this represents Phase I. Additional studies Phase II and Phase III are pres-

ently being correlated in lake and ocean water and will be reported later. The remarks that will be made here will be for chlorinated water and represent two summers of observation. Bausch and Lomb Soflens were used throughout.

Eight volunteers were tested at various times in 186 trial periods.

Vision and subjective symptoms were recorded. Examinations of the lens on the wearer, and the wearer after removal of the lens, were performed with the usual ophthalmological techniques. Vision and slit lamp examinations with a hand slit lamp were performed at the pool side. Observations were made at 3, 10, 20 and 30 minute periods while swimming, during the period after swimming, and 10 and 30 minutes after removal of the lenses.

The experiments consisted of swimming the crawl for 100 yards, swimming underwater for 100 yards with the eyes open, underwater somersaults with open eyes, diving into the pool with the eyes open, and the effect of vigorous splashing into the eyes with the water. After each procedure the candidates were evaluated as to visual acuity subjective symtoms, objective signs, ease of removal of the lens, and any effect after removal of the lens.

Laboratory studies were performed on both the lens and the pool water. The chlorine content of the lens and the clarity of the lens, were noted. Cultures of the eye and the pool were taken at pool side on blood agar plates. The osmolarity of the pool water was measured (Table 26-1).

In addition, 34 of our regular soft lens patients were given protocol sheets and asked to complete and return these to us after swimming in chlorinated pools. From these experiments we found the following:

1. There were minimal symptoms of stinging in a few, but most candidates were symptom free except for some mild redness of the eyes from the chlorine. These symptoms were no greater than without the lenses. Within 3 to 4 minutes in water the lenses adhered firmly to the cornea, and this adherence became stronger with increased duration of exposure to water. There was an absent slide factor on blinking, and in effect the lens could not be

*Reprinted from Stein, H.A., and Slatt, B.J.: Contact and Intraocular Lens Med. J. 3(3):24-26, 1977.

Table 26-1. Osmolarity

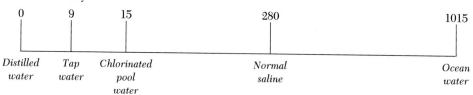

Table 26-2. Lens loss during swim tests

Swim test periods		Lens loss
Without adaptation	84	6
With adaptation	102	0

dislodged by a finger. It became firmly adherent to the cornea. This would of course make removal of these lenses dangerous with possible epithelial denuding if the lenses were to be vigorously removed. However, when the candidate continued to wear the lenses out of the water they loosened from the cornea readily, and the normal lag on blinking returned. This required about *30 minutes*. At no time was there a change in vision. The time could be somewhat hastened by instillation of normal saline. We felt this firm adhesion of the lens to the cornea in chlorinated pool water was due to the hypotonicity of the lens induced by water, with an osmotic attraction of the soft lens to the cornea.

2. We tried to evaluate the loss factor present which is so common with hard lenses and makes swimming almost contraindicated with hard lenses. In those candidates with soft lens who entered the pool without any precautions, there were six lenses lost out of a total of 84 trials (Table 26-2). Of 102 trial test periods in those who used the precaution of splashing pool water in the eye before entering the water there were no lenses lost. The lenses became hypotonic and adhered firmly to the cornea.

3. There was no clinical or laboratory damage to the lenses.

4. While wearing the lenses swimming, there was no deterioration in vision or slit lamp abnormality of the cornea, nor any aftereffects when the lenses were removed.

5. Contamination of swimming pools does occur. The World Health Organization terms a pool heavily polluted if more than 200 coliform bacteria per 100 ml. of water appears. Ontario uses a more strict criterion to close down pools and beaches. Samples of pool water periodically show low counts of staphylococci, streptococci and *Pseudomonas aeruginosa*, and these organisms are more chlorine resistant than the coliform bacteria, including fecal coliform bacteria. Such low counts of these bacteria are however not particularly associated with any increase in eye, ear, nose and throat infection. However, where *Pseudomonas aeruginosa* is found, even in light amounts, health authorities usually shock treat the public pools with additional chlorine.

Although we found occasional scant growths of *Pseudomonas aeruginosa* in pool water, from private as well as public pools, we did not find any clinical infection in our volunteers or regular soft lens patients on protocol.

Comment. Our experiments showed that there was a minimal lens loss factor or eye irritation when patients swam in chlorinated pool water with soft lenses. A firm bond between the soft lens and cornea developed, which necessitated that the lens remain in the eye for at least 30 minutes following swimming.

The major concern was the contamination of waters tested. None was free of contamination and all harboured colonies of *Pseudomonas aeruginosa* and coliform bacteria. If a patient has a small corneal abrasion such as from a tiny foreign body under the lens, then the contamination of the lens could theoretically result in a serious ocular infection. It is for this reason, and not lens loss, that we cannot recommend the unqualified use of soft lenses for swimming.

If the patient wears watertight goggles or mask, then soft lenses can be used to relieve the swimming blindness. Only if the person swims in chlorinated or lake water that upon repeated testing is found to be free of contamination with bacterial organisms, then swimming without any device can be recommended. This does not apply to ocean swimming where a large lens loss factor would occur because of the lack of binding of the lens to the cornea.

Soft contact lenses for scuba divers

Over 2 million people in Canada and the United States are aficionados of scuba diving (the acronym for self-contained underwater breathing apparatus). The use of soft contact lens has been tested and approved for scuba diving. They give good vision in divers and do not present any hazards. There is minimal lens loss. The lens loss seems to occur at shallow depths. At 30 feet, no lens loss is encountered. There is tolerance for these lenses despite the low water temperatures in which they are used. Bacterial contamination of these lenses has not been a problem. However divers' eyes are somewhat protected by the face mask worn during diving

NYSTAGMUS

Persons with nystagmus, particularly of the congenital type, see very poorly with glasses. The oscillations of the eyes under the spectacles produce a constant parallax. With contact lenses, vision disturbance that was created by eyes constantly in motion against fixed spectacle lenses is vastly improved.

The visual gains are truly remarkable; frequently visual acuity can be improved from 20/200 to 20/50 or 20/30.

As fixation is improved by the corrective lens moving with the eye, the actual amplitude of oscillations is decreased. This is particularly noticeable under dim illumination. Also many people with nystagmus seem to have a large degree of astigmatism, which makes correction by anything but a rigid lens a futile endeavor.

The only precaution in the fitting of such lenses is to employ larger-diameter lenses that are gas permeable.

Comment. Improvement is most apparent in those persons who have pendular nystagmus

without foveal aplasia. Those with albinism, aniridia, and achromatopsia do not make good visual gains with contact lenses.

COLORED SOFT LENSES

Colored lenses are used to cover unsightly blind eyes. These lenses must be larger than regular hard lenses to completely cover the iris so that telltale scars are not visible to spoil the cosmetic effect. Colored soft lenses are available today in a variety of tints. For the majority, these lenses are entirely cosmetic, enhancing or changing the color of the iris. Until recently most of the tints eventually leached out of the lenses. Today, however, it is technically possible to produce a colorfast lens.

Frequently persons such as actors ask for tinted lenses to change the color of their eyes for cosmetic or professional purposes. Some iris colors can be easily changed. A gray iris can be altered to appear the color of any lens tint, whereas darker irises, such as brown, cannot be lightened or changed to another color. The best cosmetic effect is achieved when the lens is the same color as the iris and merely enhances its color. If radical changes in color are made, the lens diameter must be increased to avoid appearing unnatural or conspicuous. A small, dark blue lens on a light gray eye may look ridiculous.

It is also important to note that a tinted lens when placed on the eye looks richer and more saturated with color. This phenomenon occurs because light travels through the lens twice. The second passage is the result of reflected light bouncing back to the observer from the lens wearer's iris.

The medical advantage to the development of colored lenses is the ability to cover an unsightly scarred eye with a new iris-pupil combination (Fig. 26-3). The lenses have a central black pupil with an iris that matches the fellow eye. In addition, other uses for a colored lens are to protect an albino or a patient with aniridia from the intensity of light. A shaded lens may be used as an occluder lens to improve an amblyopic fellow eye.

Comment. Light tints in regular soft lenses are helpful when one is looking for the lenses when they are lost or in the carrying case. Deeply tinted lenses should not be used for regular wear because they reduce contrast and

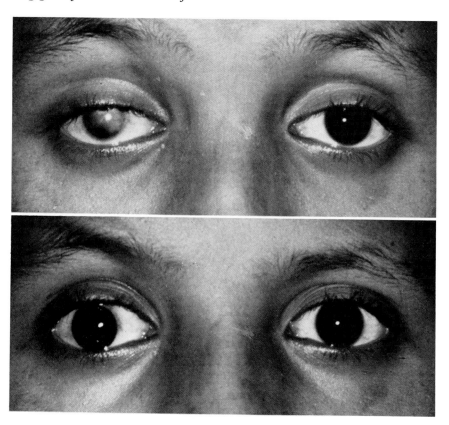

Fig. 26-3. Scarred cornea covered by tinted cosmetic contact lens. (Courtesy Western Technologies, Inc., Phoenix, Ariz.)

decrease visual acuity, especially in dimly illuminated situations, as in driving at dusk or reading menus in restaurants.

CONTACT LENSES FOR CHILDREN

Contact lenses are being used to treat children under 1 year of age. These children are usually aphakic, and lenses are a must if their aphakia is monocular.

They have also been used as an occluder in which the lens is overplussed to create blurred vision in the fixing eye.

Other medical uses of contact lenses in children include the treatment of aniridia, albinism, and achromatopsia. These lenses usually have a deep peripheral tint outside the optic zone to offset partially the effects of photophobia and glare.

With aniridia there is no iris. With achromatopsia, there is an absence of a cone population, and so protection against excess light is mandatory. With albinism, the iris pigment is missing as shown with transillumination, and these children are virtually incapacitated by light. At times, a contact lens is worthwhile for the treatment of unilateral myopia with amblyopia.

If the child is aphakic, K readings can be done in the operating room using a Terry keratometer. The K readings are helpful but not crucial, and one need not use a general anesthetic just to obtain a K reading.

These lenses should be fitted flat so that there is adequate movement. Small lenses must be custom ordered so that they may be inserted into the narrow palpebral tissues. The power of the lens is estimated by retinoscopy. If there is frequent lens loss in infants, the lens ordered should be 15 to 16 mm in diameter.

Gas-permeable lenses and soft lenses are both advocated. The rigid lenses are more easily handled by parents, and one can use devices that aid in insertion and removal. Also, these lenses have superior optic properties and are more durable. They do not get torn, and they do not spoil the way a soft lens can because of protein accumulation.

To go through this exercise, the parents must be highly motivated and intelligent. The failure rate under the best of conditions is high. Part of the reason is the very early date in which some children are fitted. For infants with congenital cataracts, surgery in some centers with the application of a contact lens is now being done on the first day of an infant's life. Special custom-ordered lenses of 25 diopters or more are often required for the small infant.

There is great difficulty in fitting a contact lens for children. Despite gloomy reports of the past, better fitting techniques on very young children, even 1 month old, have yielded new triumphs with this disorder.

It is reasonable to ask, Why not intraocular lenses for children? They would eliminate handling problems, high cost of maintaining lenses through loss or breakage, infection, and the unending commitment of parents to an eye. Indeed, this method may be the best route to choose for the long-term correction and comfort. However, there are no 40- or 50-year-old studies to employ for guidance. Therefore there is some risk that these lenses employed safely in adults for 10 to 15 years may not be adequate for children. Also a child's eye grows in size developmentally with the rest of the body. It is not reasonable to operate every once in a while to change the size of the intraocular lens.

Fitting

The fitting of any type of contact lens may be done with the Terry keratometer and the child under general anesthesia. In this manner, a lens fitted closely to the topography of the cornea can be selected. Because these lenses are thicker and larger than regular lenses, the fitting should be flat so that the lens will move. An aphakic lens dropped by gravity and hanging low on the lower limbus and beyond is unacceptable. The lens should move freely so that molding of the cornea does not occur, and the lens is properly centered to that the pupil is directly under the optic section of the lens.

Comment. In children under 18 months of age, general anesthesia may not be needed. The child can be restrained for both the keratometer and the final over-refraction by retinoscopy.

With silicone lenses a suction force is created by the flat-fitting lens and the cornea. To remove the lens, one must move the lens over to the limbus where the suction effect is released. The lens can then be removed with a suction cup. It is applied to the surface of the lens, which now can be safely removed from the eye.

Hydrophilic lenses have been used for children. They are flaccid so that the chance of abrading the cornea are minimal. Also their suppleness and hydration makes them very comfortable, and so tolerance is not an issue. The range in which a single lens can fit many eyes makes precise measurements of corneal topography unnecessary. The lens are fitted flat and if one to 2 mm of lens motion is found, no further fitting alterations need be done. The recent extended-wear hydrophilic lenses that are permeable to oxygen either by virtue of their thinness or higher water content, about 70%, relieve the burden of parents having to insert or remove these lens on a daily basis.

Silicone lenses for children

Advantages

Best permeability and best thermal conductivity
Better acuity than with hydrogel lenses
Stable in power
Medications can be given with the lens in place
Minimal lens loss cause of the tighter fitting characteristics
Minimal flexure
No interstices for bacterial growth in the lens itself

Disadvantages

Protein debris on the lens can be excessive
Loss of surface coating, which makes the lens hydrophobic
Corneal vascularization
Corneal infiltrates
Flat fit makes removal of lens hazardous if done the regular way

Yet, despite these advantages, there are complications even with extended wear hydrophilic lenses. Spheric lenses do not correct astigmatism, which may require a spectacle overcorrection or an acceptance of smaller visual-acuity goals. Toric soft lenses are too complicated to regulate for an infant. The large size of these lens make them difficult to insert and remove in a child. Despite extended wear, these lens must be removed and cleaned periodically. A hazard of their wear is that corneal edema with vascularization can occur without visible evidence of this happening. Periodic slitlamp assessments are vital either directly or under anesthesia. Practical objections also include the high initial cost, a greater loss and breakage rate, and the need for frequent changes because the cornea changes its size in the first 4 years.

Hydrophilic-lens enthusiasts point out that the astigmatic portion of visual loss is minimal and it is not common under the best of circumstances to achieve 20/20 in a unilaterally aphakic child. Pediatric lenses are available and present in most power selections. The need to change the lenses in terms of fit and power would be necessary despite the type and plastic utilized. Inflammation in soft lenses is usually related to soft lens solutions, particularly nonpreserved saline solution that has not been changed daily and contaminated distilled water. Dirty cases and screw-top vials are also a source of bacterial contamination. The likelihood of infection occurring in an adult-supervised soft lens is minimal because the care systems would be closely monitored.

Comment. If autoclaving of the lenses is done periodically, the infection rate is minimal. We have not had any infections, but we have only run a small number of cases with a pediatric hydrophilic lens.

The ease of fitting and the ability to use the hydrophilic lenses over an extended time makes this lens a top choice. Lenses are now being inserted after cataract surgery that is currently being advocated at one day of life!

Fitting without K readings

One can fit both soft and rigid lenses without K readings by noting the high molecular weight fluorescein patterns and lens movement.

A trial lens of power +10.00 to +11.00 D is employed.

Fluorescein is placed in the lower cul-de-sac. Apical touch means the lens is too flat, and a bubble under the lens indicates the lens is too steep.

Err on the flatter side.

The lens movement with the lens passively rotated by the patient's lids should be free and unencumbered.

Refraction should be done with the lens in place. This eliminates vertex calculations and takes into account the positive tear meniscus, which can result in 2.00 or more diopters of power. Our best results occur when the lens is freely movable. Some fitters do fit steeply and because of this obtain a larger tear pool effect, giving extra plus power.

The final lens should be over-powered by 1.50 to 2.00 D to provide the child with best vision at the near range because this is the most useful distance.

Silicone lenses may be preferred because they provide better optic characteristics than soft lenses do and can be worn in an extended fashion. With silicone-acrylate lenses it is important to utilize only those lenses with a high silicone content that are permeable to oxygen at the thickness required for an aphakic lens.

Which lens to choose

Obviously each lens system requires parental management. The rigid lens system is the most demanding because of daily routines. The parent must accept the long-term duty of caring for the lens until the child is able to do this job without assistance.

The intraocular lenses would solve most of the problems of any aphakic contact lens system. At this moment, no one is advocating this method for routine use until more data are accumulated.

We like the pediatric hydrogel extended-wear lens. It relieves the family of the daily task of handling lenses. Its lack of durability is a problem because in many cases the lens may survive only 6 months to 1 year. Cost is also a consideration. Yet, despite these imperfections, our best results come with the use of hydrogel lenses.

It is important to remember that despite poor acuity, such as 20/60, the overall visual gains make the enterprise still valid.

Comment. We have used the hydrogel lenses for extended wear and then switched to gas-permeable lenses when the child was old enough to handle a daily-wear lens without difficulty.

ORTHOKERATOLOGY

Orthokeratology has been advanced as a system for "sight without glasses." The premise behind the system is that progressive flattening of the cornea through the use of a series of flatter-fitting lenses will eliminate myopia. The assumption is made that the degree of flattening will be uniform in all meridians. Certainly this is not always the case because there are many instances of flat-fitting lenses being worn over a long period of time resulting in a toric cornea.

The advocates of this technique point to its usefulness in treating certain groups of people who require good vision but cannot wear contact lenses. This group includes pilots, airline stewardesses, fire fighters, athletes engaged in competitive sports, policemen, and people who do a great deal of swimming. This method of doing away with glasses is certainly not any bolder than thermokeratoplasty or Barraquer's surgical keratoplasty (keratomileusis) or serial radial cuts in the cornea (radial keratotomy).

Orthokeratology fitting sets are available. American Optical Corporation employs the May-Grant method, which uses a fitting set of 370 lenses with a base-curve range of 38.00 to 47.00 D and a power range of $+0.50$ to -4.00 D. Corneal curvature changes are effected when between 70% and 80% of the corneal surface is covered. Larger-diameter lenses are used with a range varying from 8.5 mm for the steepest curves to 10.2 mm for the flattest base curves. The thickness of the lens is within the ordinary range of rigid lenses, that is, about 0.15 mm, depending on the power of the lenses. At present, gas-permeable lenses are being used to relieve the effects of corneal hypoxia. These lenses have made the procedure safer and the wearing of these lenses more comfortable.

The lenses are reassessed approximately every 6 weeks with particular attention given to refraction through the lenses, new corneal readings, and slitlamp evaluation of the cornea.

When changes of corneal curvature occur, a new lens is given, predicated on the new, flattest corneal curvature. An appropriate power reduction should normally ensue. A patient may need five or six pairs of lenses the first year, three or four the second year, and two or three more the third year.

A proper fit is one in which the lens has a tangent touch to the flattest meridian of the cornea. As a general rule, five to seven pairs of lenses are required to achieve a flattening effect. Among persons with myopia who practice this technique it is estimated that 85% with 20/100 vision will develop 20/20 vision in 1 year, 70% with 20/200 vision will develop 20/20 vision in 2 years, and 55% with 20/300 vision will develop 20/20 vision in 3 years. The procedure is most applicable to myopic people and is only practical with those with moderate degrees of myopia, -3.00 D or less.

A retainer, plano lens has to be worn during the day with a minimum wearing schedule to keep the cornea flat. Some patients can eventually be weaned from the retainer, whereas most require it indefinitely once a week or once a day. A recent study of 150 Air Force cadets in Colorado Springs who had orthokeratology performed on them and were followed revealed that none of them showed significant permanent changes. It was not uncommon for the cadets to have their vision improved from 20/100 to 20/40. However, most of these changes were transient unless a retainer was employed. But induced cylinder and corneal abrasions were no more frequent than in the average contact lens wearer.

The experience with orthokeratology among ophthalmologists is minimal. Such complications as overwear reactions, corneal abrasions, induced corneal astigmatism, and ocular discomfort from the wearing of such large, flat lenses are possible. In fact, in medical studies done, the rate of corneal complications was no greater than with ordinary rigid lenses. So the added risk, in terms of the health of the eye, may be exaggerated. More experience with this technique is needed. The main objections to the procedure are as follows:

1. The length of time required for results is high, and so the procedure is costly.
2. The effect is not predictable. There is no way to screen who will benefit and who will not.

3. A retainer lens is required to keep the flattening effect. The treatment does not offer sight without glasses or contact lenses.
4. The scope of people who can be helped is limited to moderate myopes.
5. The improvement is not uniform. A patient frequently will obtain 20/20 vision in one eye and 20/40 vision in the other.

Medical evaluation of this technique has recently been done in which an ophthalmologist (P. Binder) and two optometrists who practice orthokeratology (C.H. May and S.C. Grant) worked together on a series of cases.

Their conclusions were as follows:

1. The procedure is essentially safe. No adverse effect was found in the orthokeratology group.

   There was some mild distortion of the keratometric mires but nothing really serious. None developed corneal warpage, and there was no increased incidence of corneal abrasion, punctate staining, or other signs of corneal disease.

   There were some optic suprises. A third of the group studied required reading glasses. Also, the quality of unaided visual acuity was worse than that obtained through glasses or contact lenses.
2. Refractive errors beyond 4 diopters were not significantly aided by this technique. Also, it was difficult to predict which patient would do well once therapy was initiated.
3. Reduction in refractive errors of 1.5 D could be done with eyes with moderate myopia (2.00 to 4.00 D) but not in eyes of minimal myopia (-1.25 D or less).
4. There was no correlation between the change in corneal curvature and the change in refraction. An analysis of peripheral corneal contours and refractive change yielded similar results.

5. The retainer lens stage was not reached by the majority of patients. Those who did achieve this plateau did so after 24 months.
6. In three of the four patients who reached retainer levels, the corneas promptly resumed their prefitting shape once the retainers were discarded.
7. A high rate of failure was attributed to patients who failed to keep appointments.
8. Disturbing optic features include a high incidence of spectacle blur, induced with-the-rule astigmatism, myopia, and a poor quality of unaided vision, often 20/40.
9. The results were unpredictable, with the maximum benefit taking place within 9 months. There were no stable parameters to predict which patients would benefit from this treatment.
10. Best results occured with myopia of 2 D and worsened as the refractive error increased, especially beyond 4 D.

Comments. Despite the rather negative tones of this report, the subject requires some analysis. There are very few reports from the medical side on the veracity of orthokeratology. We need more testing to evaluate this technique.

In terms of safety and expense, it is cheaper and safer than surgical techniques, such as radial keratometry. As the demand for sight without a device is there, it behooves us to look at this procedure and try to improve it, rather than discard it. If it can be made to function so that the effect is permanent, it just might make surgical efforts obsolete.

There is very little orthokeratology practiced among ophthalmologists. It is even limited among optometrists. The limitations of this procedure as it stands today do not make the enterprise clinically worthwhile.

APHAKIC RIGID AND SOFT LENSES

CONTACT LENSES VERSUS INTRAOCULAR LENSES

Effective functional visual return and patient satisfaction are the first considerations for the cataract patient.

Cataract patients today demand better methods of visual rehabilitation than aphakic spectacles provide. Aphakic spectacles with all their inherent aberrations, distortions, and field limitation leave much to be desired (Fig. 27-1). The method of operating on some persons for cataracts and fitting them with spectacles afterwards immobilizes their daily activity to such an extent that it often ages them considerably and substitutes one disability for another. Many cataract patients have become informed with the media coverage extended to the innovations in ophthalmology.

The patient may ask for and even insist on an intraocular lens, contact lens, or an extended-wear lens. At times the patient's knowledge is imperfect, and there are some who still demand having their cataracts removed by laser therapy or some other method not applicable to their case. Regardless of the source, the patient is much more knowledgeable about his condition and the remedies possible. The ophthalmologist who does not update his techniques soon becomes a "referring doctor."

In North America there has developed an unusual enthusiasm for intraocular lenses in the past few years. Scarcely an ophthalmologic meeting fails to give testimony to this. Paralleling this increase in enthusiasm for intraocular lenses has been also an increase in the use of contact lenses for aphakia, both gas-permeable lenses and extended-wear lenses. With the increased number of available lenses today, the ophthalmologist is able to provide a more natural type of vision for the cataract patient.

Because of the advent of intraocular lens implantation, ophthalmologists must make a judgment in advance as to the best modality to restore vision. No longer can this decision be postponed until after cataract surgery.

What factors do we use in establishing clinical judgment as to the best method for restoring vision in any one individual? It is difficult to be dogmatic because these indications are changing. At one time intraocular lenses were indicated only if the patient was very elderly, had macular degeneration, and was offered the procedure in one eye only. The indications have broadened, to say the least. The following are guidelines for patient selection for aphakic contact lenses at this time:

1. Ability to handle lenses daily or weekly
2. Ability to take care of contact lenses with proper hygienic care
3. Lack of serious corneal disease
4. Lack of sufficient tear film
5. Patient-assistance availability in times of distress
6. No serious ocular disease such as severe endothelial dystrophy

In conditions or situations in which an intraocular lens is contraindicated such as long-standing diabetes, iris abnormalities, abnormalities of the anterior chamber, bleeding tendency, or any patient reluctance, a contact lens provides a safe effective alternative method for

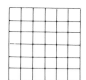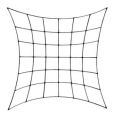

Fig. 27-1. Distortion by a strong convex aphakic lens that distorts a square to a pincushion shape. (From Stein, H.A., and Slatt, B.J.: The ophthalmic assistant, ed. 4, St. Louis, 1983, The C.V. Mosby Co.)

visual rehabilitation. The ophthalmic surgeon should be prepared to present a fair picture to each cataract patient about the advantages and disadvantages of whichever modality is chosen.

Most studies show that if the patient has an intraocular lens in one eye and a contact lens in the other the intraocular lens is preferred. As the patient's handling ability deteriorates with aging, this feeling is reenforced.

The fastest spreading operation today for the treatment of cataracts is the one followed by implant within the anterior or posterior chamber. A lens implant is our procedure of choice for the treatment of aphakia. A contact lens is used only in those cases in whom an implant is not feasible.

Despite the shrinking population using contact lenses for the therapy of aphakia, a sizable percentage of patients will always need aphakic contact lenses to give them the best in therapy.

While randomized selected studies have shown that there is much less risk of serious problems with contact lenses over intraocular lenses, the improved life style with intraocular lenses may be a significant trade-off. The question is not the relative merits of intraocular lenses over contacts or vice versa, but that both modalities represent a technologic advance that has made the consequences of cataract surgery in this decade far more pleasant than in the past.

In this chapter we basically cover the daily-wear lens and leave the detailed use of extended wear lenses to a later chapter.

SELECTION OF LENSES

Every ophthalmic resident learns early the enormous visual advantages that contact lenses possess over a spectacle correction for the treatment of aphakia.

The rigid lens offers good optic performance

and can completely cover any astigmatism. Since the prime purpose of doing a surgical procedure on a cataractous lens is to improve visual acuity, the superior vision of a rigid lens makes it most desirable. Another advantage of a rigid lens is its small size, which makes it easier to insert into the small, recessed palpebral openings of the aphakic patient. A rigid lens can be felt, a feature of great importance to the bilateral aphakic patient, and can be removed with lid manipulations.

A soft lens is difficult to see swimming around in a solution, is likely to flip inside out when it is applied to the eye, and must be removed directly by pinching it off the cornea, a feat that many elderly patients find frightening.

What makes the situation worse is that these lenses are not very tactile. In essence, what an ophthalmologist does when prescribing an aphakic soft lens for both eyes is to ask an elderly person to use a device that he or she can neither see nor feel and is apprehensive about in the first place.

The major disadvantage of any lens, be it rigid or soft, is that it must be handled. For the elderly patient with arthritis, a tremor of the head or finger, Parkinson's rigidity, or poor central acuity resulting from macular degenerative changes, an intraocular lens is perhaps the only choice. For the elderly patient over 70 years of age an intraocular lens is a better suggestion because it is well known that the number of lens dropouts increases dramatically with increasing age. Elderly patients cannot cope with lens insertions, running out to purchase solutions, or the fear, especially if they live alone, of one day being unable to remove their lenses. Also elderly people who have never worn contact lenses view such an enterprise with considerable apprehension and repugnance. Bilaterally aphakic patients, unless they use a special spectacle accessory device, cannot see to find their lenses.

The ideal aphakic lens wearer is a relatively young person, less than 70 years of age, in good health, with monocular aphakia. (However it can be argued that a young aphakic patient invariably becomes an older aphakic patient and that most persons with monocular aphakia develop binocular aphakia.)

Comment. Our preference for daily-wear contact lens is a gas-permeable rigid aphakic lens. The optic performance is better, the handling is easier, and the touch of the lens is more sure. The only thing the practitioner has to know is the oxygen permeability of the lens selected at aphakic levels of lens thickness.

DAILY-WEAR APHAKIC SOFT LENSES

The daily-wear soft lens is best used for the unilateral aphakic. If the aphakic person is soon to become bilaterally aphakic, extended-wear lenses should be considered or a lens implant or spectacles.

Prefit evaluation

The time to fit a lens is quite variable because the cataract surgical procedures are no longer uniform. An eye with a small incision from phacoemulsification can be given a soft contact lens in the first postoperative week. An extracapsular cataract extraction done with a larger incision will have to wait until the inflammatory reaction and the corneal parameters have settled. An intracapsular cataract extraction done under a microscope and with many interrupted sutures or a fine running nylon suture may be ready in 2 to 3 weeks, especially if the incision is less than 150 degrees.

A good guide to the fitting time is to wait until there is no further corneal edema. Corneal edema is best assessed with the pachometer. The measurement consists in alignment of the displaced image of the anterior corneal surface with the image of the posterior surface. The readings are usually made in millimeters. The average corneal thickness is 0.507 to 0.505 mm. A thickness of 0.6 mm should be considered as suspect and more than 0.7 mm as showing pronounced corneal edema.

A contact lens by itself can cause corneal edema. An aphakic lens placed on a normal nonoperated cornea can cause a 4% to 8% increase in corneal thickness. One must keep in mind that an aphakic lens is the thickest contact lens employed. A -10 D myope has the thin portion over the visual axis, whereas a $+10$ D hyperope or aphakic person has the thickest portion of the lens over the corneal cap and visual axis. So a soft lens used for aphakia causes an increase in corneal edema over the most critical part of that structure. Even if highly permeable lenses are used, the permeability at aphakic levels of lens thickness may not be great.

Because most private ophthalmic offices do not have a pachometer, there are other methods to consider. The corneal keratometer measurements should be clear, undistorted, and stable with two readings taken 1 week apart. The aphakic person often is unable to fixate well, and a small fixation light attached to the keratometer or the light of the topogometer may be helpful to obtain central K readings. The retinoscopy reflex should be undistorted and the refraction stable over a 2-week span. Slitlamp findings of vertical striae, dry spots on the cornea, and epithelial edema shown with sclerotic scatter or retroillumination can also yield good data as to the state of corneal repair.

Another problem with the early fitting of an aphkic contact lens is loss of endothelial cells. It has been shown that an aphakic soft lens placed on an eye can cause a dropping or falling out of endothelial cells after one day's wear. So, when one is fitting the lens, it is important to begin when corneal edema is virtually absent.

Comment. Persistent corneal edema should be detected and treated. It may be attributable to endothelial cell loss, vitreous touch, and so on. A contact lens placed over such an eye can only aggravate the condition.

Fitting technique

The vertex distance of the refraction should be rcorded, since a proper account of this must be taken into consideration in determination of the power required in the final lens. In general, because of the greater weight of the aphakic soft lens, the diameter of the soft lens must be made larger to stabilize the lens for proper centration. This fact is particularly true if there is significant astigmatism present.

As with most lenses, the prescription should be converted to minus cylinders. If the cylinder is less than 0.50 D, it can be disregarded. If the cylinder is greater than 0.50 diopters, take one half the cylinder and add it to the sphere (the spheric equivalent). If the cylinder is 1.50 diopters or greater, incorporate this additional cylinder into the bifocal spectacles. The vertex distance must be accounted for because it can change the final power by as much as 1.00 to 1.50 diopters. Convert the patient's K reading into millimeters. The initial K reading is only a guide to lens selection. The lens should be placed in the eye and allowed to settle for 20 to 30 minutes. At his point an over-refraction can be done to yield the final prescription.

If the lens does not move 1 to 2 mm with a blink, a flatter lens should be chosen. The regular soft aphakic lens does not have great permeability features, and so adequate tear exchange must be present. Also with time, deposits tend to tighten a lens by increasing its radius of curvature and making its contour steeper.

The base curves most commonly used for aphakic patients are 8.1 to 8.4 mm. The base curve should be flatter than the radius of curvature in the central region. The lens should rest on the apex of the cornea, vault the region of the limbus, and rest again on the peripheral portion of the sclera.

Myths about soft aphakic lenses

The soft aphakic lens is as durable as its rigid counterpart. The soft aphakic lens does well to last 1 year. The deposits are heavier and more varied and include mineral and lipids as well as protein. A rigid lens does not accumulate tenacious adherent deposits that are hard to remove with simple cleaners.

The incidence of infection is the same for an aphakic person wearing a soft lens as it is for a phakic person. The aphakic person has a higher incidence of bacterial conjunctivitis. The tear film is likely to be reduced. There may be corneal erosion from xerosis. This means that the concentration of the tear antibacterial enzyme, lysozyme, is also reduced. With increased protein precipitates and lower defense mechanisms, the setup is for a greater incidence of bacterial conjunctivitis.

Because the soft lens is so thick in the aphakic person, the vision is good because the astigmatism is masked. If there is significant astigmatism, 2.00 D or greater, the aphakic person with a healthy retina will not see 20/20. In fact, if there is no astigmatism, the aphakic person with a soft lens will not see as well as an aphakic person with a rigid lens. The contrast gradient with any soft lens is reduced when compared to that vision yielded through a rigid lens.

The vision with a soft lens may be brought up to rigid-lens efficiency with the use of spectacles. Patients who switch from rigid lenses to soft lenses will invariably complain of hazy vision even if the recorded vision is 20/20 in each eye with both sets of lenses.

An aphakic soft lens may last 6 months to 1 year. Its life is shortened by the following:
1. Deposits, which interfere with clarity of vision.
2. Splitting by the fingernail or poor placement in the case.
3. Loss because this lens is impossible to see or feel, especially when storage is in a liquid medium.
4. Displacement because this lens can be decentered without causing pain, and so this event may not be noted early.

The success rate for a soft aphakic lens is high. This is true in a 1-year projection, but it is dismal 5 years later. From 80% satisfaction in the honeymoon year, the rate of wear drops down to 30% in good hands. This occurs with bilaterally aphakic people.

Extended-wear soft lenses solve all the problems of daily-wear lenses. They eliminate some handling, and that is the best of its remedy. Deposit formation may be so intense and rapid that a lens may have to be replaced every 3 to 6 months.

Neovascularization of the cornea is the same whichever lens is applied. The aphakic soft lens wear is the most prone to neovascularization of the cornea. This is true whether the patient wears daily or extended-wear lenses. Corneal edema under a soft lens can be as much as 10%. With a rigid lens, corneal edema is apical in location and so limbal blood vessels cannot penetrate the compact peripheral stroma. With a soft lens, the entire cornea is edematous.

The success rate of hydrogel fitting is directly related to the motivation and patience of the fitter and his patient. Although this is true, motivation alone will not conquer handling problems, mucous strands, xerosis, infection, vascularization of the cornea, cleaning problems, cost, and repetitive visits to the fitter.

DAILY-WEAR RIGID APHAKIC LENSES

An aphakic lens can be fitted when the K readings and refraction have stabilized. At least two similar K readings should be obtained before a lens is ordered. With the present refinements in surgery, measurements can frequently be made by the fourth week after surgery, with patients obtaining the lenses by the fifth or sixth week. It is well to remember that a round pupil extraction eliminates the flare often encountered after keyhole or full iridectomies. With phacoemulsification techniques a lens may be applied to the cornea within a week. In general the smaller the size of the surgical wound, the earlier the lens can be applied to the eye.

Motivation of the aged patient may be enhanced when patients are given their spectacle correction in a trial frame and they are allowed to take a short stroll with assistance outside the office. The same procedure should be done with a trial contact lens. The results are most gratifying.

Fitting technique

Aphakic lenses are best ordered through a trial set. Some of the advantages are that patients can be introduced to a lens without making a firm commitment to order one. Since the initial discomfort of a rigid aphakic lens is not so severe as a cosmetic lens fitted to a normal cornea, patients gain confidence as to their suitability for lens wear. The fitter gains a more dynamic overview of the lens-cornea relationship. Vertex-distance allowances do not have to be made because they are taken care of in the over-refraction. Also, the effects of lens size, lid adherence, and lens centration can all be assessed in a glance with trial lenses.

The guide for lens selection is keratometry. This is somewhat difficult in the aphakic patient because fixation is not accurate and because of the poor, uncorrected visual acuity. However a lighted fixation target mounted on the keratometer overcomes this particular

problem (Fig. 27-2). Before a lens is ordered, the mires should be clear and free of distortion and the K readings should be stabilized.

It is important that measurements of power of aphakic lenses be done in the same way in the office as in the laboratory. Front-vertex power is measured when the concave surface faces the examiner in the lensometer. The back-vertex power is assessed when the convex surface faces the examiner. With aphakic lenses over 10.00 D there may be up to 2.00 D of difference between the front- and back-vertex powers.

Many fitters advocate overplussing one eye by 0.50 D to give the patient good vision in the intermediate zone and adding excessive power in the other eye by +1.50 D to facilitate reading. This is an excellent idea for many elderly patients whose functional distance vision is no greater than the size of a room. Of course, if the patient drives a car, he or she should be given the best possible distance correction.

If the astigmatism exceeds 1.50 D, the lens should be fitted about 0.1 mm steeper than the flattest K. If the astigmatism is 3.00 D or greater and centration is poor, a toric peripheral curve is best, since toric base-curve lenses are generally unsatisfactory.

The choice of final lens should be based on the centration, movement, and fluorescein pattern. The lens should center well, ride slightly up after the blink, and then gradually drop 1 to 3 mm.

Problems in fitting

The proper fitting of the person with aphakia is a highly complex matter of (1) the tendency of high-plus lenses to ride down and be moved excessively by the lids because of their greater thickness and weight and their more forward center of gravity, (2) often flaccid or lax lower lids of older patients, unable to support the weight of some low-riding lenses, that may allow the lenses to dig into and irritate the lower limbus, (3) pupillary irregularities such as keyhole or upward-displaced pupils, which are still quite common, and (4) high degrees of corneal cylinder astigmatism against the rule often found after cataract surgery.

To avoid visual disturbances such as flare, ghost images, or double vision, it is imperative to position the lens so that the optic zone covers the entire exposed pupil at all times.

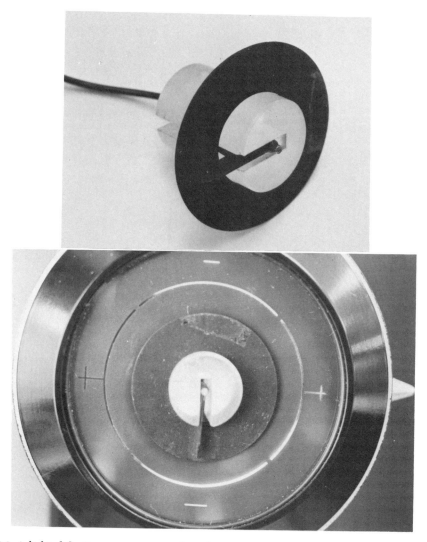

Fig. 27-2. A lighted fixation target mounted on the keratometer adds guidance for fixation for the bilateral aphakic patient.

Types of rigid aphakic lenses

There are basically two types of rigid aphakic lenses: the minus-carrier lenticular lens and the single-cut lens. The correct selection depends on the pupil and the lid characteristics of each individual case. For example, a keyhole pupil requires a lens, which usually rides somewhat above center, to completely cover the exposed pupil. If there is a mild postoperative ptosis so that the upper lid extends down far enough to cover virtually all the exposed su-

perior pillars of the cut iris, this factor need not be considered.

Lenses with larger optic zones are necessary for larger pupils and for conditions such as astigmatism against the rule or decentered corneal apical caps that tend to displace lenses laterally.

For flaccid lower lids, thick lens edges may be desirable to better support the weight of low-riding lenses or the lenses may be designed to ride up, held there by the upper lids.

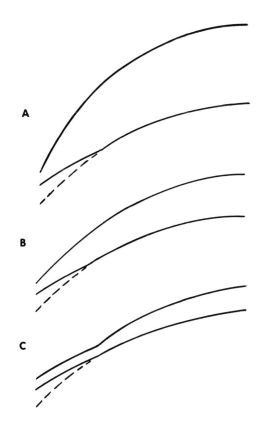

Fig. 27-3. A, Single-cut plus lens; **B,** regular lenticular construction for plus lenses; **C,** minus-carrier lenticular construction for plus lenses. **A** through **C** have the following common parameters: central posterior radius (base curve), 7.5 mm; posterior optic zone, 7.5 mm; posterior peripheral radius, 9.0 mm; lens diameter, 10.0 mm; central anterior radius, 6.0 mm; edge thickness, same for all. **B** and **C** have the following similarities and differences: (1) The anterior optic zone is 7.5 mm for both, and both are of a lenticular construction with the carrier radius (anterior peripheral radius) flatter than the anterior central radius. (2) The carrier radius of **B** is concentric to the posterior central radius (7.5 mm), whereas the carrier radius of **C** is concentric with the posterior peripheral radius (9.0 mm). The relationship of the carrier radius of 9.0 mm to the base curve radius of 7.5 mm is approximately −10.00. The major advantages of the minus-carrier lenticular construction over the regular lenticular lens construction are (1) minimum thickness, **A** through **C**; (2) more upper lid "hold" on the lens resulting from the flatter carrier; and (3) diameter reductions that can be made without affecting the edge thickness or the posterior curve. By consistently making the carrier radius concentric to the posterior peripheral curve(s) the only variables that affect the thickness are the power and the anterior optic zone.

Minus-carrier lenticular lens (Fig. 27-3)

Indications. The following are indications for minus-carrier lenticular lenses:

1. Low-riding aphakic lens
2. Corneal curvature flatter than 45.00 D
3. Astigmatism against the rule greater than 1.50 D
4. Large palpebral apertures, especially accompanied by lax lower lids
5. Round pupil extractions

This lens has a flat carrier curve that increases the upward vector component of the upper lid pull on the lens. The flat carrier curve functions to reduce the weight of the lens, and as a result the tendency to sag is diminished (Fig. 27-4). This lessened diminishment is achieved when the lens is designed with a small, anterior optic zone, preferably 7.0 mm in diameter.

Such an expedient is helpful to compensate for the excessive center thickness of the lens, which, of course, is determined by its power. For example, a +2.00 D lens, 8.5 mm in diameter, would have a center thickness of 0.045

Specifications for minus-carrier lenticular lens

Base curve: Trial set best; starting base curve should be 0.25 to 0.50 D steeper than K for initial lens; for each diopter greater than K 0.25 D should be added to base curve
Diameter: 9.0 to 9.5 mm; diameter should be increased for (1) flatter corneal curvature, (2) large corneas, and (3) lax and low lower lid margins
Edge thickness: 0.3 to 0.45 mm; varies largely with diameter and size of optic zone
Optic zone: 7.0 to 7.5 mm; smallest size consistent with good vision is best; optic zone should be 2 to 3 mm larger than pupil size and usually 1.5 to 2 mm smaller than diameter
Peripheral curve: 5.00 to 6.00 D flatter than the primary base curve
Power: Best determined by refraction over a trial lens
Radius of carrier: 1 to 3 mm flatter than base curve

334 *Fitting guide for more advanced fitters*

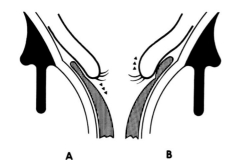

Fig. 27-4. A, A lenticular lens has a convex peripheral ridge, which the lid tends to push down. **B,** A minus lenticular lens. The lid tends to lift such a lens by its hold on the peripheral wedge.

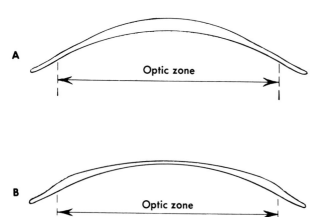

Fig. 27-5. Lenticular lenses. **A,** High-plus lenses tend to ride low because of their bulk and weight. **B,** The minus-carrier lenticular lens is thinner than a conventional lenticular lens and is well supported by the upper lid acting on the peripheral carrier.

mm as compared to a +10.00 D lens, 8.5 mm in diameter, which would have a center thickness of 0.22 mm. An aphakic lens is frequently five times thicker than a corresponding low-powered plus lens.

The ordinary lenticular lens has been pushed into obscurity by the minus-carrier lenticular lens (Fig. 27-5). The former lens was difficult to manufacture, and it frequently caused lid irritation as the upper lid passed from the relatively flat curve of the carrier portion to the steep curve of the optic portion of the lens. Also the downward force exerted on the lens as the upper lid collided with the steep curve of the anterior optic zone tended to push the lens down.

The minus-carrier lenticular lens is well supported by the upper lid and can be held in po-

sition about 1 mm above the corneal center. Since this lens is much thinner than a conventional lenticular lens, there is less tendency for it to drop over the lower limbus (Fig. 27-6).

Comment. This relatively large lens is most suitable for large, flat eyes. One advantage of its size is that insertion and removal are easier for the aphakic patient. It centers well, an asset to the elderly patient with lax lower lids.

It is unsuitable for keyhole pupils because the transition zone of the minus carrier may cross the pupil, causing flare or visual disturbances (Fig. 27-7). The fitting must be precise so that the posterior peripheral curves conform to the contours of the cornea. Usually an intermediate as well as peripheral curve is required.

Tinted lenses are quite helpful for aphakic lenses. Blue or gray tints are usually recommended. Aphakic patients frequently complain of halos around lights and reflections from artificial illumination. The annoying sensitivity to light may be caused by poor lens optic properties or internal lens reflections of the lens and the absence of the patients' own lens, which previously absorbed most of the visible wavelengths of incident light. The crystalline lens of the eye is a light filter; when it is removed the retina is struck by light never before experienced.

Single-cut lens. The single-cut lens should be used for patients with a full or keyhole pupil in order to diminish flare (Fig. 27-8). There is no carrier segment on the periphery of the lens that can create ghosting and flare with keyhole pupils (Fig. 27-9). The small dimensions of this lens also mean that the edge thickness can be made smaller than the edge of any lenticular lens. This is quite desirable since it makes the lens more comfortable. Though smaller in

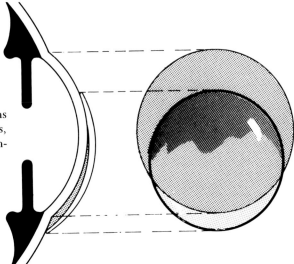

Fig. 27-6. A major disadvantage of any lenticular lens is that it tends to ride low. When the person reads, the depression of the lens over the limbus is accentuated.

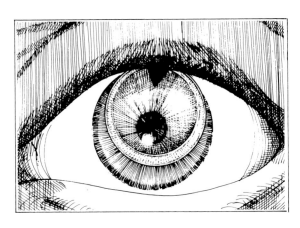

Fig. 27-7. The minus-carrier lenticular lens is best used for round pupil extractions. The peripheral portion of the lens creates flare in patients with sector iridectomies.

Specifications for single-cut lens

Base curve: Fit steeper than K by 0.50 D; fit spheric lens for 1.00 D or less of astigmatism
Central thickness: 0.35 mm centrally
Diameter: 7.5 to 8.5 mm; the difference between a 7.5 and an 8.5 mm diameter lens can mean a difference in 40% of the weight of the lens
Edge thickness: 0.1 to 0.2 mm thick; the average is 0.125 mm
Optic zone: 7.0 mm; this varies with the pupillary size; with complete iridectomy an 8.0 mm size may be optimal
Peripheral curve: Usually only a single peripheral curve is needed that is 6.00 to 7.00 D flatter than the base curve
Power: Best determined by refraction over a trial lens

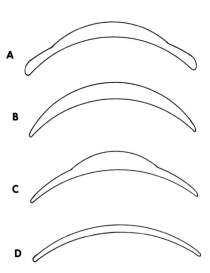

Fig. 27-8. Aphakic lens designs. **A,** Minus-carrier lens; **B,** single-cut lens; **C,** lenticular lens; **D,** microthin single-cut lens.

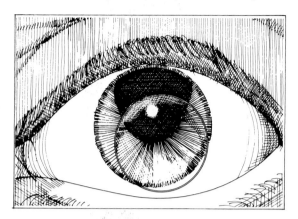

Fig. 27-9. Single-cut lenticular lens. This lens should be used in patients who have had a sector iridectomy.

Specifications for aphakic (Welsh) lens

Central thickness: 0.35 mm, approximately, depending on the power
Diameter: 7.5 mm
Edge thickness: 0.125 mm
Flat peripheral curve: 12 to 13 mm radius and 0.2 mm from the edge
Minimal blend: 0.1 mm to smooth the junction
Optic zone: 6.7 mm

overall dimension, the optic zone of the lens is quite large and compares favorably to that of a lenticular lens. A key advantage of this lens is the absence of a sharp juncture between the central and carrier front-surface curves, which eliminates the annoying lid bump.

The following are indications for the single-cut lens:

1. Small palpebral apertures
2. Steep corneas—more than 45.00 D
3. Low-riding lenses

One difficulty with the single-cut lens is its convex edge, which is easily pushed down by the descending lid. This lens also tends to drop with astigmatism with the rule. The major disadvantage is lens removal; the elderly aphakic patient experiences great difficulty in removing this small, steep lens from the cornea.

Modification. A modification of the single-cut lens is the 7.5 mm diameter aphakic lens designed by Dr. Robert Welsh. This lens is particularly successful when the steepness of the cornea is 45.00 D or greater. This lens centers well, is quite comfortable, and creates a minimum of spectacle blur. This small, lightweight lens can be worn continuously on selected patients, who must be previously day adapted before full-time wear and seen on a daily basis initially to ensure that the cornea tolerates the lens. Some persons with aphakia learn to displace their lenses onto the sclera and wear their hard lenses continuously on this basis.

This lens is often fitted steep to make the fit tighter. If the total power is 10.00 D, by making the base curve steeper than K by +2.00 D, one can create +2.00 D of power in the lacrimal layer, and the final lens power need only be +8.00 D.

The small, thin lens frequently creates handling problems, particularly upon insertion and removal. The thin edge, which makes it more pleasant to wear, also makes it more difficult to remove. Frequently a second party is required to assist the aphakic patient in manipulating the lens. It is also more prone to warp. Despite these drawbacks, the single-cut lens is the lens of choice for a steep cornea, that is, any cornea greater than 44.00 D. This lens is comfortable, and because of its light weight is less likely to cause corneal edema or sag.

Comment. Single-cut lenses are thinnest at the edge and may tend to break or chip at this point. Handling problems in the aphakic patient increase the possibility of breakage. A common mishap is fracturing the lens at the edge when one is placing the cover on a decentered lens in the storage case.

INSERTION OF APHAKIC LENSES

As mentioned previously, aphakic lens candidates are more likely to be successful if they are less than 70 years of age because they are usually better able to handle a lens. After the age of 70 years the elderly patient is more likely to have osteoarthritis, a tremor of the hand, and some loss of proprioceptive facility, which make manipulation of a lens exceedingly difficult and frustrating.

The bilaterally aphakic patient has a real problem in finding the lens. Unless the person is guided by spectacles, the lens must be found by feel. This is really not much different from giving a blind person contact lenses.

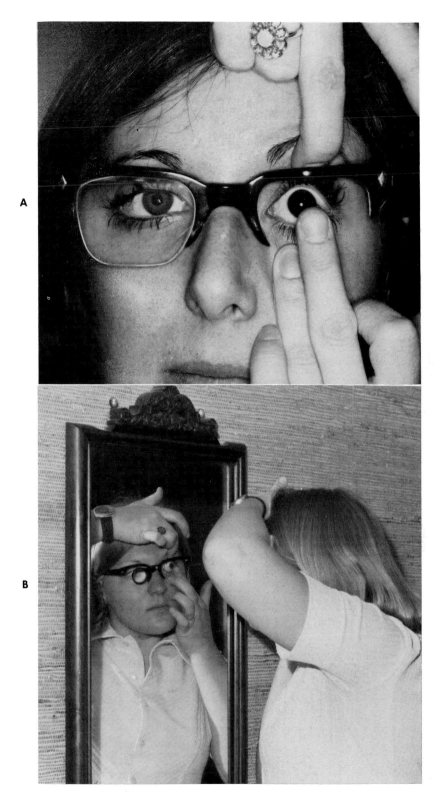

Fig. 27-10. A, Special frames to aid the aphakic person in the insertion of lenses. The glass is removed from one side and the plastic is bowed forward to permit the finger to grasp the upper eyelid. **B,** Spectacle aid device for bilateral aphakic patients. The empty frame allows for insertion of the lens. Guidance to and fixation come from the opposite optically corrected side.

For those patients who cannot manage a lens by conventional techniques, the use of reading aphkic spectacles with one frame blank or the aphakic lens attached on a flip hinge (Fig. 27-10, *A*) is a helpful device (Fig. 27-10, *B*). The patient can insert the lens through the blank side of the frame while guided by the other eye, which has the advantage of a spectacle correction of +12.00 to +16.00 D.

Insertion aids, such as magnification mirrors, are helpful as plastic fingers are. The best technique is the blind one. The patient should be shown that the eye can be found with one's proprioceptive abilities and not with vision; that is, it is quite easy to touch the tip of one's nose with the eyes closed. At times the upper lid will have to be lifted to allow enough room for the bulky soft lens.

For the patient with a tremor the lens can be placed on the middle finger while the index finger below retracts the lower lid. The index finger then gives support to the lens-carrying finger.

REMOVAL OF APHAKIC LENSES

Removal of the lens is also a chore. The lids are lax and the lid margin of the upper lid may buckle when the lid is laterally snapped to remove the lens. Also, such patients frequently live alone because of the death of a spouse, and so secondary aid is not always present. Ancillary services may be more of a hazard than a help. For example, a suction cup is a danger-ous aid for elderly patients living alone because they may apply the cup directly to the cornea when without their knowledge the lens has become decentered. An eyecup with water inserted in the lower fornix can be the salvation of patients with lax lids trying to get lenses out of their eyes (Fig. 27-11). The lens can also be washed out with saline irrigation or by dunking of the head in a basin of water with the drain closed.

Make up office pamphlets with information on what to do if emergencies arise. What is drilled in the office may disappear in the mind of elderly persons. Their memory may not be great. The pamphlet may help the patient cope with red eyes, abraded corneas, signs of infection, lost lenses, and so on.

Comment. Their are two anachronisms in this section. The keyhole pupil, or full iridectomy, is virtually obsolete. Also rigid PMMA lenses have given way to rigid silicone lenses.

GAS-PERMEABLE LENSES FOR APHAKIA

Our favorite aphakic gas-permeable lens has been the silicone-acrylate combination material, which is described in detail in Chapter 21.

One of the major disadvantages of using a gas-permeable lens is that the lens may become tight. With pure silicone lenses, the elastomer is not a barrier to water vapor. The tear pool behind the lens may evaporate. The lens becomes adherent, and the elastic property of the material only aggravates the tenacious ad-

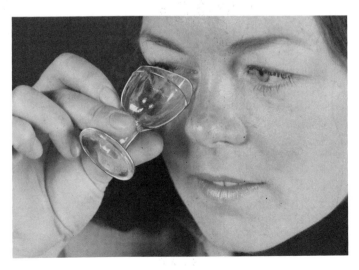

Fig. 27-11. Emergency removal with eyecup filled with water.

herence of the lens to the cornea. A negative suction cup effect is introduced. A cycle of events is introduced because the pressure on the tear film by the lid and lens only serves to squeeze out more tears. When the lid is in the up position, the lens shapes itself to the cornea and blocks the inflow of tears, producing a one-way valve effect.

Also some gas-permeable lenses do not permit enough oxygen permeability at the thickness required for an extended wear aphakic lens. For example, the CAB lens at 0.30 mm center thickness really cannot support the oxygen needs of the cornea under the closed lid. If these lenses are to be used for extended wear, the lens should have adequate gas permeability with respect to the thickness of the lens, the temperature zone in which it is going to be worn, and the adequacy of the tear film.

A problem with aphakic lenses of any material that is rigid, is that these thicker lenses tend to ride low. If the upper edge of the lens is not covered by the upper lid, the major remedy for discomfort is lost.

Fitting the silicone-acrylate lens*
(Table 27-1)

Although single-cut and lenticular designs may be equally effective in many patients (Fig. 27-12), the elderly aphakic patient will find the larger lenticular contact lens easier to handle. Therefore, the initial trial lens should have a large-diameter, lenticular myoflange (minus carrier) design (Fig. 27-13), and a base curve that provides the fluorescein pattern of minimal apical clearance.

1. If the initial trial lens positions sufficiently high so that the upper lid covers the superior portion of the carrier throughout

---

*Modified from Rosenthal, P.: The Boston Lens: theory and practice, Wilmington, Mass., 1979, Polymer Technology Corp.

Table 27-1. Aphakia trial set for the silicone-acrylate lens

Diameter (mm)	Central posterior curve (mm)	Power (D)	Intermediate optic zone (mm)	Design-carrier
8.7	7.20-8.20	+14.00	7.7	Single cut
9.2	7.20-8.20	+14.00	8.0	Single cut
9.8	7.30-8.50	+14.00	8.2	Lenticular EOZ* 8.0 mm—6.00 D
11.0	7.50-8.50	+14.00	9.0	Double lenticular EOZ 8.0 mm—3.00 D
				EOZ 9.5 mm—15.00 D

*EOZ, Exterior optic zone.

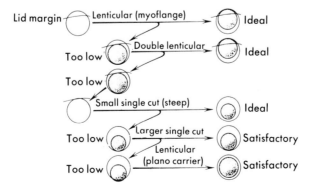

Fig. 27-12. Fitting the aphake. (Courtesy Polymer Technology Corp., Wilmington, Mass.)

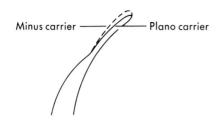

Fig. 27-13. Profile of lenticular-design aphakic or hyperopic contact lens. (Courtesy Polymer Technology Corp., Wilmington, Mass.)

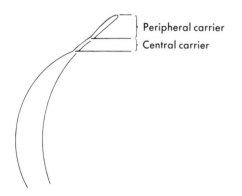

Fig. 27-14. Double lenticular design for aphakic contact lens. (Courtesy Polymer Technology Corp., Wilmington, Mass.)

the blink cycle, it is the design of choice.

2. If the initial trial lens slips below the margin of the upper lid despite the fact that the upper lid covers the superior portion of the cornea, evaluate a larger double lenticular design (Fig. 27-14). If the superior portion of the carrier remains tucked under the upper lid, it is the design of choice.

3. If the lenticular and double lenticular designs position too low or if the upper lid does not cover a sufficient area of the cornea to hold a lenticular lens in a satisfactory position, evaluate the fit of steeper single-cut lenses.

4. If single-cut lenses, regardless of diameter, position too low for satisfactory vision or' slide off the cornea as the patient blinks in upward gaze, a lenticular design having a tapered plano carrier or tangen-

tial periphery may be the best lens for that patient.

EXTENDED-WEAR RIGID LENSES FOR APHAKIA
PMMA lenses

PMMA (polymethylmethacrylate) lenses have been used in the past as extended-wear lenses though they are not recommended for this use. They have no permeability features and act as corneal insulators. The tolerance to these lenses is not predictable. Some patients can use them, but most get hypoxic changes.

When they are not tolerated, the cornea may become very edematous with vertical striae in Descemet's membrane, iritis, and pronounced conjunctival injection and lid swelling. It may be a dangerous experiment. Welsh was able to fit 80 to 200 aphakic eyes with hard PMMA lenses of his own design. These lenses were worn as extended-wear lenses. His experience has not been shared.

Welsh no longer uses extended-wear PMMA lenses though he pioneered this aspect of contact lens therapy.

CAB lenses

Cellulose acetate butyrate is permeable to oxygen and carbon dioxide, is a thermal conductor, and has a lower surface tension and lower wetting angle than polymethylmethacrylate does. The optic performance is fine, and the lens is comfortable. The permeability of this lens at the thickness required for an aphakic lens is too small to permit sufficient oxygen to reach the cornea under the closed lid. The CAB lens at 0.3 mm thickness delivers only 2% equivalent oxygen whereas the suggested safe tolerance level is between 7% and 10% for extended wear. Pachometry studies have shown that CAB-covered corneas had a thickness of 0.55 mm whereas the nonaphakic eye had a thickness of 0.32 mm. This lens should not work, but it does according to reliable resources. Some investigators have indicated this type of lens can be worn as an extended-wear lens in four out of five cases.

Comment. A new type of thin CAB lens has been introduced. This type should have better permeability features than the earlier type. At this point, no one has accumulated much clinical experience with this lens.

Silicone lenses

Potentially the silicone lens has the best opportunity for extended wear. For the past 5 years it has remained the lens of the future. But at this writing, the time has arrived for extended-wear use.

This lens should be ideal because it is at the top of the list of everyone's permeability charts. Even at 0.3 mm thickness, it provides almost 20% equivalent oxygen performance, way above the level required for maintaining the oxidative need of the cornea under a closed lid.

The good features are its optic performance and its ability to render the cornea free of any hypoxic changes. The lens is large in terms of a rigid lens and varies from 11 to 12.5 mm. The large size and firmness of the lens is a definite aid to the bilaterally aphakic who employs touch to handle the lens. The 11.3 mm lens is the most popular because the larger lens tends to be a little tight.

On the negative side is the discomfort of the lens. It feels more like a rigid lens than a hydrogel lens. Also some of the early silicone lenses have a tendency to decenter. At this time, great improvements have been made in centration, which in turn means a more comfortable lens.

Another drawback until recently was the tendency of the lens to cling and adhere to the cornea. In some cases the adherence was so strong that this phenomenon developed the epithet of the "sucked-on lens syndrome." The newer type of silicone lenses does not adhere to the cornea with such tenacity.

In addition to their own built-in problems, the silicone lens shares the complications of any extended-wear lens. These include giant papillary hypertrophy, corneal erosion, vascularization of the cornea, and contact-lens spoilage from mucus, protein deposits, and lipids.

The other consideration as with any extended-wear lens is cost. They have to be replaced frequently; 1 year is often the limit. But this applies to all types of extended lenses. There is the cost of cleaning, disinfecting, storing, and rinsing, as well as the use of adjuncts such as artificial tears to consider.

The two silicone lenses that are most readily available in the North American market are a silicone resin lens, Silcon, and a silicone elastomer lens, Silsoft. In Chapter 22 Morgan discusses in detail the fitting of these lenses in aphakic patients.

Comment. With a choice between an intraocular lens and an extended-wear lens the majority of patients will prefer an intraocular lens even when the vision is better in the eye covered by an extended-wear lens. There is, however, a considerable difference in success between a unilaterally aphakic person and a bilaterally aphakic person with respect to wearing aphakic contact lenses. In our hands 88% of unilateral aphakes were wearing thin lenses 3 years after surgery. Only 30% of bilateral aphakes wanted to cope with aphakic contact lenses in a similar period. The important factors for the bilateral aphakes include diminished manual agility in handling lenses, inability to cope with routines of cleaning, illness, cost, frequent lens replacements, fear of injuring an eye, and general difficulty in going to and from the ophthalmologist's office.

EXTENDED-WEAR LENSES

Today advanced lens technology is addressing itself to the problem of improving lenses that can be worn for extended periods of time without the need for daily handling. Advances in lens material and design combined with more sophisticated techniques in determining the response of the cornea to a lens worn on a 24-hour basis have made this possible. The news media have perhaps helped in increasing the demands of the public by making them aware that there are methods that will permit them to see without the trouble of insertion and removal and the accompanying care required. These methods are radial keratometry, surgical refractive keratoplasty and extended-wear contact lenses.

Extended-wear lenses have become a reality since the previous edition of this book. Two factors have influenced this development. One has been the manufacturing technologic advance in producing thinner and thinner soft lenses to provide a more comfortable lens with thinner edges that do not irritate the eyelid. This has resulted in the ability of the lenses to transmit oxygen. It has been clearly shown that if one halves the thickness of a soft lens, one will double its oxygen transmission. A second factor that has resulted in the availability of extended-wear lenses has been the ability to polymerize soft lens materials and manufacture lenses that will absorb more water in their substance. For every 10% increase in water absorption of these materials there is a corresponding 50% increase in oxygen transmission; thus if water content increases 20%, the oxygen transmission doubles.

Unfortunately the news media ignore the problems and attendant risks involved and appeal only to the imaginative, emotional response of the individual. This produces considerable pressure on the surgeon and contact lens fitter.

We have worked with aphakic patients, particularly the very young and the elderly; of the latter, only 30% can manage daily-wear lenses because of handling problems. The best result of other clinical investigators over a 2-year period still is less than 55% for aphakia. The direction and emphasis in ophthalmology have been to provide a better method of visual rehabilitation for the aphakic person either with contact lenses or with intraocular lenses than do present spectacles with their inherent problems (Fig. 28-1).

To some extent the growth and popularity of extended-wear lenses have been delayed by adverse publicity on isolated problems, by the practitioners' reluctance to handle the extra visits required, by the patients' reluctance to accept the higher fee necessary, by the fitters' reluctance to be faced with some medical problems that he or she may not be able to handle, and by the risk of the rare sight-threatening complications.

The extended- or prolonged-wear lens for the aphakic person has presently reached a

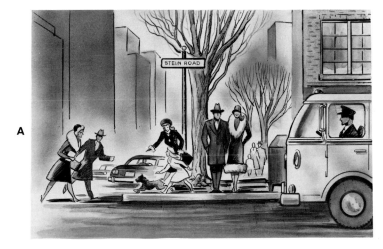

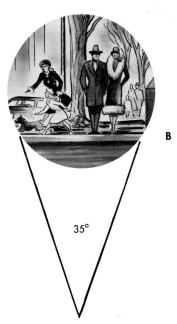

35°

Fig. 28-1. The aphakic person with a contact lens sees the entire field of vision, **A**, whereas the aphakic person with spectacles sees a limited central field, **B**. This is a definite hazard in driving.

state where the benefits outweigh the risks involved, and it rivals the intraocular lens as a safer alternative.

Both rigid and flexible lenses have been reported of value as an extended-wear lens for aphakia. Welsh, with his small polymethylmethacrylate lenses, and Garcia's report on CAB lenses show a statistically significant percent of success. Newer gas-permeable polymethylmethacrylate lenses are presently being tried on an investigational basis and offer considerable promise. Silicone offers great potential for 24-hour lens wear if satisfactory manufacturing capability can be introduced to create a long-lasting hydrophilic surface.

More significant have been advances made with hydrogel lenses. Information on corneal physiology has shown that the oxygen requirement of the cornea during sleep is less than one half that required when the eyes are open. It has also been shown that a change of dimension of the following two factors results in better oxygen transmission of a lens: (1) the thinness (Fig. 28-2) and (2) the water content of the lens. Measurements show that the oxygen transmission of a lens measured at body temperature is 15% to 40% greater than that of a lens measured at room temperature (Table 28-1); consequently laboratory methods of measuring gas transfer of a lens do not truly reflect its behavior on the eye.

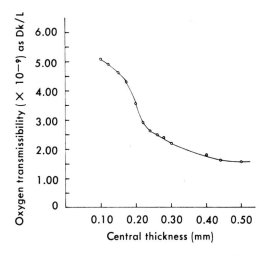

Fig. 28-2. Curve to illustrate the nonlinear relationship between the central thickness and the oxygen permeability of hydrophilic lenses at 20° C. The thinner the lens, the greater the oxygen transmission. (From Feldman, G., and associates: Contact Lens J. **10**(3):13-20, Dec. 1976.)

Generally lenses that have power are constructed with either a thicker center or a thicker periphery depending on whether they are plus or minus lenses. Thus any given contact lens will have a variation of oxygen being transmitted across its surface. Because of this, the information that is truly significant is how much total oxygen reaches the corneal side of a contact lens. This is based on the average thickness of the lens. The factor of tear exchange and venting comes into play in which additional oxygen is provided from the tear film on flexure and movement of the lens.

The thickness of an aphakic lens often causes problems. In order to incorporate adequate power into a lens of +10.00 D the lens must be at least 0.4 mm thick in the center, whereas a −4.00 D power can have a central thickness of only 0.03 mm. This also means that the aphakic lens is heavier and must be made in a larger diameter for stabilization. Its thickness also makes it less permeable to oxygen (Fig. 28-3). Thus to create an ideal oxygen-permeable hydrogel lens, one cannot significantly reduce the thickness of an aphakic lens because

of the power requirement, which makes it necessary for the lens to be at least three times thicker than a myopic lens.

Two types of hydrogel lenses have evolved: (1) those with water contents less than 60% that are designed for daily wear and (2) those with higher water contents that are designed for extended wear. The added water composition provides two elements that favor extended wear: (1) increased oxygen transmission so that there is adequate oxygen to a thermally elevated cornea lying under a closed eyelid, and (2) greater heat dissipation from the cornea.

Both the thinner, myopic, hydrogel lens and the thicker, hydrogel, aphakic lens can be safely worn on an extended-wear basis by a certain number of persons, regardless of the water

Table 28-1. Comparison of expansion rate and oxygen permeability of four polymers of varying water content as hydrogel lenses at a standard thickness of 0.2 mm*

Polymer	Average water content (%)	Average expansion rate (%)	Oxygen permeability, DK ($\times 10^{-11}$)		
			21° C	27° C	35° C
A	43.8	16.8	2.50	3.33	4.30
B	53.1	25.8	6.81	8.23	10.21
C	63.2	36.4	9.71	11.82	14.24
D	71.3	46.7	14.28	15.33	17.77

From Feldman, G., and associates: Fitting characteristics and gas permeability of thin hydrogel lenses, Contact Lens J. **10**(3):13-20, Dec. 1976.
*Note that the higher the water content the greater the oxygen permeability.

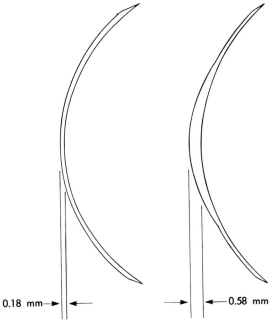

Fig. 28-3. Comparison of a regular soft lens, *left*, with an aphakic lenticular lens, *right*. Note the considerably thicker central portion of the aphakic lens that contributes to corneal edema.

0.18 mm→ ←   → ←0.58 mm

content of the lens. The problem is how to define the number of persons who are at risk. Even after daytime adaptation and continual monitoring, significant lens deposits and corneal changes will occur in a number of patients.

Although corneal changes are minimal with well-fitted lenses, coating of these lenses does become a significant problem in the elderly. With coating of lenses, there are some physiologic factors that decrease vision, impair corneal performance, and irritate the tarsal conjunctiva. Consequently, extended wear lenses are not "fit-and-forget" lenses. The patient must be routinely monitored to avoid medicolegal implications if problems arise.

PHYSIOLOGIC CONSIDERATIONS

The aim to wear a lens 24 hours of the day for several days must take into consideration a number of physiologic problems that arise when the eyelid is closed and there is no longer adequate tear exchange through blinking. In this situation, with the closed eyelid, atmospheric oxygen is snuffed out and the cornea must obtain its oxygen supply directly from the overlying tarsal conjunctival plexus of vessels. At least 5% of atmospheric oxygen equivalent is necessary for adequate oxygenation of the cornea for maintenance of corneal glucose reserves at an adequate level.

Some nocturnal changes that occur when the eye is closed are outlined below:

1. Richard Hill has pointed out that the oxygen supply normally is decreased by a third in the nighttime closed-eye environment compared to the daytime closed-eye environment oxygen supply. Furthermore, there is still a further oxygen reduction to the cornea under a contact lens.

2. There is nocturnal swelling of the cornea as supported by pachometric evidence (Fig. 28-4). As the cornea thickens, the lens may no longer fit with a thicker cornea and may reveal tight signs.

3. Even during the waking day, with normal blinking there is only 1% to 5% tear exchange under a soft lens as compared to 20% tear exchange under a rigid lens. Thus one is most dependent on the oxygen transmission of the material of extended wear lenses.

4. The temperature of the cornea increases 3 to 4 degrees C with closed eyelids. The cornea in turn requires more oxygen with a higher temperature.

5. There is diminished tear production during sleep. As a result, the soft contact lens dries out, leading to edge lift-off and ejection

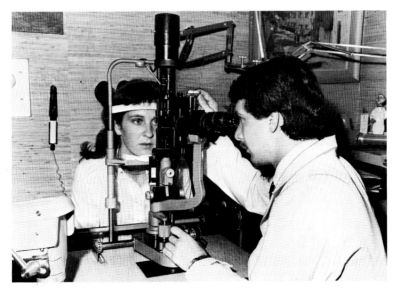

Fig. 28-4. The thickness of the cornea may be measured with a pachometer. Corneal swelling over 6% to 8% is usually pathologic. (From Stein, H.A., and Slatt, B.J.: The ophthalmic assistant, ed. 4, St. Louis, 1983, The C.V. Mosby Co.)

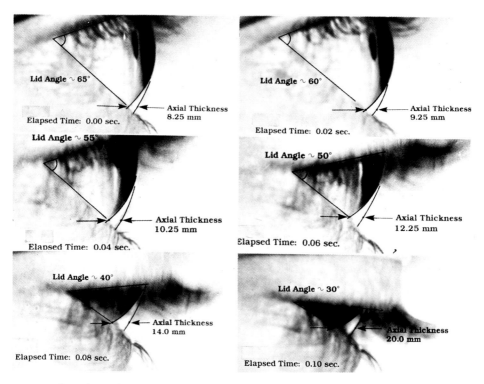

Fig. 28-5. Softcon lens photographed by high-speed film sequences (50 frames/sec), showing lens tear pumping action. (Courtesy Dr. Lester E. Janoff and American Optical Corp., Southbridge, Mass.)

of the lens by the lower eyelid. Consequently there is a higher loss rate in the elderly and in children who frequently rub the eyes on arising.

6. The pH of the tears shifts to acid at night because of the buildup of lactic acid. The soft lens shortens its radius and tightens up when in an acid medium. This can be shown in tests in a beaker with changing pH. The significance of this is that a well-fitting lens may become too tight at night and when one arises in the morning. This may account for the tight lens syndrome described under the discussion on complications.

7. In dry environments, a lens can lose 20% of its water content. This is more significant in the low water and thin lenses. Not only may the lenses steepen, but also Hill has shown that there is a decrease in equivalent oxygen performance and a resulting corneal edema.

8. Korb and Holden have shown that the aphakic cornea requires only about 50% of the oxygen that a phakic cornea requires. Conse-

quently, aphakes can get by for extended wear with the thicker lenses required for aphakic power considerations.

9. The tear pump action, even with extended wear lenses, plays a role in corneal oxygenation. Although the eye does not blink at night, there are still roving and rapid movements of the eye, at least during sleep, that will result in tear exchange and removal of debris. During the day, the beautiful high-speed photographs of the eye (Fig. 28-5) illustrate that during blinking the tear reservoir at the periphery of the lens and cornea is expelled, creating a partial vacuum in the area of the vault.

OXYGEN CHARACTERISTICS

The greater the oxygen transmissibility of a lens, the better the lens performance will be for achieving extended wear with minimal corneal interference. However, one must look at terminology carefully. The oxygen transmission of a lens represented by $\dfrac{DK}{L}$, where D is the

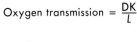

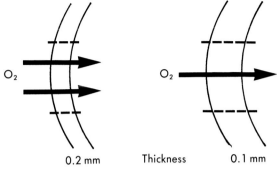

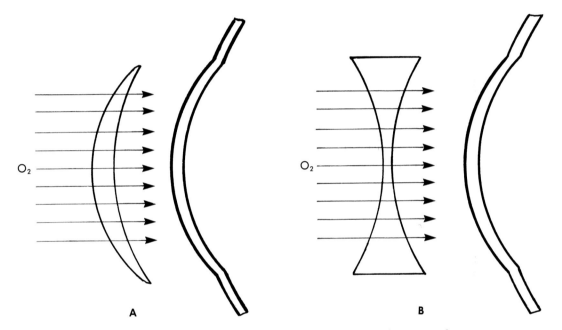

Fig. 28-6. Oxygen transmission of any contact lens will vary with the thickness of the material. The thinner the lens, the more oxygen will be transmitted. This is directly proportional.

Fig. 28-7. Equivalent oxygen performance (EOP) represents the total amount of oxygen passing through the entire contact lens. **A,** EOP of a plus lens, which is thicker in the center. **B,** EOP of a minus lens, which is thicker in the periphery.

diffusion coefficient of a material, K is the solubility constant, and L is the lens thickness. This is a laboratory measurement and is a satisfactory way to compare one material over another (Fig. 28-6). Of more importance clinically is the EOP, or equivalent oxygen performance (Fig. 28-7). This is a value relating the percentage of oxygen reaching the cornea to atmospheric oxygen percentage. One can see from the illustration that in high-minus lenses, there is inadequate oxygen transmitted through the lens through the thicker periphery. Similarly

with high-plus lenses, there is less oxygen passing through the lens centrally.

Another factor to consider is tear exchange—the extended-wear lenses, particularly the thinner lenses, may have to be fit somewhat tighter to prevent wrinkling and visual aberrations. If the permeability of the lens is adequate, this can be performed without difficulty or compromise to the cornea. Generally speaking however, one always should be on guard for a situation of stasis of the lens because of the tightening and dehydration.

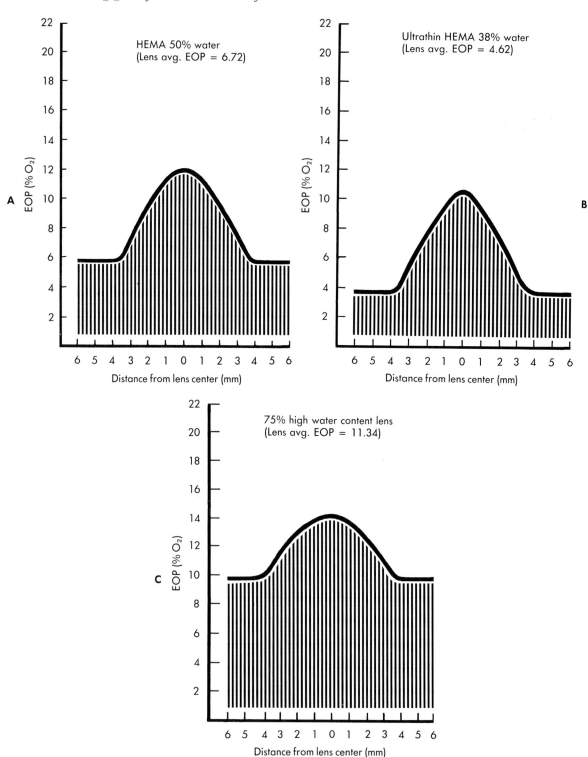

Fig. 28-8. The equivalent oxygen performance of −3 D lens. **A,** Standard HEMA minus lens of 50% water with center thickness 0.06 mm. **B,** Ultrathin 0.03 mm center thickness lens of 38% water. **C,** High-water-content (75%) lens with center thickness 0.15 mm. Note the relatively better EOP of the high-water-content lens, particularly at the periphery of the lens. (Courtesy CooperVision, Inc., Optics Division, Irvine, Calif.)

With many of the soft hydrogel lenses there is a trade-off as to how thin they can be made with the high- or low-water-content variety without breakage and damage easily occurring to the lenses. However, the lenses have become better polymerized today so that lens damage is not a major factor even with the very thin or high-water-content lenses.

Remember that for every halving of the thickness of a lens, the equivalent oxygen performance (EOP) is doubled. On the other hand, for every 10% increase in water content of a soft lens, the oxygen performance is increased 50%. So a 60% water-content lens has 50% more oxygen performance than a 50% water-content lens, and a 70% water-content lens has double the oxygen performance that a 50% water-content lens has. This factor may be very significant in the thicker parts of a lens such as the center of a high-plus lens or the periphery of a high-minus lens (Fig. 28-8).

Comment. Inadequate tears can really be a spoiler of extended-wear lenses. There is often a shift residual tears to the lens based on osmotic flow. Lack of tears causes great protein deposition, which in turn may change the shape of the lens, makes it tighter and more myopic than before, reduces the oxygen permeability of the lens, and reduces visual acuity.

APHAKIC VERSUS MYOPIC EXTENDED WEAR

The therapeutic need for a contact lens for visual rehabilitation of an aphake is without question. Even with the explosive influence of the intraocular lens in today's management of aphakia, there still exists a real need for an extended-wear lens that can rival the intraocular lens for visual effectiveness and safety. Of the 500,000 cataract operations performed annually in the United States, only about 40% to 50% had intraocular lens implantations in 1981, with many of the remainder consisting of one-eyed patients, corneal and anterior segment disorders, advanced diabetes or glaucoma, and a host of other absolute and relative contraindications. Coupled with this is the reluctance of many surgeons to subject their patient to intraocular lens surgery that they believe would carry a higher statistical risk of complications than a regular procedure would. So the extended wear lens offers a solution for many patients and many ophthalmologists.

Considerations for the aphakic person are different from those for the myope. Usually the aphakic patient is much older with poor tear function and inadequate tear constituents. In addition, the declining proprioceptive fingertip fibers, slight tremor of the hand, and poorer visual acuity may make insertion and removal more difficult for the elderly. In addition, the aphakic lens is usually three times thicker than the myope's lens, and it transmits less oxygen. Studies by Korb, however, have shown that the cornea of an aphakic requires only half as much oxygen as that of a phakic individual. Thus one may get by with a lens that is not so oxygen permeable for aphakia.

Success for extended-wear lenses is enhanced in aphakia with careful selection of patients. The following persons are best suited to the lenses:

1. Poor sleepers who wake up several times during the night
2. Persons who are previously adapted
3. Persons with good tear production
4. Persons with low-power aphakic prescriptions so that the lens can be made thinner centrally.

Comment. Aphakic persons have a greater need for an extended-wear lens than a young myope does. The pity is that such a lens has so many problems for the aphake and very few for the young myope.

In myopia, the problems are much simpler. The lens may be made extremely thin (0.035 mm). Generally, these persons are young, have healthy tear constitutients with adequate tear flow, do not have marginal corneal degenerative or dystrophic changes, and generally are alert and sensitive enough to recognize and report early signs of irritation. In addition, being generally younger in nature, they are more skillful in following the routines of care and being able to remove the lens in case of trouble. Wilson has outlined some of the reasons why myopic extended-wear lenses are much more successful than aphakic extended-wear ones.

Advantages of cosmetic lenses over extended-wear lenses

1. Initial fit equals final fit
2. Easier to handle

3. Lens thinner and with better oxygen performance
4. Healthier cornea
5. Better tear constitutients
6. Better tear flow
7. Less prone to infection
8. Fewer failures with selected patients

PATIENT SELECTION

For myopic extended-wear lenses our first choice for patients are those who have already been soft contact lens wearers. These patients are well motivated, know how to take care of soft lenses, and are most appreciative of the minimal care requirements for extended wear. They are also so indoctrinated with the care of contact lenses that they are not likely to forget the care routines once fitted. In the event of irritability from any source, such as fitting change, dust, or foreign body, they are usually sufficiently aware as to how to remove the lenses.

Other persons suitable for myopic extended-wear lenses are those that have some hand abnormality or medical condition that makes putting on and off a pair of spectacles a real chore. We have seen patients with multiple sclerosis who have almost injured their eyes upon applying spectacles.

There are three types of patients who may develop problems with extended-wear lenses:
1. Dry-eyed patients
2. Patients with lid-margin disease
3. Patients with ocular infections

The eyes dry more frequently during sleep and may cause more of a problem with extended-wear lenses than with daily-wear lenses. If mild, it may be overcome by the use of artificial tears. If unmanageable, it indicates that extended-wear lenses should be discontinued.

Nocturnal lagophthalmos or lagophthalmos occurring after ptosis or blepharoplasty surgery may result in drying. Dry climates such as Arizona may further produce a problem and compromise extended-wear fitting.

Blepharitis or meibomianitis may also compromise extended-wear lenses, since *Staphylococcus*, frequently a causative organism, may produce conjunctivitis, keratitis, and corneal ulceration. Extended wear can be undertaken only when the lid margins are clear.

Comment. Evaporation of water from a hydrogel lens is common in an arid environment. Places like Arizona, the interior of an automobile, some older office buildings and schools, and so on can cause the anterior surface of a lens to lose some of its hydration. Instead of having regular anterior surface optic characteristics, the surface becomes wavy and the vision variable. It is a common cause of 4 P.M. visual focusing problems.

AVAILABLE LENSES

Up to now, there have been a number of lenses that appear to have a capability for extended wear, listed as follows:

Hydrogel lenses
  High-water-content lenses, >70%
  Ultrathin lenses, <0.05 mm
Silicone soft lenses
Gas-permeable rigid lenses
  Silicone-acrylate
  Silicone resin
  CAB (cellulose acetate butyrate)
  Styrene

Any or all of the above lenses may effectively be used. One must learn to develop an experience with one or more of the lenses, recognize the problems that arise, and learn how to correct them. The fitting and the selection of patients has to be ideal so that one can maximize the number of patients wearing extended-wear lenses and minimize the number of unscheduled return appointments.

Our preference for an extended-wear lens at present is for a high-water-content lens, such as Permalens, Sauflon, or Duragel, or the very thin lenses with 0.03 mm center thickness. Remember that one must be concerned with oxygen flow through the peripheral portion and not just the center of a contact lens. Fig. 28-9 illustrates the larger percentage of corneal cells in the periphery of a cornea. If the lens is myopic, in the higher powers there will be a thicker lens profile in the periphery. The CSI lens designed by Korb was essentially designed to provide a thinness to the periphery of the lens (Fig. 28-10). Fig. 28-8 illustrates the oxygen performance through the periphery of a Duragel 75% water-content lens as compared to a 50% water-content hydrogel lens and an ultrathin 38% water-content lens. New molded

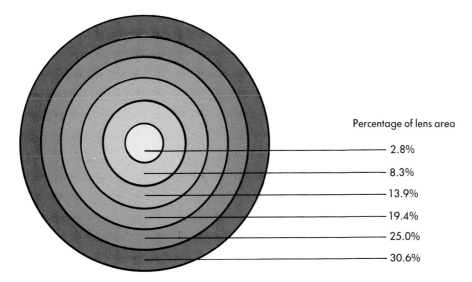

Percentage of lens area

2.8%

8.3%

13.9%

19.4%

25.0%

30.6%

Fig. 28-9. Relative percentage of the cornea covered by a soft contact lens. Note the high percent of the peripheral corneal cells, which may be embarrassed further if there is insufficient peripheral oxygen transmissibility. (Courtesy CooperVision Inc., Optics Division, Irvine, Calif.)

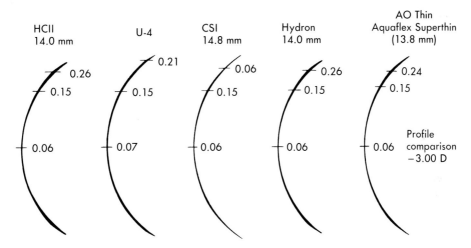

HCII 14.0 mm	U-4	CSI 14.8 mm	Hydron 14.0 mm	AO Thin Aquaflex Superthin (13.8 mm)
0.26	0.21	0.06	0.26	0.24
0.15	0.15	0.15	0.15	0.15
0.06	0.07	0.06	0.06	0.06

Profile comparison −3.00 D

Fig. 28-10. Profile comparison of a −3 D lens. All lenses have the same center thickness, but the CSI lens has a thinner periphery.

high-water-content lenses appearing on the market today offer increased durability.

Comment. Although new systems of molded soft lenses may provide an increased durability to the lens and a reduction in cost, the ultimate achievement will occur when the material can be made dropout resistant.

FITTING

Because lens designs change rapidly and new series, diameters, and base curves change so frequently, the practitioner is advised to consult the manufacturer of the lens of his choice for detailed parameter information.

Certain basic principles and guidelines to follow:

1. Decide whether one is fitting high-water-content lenses, such as Permalens, Sauflon, Duragel, TC 75, and Scanlens 75, or low-water-content thin lenses, such as O_4, CSI, Cibasoft thin, Hydrocurve II, and Hydron, or whether one wishes to use silicone or the gas-permeable rigid lens.

2. Fit the flattest lens that will give good comfort and vision.

3. No matter how sloppy and loose the lens

may appear, if the patient sees well and is comfortable it is safer to leave it. Ultimately there may be a tightening up of the lens.

4. Avoid fitting a lens too tight with little movement. Although with extended-wear lenses during daytime use one may safely get away with this, bear in mind that the buildup of lactic acid during sleep may tighten the lens and produce limbal compression.

5. In case of a red eye be sure to give adequate instruction in removal of the lens. Serious complications can be avoided by early lens removal.

6. Be sure the patient can handle the lens well and knows the care systems for looking after the lenses.

7. In aphakia, if poor vision is a problem, try to select a lens with a large optic zone. Frustration with one manufacturer's lens because of the optic zone or edge design does not mean another lens will not work.

8. In myopic extended wear, the initial fit is usually the final fit. In aphakia, there may be a tightening up of the lens within a week, and so the lens may have to be changed in fit.

9. The myopic lens, being thin, may drape over the periphery of the cornea and entrap tears centrally. This may produce a plus tear film (Fig. 9-6) requiring more minus power for correction. If this occurs, a flatter lens rather than a power change is required.

10. In power, the thicker hyperopic lens may stand away from the paracentral portion of the cornea, creating a minus tear film (Fig. 9-6, *B*). This may result in 1 to 2 D more plus power required after the patient has been wearing the lens a week.

11. Lenses may give a pseudotight appearance on gross observation. One may apply, under slitlamp obervations, light finger touch on the lower lid to displace the lens upward. The lens should move easily and drop quickly, an indication of a safe fit. The old rule of a 0.5 to 1 mm lag may not necessarily apply to the extended-wear lenses, which require only minimal tear exchange.

A. Nesburn in a meeting outlined some fitting characteristics that are worth repeating, as follows.

Characteristics of a flat fit

1. Excessive movement and frequent dislocation of the lens occur.
2. Through a dilated pupil, a retinoscopic reflex is crisp centrally and distorted peripherally.
3. There may be conjunctival injection.
4. There is awareness of the lens.
5. Visual acuity is variable.

Characteristics of a steep fit

1. There is no movement of the lens when blinking.
2. The lens does not move easily when one attempts to move off center.
3. The limbal vessels may be congested.
4. The cornea may show microcystic edema or even gross edema.
5. If the pupil is dilated, the retinoscopic reflex will be distorted on blinking.
6. There is lens awareness.
7. The vision acuity is variable and will change with blinking

MANAGING AN EXTENDED-WEAR PRACTICE

There are two basic systems in managing an extended lens wearer. The majority of practitioners chose the method in which a single lens per eye is purchased, the patient either wears the lens for a definite period (such as 2 weeks to 2 months) or wears the lens without changing it until a sufficient coating of the lens occurs or problems arise so that a change of lens is required. An alternate method is to provide two lenses per eye initially and when the patient returns for monitoring the unused one is inserted and the previous lens is kept to be professionaly cleaned. Either method is suitable. One system may lend itself more for one patient than for another.

Management of extended wear

↙   ↘

Replace lens when required	Switch two lenses each visit and clean one

Once one has arrived at the initial lens selection either through an ordering system for diagnostic lenses or from an inventory system, one has to then decide on whether one will engage the patient in care systems for their extended-wear lenses.

Hartstein believes that extended-wear lenses are best left alone without removal until they cloud sufficiently from deposit formation. This of course minimizes hand-to-eye contamination and exposure to lens disinfectants with possible allergic reactions. On the other hand, we believe in removal and cleaning every 2 weeks or at least every month. Our studies on 386 lenses studied showed that lenses with no cleaning lasted on the average 5 months, lenses cleaned monthly or every 2 months lasted 9 months, and lenses cleaned weekly lasted 1 to 2 years. We believe a clean lens significantly improves comfort of the lens, clarity of vision, and prolongation of lens life.

Our routine for a new extended-wear lens patient, where possible, is to select the correct extended-wear lens from our inventory of lenses. The patient is then started on a daily wear handling routine for 7 days and then reports to the office on the morning of the eighth day, having slept with the lenses the night before. By going on a daily-wear routine first, the patient, we believe, complains less because of corneal and lid adaptation and learns how to insert and remove the lenses while being still sufficiently motivated. Myopic lenses are generally stable in fit and power and require no change.

At the 24-hour overnight check, visual acuity should be noted. A slitlamp examination will evaluate the fit, the movement of the lens, and the state of the cornea. Careful attention to corneal clarity is important. Epithelial edema with a drop in vision can best be visualized by retroillumination with a slitlamp beam. Stromal edema can best be detected by wrinkling of Descemet's membrane, particularly in the central part of the cornea. The limbal vasculature should be examined carefully.

Once the patient is examined on the eighth day after overnight wear, he is permitted to wear the lenses for 2 weeks and visits with us at the end of this period provided that there is satisfactory ocular performance of the eye lids. lenses are then examined along with the eyes, and the patient is permitted to continue wearing lenses as long as he continues wit the recommended care systems. Patients return at 3- and 6-month intervals. All are informed that we are problem oriented, and so they are asked to return, particularly if vision has decreased, they develop a red eye, or the lens becomes uncomfortable.

Comment. The merit of keeping the lenses in as long as possible is freedom from hand and chemical contamination. But why wait until the lens is cloudy and the eye red?

CARE

As noted previously, we believe that the extended-wear lens should have some form of cleaning. Adequate cleaning followed by disinfection increases the life of any lens and in particular extended-wear lenses.

The effects of coating of a lens are multiple:

1. Vision is decreased, often significantly, in the aging process of the lens and in the aged.
2. The increase in the mass of the lens alters the heaviness of the lens and so it rides low. This is more predominant with the high-plus lens.
3. The adhering deposit produces an antigen, which in turns gives rise to giant follicular conjunctivitis.
4. With deposits there may be a tightening of the lens and thus a parameter change. Vaulting at the corneal apex occurs, and so the power of the lens is reduced. A hyperopic lens requires more plus whereas a myopic lens requires more minus.
5. There is a decrease in the oxygen transmission of a deposit-ridden contact lens.

A number of systems for cleaning an extended-wear lens are available:

1. Enzymatic cleaning may be used. With high-water-content lenses there may be residual enzymatic activity in the lenses that may be mildly toxic to the cornea. We recommend reducing the enzymatic contact time to perhaps only 1 hour, cleaning with surfactant, rinsing well, and storing in normal saline solution.
2. Hydrogen peroxide, 3%, is an effective oxidation method that aids cleaning and also disinfection of a lens. The hydrogen peroxide penetrates the lens matrix causes lens expansion, and loosens parti-

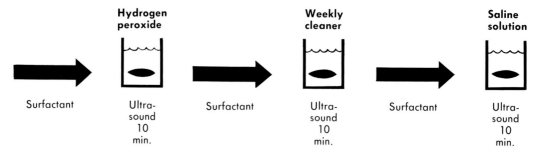

Fig. 28-11. Ultrasound method of cleaning a heavily coated lens through a system using hydrogen peroxide followed by cleaning in a weekly cleaner or enzymatic cleaner followed by purging with ultrasound in a saline bath.

cles within the lens and on the lens surface.

3. Ultrasound acts as a catalyst in speeding up any chemical used on a contact lens. It also generates heat, which also accelerates the cleaning process. Currently we recommend the ultrasound cleaner manufactured by BPI,* a biphasic unit that is gentle enough to clean a soft lens without damaging the plastic. This is an in-office unit to rejuvenate old lenses. Home units for prophylactic cleaning are available. Our system is to use any surfactant cleaner and place the lens in 3% hydrogen peroxide with ultrasound, followed by a further 10 minutes in a weekly cleaner or enzyme tablet for 10 minutes, followed by 10 minutes in normal saline solution (Fig. 28-11).

4. A variety of surfactants for soft lenses is available. These agents solubilize the residue accumulated and mobilize the surface deposits that have accumulated. We have been especially pleased with some of the more recent all-purpose surfactants, which appear to give superior cleaning results for all lenses and reduce the need for the enzyme tablet.

Although the cleaning system is only minimal for extended-wear as compared to daily-wear lenses, there has been a considerable decrease in the adverse response, toxic and allergic, that so frequently arises from daily use of thimerosal- and chlorhexidine-based products. It is most uncommon to see this phenomenon with extended-wear lenses.

*Brain Power Inc., Miami, Fla.

COMPLICATIONS AND PROBLEMS WITH EXTENDED WEAR

The majority of problems that were initially seen in the early days of extended wear have, in fact, faded with improvements in lens plastic, lens designs, and better care systems for extended-wear lenses. With the development of high-water-content lenses, very thin lenses, silicone lenses, and silicone-acrylate lenses, all possessing reasonable permeability (DK) values and adequate oxygen performance, we have today reasonably successful lenses for extended wear. To this we have a better understanding of who should and who should not wear extended-wear contact lenses.

In fitting extended-wear lenses one should be alerted to the following possible complications, which are then discussed more fully:

Early complications
1. Blurring vision
2. Acute keratopathy
3. Diffuse corneal edema
4. Tightening of lens
5. Lost lenses

Late complications
1. Lens problems
   a. Protein, lipid, or mineral buildup (hazy vision, corneal edema)
   b. Lens displacement
   c. Fungus invasion
   d. Glued-on lens syndrome
2. Patient problems
   a. Corneal vascularization
   b. Keratoconjunctivitis
   c. Corneal edema
   d. Corneal steepening
   e. Patient dropouts

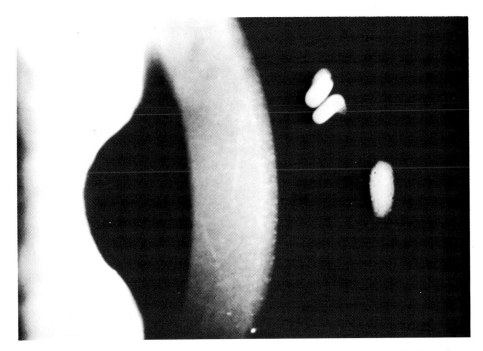

Fig. 28-12. Vertical striae are frequent occurrence during first 2 weeks of extended wear. Patient should be observed to determine that condition does not worsen and disappears within that time. Recurrence after several months of extended wear signals the fitter that the lens has become soiled. (From Feldman, G.L.: In Hartstein, J., ed.: Extended wear contact lenses for aphakia and myopia, St. Louis, 1982, The C.V. Mosby Co.)

Early complications

The following problems are sometimes seen with extended aphakic hydrophilic lens wear:

Blurring vision. A decrease in vision and morning blur may initially be adaptive symptoms caused by corneal hydration in the early days. This can be tolerated for 1 to 2 weeks because it is often a normal adaptive system, but, if it persists, a lens change in either a flatter fit or a new material is required. This early blurring of vision may also be caused by relative dehydration of high-water-content lenses during a dry state at night and may be helped by a nighttime and morning lubricating drop. The early manifestation may be fine vertical striae in Descemet's membrane (Fig. 28-12).

Acute keratopathy. Acute keratopathy is a serious complication that can occur at any time within the first 24 to 72 hours of wear. The cornea becomes edematous, with edema being present from endothelium to epithelium. Wrinkles may form in Descemet's membrane. The full diameter of the cornea is involved, not just the corneal cap as seen with rigid-lens overwear reactions, this last being limited in depth as well as in diameter.

There is pronounced ciliary injection, extensive swelling of both upper and lower lids, and some flare and cells in the anterior chamber. The patient is often prostrate with pain, similar to a rigid-lens overwear reaction.

This type of reaction occurs in normal aphakic corneas with no vitreous touch or endothelial dystrophy. This reaction may occur in aphakia but is uncommon in myopia. It is also uncommon if suitable extended-wear lenses are used.

Diffuse corneal edema. Diffuse corneal edema is a reaction to the presence of a hydrogel aphakic lens without the acute congestive components. The cornea becomes edematous and steamy, there is some circumcorneal injection, vision is impaired, and the patient is uncomfortable. Under these conditions the lens cannot be tolerated, since visual performance is too poor, and in the milder forms corneal vascularization eventually develops. Again, this reaction is rare if lenses that are designed for extended wear are chosen. However, overzealous practitioners still experiment with lenses for extended wear that are not in the manufacturer's design for extended wear.

In postcataract surgical cases in which we personally have attempted extended wear, we generally wait until the K readings are stabilized, the cornea is free of edema, there is no sign of postoperative inflammatory response, and the endothelium appears normal by slit-lamp assessment before insertion of the lenses. In the early years of extended-wear lenses we have attempted large fenestrations of HEMA lenses. We also made a minihydrophilic aphakic lens with a diameter of 9.5 mm, but this lens centered poorly, was uncomfortable, and did not facilitate extended wear. Each attempt at modifying a conventional lens for extended wear was poorly received. Fortunately with today's technology excellent oxygen-transmission lenses for extended wear have been developed.

Tightening of lens. The lens may become dehydrated during sleep, and this dehydration may lead to a tightening of the lens when the wearer arises in the morning. This tightening may cause limbal compression and a ciliary injection (Fig. 28-13).

Late complications

The following lens problems are frequently late complications of extended hydrophilic lens wear.

Protein and lipid buildup. Protein or lipid deposits on the surface of the lens occur anywhere from a few days to 1 year. Once protein is tenaciously deposited on the lenses, there is often hazy vision, an effective loss of clarity, and a change in the base curve of the lens (Fig. 28-14).

Mineral deposits. Calcium deposits, seen as white discrete surface deposits on a lens, frequently grow in size. They may grow sufficiently in size to penetrate the pore structure of the lens so that when they are removed they leave large holes in the matrix. These holes in the matrix are often sufficiently large to permit bacteria to enter the substance of the lens.

Lens displacement. Lens displacement is a frequent complication in aphakia, since elderly patients often rub their eyes, especially when they wake up. The mechanical displacement of the lens often results in a lens that is wrinkled or folded, lying in the upper or lower fornix. Sometimes these lenses split when the eyes are rubbed, and occasionally they are lost. In children the problem is even more common. Chil-

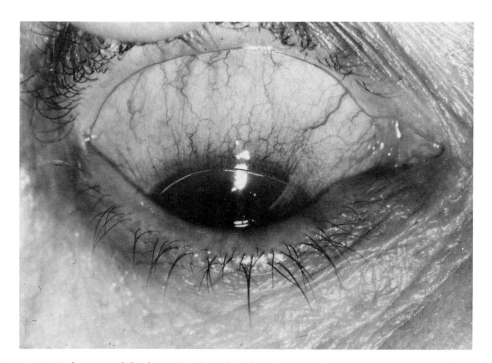

Fig. 28-13. Tightening of the lens. The lens dehydrated when the wearer was asleep, and it became immobile and caused limbal compression when he arose in the morning.

dren require larger lenses (15 mm diameter) because they frequently rub their lenses out.

Infections. Infections are very rare with extended-wear lenses. Extended-wear lenses actually minimize the hand-to-eye contamination that may occur with daily-wear lenses. There have, however, been isolated reports but not with the same degree as with rigid and soft daily-wear lenses. The only exception may be the possibility of spores of fungi, which may land on the soft lens, become adherent, and grow. Although they may destroy the outer surface of the soft lens, they do not invade the cornea, and no serious eye damage has been reported.

Corneal vascularization. Vascularization with today's lenses are very uncommon in our hands (Fig 28-15). It occurs if one selects improper lenses that are not designed for extended wear or if the patient is not carefully fitted so that the lenses are tight. It may occur if there is excess deposit formation on the lens, which alters the parameters of the lens. When seen, the vascularization is usually confined to the limbal area but may extend either superficially into the cornea or extend deep into the stromal area. Signs of deep stromal invasion are indicative of severe hypoxic changes and call for either steroid treatment along with a new and better-fitting lens or else complete discontinuance of extended-wear lenses. Usually in this case the vessels regress, and ghost vessels remain.

One should make some notation of the normal extent of vascularization that may be present at the superior limbus. If this is not identified, the fitter may believe that he or she has a lens-induced complication, which of course may not be true.

Marginal subepithelial infiltrates. Small round lesions occurring under the peripheral epithelium may occasionally be seen not only with daily-wear but also with extended-wear lenses. They may be small localized abcesses of *Staphylococcus aureus*. Alternatively they may be an allergic response of the cornea to antigen protein adherent to the contact lenses. Epithelial infiltrates have been reported by Josephson, Holden, and Zantos. Josephson has shown that lens-induced infiltrates may take up to 2½ months to resolve.

Minor corneal edema. Corneal edema is often undetected with the slitlamp microscope until there is at least an 8% increase in thickness as measured with the keratometer. Below this level early cases of corneal hypoxia can be detected by vertical striae.

Glued-on or "sucked-on" lens syndrome (tight-lens syndrome). The glued-on lens syndrome, reported by Wilson and associates, involves a tight, nonmovable lens that is associated with red eye (Fig. 28-16). Its cause is still

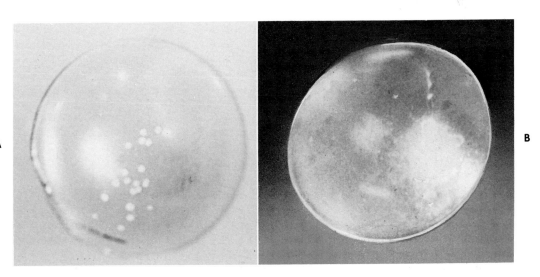

Fig. 28-14. A, Deposits on a soft lens. **B,** Protein buildup on a soft lens will vary with the duration of wear, the method of sterilization, and the tear composition and concentration of individual patients. (**A** from Stein, H.A., and Slatt, B.J.: The ophthalmic assistant, ed. 4, St. Louis, 1983, The C.V. Mosby Co.)

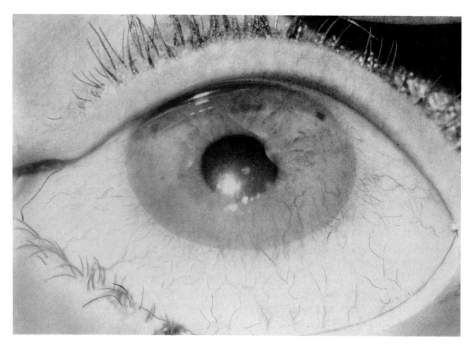

Fig. 28-15. Vascularization after use of low-water-content standard-thickness lens as an extended-wear lens.

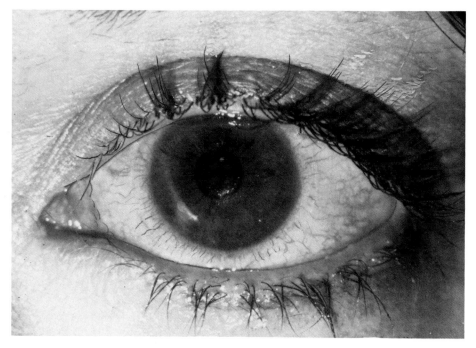

Fig. 28-16. Glued-on lens syndrome. Lens became adherent to the cornea and could not be dislodged causing corneal complications.

controversial, but it may result from chemical or pH changes that alter the steepness of the lens. It may be relieved by the use of alkaline drops such as Balanced Salt Solution.

Wilson postulates a shift to an acid PH because of lactic acid buildup at night with consequent tightening of the lens and trapping of mucus and debris under the lens. The treatment is to culture the conjunctiva, remove the lens for a week, and treat with antibiotics. After that insult, the patient should be placed in a morning and nighttime regimen of using an alkaline drop such as Blinks or Balanced Salt Solution. We have personally found this syndrome very uncommon in our practice.

Microcysts and vacuoles. With long-term wear of extended-wear lenses, Zantos and others have reported vacuoles and microcysts present in the midperiphery of the cornea in at least 40% of patients. These may clinically be indistinguishable from Cogan's microcystic dystrophy. They may be a result of prolonged low-level anaerobic cell respiration and the resulting lactic acid buildup. They clear in time when the lens is removed.

Fungal infection. The classic fungal infection of a slow-growing infiltrate with small hypopyon and perhaps slight hemorrhage in the anterior chamber requires a rigid response in management. Usually the laboratory must be extra helpful in providing adequate fungal cultures.

FURTHER COMPLICATIONS AND WHY THEY OCCUR

1. The eye needs at least 5% EOP (equivalent oxygen performance) to be sufficiently effective for corneal oxygenation.

2. A large percentage of corneal cells lie at the outer peripheral ring, and consequently neovascularization occurs in this area if there is insufficient EOP for this portion of the cornea. This can be obstructed by the thickness of a myopic lens at the periphery.

3. Contamination of a lens and infection is more likely to occur with daily-wear lenses, when the patient does not follow the recommended manufacturer's method of cleaning and disinfection. Extended-wear lenses minimize the handling problem, and consequently microbial contamination.

4. The deposits in extended-wear lenses according to Allansmith are diffusely coated, whereas daily-wear lenses show peaks and valleys in the coating. The deposits in extended-wear lenses are flatter and result in a smooth refracting surface. Within 8 hours 95% of the lens is covered. These deposits can be up to 1 μm in depth. However, the oxygen permeability is not decreased.

5. Some authors (Binder, Allansmith) contend that deposit formation on lenses does not impair the oxygen transmission. However, Richard Hill believes that there is a progressive decrease in oxygen transmission as deposits form on lenses. Once the lenses are cleaned, there is an increase gained in oxygen transmission. Koetting has shown that the BUT (tear-film breakup time) is less than 15 seconds and a coating will develop on continuous-wear lenses and shorten the life of the lens.

6. Binder and Worthen have shown that prophylactic antibiotics are not necessary with continuous-wear hydrophilic lenses.

7. Hill has indicated that a lens in areas of low humidity loses 20% of its water content in 5 minutes. He has shown that if the water content is lower there is a significant decrease in the EOP value and a reduction in oxygen flowing through the lens.

8. Farris and Gildar have developed a tear irregularity–determination test for dry eyes. In this a micropipette is used to collect a fine tear sample to be frozen and analyzed for the osmolarity content. He has shown that this is a more sensitive test for keratoconjunctivitis sicca than rose bengal staining.

9. Swimming may be a problem. Removal of extended-wear lenses is often impractical. We have reported on studies in which swimming in pool and lake water can be performed provided that the swimmer splashes water in the eyes for 1 minute and also does not remove the lenses after leaving the water. In ocean water the lenses may easily be lost, and swim goggles are advised.

10. The cost initially for obtaining extended-wear lenses may be higher, but the maintenance cost is considerably less than that for daily-wear lenses even when one adds the cost of replacing lenses.

11. Because disinfection of extended-wear lenses is considerably reduced, there is less chance of chemical toxic or allergic corneal insult.

12. Patients with filtering blebs may displace lenses and create a problem. There is an additional risk of irritating the bleb and giving rise to bacterial infection.

13. Avoid fitting patients with extended-wear lenses who live in remote areas that are inaccessible to eye care.

14. In aphakia large postoperative astigmatism may be a limiting factor unless the patient understands that an over-corrective spectacle lens will be worn.

15. All topical eye solutions and surfactants may be used with the contact lens; ointments should be avoided because they blur vision.

CONCLUSION

The thrust in this decade is the normalization of myopia. Radial keratotomy surgeons and orthokeratology specialists have created a large demand. We have witnessed the technologic advance in a better and safer contact lens that can be worn on an extended basis. In addition better care products for these lenses have improved to the point where extended-wear lenses are a feasible alternative to these other modalities for the correction of myopic and hyperopic refractive errors.

Although the prospect of fitting the young myopic person with extended-wear lenses is much better than that of the aphakic person because of the thin lens centers, healthier corneas, and better tear film often found in myopic persons, the risk-to-benefit ratio warrants its use in fitting the aphakic. We have now reached a stage where a prolonged extended-wear lens for aphakia has become a reality and emphasis needs to be placed on better monitoring and delegation of systems to ancillary personnel.

As lens technology advances, even more improved systems will undoubtedly be developed for visual restoration and be made available. Although careful monitoring of prolonged-wear aphakic patients is still the guideline of a careful and responsible fitter, the monitoring technique presently established may become more streamlined as confidence develops in extended-wear lenses. The safety of the lens system for prolonged wear may ultimately provide a safer alternative and sharper spectacle-free final visual acuity than the intraocular lens does for the aphakic person. It may be a safer alternative for the myope than refractive keratoplasty is.

CHAPTER 29

BANDAGE LENSES

James V. Aquavella
Harold A. Stein
Bernard J. Slatt

Therapeutic use of bandage
lenses

General principles of bandage
lenses

Other uses of therapeutic soft
lenses

THERAPEUTIC USE OF BANDAGE LENSES

JAMES V. AQUAVELLA*

The term "hydrophilic *bandage* lens" is utilized when the lens is fitted primarily as a therapeutic modality, in contrast to the fitting of a corrective lens when the goal is solely for the elimination of refractive error. In most instances the bandage lens will have plano (zero) power; however there are many situations when it is desirable to include refractive power though the lens is being utilized primarily for bandage purposes. Even if refractive power will ultimately be indicated, a thin plano lens should be tried first.

Although a wide variety of hydrophilic lenses is currently available, two basic manufacturing techniques are utilized—the spin-casting and the lathe-cutting techniques. The various hydrophilic lenses vary in design and polymeric constitution. For bandage purposes the primary concerns are the properties of flexibility, permeability, and architectural configuration of the lens. These properties will vary with the observed thickness, diameter, and curvature of the finished bandage lens.

Indications for therapeutic lenses

Indications for therapeutic lenses may be divided into medical and surgical and are listed in the outlines on this page.

*M.D., F.A.C.S., Director, Department of Ophthalmology, Park Ridge Hospital; Medical Director, Rochester Eye Bank; Clinical Associate Professor of Ophthalmology, University of Rochester, Rochester, N.Y.

Medical indications for hydrophilic bandage lens therapy

Chronic corneal edema (bullous keratopathy, Fuchs' dystrophy)
Abrasions, erosions, ulcerations
Keratitis filamentosa
Chemical keratitis (including alkaline burns)
Neurotrophic keratitis
Neuroparalytic keratitis
Herpetic keratitis (stromal disease)
Dry-eye syndromes (keratitis sicca, benign mucosal pemphigoid, Stevens-Johnson syndrome)
Ectatic dystrophies (keratoconus)
Anterior membrane corneal dystrophies
Lid problems (entropion, trichiasis, defects)

Surgical indications for hydrophilic bandage lens therapy

Postoperative discomfort
Lacerations
Perforations
Penetrating keratoplasty (especially in infants and alkaline burns)
Lamellar keratoplasty
Keratectomy
Thermokeratoplasty
Cyanoacrylate adhesives

Fig. 29-1 represents an eye with severe painful bullous keratopathy after perforating injury with subsequent cataract extraction and glaucoma procedure. The eye is painful and there is no hope of visual rehabilitation. A hydrophilic bandage lens is a simple, nonsurgical option. A relatively tight fit with only 1 to 2 mm of motion will afford better pain relief. If unsuccessful, enucleation may be considered.

Fig. 29-2 is a case of Fuchs' dystrophy with secondary bullous keratopathy and a visual acuity limited to counting fingers. In Fig. 29-3 we see the appearance of the eye with a hydro-

philic bandage lens in place. Note the reduction in edema and the regularity of the surface. The acuity was only improved to 20/200, and penetrating keratoplasty was subsequently successfully performed. A therapeutic trial with hydrophilic lenses in such a case is often indicated because of its simplicity. In this particular instance there was no significant discomfort and the rationale for lens application was strictly related to an attempt to improve the acuity. A relatively flat fit will afford optimum acuity.

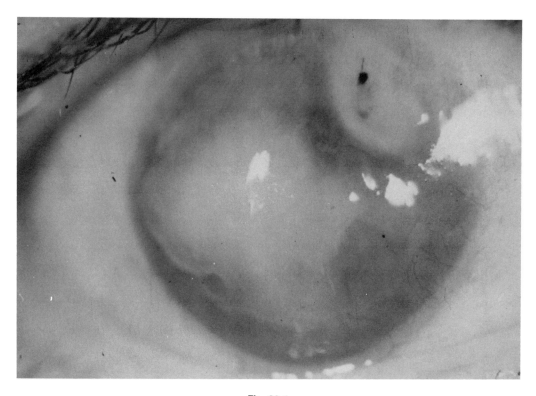

Fig. 29-1

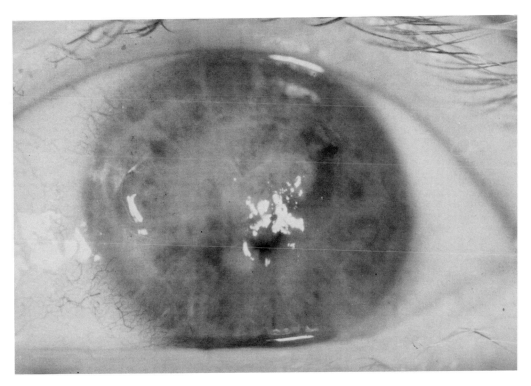

Fig. 29-2

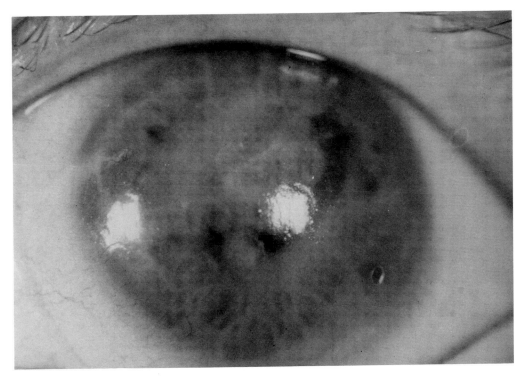

Fig. 29-3

In Fig. 29-4 a case of aphakia with endothelial decompensation and epithelial edema can be seen. Fig. 29-5 reveals the appearance of the eye with a thin hydrophilic bandage in place. The visual acuity in this instance was improved (with spectacle over-correction) from 20/200 to 20/60. Our experience has shown that flat-fitting high-water-content lenses will provide best results in these cases.

Fig. 29-6 shows another case of aphakia with endothelial decompensation and secondary edema. In this particular instance the bandage lens was not efficacious in reducing corneal edema. Our preference in such a case is to begin treatment with frequent instillation of hypertonic saline solution alone. If the intraocular pressure is elevated, topical or systemic glaucoma medication is also utilized. Only when these conventional means have not resulted in improvement do we resort to a trial with a hydrophilic lens. We generally prefer the use of a thin, relatively high fluid content lathe-cut lens with plano power. The patient should be comfortable and, if able, may insert and remove the lens on a daily basis. Hypertonic saline solution is prescribed for use over the lens. Refitting and attempts at over-refraction are performed; if substantial improvement is to be obtained, it will usually occur in 1 month to 6 weeks. At this point over-refraction utilizing a K reading taken from the front surface of the hydrophilic lens is performed. The aphakic patient may then be fitted with a pair of aphakic spectacles. If an aphakic lens is utilized, the patient should be watched very closely. Because of the increased thickness in the aphakic lens and subsequently reduced oxygen permeability, there are cases in which the eye will not support the use of the aphakic bandage lens but will do nicely with the thin plano lens system.

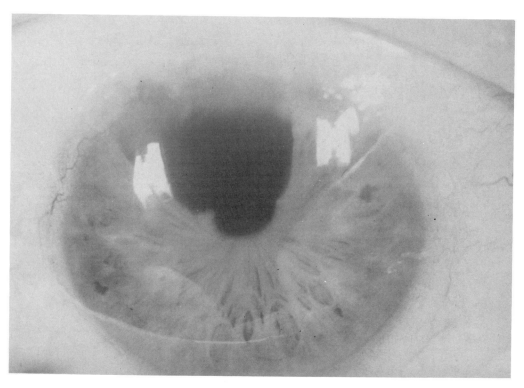

Fig. 29-4

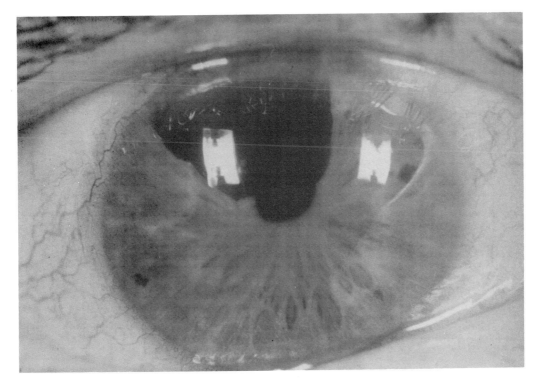

Fig. 29-5

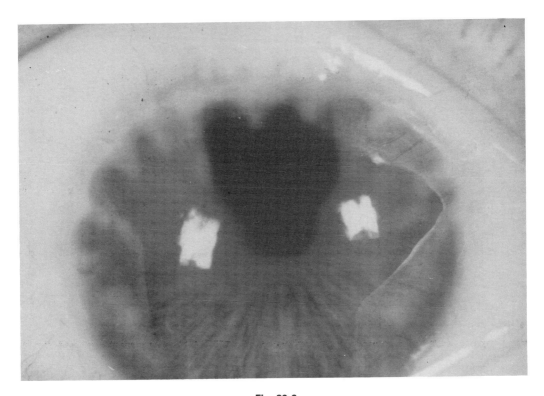

Fig. 29-6

Fig. 29-7 reveals an eye with an old scarred cornea with the presence of a recurrent erosion. Note the irregularity of the epithelial surface indicated by the light reflexes. In fitting such a patient one should try not to utilize a local anesthetic so that the patient's comfort may be readily ascertained. One should have available a variety of lenses. We currently prefer the Permalens or Sauflon lenses. The CSI thin bandage lens is also highly desirable. On occasion a thin Softcon or Hydrocurve lens will work best. The principle in fitting the eye will depend on the specific location of the eroded area. Ideally, the lens should clear the eroded area, and a slightly steep fitting situation is indicated at least in the first few days. In addition one would hope to achieve a fit that would demonstrate only 1 or 2 mm of movement. Excess movement in erosion cases can sometimes result in increased discomfort. If the lens applied is very steep, 24 to 48 hours of increased stromal edema may result when one checks the appearance of the eye with the slitlamp. Consequently, a slightly flatter fit situation may be indicated. In most cases of erosions and abrasions the patient may be expected to have considerable discomfort periodically, even with the lens, for the first 48 to 72 hours. For this reason it is often wise to instill cycloplegics and to warn the patient that he or she will feel discomfort for the first few days.

If the lens has been utilized in a case of recurrent erosion, one should recall that 4 to 6 weeks are necessary for newly formed epithelial cells to produce an adequate basement membrane. In many cases, if the vision is adequate, the lens can be allowed to remain in place for 6 months to 1 year. We prefer to utilize topical instillation of artificial tear solution three or four times daily in such cases of long-term wear.

Fig. 29-8 represents the appearance of a 25-year-old patient with a combination of neurotrophic and neuroparalytic keratitis in a totally dry eye. She was fitted with a hydrophilic lens with parameters of plano power, 14.0 mm diameter, and 8.1 mm radius of curvature. There was no contact between the posterior surface of the lens and the ulcerated area. It was necessary for artificial tear solutions to be instilled every ½ to 1 hour. Occasionally antibiotics and steroids were utilized for long periods of time. With this regimen visual acuity of 20/30 was achieved. One should realize that all of the dry-eye conditions are prone to secondary infection and inflammatory episodes. In addition, they are among the most difficult conditions to treat with or without hydrophilic lenses. Nevertheless in many cases the risks are relatively minor and the potential reward is great.

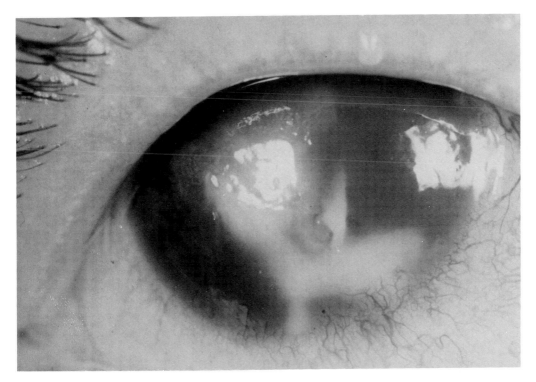

Fig. 29-7

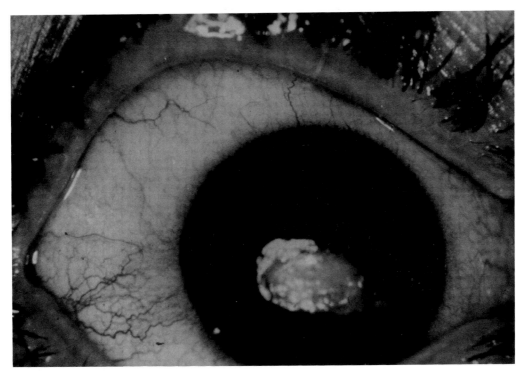

Fig. 29-8

Fig. 29-9 shows the blepharitis that often accompanies keratitis sicca. In Fig. 29-10 we see the degree of corneal involvement in the same patient as seen in Fig. 29-9. With the application of a hydrophilic lens and frequent artificial tear solution, accompanied by application of prophylactic antibiotics, the visual acuity as well as the physical appearance of the lesion improved within 2 weeks. Fig. 29-11 shows the eye after only 2 weeks of therapy. Lid scrubs, systemic antibiotics for severe blepharitis, topical antibiotics and steroids, and copious irrigation with artificial tear solutions are all necessary in these cases. Lenses used in patients with dry eyes should be disinfected and cleaned more frequently than when there is a normal tear flow. On occasion the dry-eye patients will develop deposits on their lens in very short periods of time. This can be managed by the use of frequent friction cleaning, by the use of the enzymatic hydrophilic lens cleaner, and often by the dispensing of two lenses for the patient. In some instances neovascularization will present a problem, and modified wearing schedules may very well be necessary. In all instances one should eliminate the environmental conditions that may result in further drying. Punctate occlusion, moist chamber goggles, and ocular inserts also may be indicated as part of a comprehensive therapeutic plan.

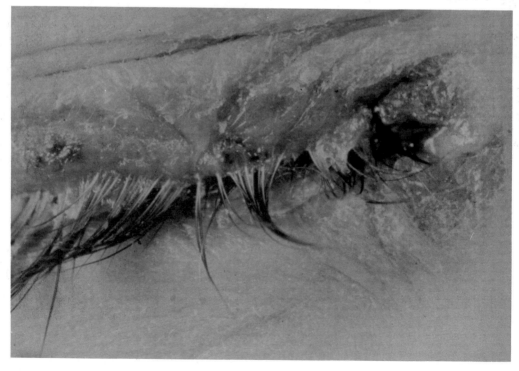

Fig. 29-9

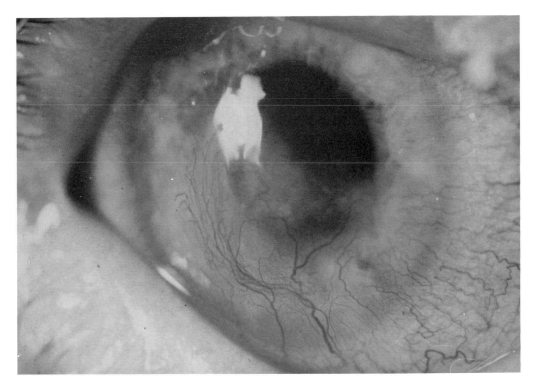

Fig. 29-10

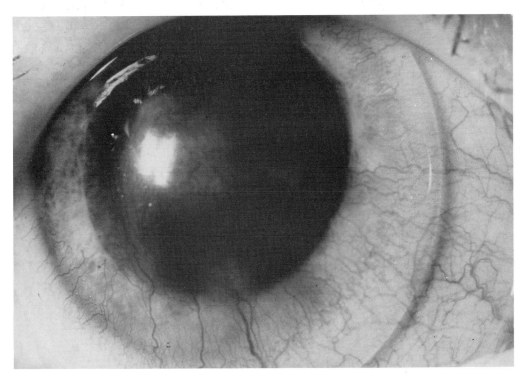

Fig. 29-11

Fig. 29-12 shows an acutely inflamed eye with marginal ulceration. This lesion was very painful and was believed to be nonherpetic. The condition responded quickly to treatment with a hydrophilic bandage and topical instillation of both antibiotics and steroids. The ability of the hydrophilic lens to ensure all-over wetting in such irregular lesions is paramount in the therapeutic efficacy. A large-diameter lens to bridge the lesion will be comfortable.

Fig. 29-13 shows the appearance of an eye with severe marginal degeneration that is being treated with a thin lens. Note the serpiginous peripheral ulceration. Not all of these cases respond to hydrophilic lens therapy, but the use of the lens combined with other therapeutic modalities is often extremely helpful.

In Fig. 29-14 is an eye with exposure keratitis with the inferior lateral third of the cornea severely affected. The lesion responded rapidly with application of a hydrophilic lens and topical administration of antibiotics and steroids. A partial lateral tarsorrhaphy was performed after the inflammation had subsided. Very often a partial lateral tarsorrhaphy will be helpful in maintaining seating and hydration of the hydrophilic lens. Without proper lid action it is difficult for the lens to be maintained in its proper position and there is more of a tendency for the lens to dry.

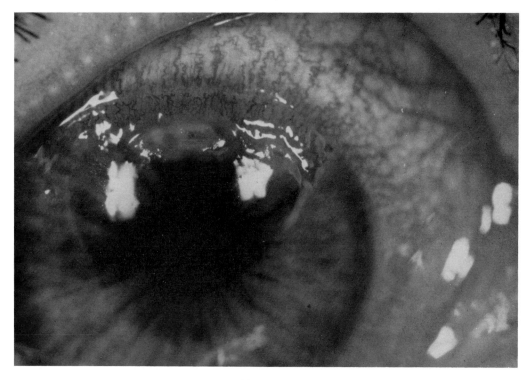

Fig. 29-12

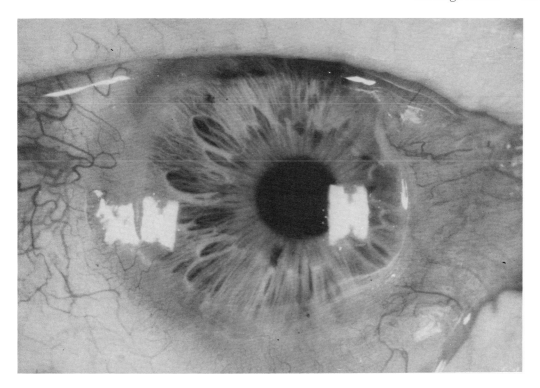

Fig. 29-13

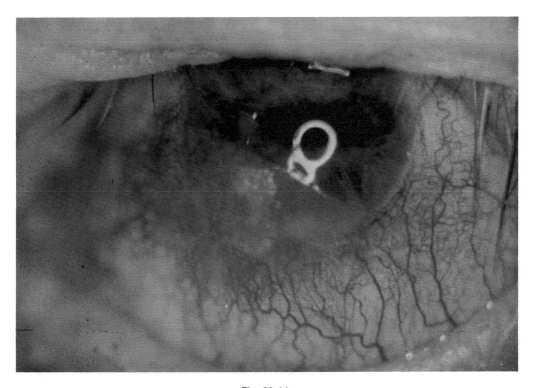

Fig. 29-14

Fig. 29-15 shows a rather extensive recurrent erosion. In treating such lesions with hydrophilic bandage lenses, it is often wise to obtain cycloplegia to prevent the development of secondary ciliary spasm. Large, rather tight lenses to relieve pain are preferred.

In Fig. 29-16 we see an almost totally opaque cornea as the result of an alkaline burn. However, the central corneal area is very thin and irregular and the application of the hydrophilic bandage lens improved the acuity from seeing hand motions to 20/80.

For the surgical indications for hydrophilic bandage lenses see the outlined indications on p. 361.

Fig. 29-17 demonstrates the use of a hydrophilic bandage lens in a patient who had an excision of a hypertrophic filtering bleb. A partial peripheral keratectomy was necessary, and the application of a bandage lens resulted in a comfortable eye during the postoperative period. The lens can be applied on the operating table.

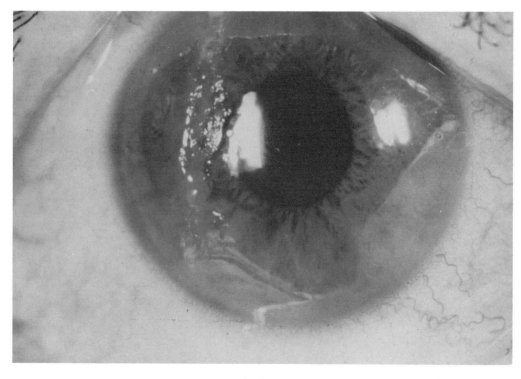

Fig. 29-15

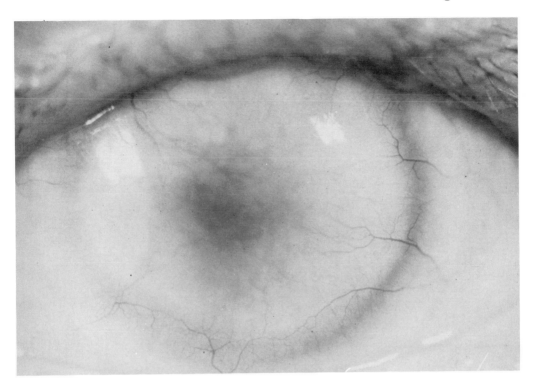

Fig. 29-16

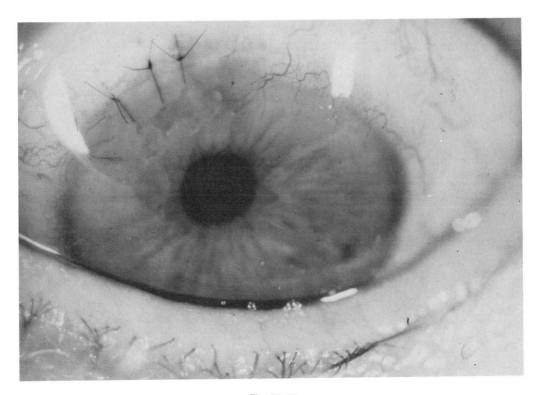

Fig. 29-17

Fig. 29-18 demonstrates the use of a hydrophilic bandage lens in a case of spastic entropion with secondary corneal ulceration. Although surgical intervention is certainly indicated to restore the normal function of the lower lid, application of the hydrophilic bandage assists in obtainment of a comfortable eye until the surgery can be performed.

Fig. 29-19 illustrates the use of a hydrophilic bandage lens before keratoplasty. This patient, with a severe alkaline burn, had a very irregu-

lar calcified corneal surface with secondary inflammation and blepharospasm. The application of a hydrophilic lens combined with topical medication helped to quiet the eye before surgery.

Fig. 29-20 shows the postoperative appearance of a 10 mm graft in a case of keratoconus. Notice the paracentral area of corneal drying as a result of inadequate wetting of the surface associated with the plateau effect produced by the running monofilament nylon sutures.

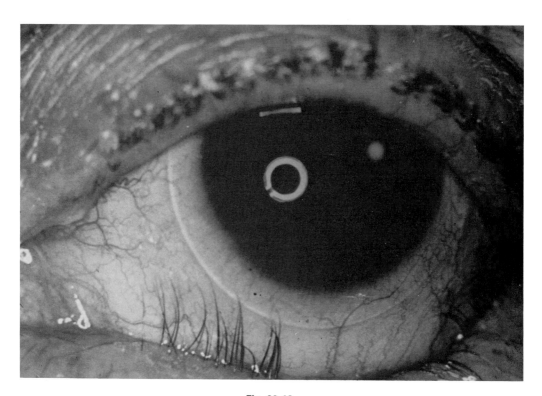

Fig. 29-18

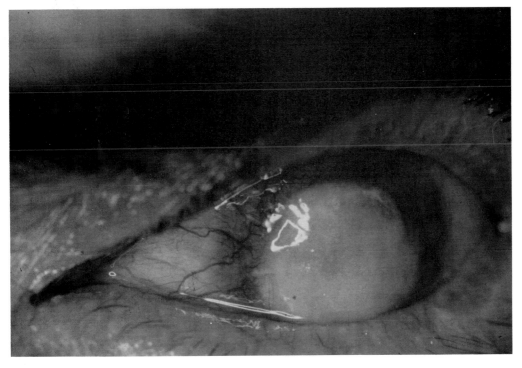

Fig. 29-19

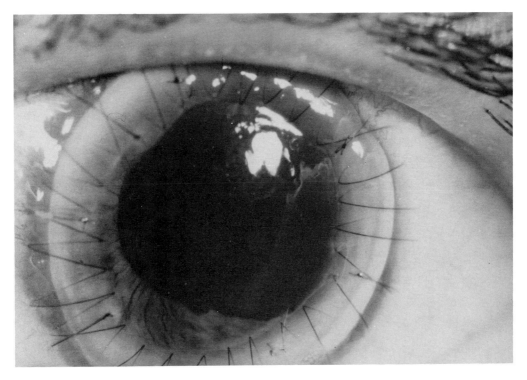

Fig. 29-20

In Fig. 29-21 we see the same case after application of a large lens ensuring the adequate wetting of the surface of the graft.

Fig. 29-22 shows another postoperative corneal graft in which the application of a hydrophilic lens has assisted in obtainment of proper wetting of the surface of the graft. The high-water-content, thin lenses are most useful in postoperative keratoplasty.

Fig. 29-23 shows the appearance of an eye after severe chemical injury with deep central ulceration and peripheral vascularization. The hydrophilic lens was utilized both preoperatively and postoperatively. In transplants performed in dry eyes and in eyes with chemical keratitis, the application of a hydrophilic bandage lens for the postoperative period assists in the preservation of the grafted epithelial cells.

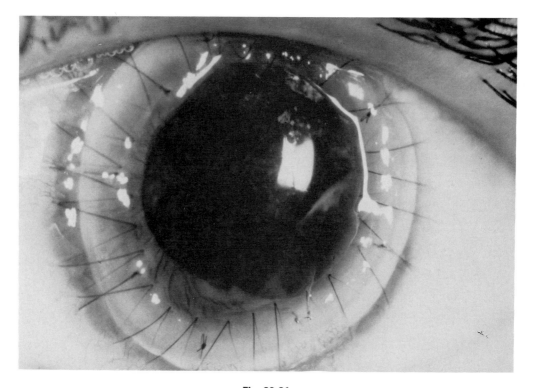

Fig. 29-21

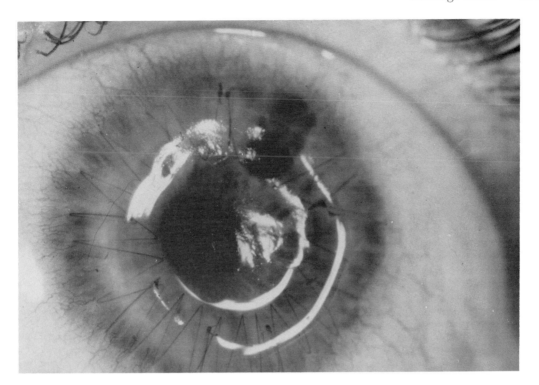

Fig. 29-22

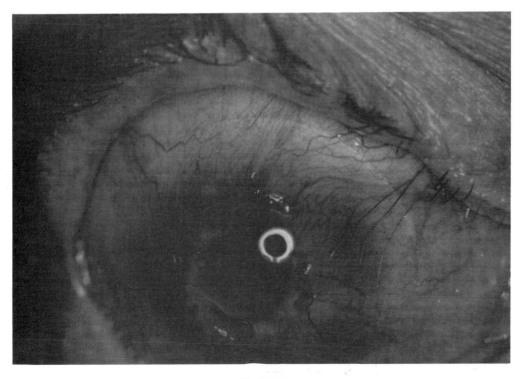

Fig. 29-23

Fig. 29-24 shows a well-centered lens that has been fitted in a case of keratitis sicca. Generally speaking, in cases where it is important to preserve maximum visual acuity while the bandage lens is being worn, a well-centering lens with virtual contact between the posterior surface of the lens and the anterior corneal surface will usually afford maximum acuity.

Fig. 29-25 demonstrates a lens that is decentered inferiorally. Although such a lens may be perfectly adequate to control discomfort in bullous keratopathy, we should ensure that the lens does not have a tendency to become displaced with a blink and with ocular rotations. However, in a case of recurrent erosion a lens that is loose may move excessively on the corneal surface and produce secondary irritation and occasionally blepharospasm.

Fig. 29-26 shows a lens that is so flat that the peripheral lip of the lens has become everted. If the edges of the bandage lens tend to flare, they can produce discomfort. It is important to inspect the periphery of the bandage lens with a slitlamp to determine that the lens is neither flaring or gripping so tightly as to produce a suction-cup effect.

Comment. Another cause for an eventful edge of a lens is that the lens was applied to the eye inside out.

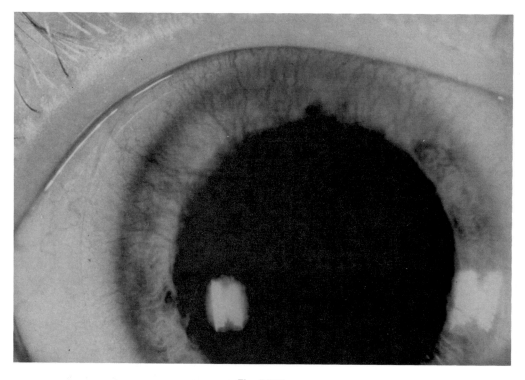

Fig. 29-24

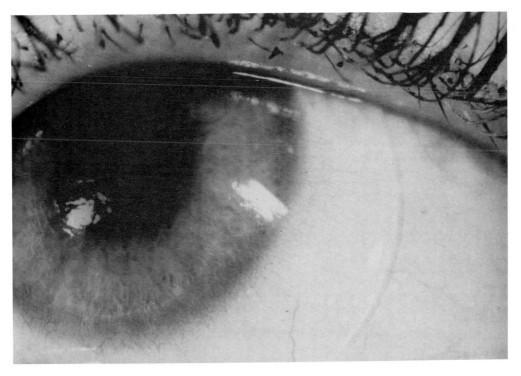

Fig. 29-25

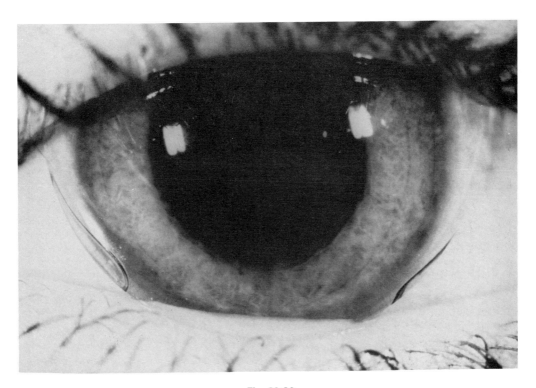

Fig. 29-26

Table 29-1. Thickness of Bausch & Lomb lenses

	Plano T*	*Plano U$_4$*	*Plano O$_4$*	*O$_4$ series (−2.00 D)*
Thickness	0.10 mm	0.07 mm	0.06 mm	0.03 mm
Diameter	14.7 mm	14.5 mm	14.5 mm	14.5 mm

*Capital letters mean thickness; subscript numbers mean diameter.

GENERAL PRINCIPLES OF BANDAGE LENSES

HAROLD A. STEIN

BERNARD J. SLATT

Bandage lenses are those contact lenses used for therapeutic purposes on a cornea to enhance epithelial regeneration and corneal healing. They provide sufficient oxygenation to the cornea so as to minimally disturb corneal physiology. In addition, bandage lenses are used to provide ocular comfort and a barrier to the cornea from the eyelids, lashes, and environmental conditions.

Because the thickness affects the oxygen permeability of a contact lens, the thinner the lens, the greater its oxygen permeability is. Since the pioneering days of Bausch & Lomb with the plano T series and the Softcon lens with a 55% water content, great strides continue to be made in achieving a better contact lens with a better oxygen permeability and consequently providing a greater oxygen supply to the cornea.

A comparison of the relative thickness of the Bausch & Lomb lenses is shown in Table 29-1. It is noteworthy that if a very thin lens is required the lenses of the plano O series have a center thickness of 0.06 mm. The standard O series are half this thickness, 0.03 mm, and are often used when an even greater amount of oxygen is required. They are however more flimsy in handling with a greater tendency to wrinkling and edge rolling. If the standard O series of Bausch & Lomb are used, or the ultrathin series of other manufacturers, it is more practical to select a −2 or −3 D from an inventory set.

The CSI (Crofilcon) lens may be used as a bandage lens and has the advantage of uniform thickness throughout the lens body. It is available in a 14.0 mm diameter, three base curves (8.6, 8.9, and 9.35 mm), and in lower minus powers.

High-water-content lenses, usually 8.1, 14.0 plano, with 70% to 80% water, have an additional advantage in the therapeutic range by providing moisture to the cornea, and minimizing dehydration of the cornea in dry-eye syndromes. In addition, for every 10% increase in water content of a soft hydrogel lens, there is a 50% increase in the equivalent oxygen performance so that a 60%-water hydrogel lens, having 20% more water than a standard 40%-water lens, has 2 times the equivalent oxygen performance at the same thickness. This factor may be extremely important in the selection of high-plus therapeutic lenses for bullous keratopathy of aphakia or marginal aphakic corneas in which the thickness cannot be sacrificed because of power requirements of the lens.

Conditions that lend to therapy with a bandage soft lens include both corneas with broken epithelial surface (minimal movement lens) and corneas with intact epithelial surface.

Corneas with broken epithelial surface

Conditions in this category with which a minimal movement lens should be used include the following:

1. Recurrent corneal erosion
2. Painful bullous keratopathy with ruptured bullae (Fig. 29-27)
3. Corneal ulcerations (Figs. 29-28 to 29-31)
4. Thermal burns (Fig. 29-32)
5. Corneal lacerations with sharp, well-opposed margins
6. Severe forms of vernal conjunctivitis (Fig. 29-33)
7. Perforated cornea

Therapeutic lenses may be left in place day and night for months. In particular, patients with painful bullous keratopathy are so relieved to have their lenses that often they are frightened to take them out. Such patients should return every 1 to 2 months to the practitioner for removal, thorough cleaning, and disinfec-

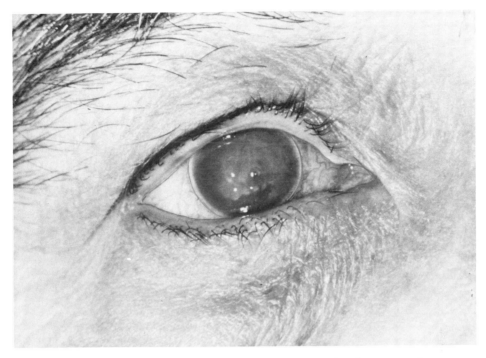

Fig. 29-27. Painful bullous keratopathy relieved by a soft bandage contact lens.

tion or replacement of the lenses. Replacement is usually the least practical. Otherwise the lenses become coated with mucus debris and mineral deposits and may form a bacterial culture medium. In addition protein deposits can cause anoxia of the cornea or change the fitting characteristics of the lens by making it steeper.

A soft lens makes an excellent splint for small corneal lacerations and perforations until healing takes place. The corneal epithelium requires an intact basement membrane for tight adhesion of the new epithelium; the soft lens will aid in this formation.

Corneas with intact epithelial surface

A lens with normal movement should be used if the corneal epithelium is intact. Better vision is obtained and the movement of the lens aids in tear exchange.

Conditions that respond to a normal moving lens include the following:

1. Dry-eye syndrome (Fig. 29-34)
2. Keratoconus
3. Corneal dystrophies
4. Entropion, trichiasis, etc., to prevent lash irritation of cornea
5. Neuroparalytic keratopathy

6. Ptosis with paralysis of superior rectus muscle (Fig. 29-35)
7. Aphakia with marginal corneas

Ancillary medication must frequently be employed with the soft lens in place. The medication must be water soluble; therefore substances that are soluble in oil, are in suspensions, or are in gels cannot be used. If steroids are to be employed, it is important to use soluble steroids rather than those in suspensions, since the latter settle out on the soft lens surface.

Cycloplegics should be used for painful corneal disease, antibiotics for corneal ulcers of a bacterial origin, and tear supplements for dry-eye syndromes.

Standard drops containing preservatives are employed. Freshly prepared solutions without preservatives are easily contaminated. Preservative concentration in the presence of routine drop administration is not a clinical concern. All epinephrine and epinephrine-like drops should be avoided because they discolor the soft lens.

A plano lens is the most desirable bandage lens, since it is thin over the entire extent of its diameter whereas a lens with plus or minus

Text continued on p. 387.

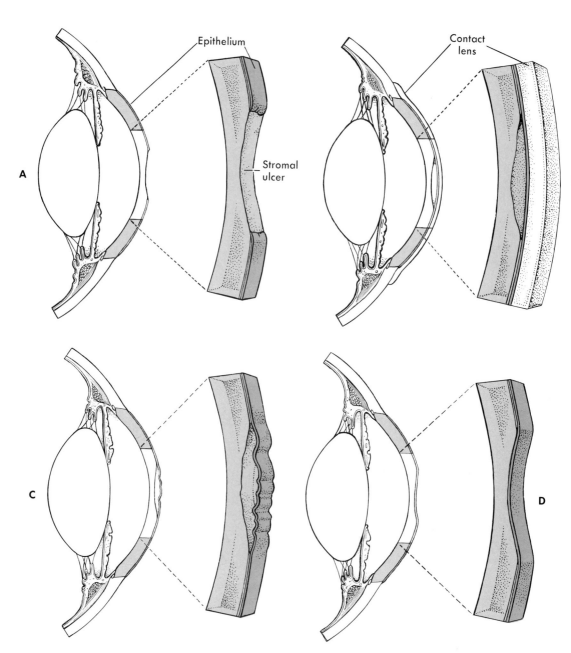

Fig. 29-28. Use of a soft lens to aid healing of a central stromal ulcer of herpes simplex origin, **A,** is depicted schematically. After the lens has been in place for some time, new epithelium bridges the ulcer site, **B.** When the lens is removed, **C,** the regenerated epithelium may initially appear as a flaccid bulla. Eventually regenerated tissue settles into the ulcer crater and adheres to the surface of the cornea, **D.** (**A** to **D** from Baum, J.L.: Hosp. Pract. **8**(8):89-95, Aug. 1973, and modified from Leibowitz, H.M., and Rosenthal, P.: Arch. Ophthalmol. **85**(2):165, 1971.)

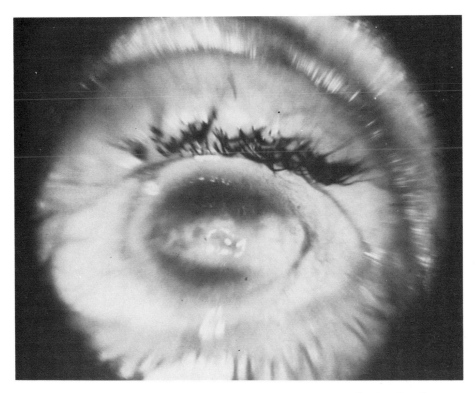

Fig. 29-29. Central corneal ulcer that responded to treatment with a bandage lens.

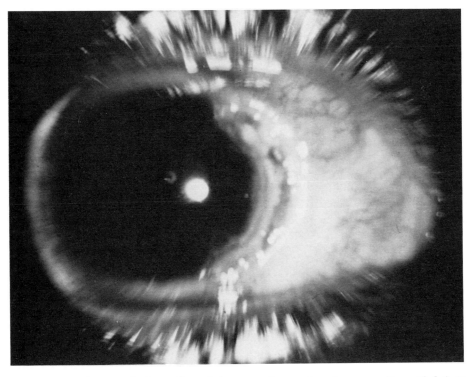

Fig. 29-30. Mooren's corneal ulcer. The soft lens may be employed temporarily until definitive therapy can be employed.

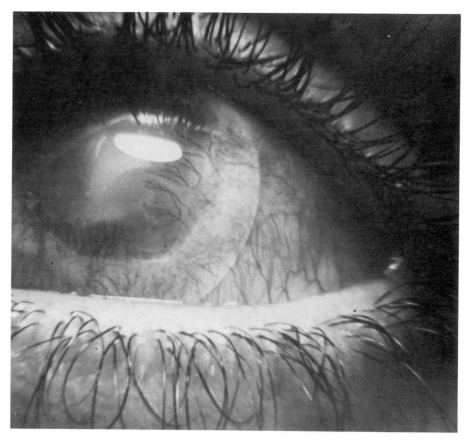

Fig. 29-31. Alkali burn of the eye. The soft lens provides a basis for the regeneration of epithelium to occur over the necrotic, ulcerated cornea.

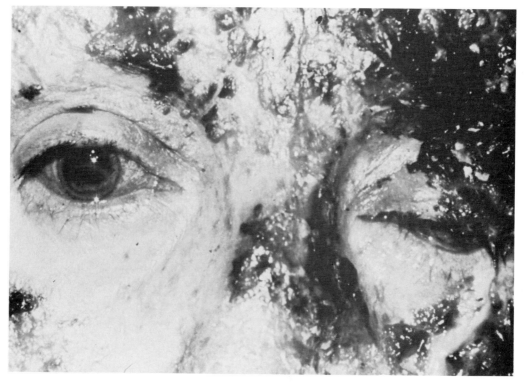

Fig. 29-32. Thermal burn around the eyes. The bandage lens can be used to heal the ulcerated cornea and prevent corneal exposure from lid retraction induced by scarring.

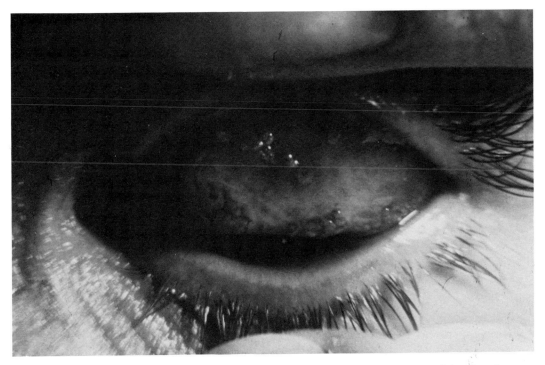

Fig. 29-33. Vernal conjunctivitis. Severe form with corneal ulceration requiring soft bandage lens for comfort and healing of the corneal ulcer.

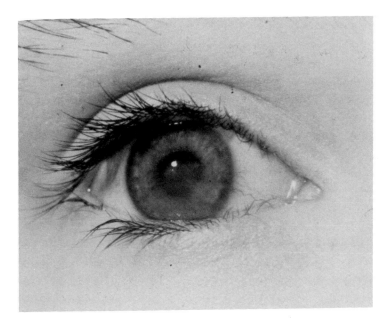

Fig. 29-34. Riley-Day syndrome. The soft lens protects the cornea from drying and erosion.

Fig. 29-35. The soft lens may be employed for corneal protection after surgery for ptosis where there is associated paralysis of the superior rectus muscle.

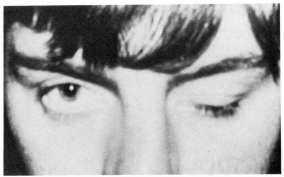

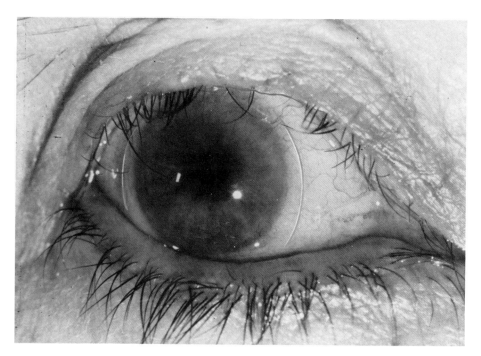

Fig. 29-36. Trichiasis of the upper lid after surgical removal of a carcinoma. The bandage lens protects the cornea from irritation.

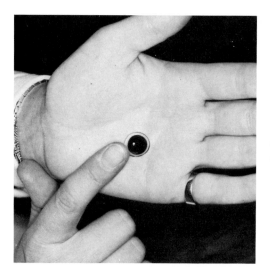

Fig. 29-37. Colored soft lens to cover cosmetically disfigured eyes. (From Stein H.A., and Slatt, B.J.: The ophthalmic assistant, ed. 4, St. Louis, 1983, The C.V. Mosby Co.)

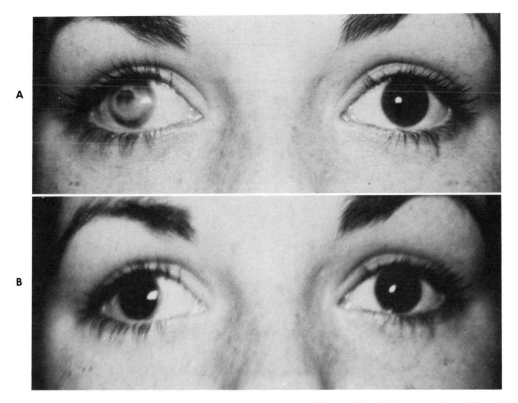

Fig. 29-38. Scarred, unsightly corneas, **A,** may be covered by a colored, therapeutic soft lens, **B.**

power has a thicker center or periphery. In aphakics, however, with marginal corneas, or bullous keratopathy, where power requirements may be necessary, high-water-content lenses are more valuable in our hands.

Fitting the bandage lens

Bandage therapeutic lenses may be fitted with minimal or no movement as in the case of those corneas in which there is a broken epithelial surface. One may select these lenses steeper simply by increasing the diameter. The clinical appearance in the slitlamp is most usable in this determination because the flatness of a cornea with ulceration cannot be detected by keratometric reading. If there is lens movement in a denuded epithelial cornea with a conventional plano lens, a low-power lens with a known diameter and base curve should be selected.

In those eyes in which the cornea has healed or the surface is intact, so that there is barrier protection from trichiasis or entropion (Fig. 29-36), the lenses should have some movement,

0.5 to 1 mm, to permit some tear exchange and transfer of metabolic products.

OTHER USES OF THERAPEUTIC SOFT LENSES

1. Filling the plateau created by a graft immediately after a corneal transplant.
2. Covering a disfigured eye (Fig. 29-37). Meschel has pioneered tinting of soft lenses as a shell and produced irises on soft lenses. Several soft lens companies in Canada, Europe, and Japan have available colored soft lenses with black pupils that can cover a disfigured eye (Fig. 29-38). In addition a photographic process can be used to match the color of the soft lens with the iris of the fellow eye. These are referred to as iris-print lenses. Some practitioners have used epinephrine to turn a soft lens brown, but these lenses are not nearly so effective as lenses that are manufactured for this purpose.
3. Protecting the cornea during retinal and orbital surgery.

4. Used as a cutaway pie for insertion of sutures in corneal transplants. Here a pie shape is cut away and used to splinter the corneal graft and maintain the anterior chamber while the cornea is sutured.

   Comment. A soft lens is not a panacea. Sometimes it does not work in conditions in which it is expected to work. Our best therapeutic use of the soft lens appears to be its use for indolent corneal ulcers and for bullous keratopathy. The use of the soft lens may, in many cases, temporize the problem of corneal disease and preserve future options of therapy.

5. The treatment of amblyopia in young children by soft lenses has been reported. A high-plus lenticular lens placed over the best seeing eye acts as a blurring lens and permits the amblyopic eye to develop its visual potential. The soft lens is used for daytime wear in children, and the parent is instructed in its insertion and removal.

6. Although soft lenses cannot usually seal a hole in a ruptured glaucomatous bleb, they may be employed as an efficient mechanism to seal a leaking postoperative cataract wound and reform the anterior chamber.

7. Bandage lenses have only limited value in neurotrophic keratitis and mild cases of keratoconjunctivitis sicca. Usually they must be supplemented with artificial tears and antibiotics.

8. In keratoconus, a thin plano therapeutic lens may be used as part of a piggyback system in which a rigid lens is placed in front.

CHAPTER 30

PRACTICAL PROBLEMS AND THEIR SOLUTION: CASE ANALYSIS

Keith W. Harrison*
Jean-Pierre Chartrand‡

The purpose of this chapter is to illustrate some common problems associated with contact lens wear. All cases cited are patients that have been seen and treated in our office. It is our belief that one of the most important aspects of a successful practice is effective troubleshooting. The practitioner who is able to solve the patient's problems will not only keep that patient but also will receive word-of-mouth referrals. The unsuccessful troubleshooter will not only lose the "problem patient" but also potential new patients.

PATIENT 1

22-year-old woman
Spin-cast soft lenses (Bausch & Lomb)

OD -2.75 U$_3$ K OD 45.00/44.62
OS -3.00 U$_3$ OS 45.00/44.75

Subjective complaint

Lens never looks clean, always smeary surface regardless of amount rinsed.
Enzyme cleaning of little help.
Visual acuity not so good as it should be.

Objective findings

Fit very good.
Lens has light-to-moderate accumulation of lipids.
Fig. 30-1.

*Keith W. Harrison, M.O.C.L.A., Lecturer and Instructor, Contact Lens Certification Program, Seneca College of Applied Arts and Technology, Willowdale, Ontario.
‡Jean-Pierre Chartrand, M.D., Department of Ophthalmology, Lakeshore General Hospital, Dorval, Quebec.

Treatment

The patient had previously been using a cold disinfection system and in our opinion strict adherance was questionable.
The patient was put on a heat regimen using a daily surfactant cleaner (Pliagel) and the Barnes-Hind weekly cleaner.

Result

After 2 weeks of using this new system, the patient had no further complaints and the lenses appeared to be much cleaner. The patient also commented that the lenses "felt" cleaner than they had previously.

Comments

This case is important by drawing attention to the fact that all debris is not protein. Cleaners and enzymes that clear only protein will have no effect on this type of deposit.

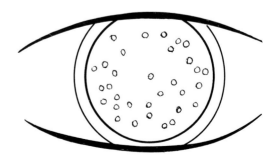

Fig. 30-1. Fat lipids on lens surface. This type of "deposit" will move about during blinking and when the lens is rinsed.

PATIENT 2

76-year-old man with aphakia in right eye
Trans Canada Contact Lens Company, TC 75, extended-wear lenses

8.4 mm 14.0 +13.75   *K* 43.50/42.50

Subjective complaint

Lens coats over and becomes blurred and uncomfortable within 2 to 4 weeks, a process necessitating removal and cleaning.

Objective findings

Moderately dry eye.
Tear-film breakup time 9 to 12 seconds, causing lens dehydration.
Fig. 30-2.

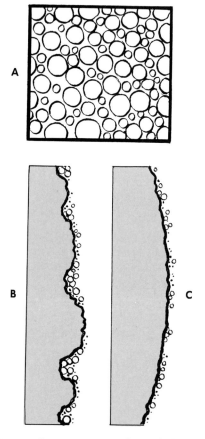

Fig. 30-2. A, Pore structure of a soft lens (highly magnified). **B,** Cross section of the surface of a soft lens that holds debris because of its dehydrated state. **C,** Cross section of surface of a fully hydrated lens. The debris runs over the surface without binding.

Treatment

Before retiring, he rinses each night with an eyecup filled with normal saline solution for 30 to 60 seconds.

Result

The period of time between cleanings increased from 2 to 4 weeks to 3 to 4 months.

Comment

We have advocated the use of lubricating drops for our extended-wear patient for some time now. However, the effects of the drops are sometimes short lived and possibly improperly instilled. The eyecup used at night seems to be easier and more effective. Many of our patients use both. However, we now advise all extended-wear aphakes to wash with an eyecup wash nightly. We have also noticed with lubrication a reduction of tight lens reactions in our extended-wear patients.

PATIENT 3

27-year-old woman with severe keratitis in both eyes
Bausch & Lomb Plano T Bandage lenses

K OD 42.75/43.00
    OS 42.75/42.87

Subjective findings

Lenses feel dry and scratchy at end of day. Must wear fluid-filled goggles for sleeping.

Objective findings

Severe keratitis; dry eye.
Fig. 30-3.

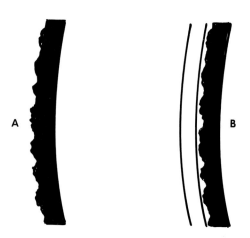

Fig. 30-3. A, Cross section of corneal epithelium denuded by keratitis. **B,** High-water-content bandage lens covering and protecting the epithelium.

Treatment

Refitting with high-water-content lenses, TC 75 both eyes, 8.4 14.0 plano.

Lubricant drops twice a day onto lenses worn on an extended-wear basis, removed and cleaned weekly.

Result

Increased comfort. Virtually all drying problems were eliminated. There is no longer the need for fluid-filled goggles.

Comment

Although generally it is not true that the drier the eye, the drier the lens required, the patient responded to a high-water-content lens as a bandage lens and was extremely pleased with the result. One of us (B.S.) would have preferred to use a rigid gas-permeable lens along with a tear supplement.

PATIENT 4

21-year-old woman
Bausch & Lomb

OD $-2.75\ U_4$ K 43.00/43.75
OS $-2.75\ U_4$ 43.00/43.50

Subjective findings

Foreign-body sensation in both eyes, photophobia, and so on.

Objective findings

Foreign-body epithelial insult on both eyes. Many small fibers on and about the lenses.
Fig. 30-4.

Treatment

Lenses were removed for 48 hours, and the corneas were clear. Upon reinstructing the patient on care and handling, it was discovered that she was refilling her sample-size bottle of Boil n' Soak saline solution. The paper label was deteriorating, and the paper fibers from the bottle

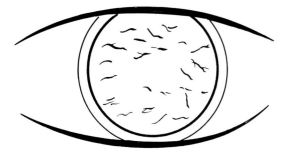

Fig. 30-4. Paper fibers on lens.

label was the root of the problem. This practice was discontinued and the problem was eliminated.

Comment

Inspection of the patients care system, case, and so on can be of great value in problem solving.

PATIENT 5

18-year-old woman
Rigid gas-permeable lenses, Boston material
Special prescription

OD $-3.00\ -2.50 \times 180$ K 42.12/45.00
OS $-3.25\ -2.75 \times 175$ 42.00/45.25

Lenses worn

OD 7.90 9.2 -3.75
OS 7.86 9.2 -4.00

Subjective complaint

Poor visual acuity.

Objective findings

Visual acuity with spectacles 20/20$^-$ in both eyes.
Visual acuity with contact lens 20/30 in both eyes
Over-refraction of contact lenses was

plano -1.00×180 20/20$^-$
$-0.25\ -1.00 \times 180$ 20/20$^-$

The fit of the lenses appeared good and the corneas were clear.

K readings taken over the lenses indicated a 1.00-diopter flexing of the lenses on the eyes.

The center thickness of the lenses was measured and found to be 0.11 and 0.10 mm, respectively.

Treatment

New lenses of the same specifications with a 0.14 mm center thickness were ordered.

Result

Visual acuity improved to 20/20 and 20/20$^-$.
The thicker lenses continue to hold their shape and do not mold to the corneal toricity.

Comment

The emphasis on this lenses in the rigid gas-permeable materials has brought with it an inherent soft lens problem, lens flexture. To fit moderate-to-high amounts of corneal astigmatism with gas-permeable lenses, slightly increased center thicknesses (0.03 to 0.05 mm) can be of considerable benefit. The effects of reduction of transmissibility caused by increased lens thickness appears to be negligible.

PATIENT 6

29-year-old woman
Bausch & Lomb

OD −7.00 U₃   K 43.50/43.62
OS −7.50 U₃   43.37/43.62

Subjective complaint

Imbalance at near blurring at the periphery.

Objective findings

Good fit, excellent centering large pupil 7.0 mm.

Treatment

U₄ lenses of the same power were tried and much the same problem persisted. Refitting with lathe-cut Hydron 0.06 lenses:

OD 8.4 14.0 −7.00
OS 8.4 14.0 −7.50

Result

Elimination of imbalance at near range and better general subjective response.

Comment

It would appear that the higher the correction with a spin-cast lens the greater the peripheral distortion attributable to its asphericity. In this case the large pupil seemed to accentuate the problem, and therefore the larger more defined optic performance of the lathe-cut lens was more satisfactory.
Fig. 30-5.

PATIENT 7

62-year-old man, monocular aphake

OD +10.25 −1.25 × 85   20/25   +2.75 add
OS − 6.25   20/50   +2.75 add

Cooper Permalens
  OD 8.0 14.0 +11.00   K 44.00/42.25

Subjective complaint

Patient wanted best acuity possible with both eyes, did not want the left eye to be fitted, and wanted to use present spectacles if possible.
Present spectacles

−6.50 sph +2.50 add
−6.25 sph +2.50 add

Objective findings

The fit of the Permalens was very good and need not be changed.

Treatment

A Permalens of the same fit but overcorrected to a +18.50 D was ordered.

Result

Visual acuity with the original minus spectacles over the lens gives 20/30 and reasonable binocularity. It seems to satisfy the patient and fit his needs.

Comment

Overcorrection and compensation of the monocular aphakic myope can save a great deal of work and aggravation. Upon the eventual extraction of the second cataract, the initial lens can be changed for optimum acuity.

PATIENT 8

24-year-old woman
Previously unsuccessful with Union lenses and Bausch & Lomb U₄ soft lenses, the latter being worn intermittently for 1 year

Subjective complaint

All previous lenses caused irritation and inability to wear more than 4 to 5 hours.

Objective findings

K OD 44.37/44.12
  OS 44.12/44.62

Spectacle prescription

−3.50 −0.50 × 5
−5.25 −0.50 × 180

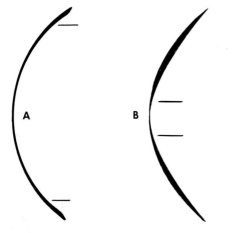

Fig. 30-5. A, Lathe-cut lens has a large usable optic zone. **B,** Spin-cast lens in the higher power range has a restricted usable optic zone.

Gutter dellen in both eyes

OD 11 to 7 o'clock
OS 1 to 5 o'clock

Tear-film breakup time 8 to 12 seconds

Treatment

High-water-content lenses (Duragel 75) were fitted for daily wear.

Result

Initial results were good, but the lenses steepened excessively after 3 weeks of wear. Flatter lens were subsequently fitted, and the patient now wears her lenses 10 to 14 hours daily with only the occasional dryness problems.

Comment

A high water content can compensate for the moderately dry eye and the transfer of enough oxygen to satisfy a moderately healthy cornea.

PATIENT 9

24-year-old woman
Wearing extended-wear Duragel 75

OD 8.8 14.0 −4.75 20/20   K 42.12/42.50
OS 8.8 14.0 −4.50 20/20   42.00/42.25

Subjective complaint

Excessive drying and lenses becoming "greased" over.

Objective findings

Some tightening late in the day because of dehydration; lenses coating heavily with oil and fat deposits.

Treatment

Refitting with ultrathin 38% H_2O lenses
Cibathin 0.035 center thickness

OD 8.9 13.8 −4.75 20/20
OS 8.9 13.8 −4.50 20/20

Result

Elimination of deposit formation and dryness complaints. Patient wears lenses for 1 week at a time before cleaning.

Comment

It is possible that in some instances for extended wear an ultrathin lens may be preferable to a high-water-content lens. A large thin lens decreases the interaction between the lids and the lens.

PATIENT 10

58-year-old woman, monocular aphake rigid lens, Boston material

42.00 9.4 +14.00 20/25   K 41.50/40.25

Subjective complaint

Constant irritation, gritty sensation

Objective findings

Recurrent keratitis
Lens low—inability to get lift even with flatter lens

Treatment

Refitting with a soft lens, heat-care regimen Union II

13.8 +14.00 20/25

Result

Increased comfort and wearability

Comment

Greater corneal coverage combined with a bandage effect of the soft lens can be of great benefit for the patient with a marginally dry cornea.
Gas-permeable lenses that fit low frequently cause severe 3 and 9 o'clock staining.

PATIENT 11

28-year-old woman
Spin-cast lenses, Bausch & Lomb

OD −2.50 B₃   K 43.00/43.25
OS −2.50 B₃   43.00/43.25

Lens age: 1¼ years

Subjective complaint

Injection in both eyes.
Six-hour maximum daily wear.

Objective findings

Mild injection in both eyes.
Visual acuity 20/30 OU fluctuating.
Lenses heavily coated, riding low.
Mild keratitis along lower edge of lens, arcuate stain.
Lids everted show early giant papillary conjunctivitis
Refracts −2.50 sphere OU 20/20

Treatment

Discontinue lenses.
Steroid drops three times a day for 2 weeks.
Refit with ultrathin lenses, Bausch & Lomb −2.50 Uₛ OU.

Heat disinfection system with nonpreserved saline solution.

Result

Visual acuity 20/20 OU.

Complete clearing of upper tarsus within 2 months.

Twelve-hour daily wearing time

Fig. 30-6.

Comments

It is imperative when checking a contact-lens wearer that the lids be everted and observed. Some 50% of soft-lens wearers may exhibit papules of varying degrees on the upper tarsus. Old or coated lenses can trigger a reaction of this sort. These lenses appear to reduce tarsal friction with the lens surface and lessen the recurrence of the giant papillary conjunctivitis.

In many instances, nothing will help because giant papillary conjunctivitis is believed to be an autoimmune response to the patient's own protein. Other alternative therapy that can be tried is switching to gas-permeable lenses, stop wearing lenses for 3 months, more vigorous cleaning of soft lenses, and switching to heat disinfection.

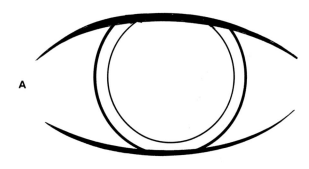

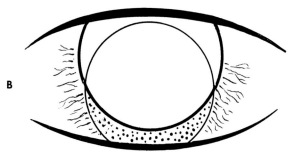

Fig. 30-6. A, Coated B₃ lens riding low causes inferior arcuate staining. **B,** New lens centering well provides good comfort, vision, and physiologic function.

PATIENT 12

32-year-old man
Lathe-cut soft lenses, Aquaflex II

OD Vault II 13.0 −4.50   *K* 41.00/41.75
OS Vault II 13.0 −5.00   41.12/41.75

Subjective complaints

Irritation.

Mild to moderate injection.

Objective findings

Keratitis.

Neovascularization from 9 to 12 o'clock position.

Good centering and movement.

Treatment

Refitting with high-water-content lenses
TC 75

OD 8.4 13.5 −4.50
OS 8.4 13.5 −5.00

To be worn on a daily-wear basis

Result

Vessel regression.

Elimination.

Increased comfort.

Comment

Keratitis and neovascularization are signs of poor oxygen supply or a cornea with a high oxygen demand. Higher-water-content lenses are able to supply better the respiratory needs of this type of cornea. Close, long-term aftercare is required to maintain a patient of this nature. Extended-wear lenses can be excellent problem solvers when applied on a daily-wear basis.

PATIENT 13

31-year-old woman
Not presently wearing lenses
Spectacle prescription

OD −6.00 −1.50 × 90 20/20   *K* 43.00/41.25
OS −5.75 −2.00 × 90 20/20   43.50/41.50

Subjective complaints

Previously unsuccessful with both rigid and rigid gas-permeable lenses.

Very aware of the rigid lenses.

Objective findings

Ocular exam within normal limits.

Treatment

Fitting with large standard-thickness lenses
TC 50-S

OD 8.7 14.5 −6.25
OS 8.7 14.5 −6.25

Result

Visual acuity with the lenses is 20/25⁻ and 20/30
Binocular vision is 20/25.
All-day comfortable wear.

Comment

Do not mask significant astigmatism. But in higher refractive errors the presence of stigmatism is better tolerated. For this woman the loss of one or two lines of vision was acceptable.

PATIENT 14

72-year-old man with aphakia in right eye
Rigid gas-permeable lenses, Boston material

   43.00 9.2 + 12.25   K 44.00/42.75
   Single-cut, center thickness 0.56 mm

Subjective complaints

Awareness of lens.
Some blurring of visual acuity when blinking.

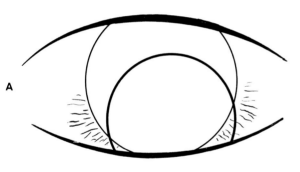

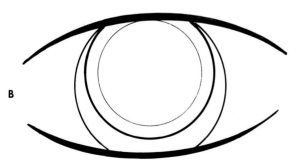

Fig. 30-7. A, Single-cut lens riding low causes irritation. **B,** Thinner, lighter lenticular lens centers well with the eyelid holding the lens. The lens also has a minus carrier to help the lifting action by the eyelid.

Objective findings

Low-riding lens.
Visual acuity 20/25⁺ fluctuating.
Some greasing of lens.

Treatment

Refit with Boston Lens II.

   43.00 9.4 + 12.75
   Lenticular minus carrier
   Center thickness 0.40 mm

Result

Good centering.
Stable vision.
Better wetting.
Fig. 30-7.

Comment

In general, lenticulation of aphakic lenses is indicated to reduce lens thickness and weight. A minus carrier may help the upper lid to grasp the lens edge and promote better centering as well as lid sweep during blinking.

PATIENT 15

24-year-old woman
Hydron 0.06 soft lenses

   OD 8.7 14.0 − 1.50   K 43.00/43.25
   OS 8.7 14.0 − 1.75   43.00/43.37

Subjective complaints

Intermittent red eye for the past 8 months.
Some discharge in the morning.
Steroids used previously were of little help.

Objective findings

Fit of lens good, some coating because of discharge.
Cornea clear.
Some follicles on upper and lower tarsi.

Treatment

Culture and scraping taken.

Results

Cultures show inclusion conjunctivitis.
Tetracycline orally.
Sulfonamide II drops.
Replacement of lenses with same type.
All symptoms cleared within 3 weeks.

Comment

Red-eye problems are often not lens related. Herpes simplex infection is another offender of the cornea that may be mistaken for a lens abrasion.

PART IV

GENERAL
CONSIDERATIONS
AFFECTING
A CONTACT LENS
PRACTICE

MANAGEMENT OF A MEDICAL LENS PRACTICE

DELEGATION

Many functions in the management of a lens practice may be delegated. Depending on the training, educational background, responsibility, and personality of the auxiliary personnel, several areas may be properly delegated so that the practitioner is free to spend time on the initial examination and fitting with adequate time for follow-up visits that are required.

COST

Lenses can be paid for in one of two ways. The first is an initial small cost outlay for the lenses, a fitting fee, and a visit fee for the practitioner, or a pay-as-you-go fee. In this way problem cases are charged proportionately, whereas "easy-fit" cases are charged less. The fitting fee may vary with the nature of the fit so that more difficult fittings, such as toric fitting or bifocal fitting, are charged a higher fee. Alternatively, one may use a total fee structure that can be broken down for the patient into the cost of the material and the cost of professional fitting (Fig. 31-1). The same charge can be made for each standard fitting regardless of the number of visits required during the adaptation period. This all-inclusive coverage period may vary from up to 3 months, after which a fee per visit is charged. We favor the latter method, in which the patient is free to call on the practitioner without being concerned about the extra expense. It is important that the patient fully understand that the practitioner is not selling lenses but that the professional-fee component is added for professional time in evaluations to ensure a successful fit.

The contact lens area is extremely competitive and price oriented. One must avoid misunderstanding and confusion in the public eye and, above all, leaving the patient with the feeling that the charges were excessive and that he was overcharged. Good public relations are important not only on the part of the fitter but also on the part of all personnel in contact with the patient (Fig. 31-2). One must be alert to exceptions to the rule, dissatisfied patients, and refunds. One must often customize the financial approach to patients.

OFFICE SPACE

Most ophthalmic practices gradually grow in the area of contact lenses. As a result space is often adapted from existing facilities. Once the practice is well established in contact lenses, three important areas become necessary. First is a *fitting area*, with a variety of handy lens-storage trays that are easily accessible for use. Second, an *insertion and removal area* with a sink for patient and fitter to wash their hands. This area permits the patient to practice insertion and removal until they are sufficiently comfortable with the procedure to take the

Our total fee is divided between the cost of material and a professional fee for fitting and service. This service is available for 3 months, after which a charge per visit will be made.

An inspection service will be provided at no charge at 6 months after initial visit.

Cost of lenses, case, and
initial supplies _____
Fitting fee _____
Warranty _____
Miscellaneous _____

Total _____

I have received lenses. _____

Signature

_____

Date

Fig. 31-1. Sample of breakdown of fee structure that is provided to patient when lenses are received.

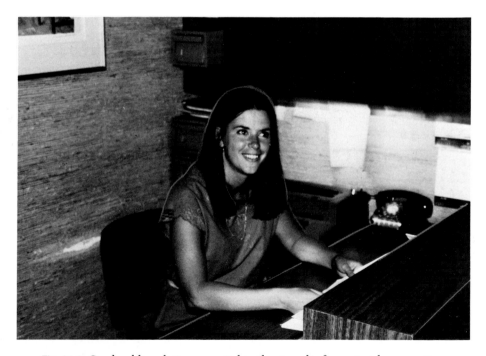

Fig. 31-2. Good public relations are vital to the growth of a contact lens practice.

```
┌─────────────────────────────────────────────────────────────┐
│                                                               │
│              Contact lens service agreement                   │
│                                                               │
│                    $25.00 1 year                              │
│                                                               │
│   Park Plaza Eye Associates hereby guarantees replacement     │
│   of lost or damaged lenses for a period of one year ending   │
│                                                               │
│            _____                        │
│                                                               │
│   Charge per lens under the terms of this warranty will be    │
│                                                    each.       │
│                                                               │
│   NAME_____         │
│                                                               │
│   ADDRESS_____         │
│                                                               │
│   Park Plaza Eye Associates, 170 Bloor Street West, Toronto,  │
│              Ontario M5S 1T9                                  │
│              Telephone 966-3333                               │
│                                                               │
└─────────────────────────────────────────────────────────────┘
```

Fig. 31-3. Sample of service agreement for contact lens replacement.

contact lenses home. This area permits ancillary personnel to spend time with the patient. Third, an area for contact lens–evaluating equipment, storage, and lens cleaning and an area for making modifications to rigid lenses.

CHARTING

Careful documentation, including a careful history, slitlamp examination, and recording of all pertinent factors should be made before fitting is begun. Important measurements and modifications must always be charted. It is often convenient to maintain separate lens records on each patient with cross-reference to standard clinical charts. A numeric system of charting with a cross-index containing patients' names arranged alphabetically is preferred.

WARRANTY OR INSURANCE

Patients are constantly worried about loss or damage to their lenses. For most patients the initial expenditure of time and money represents a sizable investment and the fear of losing a lens becomes an obsession with many patients. Their concern is justified, for insurance company profiles show a loss rate of 40% in the first year of wear, decreasing as the years go on. It is not surprising that private floaters exclude contact lenses.

Another argument for insurance is that surveys of uninsured wearers show that 40% were no longer wearing their lenses because one or both lenses had been lost and they had not bothered to replace them. Lens insurance dramatically reduces the dropout rate among wearers. Without insurance there is a tragic waste of professional time and skill, to say nothing of the patient's time and money.

In those lens areas in which insurance is unavailable or the cost excessive, we found that a simple warranty or guarantee of replacement by the practitioner at a fixed cost suffices and encourages the patient to replace the lens when it becomes chipped, scratched, or coated. The warranty may be extended to include changes required for fit and prescription changes as well as loss. A nominal replacement fee contributes greatly to the readiness of the patient to accept a new lens, particularly a soft lens, when the original lens shows the inevitable ravages of time.

Our system includes a triplicate service agreement in which one slip is given to the patient, one filed on the clinical chart, and one filed alphabetically for quick reference and for notification of expiration date (Fig. 31-3).

DUPLICATE LENSES

To reduce administrative inconvenience with rush orders for a replacement lens, every patient should have a duplicate pair of rigid lenses made up to the final prescription. This eliminates the weekend panic call before the annual school dance or speaking engagement. An extra pair of soft lenses may be ordered, but the autoclaved packed vial should not be opened because contamination of the spare pair often results from neglect in maintenance.

When duplicate rigid lenses are not provided and a loss occurs, it may be several days before the replacement lens is received. When the replacement lens arrives, if the patient continues with the same wearing schedule there is a great risk of the overwear syndrome occurring, particularly with rigid lens wearers.

The chief reason for replacing rigid lenses is loss. The chief reasons for replacement of soft lenses are deposit formation and clouding, tearing of the lens, yellowing, and roughening of the edges. There is generally a greater replacement rate for soft lenses than for rigid lenses, but the urgency factor is not so great for soft lenses because of the low loss rate.

REPLACEMENT LENSES

A systematic organized and efficient system should be developed to replace lost or damaged lenses. Many replacements for loss are often ordered by telephone, thus a way of minimizing the amount of traffic in an office. A duplicate telephone message system is invaluable as a way of minimizing errors and of re-checking the week's progress. Often patients will repeatedly call daily for lost lenses, and a systematic and quick arrival at the time the lenses were reordered and whether they have arrived may be most helpful. An alphabetic storage by surname when they arrive effectively improves the efficiency of handling replacement lenses.

INVENTORY CONTROL AND RESTERILIZATION

The proper management of a lens practice necessitates the use of some measure of inventory control of lenses in addition to a list of names of patients awaiting special-order lenses. If the inventory is not controlled, one may easily expand one's own inventory of lens considerably beyond need and in addition have all the wrong powers on hand when a lens is required.

Special lens-holding units may be used for inventory organization enabling better control of both soft and rigid stock lenses (Fig. 31-4). It is important that all lenses that are used for

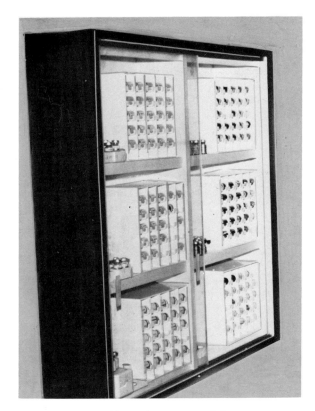

Fig. 31-4. Wall unit for storing soft lens wear.

trial fitting be properly cleaned and disinfected before being reused (Fig. 31-5).

At the beginning of a lens practice one should limit oneself to a select number of manufacturers in rigid and soft lenses whose reliability, quality control, and replacement service have been well established.

ORGANIZATION

Beside the fitter should be some lens wells in which contact lenses (from inventory lenses) can be placed during fitting. An organized system minimizes the mix-up of lenses.

A special area should be set aside for the business area and the verifying instruments in a proper lens practice. The orderly organization of this area is important. All lenses should be verified when received from the manufacturer (see Chapters 4 and 19). Proper drawers or boxes (Fig. 31-6) for lenses, clearly labelled

with power and base curve, should be maintained. A disorganized system leads to repeated confusion and time lost in rechecking the parameters of a lens to identify the stock of trial or inventory lenses. Ledger books and adequate recording of lenses and payments should be properly kept.

REFUNDS

This is a difficult area in which to have any hard-and-fast rules. In the first 6 weeks some persons will reject their lenses for justifiable reasons. It is important that practitioners listen with sympathy and understanding and put themselves in the patient's position. In those cases in which the lenses have been used only for a few days and are still adequate for replacement into the inventory after sterilization, it is usually appropriate to consider the amount of professional time and professional visits and

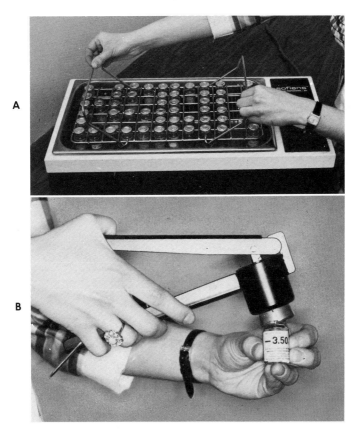

Fig. 31-5. A, Practitioner resterilizing Bausch & Lomb lenses in large carrying case. **B,** Recapping Soflens in vial for sterilization. (From Stein, H.A., and Slatt, B.J.: The ophthalmic assistant, ed. 4, St. Louis, 1983, The C.V. Mosby Co.)

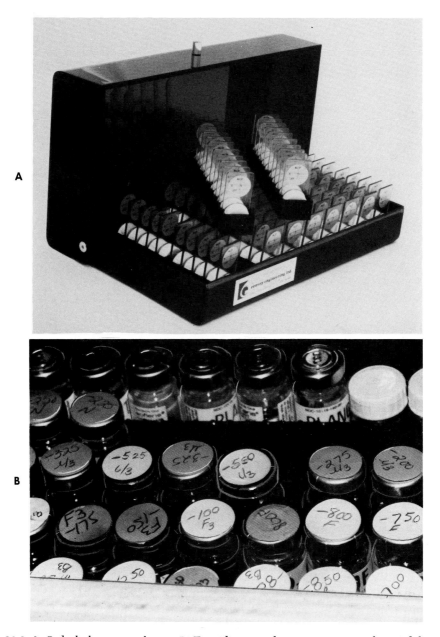

Fig. 31-6. A, Orderly lens control case. **B,** For tidiness, a drawer system may be used for storage of contact lenses. (**A,** Courtesy Convoy Engineering, Ltd., Burnaby, British Columbia.)

charge accordingly, refunding the balance of payment. This maintains the goodwill of the patient. In some of our aphakic patients a trial charge may be levied and the rest of the balance deferred for the lenses until the patients conclude that they are satisfied and wish to continue with the lenses. Most of our aphakic patients, once they have been shown the benefits of the lenses and their ability to manage more readily, will usually prefer contact lenses to spectacles.

It is important that starter supplies of cleaners, disinfecting solutions, enzyme tablets, and so on, are provided, along with a detailed description of the usage. So often patients are given purchasing slips for their local drugstore and the selected supplies are unavailable and substitutions made. This can adversely affect the success of the lenses.

INSTRUMENTATION

Many sophisticated instruments are available today for the evaluation of the patient and the lenses. In the beginning of a lens practice it is important that the practitioner have reliable and efficient diagnostic instruments for patient evaluation on both the initial and follow-up visits. As a lens practice grows, further equipment for evaluation of lenses received from the laboratory should be added and the practitioner should become less dependent on the laboratory for quality control. As the practice increases further, modifying and grinding facilities may be added to complete the picture and provide added service (Fig. 31-7).

LENS SERVICING

If a lens practice is sufficiently large, certain lens services should be provided. Such services as buffing and polishing a hard lens can be easily performed by an experienced technician with an inexpensive modification unit. A small charge may be levied to support the time involved.

Modifications are an important added feature to a contact lens practice. One can achieve instant success by slight increases in the power of a rigid lens, blending the junctional curves, flattening the peripheral curve, or making the lens diameter smaller. With the increased usage of gas-permeable rigid lenses in the present decade, in-office modifications of gas-

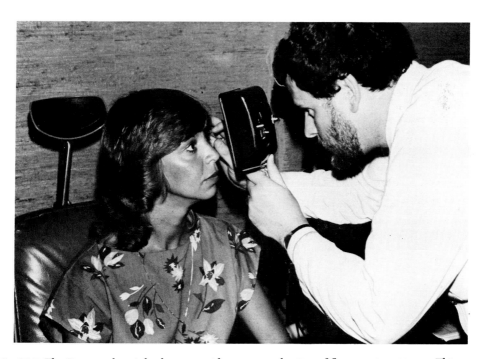

Fig. 31-7. The Burton ultraviolet lamp provides gross evaluation of fluorescein patterns. This gross assessment may be superior as an overview of the fitting pattern to the slitlamp, which may be too detailed.

PATIENT INFORMED-CONSENT FORM FOR

EXTENDED-WEAR SOFT CONTACT LENSES

The benefit to wearers of extended wear is the opportunity to attain "visual normalcy" — that is, to live like those people who have no visual handicap — for a one (1) week period. This period of wearing time can vary for different patients and can only be determined through our scheduled progress visits.

The risks associated with extended wear are similar to those of other contact lenses — insufficient oxygen for the cornea and the possibility of an eye infection. These risks are minimized with extended wear as with other contact lenses by a complete eye examination before fitting of the lenses, through instruction regarding the care of your eyes and lenses when wearing extended wear, follow-up visits to this office to monitor your eye's response to the lenses, and good JUDGEMENT on your part.

By signing this form, you are consenting to the following visits schedule to this office, which we feel are important.

24 hours check-up	6 months check-up ....
1 week check-up	1 year check-up ....
1 month check-up	Every 6 months thereafter
3 months check-up	

Our fitting fee for extended wear lenses includes all visits during the first 3 months. These visits are compulsory. Should you have any questions or problems between visits, you are to call us immediately. Failure to comply with these instructions may result in your return to a daily wear programme.

Date .... Signature ....

Fig. 31-8. Sample of informed consent form for extended-wear contact lens patients.

permeable lenses can be a great time-saver as well as practice-builder for achievement of rapid success.

Both soft and rigid lenses may from time to time require professional cleaning, and the patient should be encouraged to return for this service. Extended-wear lenses invariably build up protein and deposits that interfere with oxygen exchange and may embarrass the integrity of the cornea. The patient should return at regular intervals and should have the lenses removed and either professionally cleaned or replaced. This is most important for the elderly aphakic patient with poor tear function.

ORDERING LENSES

In the initial stages of lens practice one may wish to order on a per-case basis in which the laboratory makes new lenses and modifications without charge to the fitter. As the practice develops, fitting and ordering from trial sets is a far better method of arriving at the final lens and much sooner, and it minimizes the number of repeat office visits for the patient. As the practice grows still further, an inventory set of common powers and sizes in both rigid and soft lenses should be obtained. This further minimizes the number of office visits required, creates instant success with patients while their enthusiasm is high, and identifies the problems very early in repeat visits, providing on-site correction.

Equipment for lens practice

Necessary
  Keratometer
  Slitlamp (biomicroscope)
  Optic spherometer (Radiuscope)
  Lensometer
  Burton lamp
  Hand magnifier with measuring grid
  Millimeter ruler
  Profile analyzer
  Soft lens base curve evaluator
Additional
  Shadowgraph
  Topogometer
  Thickness gauge
  V-groove ruler
Modification
  Modification unit
  Dotting ink with marker

FOLLOW-UP OF PATIENTS

It is most important that lens patients be adequately followed up. A number of satisfied lens wearers will simply forget to return for regular examination. Lens patients require ongoing care. The rigid lens may warp and alter the corneal curvature, and the soft lens may become coated with protein causing chronic anoxia of the cornea with vascular invasion.

One may ask patients to return at regular intervals, but it is the responsibility of the practitioner to see that they actually do return. In a busy practice it is all too easy to overlook the dropouts who do not return. Thus an effective recall system, either by phone or mail, is most important. Addresses and phone numbers of patients may change, but a little detective work on the part of ancillary personnel may greatly aid in the locating of patients if for no other reason than to ensure that they obtain follow-up care either by the initial fitter or by another practitioner. We suggest a patient-agreement form be used, outlining the minimum follow-up requirements. For extended wear, this is more critical. We use informed-consent forms for aphakia to ensure return visits (Fig. 31-8).

One may gear the recall system to a set time of the year when all contact files are reviewed and those who have not returned are duly notified. Some practices use the birthday cross-reference or date of initial fit system by reviewing each chart during the month of the patient's birthday or date of initial fit, thus spreading the load over the year.

CONTACT LENS INFORMATION

The general information that a new contact patient has about contacts is often confusing and incorrect. The initial consultation should set some of this information straight and put all the questions in the proper perspective. However, sensible handouts reinforce the question's answer and often answer other questions overlooked in the initial interview. Some of these pamphlets are available from manufacturers and from the contact lens societies. They may however be customized for your own practice. Handouts are great practice builders and should be encouraged.

COSMETICS AND RIGID AND SOFT LENSES

Mascara
Face powder
Eyeliner
Eye shadow
Hair spray
Removal of cosmetics
Helpful hints

It may be beneath the dignity of the ophthalmologist to deal with cosmetic problems, but unfortunately it is not beneath the dignity of patients to present them. For this reason an appreciation of the most suitable types of cosmetics for lens wearers is as important as the correct type of solution to be used with their lenses.

Cosmetics should be applied after the lenses have been inserted. This prevents both contamination of the lens by makeup and, from the patient's point of view, disruption of her artwork by the occasional dropped tear. Also it is easier to apply a lens to a naked eye.

MASCARA

Used for lash augmentation, mascara should be used sparingly and basically only on the outer half of the lashes. The type enriched by small, hairlike fibers to produce extra lash length should be avoided because the fibers often dry and fall into the eye (Fig. 32-1). Water-soluble brands are preferred because they do not act as a foreign body if some of the pigment accidentally falls behind a lens (Fig 32-2).

Besides being a potential irritant, contaminated mascara is frequently a source of blepharoconjunctivitis in women. The product itself is free of contamination when sold; it is

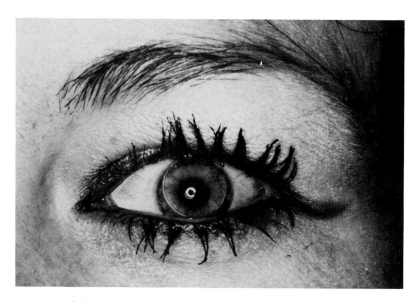

Fig. 32-1. Mascara with lash augmentors applied to the base of the eyelashes. Some of the pigment has fallen off and is deposited at 8 o'clock on the cornea.

after it is used that it becomes contaminated with bacteria and fungi. The most common contaminant is *Staphylococcus epidermidis*, whereas the most dangerous is *Pseudomonas aeruginosa*, which grows in a liquid mascara medium and can invade a small corneal erosion or abrasion.

It is prudent to culture the cosmetics, especially the mascara and its applicator, in any serious ocular infection in women who wear cosmetics. Also it is best if women discard their cosmetics after 4 months of use because of the likelihood of contamination.

FACE POWDER

Face powder comes in either a loose powder or a pressed, compact form. It contains fatty acids and magnesium silicate, which leave residues on the fingers and are thus transferred to the lens. Care should be exercised in handling face powder to avoid this problem.

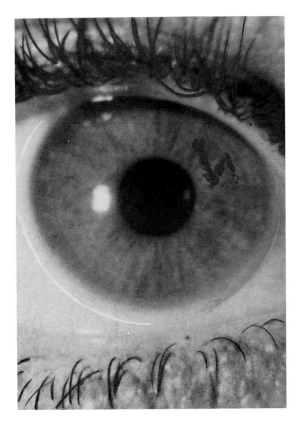

Fig. 32-2. Water-soluble mascara avoids the deposition of pigment deposits on the surface of lenses as noted in this illustration.

EYELINER

This substance, which comes in a liquid form or as a solid to be mixed with water, should be applied on the lid margin beyond the lash line. The "Cleopatra look" achieved by the application of heavy deposits of eyeliner over the entire margin of the lid should be deplored because it may cause blepharitis, styes, and chalazions (Fig. 32-3). Again, water-soluble brands are the only type that should be used.

EYE SHADOW

Iridescent types of eye shadow should be avoided. These contain such things as ground glass and oyster shells (Fig. 32-4). Greasy smudge pots and pomades should be another sacrifice for the lens wearer. The creamy-stick eye shadow or the compressed cream powder and brush-on type can be used.

HAIR SPRAY

Hair spray, used widely by both men and women, can cause a severe keratitis, erosions of the cornea, and surface opacities of contact lenses (Fig. 32-5). It comes most commonly in an aerosol form, which frequently contains lacquer. Normally persons are gazing in the mirror while applying hair spray; therefore their eyes are open. This practice should be discouraged (Fig. 32-6). The eyes should be closed and kept closed for several minutes, since the spray tends to linger. Instead of closing the eyes, it is simplest to leave the room if a spray has just been released. Even plastic spray guards or a hand, which is of help in protecting the eyes, cannot stop a vapor. Probably the best routine is not to apply hair spray while lenses are being worn; hair spray should only be used before the lenses are inserted.

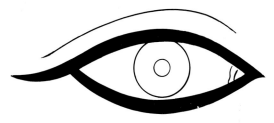

Fig. 32-3. The Cleopatra look. The eyeliner covers the lid margin, Moll's glands, and the glands of Zeis as well as the meibomian glands, which may lead to blepharitis, styes, and chalazions.

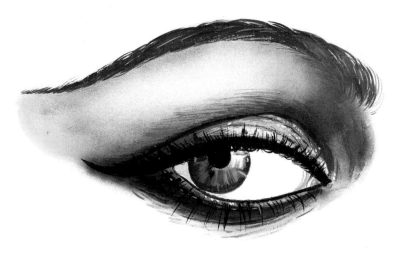

Fig. 32-4. Eye shadow with organic additives such as oyster shells frequently acts as an irritant and sensitizer.

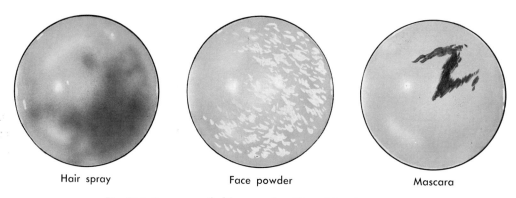

Hair spray   Face powder   Mascara

Fig. 32-5. Lenses spoiled by poor handling of facial cosmetics.

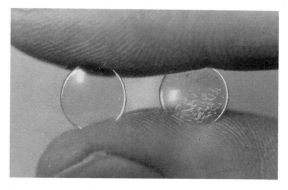

Fig. 32-6. Hair spray on a lens inadvertently exposed to an aerosol vapor.

REMOVAL OF COSMETICS

At the end of the day cosmetics should be removed after the lenses are removed because the fingers are less likely to be contaminated by the pigments, creams, and oils comprising the make-up complex. It is important to encourage women to use noncreamy or nongreasy cleansing lotions to remove their cosmetics.

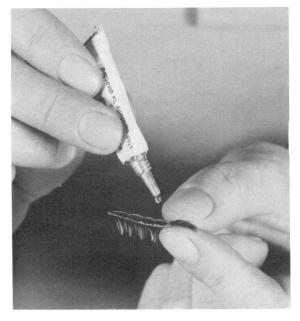

Fig. 32-7. The adhesive of false eyelashes may be an irritant and source of sensitization with repeated applications.

HELPFUL HINTS

1. Patients should be told never to swap, borrow, or lend eye make-up or applicator brushes. Trachoma and staphylococcal keratitis have been spread in this manner. Brushes should be washed frequently or, preferably, replaced by new ones.

2. Lenses should not be worn in beauty salons. The sprays and fumes in the air can damage the lenses and cause a chemical keratitis. The heat and warm air from hair dryers can cause visual hazing, discomfort, and inability to tolerate the lenses.

3. False eyelashes should be avoided. Blepharitis frequently ensues on the basis of an allergic reaction to the adhesive or lash. The adhesive may also be a direct irritant (Fig. 32-7). When the lashes are removed, they frequently take with them some of the real ones; this adds further insult to the lid margin.

If the patient requires false eyelashes for some valid reason (Singers, performers, or entertainers often require them as part of their costume), they should be encouraged to use human lashes tacked on above their own lashes (Fig. 32-8). A water-proof adhesive should be employed that has been allowed to dry slightly to a tacky stage.

4. The use of brands made by well-known cosmetic firms should be encouraged. Chances are that the quality control of the product will be better. Federal regulations regarding cosmetics are not nearly so stringent as those regarding food and drugs.

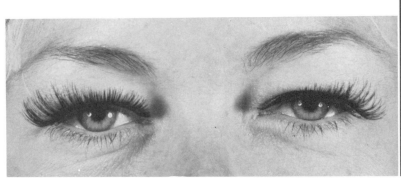
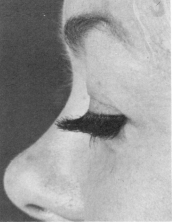

Fig. 32-8. False eyelashes should be worn above the real lashes.

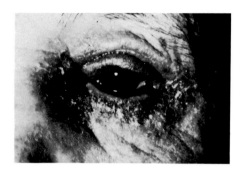

Fig. 32-9. Contact dermatitis. Reaction to face powder on eyelids.

5. Hypoallergenic compounds should be used. Approximately one woman in 10 has either a respiratory or skin allergy to perfume. Some of the oils in perfumes such as oil of lemon, oil of orange, and oil of bergamot are derived from citrus fruits; as a result people allergic to citrus fruits may also be allergic to perfumes containing such oils.

Hypoallergenic brands are designed to eliminate from their preparation obvious sensitizers such as perfumes and lanolin (Fig. 32-9). Lanolin is used regularly in cosmetics, is one of the most common allergens, and causes severe redness, itching, and blotchy skin spots.

Even hair spray may contain serious sensitizers including perfumes, lacquers, lanolin, and solvents that can cause skin rashes or respiratory symptoms.

Unfortunately trial and error must be employed to discover which hypoallergenic brand is most suitable. Cosmetic firms do not have to label the ingredients of their products; therefore the physician cannot asses a given compound on the basis of its ingredients.

SUPPLEMENTARY
READINGS

Allansmith, M.R., Korb, D.R., Greiner, J.V., et al.: Giant papillary conjunctivitis in contact lens wearers, Am. J. Ophthalmol. **83**:697-708, 1977.

Allen, H.F.: To wet or not to wet, Arch. Ophthalmol. **67**(2):119-120, 1963.

Aquavella, J.V.: The treatment of herpetic stromal disease, Eye Ear Nose Throat Mon. **51**:374, 1972.

Aquavella, J.V.: Hydrophilic bandages in chronic corneal edema, Medcom Special Studies, New York, 1973, Medcom Press.

Aquavella, J.V., and Rao, G.N.: Which lens: contact lenses currently available for extended wear in aphakia, Ophthalmology **87**(2):151-154, 1980.

Aquavella, J.V., Jackson, G.K., and Guy, L.F.: Therapeutic effects of Bionite lenses: mechanisms of action, Ann. Ophthalmol. **3**:1341, 1971.

Bailey, N.J.: The examination and verification of a contact lens, J.A.O.A. **30**(8):557-560, 1959.

Bailey, N.J.: Inspection of a contact lens with a stereomicroscope, Optom. Weekly **50**(47):2317-2319, 1959.

Bailey, N.J.: Contact lenses must be kept wet, J.A.O.A. **31**(12):985, 1960.

Bailey, N.J.: Residual astigmatism with contact lenses. Part I. Incidence, Optom. J. Rev. Optom. **98**(1):30-31, 1961.

Bailey, N.J.: Residual astigmatism with contact lenses. Part II. Predictability, Optom. J. Rev. Optom. **98**(2):40-45, 1961.

Bailey, N.J.: Residual astigmatism with contact lenses. Part III. Possible sites, Optom. J. Rev. Optom. **98**(3):31-32, 1961.

Bailey, N.J.: Residual astigmatism with contact lenses. Part IV. Corrective techniques, Optom. J. Rev. Optom. **98**(4):43-44, 1961.

Bailey, W.R.: Preservatives for contact lens solutions, Contact Lens Soc. Am. J. **6**(3):33-39, Oct. 1972.

Baker, Z., Harrison, R.W., and Miller, B.R.: Action of synthetic detergents on the metabolism of bacteria, J. Exp. Med. **73**:249, 1941.

Baldone, J.: Contact lenses in the aphakic child, Contact Lens Med. Bull. **3**(2):25-27, April 1970.

Baum, J.L.: Therapeutic uses of soft contact lenses, Hosp. Pract. **8**(8):89-95, Aug. 1973.

Bayshore, C.A.: Report of 276 patients fitted with micro-corneal lenses, apical clearance and central ventilation, Am. J. Optom. Arch. Am. Acad. Optom. **39**(10):552-553, 1962.

Bayshore, C.A.: Astigmatic soft contact lenses: a report of 140 patients, Int. Contact Lens Clin. **4**(1):56-59, Jan.-Feb. 1977.

Beier, C.G.: A review of the literature pertaining to monovision contact lens fitting of presbyopic patients: clinical considerations, Int. Contact Lens Clin. **4**(2):49-56, March-April 1977.

Benjamin, W.J., and Hill, R.M.: Ultra-thins and oxygen update, Contact Lens Forum, pp. 43-45, Jan. 1979.

Bennet, A.G.: Optics of contact lenses, ed. 4, London, England, 1966, Association of Dispensing Opticians.

Berger, R.O., and Streeten, B.: Fungal growth in aphakic soft contact lenses, Am. J. Ophthalmol. **91**:630-633, 1981.

Bergmanson, J.P., and Chu, L.W.: Contact lens–induced corneal epithelial injury Am. J. Optom. Physiol. Opt. **59**(6):500-506, June 1982.

Bettman, J.W., Jr.: Contact lens storage, wet or dry? Am. J. Ophthalmol. **56**(1):77-84, 1963.

Bettman, J.W., Jr.: Contact lens storage, wet or dry? Am. J. Ophthalmol. **62**:324, 1966.

Bier, N.: The contour lens: a new form of corneal lens, J.A.O.A. **28**(7):394-397, 1957.

Bier, N., and Lowther, G.: Contact lens correction

Sevenoaks, Kent, 1977, Butterworth & Co., Publishers.

Binder, P.S.: The physiological effects of extended wear soft contact lenses, Ophthalmology **87**(8): Aug. 1980.

Binder, P.S., and Worthen, D.M.: Clinical evaluation of continuous wear hydrophilic lenses, Am. J. Ophthalmol. **83**(4):549-553, April 1977.

Bitonte, J.L., and Keates, R.H.: Symposium on the flexible lens: the future of flexible vs. rigid lenses, St. Louis, 1972, The C.V. Mosby Co.

Bixler, D.P.: Bacterial decontamination and cleaning of contact lenses, Am. J. Ophthalmol. **62**:324, 1966.

Black, G.J.: Ocular, anatomic, and physiologic changes due to contact lens, Ill. Med. J. **118**:279-281, 1960.

Blanco, M.: A method for detection of dissolved materials in hydrophilic lenses, Contacto **20**(2):11-14, March 1976.

Boeder, P.: Power and magnification properties of contact lenses, Arch. Ophthalmol. **19**(1):54-67, 1938.

Bonnet, R., and Cochet, P.: New method of topographical ophthalmometry: its theoretical and clinical application, Am. J. Optom. Arch. Am. Acad. Optom. **39**(5):227-251, 1962.

Boyd, H. (Sampson, W.G., and Feldman, G.L., editors): Accelerated wearing scheduling, Contact Lens Medical Seminar, Springfield, Ill., 1970, Charles C Thomas, Publisher.

Boyd, H.: Analysis of 1000 consecutive contact lens cases, First Scientific Congress of the European Contact Lens Society of Ophthalmologists, London, June 1971.

Boyd, H.: Complications of contact lens fitting, Contact Lens Med. Bull. **4**:6-8, April-June 1971.

Boyd, H.: The red eye syndrome, Contact Intraocular Lens Med. J. **1**(1-2):198-199, Jan.-June 1975.

Boyd, H., Gould, H.L., and Sampson, W.G.: Enlightened concepts in contact lens medical practice, Highlights Ophthalmol. **12**(3):139-163, 1969.

Bronstein, L.: Accuracy of fluorescein for determining corneal curvature, Contacto **3**(6):170-171, 1959.

Brown, M.R.: Survival of *Pseudomonas aeruginosa* in fluorescein solution, J. Pharm. Sci. **57**:389, 1968.

Brucker, D.: The Hydrocurve lens, Contact Intraocular Lens Med. J. **1**(3):13, July-Sept. 1975.

Brungardt, T.F.: The optics of fluorescein patterns, J.A.O.A. **53**(4):305-306, April 1982.

Burian, H.M.: Optics: fusion in unilateral aphakia, Trans. Am. Acad. Ophthalmol. Otolaryngol. **66**:285-289, 1962.

Burns, R.P., Roberts, H., and Rich, L.F.: Effect of silicone contact lenses on corneal epithelium metabolism, Am. J. Ophthalmol. **71**(2):486, Feb. 1971.

Buxton, J.N., and Locke, C.R.: A therapeutic evaluation of hydrophilic contact lenses, Am. J. Ophthalmol. **12**:532, 1971.

Buxton, J.N., Hoefle, F.B., and Koverman, J.J.: Factors that influence the progress of keratoconus. In Girard, L.J., editor: Corneal and scleral contact lenses: Proceedings of the International Congress, St. Louis, 1967, The C.V. Mosby Co.

Caldwell, D.R., Kastl P.R., Dabezies, O.H., Miller, K.R., and Hawk, T.J.: The effect of long-term hard lens wear on corneal endothelium, Contact Intraocular Lens Med. J. **8**(2):87-91, April-June 1982.

Callender, M., and Egan, D.J.: A clinical evaluation of the Weicon-T and Durasoft-TT toric soft contact lenses, Int. Contact Lens Clin. **5**(5):209-221, Sept.-Oct. 1978.

Carney, L.G., and Hill, R.M.: Human tear pH diurnal variations, Arch. Ophthalmol. **94**:821, 1976.

Carter, D.B., and Brucker, D.: Hydrophilic contact lenses for aphakia, Am. J. Optom. Physiol. Opt. **50**(4):316-319, 1973.

Cassady, J.R.: Correction of aphakia with corneal contact lenses, Am. J. Ophthalmol. **68**(2):319-323, 1969.

Castroviejo, R.: Keratoplasty in treatment of keratoconus, Arch. Ophthalmol. **42**:776-800, 1949.

Cavanagh, H.D., Bodner, B.I., and Wilson, L.A.: Extended wear hydrogel lenses, Ophthalmology **87**(9):871, Sept. 1980.

Chaston, J., and Fatt, I.: Corneal oxygen uptake under a soft contact lens in phakic and aphakic eyes, Invest. Ophthalmol. Vis. Sci. **23**(2):234-239, Aug. 1982.

Chiquain Arias, V.: New resources in keratoconus and the H and D simplified fitting technique, Contacto **10**(2):4-11, June 1966.

Cosgrove, K.W., Jr.,: An ophthalmologist wearing extended wear contact lenses, Contact Intraocular Lens Med. J. **6**(4):366-371, Oct.-Dec. 1980.

Cotter, J.: Soft contact lens testing on fresh water scuba divers, Contact Intraocular Lens Med. J. **7**(4):323-326, Oct.-Dec. 1981.

Couzi, J.: Ocular hypertension with contact lenses Contactologia **3**(3):120-124, Aug. 1981.

Covington, W., and Gordon, S.: Peripheral design considerations in prescribing plus-powered contact lenses, Optom. Weekly, October 4, 1962.

Cowan, A.: Monocular aphakia, Arch. Ophthalmol. **50**(1):16-18, 1953.

Cureton, G.L.: Clinical experience with soft lens solutions, Contacto **20**(2):25-29, March 1976.

Dabezies, O.H.: Storage of contact lenses, Am. J. Ophthalmol. **59**(4):684-696, 1965.

Dabezies, O.H.: Contact lenses and their solutions:

a review of basic principles, Eye Ear Nose Throat Mon. **45**:39, Jan.; **45**:68, Feb.; and **45**:62, March 1966.

Dabezies, O.H.: Accessory contact lens solutions. In New Orleans Academy of Ophthalmology: Symposium on contact lenses, St. Louis, 1973, The C.V. Mosby Co.

Dabezies, O.H.: Soft contact lens hygiene, Contact Intraocular Lens Med. J. **1**(1-2):103-108, Jan.-June 1975.

Davis, H.E.: Technique in the fitting of bifocal contact lenses, Contacto **3**:70, 1959.

De la Iglesia, F.A., Mitchell, L., Kayal, M., and Schwartz, E.: Evaluation of hydrophilic contact lens effects on rabbit eyes, Contacto **20**(2):18-24, March 1976.

DeCarle, J.: Further developments of bifocal contact lenses, Contacto **3**:5, 1959.

DeCarle, J.: Further developments of bifocal contact lenses, Contacto **4**:185, 1960.

DeDonato, L.M.: Changes in the hydration of hydrogel contact lenses with wear, Am. J. Optom. Physiol. Opt. **59**(3):213-214, March 1982.

D'Halnens, J.: Soft lenses, Contact Lens Med. Bull. **7**(1-2):10, Jan.-June 1976.

Dixon, J.M.: Emotional symptoms in contact lens patients, Contact Intraocular Lens Med. J. **7**(4):327-330, Oct.-Dec. 1981.

Dixon, J.M.: Ocular changes due to contact lenses, Am. J. Ophthalmol. **58**(3):424-441, 1964.

Dixon, J.M., and others: Complications associated with the wearing of contact lenses, J.A.M.A. **195**:901, 1966.

Dixon, J.M., and Lawaczeck, E.: Corneal vascularization due to contact lenses, Arch. Ophthalmol. **49**(4):473-474, 1953.

Dixon, J.M., and Lawaczeck, E.: Corneal dimples and bubbles under corneal contact lenses, Am. J. Ophthalmol. **54**(5):827-831, 1962.

Dixon, J.M., and Lawaczeck, E.: A mechanism of glare due to corneal lenses, Am. J. Ophthalmol. **54**(6):1135-1137, 1962.

Dixon, J.M., and Lawaczeck, E.: Some disadvantages of contact lenses, Eye Ear Nose Throat Mon. **43**(9):62-63, 1964.

Dixon, J.M., Lawaczeck, E., and Winkler, C.E., Jr.: *Pseudomonas* contamination of contact lens containers: preliminary reports, Am. J. Ophthalmol. **54**:461, 1962.

Dixon, W.S., and others: Unilateral aphakia and corneal contact lenses, Can. J. Ophthalmol. **8**:97-105, 1973.

Dohlman, C.H.: Complications in therapeutic soft lens wear, Trans. Am. Acad. Ophthalmol. Otolaryngol. **78**:399, 1974.

Doughman, D.J., and others: The nature of "spots" on soft lenses, Ann. Ophthalmol. **7**:345, 1975.

Dyer, J.A.: A practical nomogram for fitting corneal contact lenses, Contact Lens Med. Bull. **1**(4):8-11, 1968.

Dyer, J.A.: XIIIth Conrad Berens memorial lecture: corneal contact lenses in perspective 1948-1981, Contact Intraocular Lens Med. J. **8**(1):3-8, Jan.-March 1982.

Dyer, J.A., and Ogle, E.W.: Correction of unilateral aphakia with contact lenses, Am. J. Ophthalmol. **50**(1):11-17, 1960.

Editorial: The adjustment to aphakia, Am. J. Ophthalmol. **35**:118, 1955.

Elmstrom, G.P.: The legal aspects of contact lens practice, J.A.O.A. **35**(9):775-777, 1964.

Fatt I., and Chaston, J.: Measurement of oxygen transmissibility and permeability of hydrogel lenses and materials, Int. Contact Lens Clin. **9**(2):76-88, March-April 1982.

Fatt, I., and Chaston, J.: Relation of oxygen transmissibility to oxygen tension or EOP under the lens, Int. Contact Lens Clin. **9**(2):119-120, March-April 1982.

Feldman, G.L., Repella, D., Rafter, R., and Wilke, T.: Fitting characteristics and gas permeability of thin hydrogel lenses, Contact Lens J. **10**(3):13-20, Dec. 1976.

Filderman, I.P., and White, P.F.: Contact lens optics: applied clinical aspects, South. J. Optom. **7**(4):10-13, 16, 28-31; **7**(5):12-17, 26; **7**(6):13-17, 1965.

Fowler, S.A., and Allansmith, M.R.: Evolution of soft contact lens coating, Arch. Ophthalmol. **98**:95-99, Jan. 1980.

Franceschetti, A.: Keratoconus. In King, J.H., Jr., and McTigue, J.W., editors: The Cornea World Congress, London 1965, Butterworth & Co. (Publishers) Ltd., pp. 152-168.

Garcia, G.E.: Continuous wear of gas permeable contact lens in aphakia, Contact Intraocular Lens Med. J. **2**(1):29-34, Jan.-March 1976.

Gasset, A.R., and Kaufman, H.E.: Bandage lenses in the treatment of bullous keratopathy, Am. J. Ophthalmol. **72**:376, 1971.

Gasset, A.R., and Kaufman, H.E.: Soft contact lens, St. Louis, 1972, The C.V. Mosby Co.

Gasset, A.R., Lubo, L., and Houde, W.: Permanent wear aphakic lenses, Am. J. Ophthalmol. **83**(1):115, Jan. 1977.

Girard, L.J.: Corneal topography, keratometry, and contact lenses, Arch. Ophthalmol. **67**:753-760, 1962.

Girard, L.J., Soper, J.W., and Sampson, W.G.: Corneal contact lens, St. Louis, 1970, The C.V. Mosby Co.

Goar, E.L.: Monocular aphakia, Arch. Ophthalmol. **50**:779, 1953.

Goar, E.L.: The management of monocular cataracts, Arch. Ophthalmol. **54**(1):73-76, 1955.

Goar, E.L.: Contact lenses in monocular aphakia, Arch. Ophthalmol. **58**:417, 1957.

Goldberg, J.B.: The fallacy of the ophthalmometer in contact lens practice. J.A.O.A. **33**:593-594, 1962.

Goldberg, J.B.: Must the gas go through? Optom. Weekly **66**(34):15, Oct. 2, 1975.

Goldberg, J.B.: The conventional corneal lens: safety and efficiency, Optom. Weekly **67**(6):135-138, Feb. 5, 1976.

Gordon, S.: Some aspects of "venting" in corneal contact lenses, Encyclopedia Contact Lens Pract. **1**(11):6-34, 1961.

Gordon, S.: An evaluation of small, thin contact lenses, Optom. Weekly **55**(5):21-25, 1964.

Gordon, S.: Contact lens hydration: a study of the wetting-drying cycle, Optom. Weekly **56**(14):55-62, 1965.

Gordon, S.: Designing a minimum-thickness hard contact lens, Contact Lens Forum, pp. 41-53, June 1976.

Gould, H.L.: Management of keratoconus with corneal and scleral lenses, Am. J. Ophthalmol. **70**:624, 1970.

Grant, S.C., and May, C.H.: Orthokeratology—the control of refractive errors through contact lenses, Optician **163**:8-11, 1972.

Grayson, M.: Diseases of the cornea, ed. 2, St. Louis, 1983 The C.V. Mosby Co.

Green, W.R.: An embedded ("lost") contact lens, Arch. Ophthalmol. **69**(1):23-24, 1963.

Gregg, B.R.: Aspheric contact lenses: development and doubt, Contact Lens **2**(5):20-24, 31, 1969.

Grosvenor, T.: Clinical use of the keratometer in evaluating corneal contour, J.A.O.A. **38**(5):237-246, 1961.

Grosvenor, T.: Optical principles of soft contact lenses, Optom. Weekly **67**(3):29-31, Jan. 15, 1976.

Grosvenor, T.: Optical principles of aphakic contact lens fitting, Optom. Weekly **67**(8):27-30, Feb. 19, 1976.

Gruber, E.: Six years experience with Soflens, Contact Intraocular Lens Med. J. **1**(2):70-82, Jan.-June 1975.

Hall, K.C.: A special contact lens for complete ptosis, J.A.O.A. **30**(2):121-123, 1958.

Hall, N.C., and Krezanoski, J.Z.: Antimicrobial synergism in a contact lens soaking solution, N. Engl. J. Optom. **13**(9):229-233, 1963.

Hamano, H.: The change of precorneal tear film by the application of contact lenses, Contact Intraocular Lens Med. J. **7**(3):205-209, July-Sept. 1981.

Hamano, H., and Kawabe, H.: Standardization of soft contact lenses, Contacto **20**(4):14-19, July 1976.

Hamano, H., and Kawabe, H.: Variation of base curve of soft lens during wearing, Contacto **22**:10-14, Jan. 1978.

Hamano, H., Kawabe, H., Maeshima, J., and Kojima, S.: Statistical trends of wearers of contact lenses, Contact Intraocular Lens Med. J. **8**(1):29-37, Jan.-March 1982.

Harris, M.G., Harris, K.L., and Ruddell, D.: Rotation of lathe-cut hydrogel lenses on the eye, Am. J. Optom. Physiol. Opt. **53**(1):20-26, Jan. 1976.

Hartstein, J.: Astigmatism induced by corneal contact lenses. In Becker, B., and Drews, R.C.: Current concepts in ophthalmology, vol. 1, St. Louis, 1967, The C.V. Mosby Co.

Hartstein, J.: Practical points in contact lens fitting, Eye Ear Nose Throat Mon. **46**(8):1004-1005, 1967.

Highman, V.N.: High water content soft contact lenses for continuous wear, Contact Lens J. **5**(5):1976.

Hill, J.F.: Variation in refractive error and corneal curvature after wearing hydrophilic contact lenses, J.A.O.A. **3**(46):290-294, 1975.

Hill, M.E.: Lenses in ambience, Int. Contact Lens Clin. **9**(2):94-96, March-April 1982.

Hill, R.M.: Extended wear: closing the gap, Contact Lens Forum **4**(12):67-69, Dec. 1979.

Hill, R.M., and Carney, L.G.: Extended wear systems, Contact Lens Forum **1**(6):29-31, Oct. 1976.

Hind, H.W., and Szekely, I.J.: Wetting and hydration of contact lenses, Contacto **3**(3):65-68, 1959.

Hind, H.W., Szekely, I.J., and Krezanoski, J.Z.: Contact lens wetting and comfort, Encyclopedia Contact Lens Pract. **4**(21):32-42, 1963.

Hoefle, F.B.: Contact lens insertion and removal for aphakes, Contact Lens Med. Bull. **6**(4):19, Oct.-Dec. 1973.

Holden, B.A.: The principles and practice of correcting astigmatism with soft contact lenses, Aust. J. Optom. **58**:279-299, 1975.

Holly, F.J., and Lemp, M.A.: Tear physiology and dry eyes, Surv. Ophthalmol. **22**(2):69-87 Sept.-Oct. 1977.

Holly, F.J., and Refojo, M.F.: Oxygen permeability of hydrogel contact lenses, J.A.O.A. **43**:1173-1178, 1972.

Holly, F.J., and Refojo, M.F.: Wettability of hydrogels, J. Biomed. Mater. Res. **9**:315-326, 1975.

Hosty, F.E.: Problems encountered during the fitting and wearing of contact lenses, J. Fla. Med. Assoc. **48**:971, 1962.

Houde, W.L., and Rubin, M.L.: Extended wear lenses: an update, Surv. Ophthalmol. **26**(2):103-105, Sept.-Oct. 1981.

Ing. M.R.: Experience with extended wear hydrogel lenses for aphakia, Ann. Ophthalmol. **13**(2):181-182, Feb. 1981.

Jenkin, L.: Fitting haptic lenses by impression technique, Br. J. Physiol. Opt. **21**(3):163-168, 1964.

Jessen, G.W.: Medium and large lens fitting techniques, Contacto **2**(1):37-39, 1967.

Jessop, D.G.: Peripheral keratometric findings, Contacto 6:19-23, 1962.

Johnson, D.G.: Soft hydrophilic contact lenses, Can. J. Ophthalmol. 6:342, 1971.

Johnson, D.G.: Keratoconjunctivitis associated with wearing hydrophilic contact lenses, Can. J. Ophthalmol. 8:92, 1973.

Josephson, J.E.: Hydrogel lens wearers utilizing preserved solutions, J. Am. Optom. Assoc. 49:280, 1978.

Josephson, J.E.: Appearance of the preocular tear film lipid layer, Am. J. Optom. Physiol. Opt. 60(11):883, Nov. 1983.

Josephson, J.E., and Caffery, B.E.: Hydrogel lens solutions, Int. Ophthalmol. Clin. 21:163, 1981.

Josephson, J.E., Caffery, B.E., and Pope, C.A.: Clinical experience with tinted hydrogel lenses, Can. J. Optom. 44(3):21, 1983.

Junzo, A., and Manabu, A., editors: Menicon hard and soft contact lenses, Tokyo, 1977, Tokyo Contact Lens Co.

Kaetting, R.A., and Boyd, W.S.: Surface artifacts found on unboiled hydrophilic lenses, Int. Contact Lens Clin. 3(4):37-41, Dec. 1976.

Kamiki, T., and Kikkawa, Y.: Ozone sterilization technique of hydrophilic contact lenses, Contacto 20(3):16-18, May 1976.

Kapetansky, F.M., Suie, T., Gracy, A.D., and Bitonte, J.L.: Contact lens bacteriology, Am. J. Ophthalmol. 57(2):255-258, 1964.

Kaufman, H.E.: Problems associated with prolonged wear soft contact lenses, ophthalmology 86: 411-417, March 1979.

Kaufman, H.E., and others: The medical uses of soft contact lenses, Trans. Am. Acad. Ophthalmol. Otolaryngol. 74:902, 1970.

Kaufman, H.E., Uotila, M.H., Gasset, A.R., Wood, T.O., and Ellison, E.D.: The medical use of soft contact lenses, Trans. Am. Acad. Ophthalmol. Otolaryngol. 75:361-373, 1971.

Keates, R.H., and Falkenstein, S.: Keratoplasty in keratoconus, Am. J. Ophthalmol. 74(3):442-444, 1972.

Kerns, R.L. Contact lens control of myopia, Am. J. Optom. Physiol. Opt. 58(7):541-545, July 1981.

Kersley, H.J.: Soft contact lenses in aphaki, Contact Lens J. 5(8):29-30, 1977.

Kimura, S.J.: Fluorescein paper, Am. J. Ophthalmol. 34(3):446-447, 1951.

Kleist, F.: Appearance and nature of hydrophilic contact lens deposits, Int. Contact Lens Clin. 6(3):120-130, May-June 1979.

Koliopoulos, J., and Tragakis, M.: Visual correction of keratoconus with soft contact lenses, Ann. Ophthalmol. 13(7):835-837, July 1981.

Koller, H.P., and Caputo, A.: The use of the hydrophilic contact lens in amblyopia therapy, scientific exhibit, Am. Acad. Ophthalmol. Otolaryngol. 74(3):534, Sept. 1972.

Korb, D.R.: Edematous corneal formation, J.A.O.A. 44(3):March 1973.

Korb, D.R., and Exford, J.M.: A study of three and nine o'clock staining after unilateral lens removal, J.A.O.A. 41(3):7-10, 1970.

Korb, D.R., and Korb, J.E.: A new concept in contact lens design. Parts I and II, J.A.O.A. 41(12):1023-1032, 1970.

Korb, D., and Refojo, M.: Personal communications, Boston, 1982.

Korb, D.R., Finnemore, V.M., and Herman, J.P.: Apical changes and scarring in keratoconus as related to contact lens fitting techniques, J.A.O.A. 53(3):199-205, March 1982.

Krause, A.C.: Biochemistry of the eye, Arch. Ophthalmol. 15(3):522-543, 1936.

Krezanoski, J.: The significance of cleaning hydrophilic contact lenses, J.A.O.A. 43:305, 1972.

Krezanoski, J.: Where are we in the developments of pharmaceutical products for soft (hydrophilic) lenses? Contacto 20(1):12-16, Jan. 1976.

Krezanoski, J.: Care of soft contacts: an update, Contact Lens Forum 1(2):63-69, June 1976.

Lambert, S.R., and Klyce, S.D.: The origins of soft contact lens fit, Ophthalmology 91(1):51-56, Jan. 1981.

Lamp, M., Goldberg, M., and Roddy, M.: The effect of tear substitutes on tear film break up time, Invest. Med. 14(3):255, March 1975.

Lansche, R.K., and Lee, R.C.: Acute complications from present day corneal contact lenses: a report of fourteen new cases, Arch. Ophthalmol. 64:275, 1960.

Lebensohn, J.E.: The nature of photophobia, Arch. Ophthalmol. 12:380, 1934.

Lebensohn, J.E.: Photophobia: mechanisms and implications, Am. J. Ophthalmol. 34(9):1294-1300, 1951.

Lehmann, S.P.: Corneal areas utilized in keratometry, Optician 154(3989):261-264, 1967.

Leibowitz, H.M.: Continuous wear of hydrophilic contact lenses, Arch. Ophthalmol. 89:306, 1973.

Leibowitz, H.M., and Rosenthal, P.: Hydrophilic contact lenses in corneal diseases, Arch. Ophthalmol. 85:163, 1971.

Lemp, M.A., Holly, F.J., and Dohlman, C.H.: Corneal desiccation despite normal tear volume, Ann. Ophthalmol. 2(3):258-261, 1970.

Lemp, M.A., Holly, F.J., Iwata, S., and Dohlman, C.H.: The precorneal tear film. I. Factors in spreading and maintaining a continuous tear film over the corneal surface, Arch. Ophthalmol. 83:89, 1970.

Lenz, M.A., and Hammil, R.H.: Factors affecting tear film breakup in normal eyes, Arch. Ophthalmol. 89:103, 1973.

Lester, R.W.: Fluorescein and contact lenses, Contacto 2(4):91, 1958.

Levinson, A., and Weissman, B.: An analysis of the general fitting of hydrophilic contact lenses in Israel, Int. Contact Lens Clin. 3(4):64-70, Nov.-Dec. 1976.

Lippman, J.I.: Gas permeable contact lenses: an overview, Contact Intraocular Med. J. 7(1):15, Jan.-March 1981.

Lowe, R.F.: Recurrent erosion of the cornea, Br. J. Ophthalmol. 54(12):805-809, 1970.

Mackie, I.A.: Localised corneal drying in association with dellen, pterygia, and related lesions, Trans. Ophthalmol. Soc. U.K. 91:129, 1972.

Maltzman, B.A., and Cinotti, A.A.: Extended wear contact lenses, Contact Lens 5(3):19-25, July-Sept. 1979.

Mandell, A.M.: Contact lenses for keratoconus, CLAO Papers 2(8):August 1960 (Contact Lens Association of Ophthalmology).

Mandell, R.B.: Corneal oxygen need and gas permeable contact lenses, J.A.O.A. 53(3):211-214, March 1982.

Mandell, R.B.: Keratopography, Encyclopedia Contact Lens Pract. 3:12-51, 1962.

Mandell, R.B., editor: International Contact Lens Clinics, Chicago, 1974, Professional Press.

Mandell, R.B.: Contact lens practice, ed. 2, Springfield, Ill., 1974, Charles C Thomas, Publisher.

Martin, W.F.: Results of a research study on the vision of athletes, Optom. Weekly 55(29):23-27, 1964.

Martin, W.R.J., and Smith, E.L.: Some points in the surgical technique of keratoplasty, Am. J. Ophthalmol. 55:1199-1208, 1963.

Meschel, L.G.: Second generation soft contact lenses, Contact Intraocular Lens Med. J. 2(3):26-39, July-Sept. 1976.

Miller, D.: An analysis of the physical forces applied to a corneal contact lens, Arch. Ophthalmol. 70(6):823-829, 1963.

Miller, D.: Contact lens-induced corneal curvature and thickness changes, Arch. Ophthalmol. 80(4):430-432, 1968.

Millodot, M.: Effect of long-term wear of hard contact lenses on corneal sensitivity, Arch. Ophthalmol. 96:1225-1227, July 1978.

Mitra, S., and Lamberts, D.W.: Contact sensitivity in soft lens wearers, Contact Intraocular Lens Med. J. 7(4):315-322, Oct.-Dec. 1981.

Mizutani, Y., and Miwa, Y.: Hydrophilic silicone rubber contact lens, Contacto 21(1):15-19, Jan. 1977.

Mobilia, E.F., and Foster, C.S.: A comparison of various extended wear lenses for use in aphakia, Contact Intraocular Lens Med. J. 8(1):12-15, Jan.-March 1982.

Mobilia, E.F., Yamamoto, G.K. and Dohlman, C.H.: Cornea wrinkling induced by ultra-thin soft contact lenses, Ann. Ophthalmol. 12(4):371-375, April 1980.

Molinari, J.F.: The clinical assessment of giant papillary conjunctivitis, Am. J. Optom. Physiol. Opt. 58(10):886-891, Oct. 1981.

Mondino, B.J., Salamon, S.M., and Zaidman, G.W.: Allergic and toxic reactions in soft contact lens wearers, Surv. Ophthalmol. 26(6):337-343, May-June 1982.

Morgan, J.F.: Induced corneal astigmatism with hydrophilic contact lenses, Can. J. Ophthalmol. 10:207-213, 1975.

Morrison, R.: Small thin contact lens use, Optom. Weekly 54(18):853-855, 1963.

New Orleans Academy of Ophthalmology: Symposium on contact lenses, St. Louis, 1973, The C.V. Mosby Co.

Nony, J.C.: Retention of contact lens in upper fornix, Am. J. Ophthalmol. 56(2):309, 1963.

Obean, M.F., and Winter, F.C.: Contact lens storage, Am. J. Ophthalmol. 57(3):441-443, 1964.

Ogle, K.N., Burian, H.M., and Bannon, R.E.: On the correction of unilateral aphakia with contact lenses, Arch. Ophthalmol. 59(5):639-652, 1958.

Ohrt, V.: Acute keratoconus caused by displacement of a contact lens, Acta Ophthalmol. 34:218, 1956.

Pierce, D., and Kersley, H.J.: Hydrophilic lenses for continuous wear in aphakia: fitting at operation, Br. J. Ophthalmol. 61(1):34-37, Jan. 1977.

Podos, S.M., Becker, B., Asseff, C., and Hartstein, J.: Pilocarpine therapy with soft contact lenses, Am. J. Ophthalmol. 73:336-341, 1972.

Polse, H.A., Sarver, M.D., and Harris, M.G.: Corneal effects of high plus hydrogel lenses, Am. J. Optom. Physiol. Opt. 55:234-237, 1978.

Portfolio, A.G.: Continuous contact lens wear, Arch. Ophthalmol. 70(3):443, 1963.

Poster, M.G.: Hydro-dynamics of corneal contact lenses, Am. J. Optom. Arch. Am. Acad. Optom. 41(7):422-425, 1964.

Pratt-Johnson, J., and Warner, D.: Corneal curvature changes, Am. J. Ophthalmol. 60(5):852-855, 1965.

Precision COSMET Digest, monthly bulletins, 1976, Ullen, R., editor.

Price, M.J., Morgan, J.F., Willis, W.E., and Wasan, S.: Tarsal conjunctival appearance in contact lens wearers, Contact Intraocular Lens Med. J. 8(1):16-22, Jan.-March 1982.

Refojo, M.F.: A critical review of properties and applications of soft hydrogel contact lenses, Surv. Ophthalmol. 16:233, 1972.

Refojo, M.F.: Materials in bandage lenses Contact Intraocular Med. J. 5(1):34-44, Jan.-March 1979.

Refojo, M.F., and Holly, F.J.: Tear protein adsorption on hydrogels: a possible cause of contact lens allergy, Contact Intraocular Lens Med. J. **3**(1):23-35, Jan.-March 1977.

Rengstorf, R.H.: A study of visual acuity loss after contact lens wear, Am. J. Optom. **43**(7):431-440, 1966.

Reynolds, A.E., and Kratt, H.J.: The photo-electronic keratoscope, Contacto **3**:53, 1959.

Rich, G.E.: Fitting hydrogel lenses with photokeratography, Int. Contact Lens Clin. **4**(1):36-47, Jan.-Feb. 1977.

Ridley, F.: Contact lenses in treatment of keratoconus, Br. J. Ophthalmol. **40**:295-304, 1956.

Ridley, F.: Scleral contact lenses, Arch. Ophthalmol. **70**(6):740-745, 1963.

Ridley, F.: Contact lenses—the role of the ophthalmologist, Proc. R. Soc. Med. **57**:27, 1964.

Rietschel, R.L., and Wilson, L.A.: Ocular inflammation in patients using soft contact lenses, Arch. Dermatol. **118**(3):147-149, March 1982.

Rocher, P., and Francois, J.: Choice of total diameter of a contact lens, Contacto **12**(2):30-35, 1968.

Rosenthal, J.W.: Clinical pathology in contact lenses. In Raiford, M., editor: Contact lens management, Boston, 1962, Little, Brown & Co.

Rosenthal, P.: Corneal contact lenses: large or small, Arch. Ophthalmol. **76**:631-632, 1966.

Ruben, M.: Corneal changes in contact lens wear, Trans. Ophthalmol. Soc. U.K. **87**:27-43, 1967.

Ruben, M.: The fitting of corneal contact lenses, Trans. Ophthalmol. Soc. U.K. **87**:661, 1967.

Ruben, M., editor: Soft contact lenses: clinical and applied technology, London, 1978, Bailliere Tindall Pubs. (New York, Wiley Medical Publications).

Ruben, R., Tripathi, C., and Winder, A.F.: Calcium deposits as a cause of spoilation of hydrophilic contact lenses, Br. J. Ophthalmol. **59**:141-148, 1975.

Sampson, W.G.: The properties of ophthalmic prisms and their application in corneal contact lenses, presented at First Annual Ophthalmology Alumni Meeting, Houston, Texas, April 1964.

Sampson, W.G.: Contact lenses and the AC/A ratio: applications in accommodative esotropia, Contact Lens Med. Bull. **2**(3):9-15, 1969.

Sampson, W.G.: Curvature irregularity and its dioptric effect on corneal contact lenses, Contact Lens Med. Bull. **1**(1-2):4-7, Jan.-March 1968.

Sampson, W.G.: Correction of refractive errors: effect on accommodation and convergence, Trans. Am. Acad. Ophthalmol. Otolaryngol. **75**(1):124-132, 1971.

Sampson, W.G., Soper, J.W., and Girard, L.J.: Topographical keratometry and contact lenses, Trans. Am. Ophthalmol. Otolaryngol. **69**:959-969, 1965.

Schlossman, A.: The ophthalmological advanced fitting contact lens symposium. Part 2, Eye Ear Nose Throat Mon. **45**(1):94, 118, 1966.

Shaw, E.L.: Diagrams and pathophysiology of keratoconus, Contact Lens Med. Bull. **7**(3):56, July-Sept. 1974.

Sibley, M.J.: Tailoring solutions for new lens material, Contacto **20**(5):32-33, Sept. 1976.

Slatt, B.J., and Stein, H.A.: Why wear glasses if you want contacts? Richmond Hill, Ontario, 1972, Simon & Schuster of Canada Ltd.

Sloan, D.P.: A report on continuous contact lens wearing, Contacto **4**(4):117-122, 1960.

Smelser, G.K.: Relation of factors involved in maintenance of optical properties of cornea to contact lens wear. Arch. Ophthalmol. **47**:328, 1952.

Smelser, G.K., and Chen, D.K.: Physiological changes in cornea induced by contact lenses, Arch. Ophthalmol. **53**(5):676-679, 1955.

Snyder, D.A., Litinsky, S.M., and Gelender, H.: Hypopyon iridocyclitis associated with extended wear soft contact lenses, Am. J. Ophthalmol. **93**(4):519-520, April 1982.

Soft lens care: scientific and clinical aspects, roundtable discussion, PanAmerican Congress of Ophthalmology, April 23, 1975.

Soper, J.W.: A new lens for keratoconus, presented to the annual convention of the Contact Lens Society of America, Las Vegas, 1969.

Soper, J.W., editor: Contact lenses: advances in design, fitting, application, New York, 1974, Stratton Intercontinental Medical Book Corp.

Soper, J.W., Sampson, W.G., and Girard, L.J.: Corneal topography, keratometry, and contact lenses, Arch. Ophthalmol. **67**(6):753-760, 1962.

Spring, T.: Corneal endothelium: the effects of contact lenses and keratoconus, Contact Intraocular Lens Med. J. **8**(1):9-11, Jan.-March 1982.

Stark, W.J., and Martin, N.F.: Extended-wear contact lenses for myopic correction, Arch. Ophthalmol. **99**(11):1963-1966, Nov. 1981.

Stark, W.J., Kracher, G.P., Cowan, C.L., et al.: Extended-wear contact lens and intraocular lenses for aphakic correction, Am. J. Ophthalmol. **88**(3 Pt. 2):535-542, 1979.

Steele, E.: The fitting of aspheric corneal contact lenses, Contacto **13**(4):55-57, 1969.

Steele, E.: The fitting of aspheric corneal contact lenses, Ophthalmol. Optician, pp. 1216-1218, Nov. 15, 1969.

Stein, H.A.: Swimming with soft contact lenses, Contact Lens J. **10**(3):10-12, Dec. 1976.

Stein, H.A.: Therapeutic uses of soft lenses, Contact Lens J. **10**(3):25-28, Dec. 1976.

Stein, H.A.: Aphakia—selection of patients for contact lenses, intraocular lenses or spectacles: review of 1,000 cataract operations, Contact Intraocular Lens Med. J. **7**(3):210-218, July-Sept. 1981.

Stein, H.A., and Slatt, B.J.: Clinical impressions of hydrophilic lenses, Can. J. Ophthalmol. **8:**83, 1973.

Stein, H.A., and Slatt, B.J.: Contact lenses after cataract surgery, Can. J. Ophthalmol. **9**(1):79-80, 1974.

Stein, H.A., and Slatt, B.J.: The ophthalmic assistant, ed. 3, St. Louis, 1976, The C.V. Mosby Co.

Stein, H.A., and Slatt, B.J.: Swimming and contact lenses, Contact Intraocular Lens Med. J. **3**(3):24-26, July-Sept. 1977.

Stone, J.: Comments on orthokeratology and extended wear contact lenses, Can. J. Ophthalmol. **40**(1):4, March 1978.

Stone, J., and Phillips, A.J., editors: Contact lenses: a textbook for practitioner and student, ed. 2, Sevenoaks, Kent, 1981, Butterworth & Co. (Pubs.) Ltd.

Sutherland, R.L., and VanLeeuwen, W.N.: Soft contact lenses, Can. Med. Assoc. J. **107:**49-50, July 1972.

Sutten, V.L., and others: *Pseudomonas* in human saliva, J. Dent. Res. **45:**1800, 1966.

Swanson, K.: Dispensing contact lenses, St. Louis, 1975, Mo-Con Laboratories, Inc.

Szekely, I.J., and Hind, H.W.: Treated polyvinyl alcohol for contact lens solution, United States Patent 3, 183, 152, 1965.

Szekely, I.J., Hind, H.W., and Krezanoski, J.Z.: Accessory contact lens solutions, Encyclopedia Contact Lens Pract. **4**(20):13-26, 1963.

Tajiri, A.: Impression technique to determine edge contour of contact lenses, Contacto **4**(9):391-397, 1960.

Tannehill, J.C., and Sampson, W.G.: Extended use of the Radiuscope in contact lens inspection, Am. J. Ophthalmol. **62:**538, 1966.

Temprano, J.: Therapeutic use of soft contact lenses, Contact Intraocular Lens Med. J. **2**(3):60-67, July-Sept. 1976.

Tripathi, R.C., and Tripathi, B.J.: The role of the lids in soft lens spoilage, Contact Intraocular Lens Med. J. **7**(3):234-241, July-Sept. 1981.

Tripathi, R.C., Tripathi, B.J., and Ruben, M.: The pathology of soft contact lens spoilage, J. Ophthalmol. **87**(5):365-380, May 1980.

Tsuda, S., Tanaka, K., Takahashi, K., et al.: Corneal physiology and oxygen permeability of contact lenses, Int. Contact Lens Clin. **8**(3):11-22, May-June 1981.

Ullen, R.L.: Legal implications in fitting contact lenses, J.A.O.A. **38**(4):288-291, 1961.

Vaughan, D.G.: The contamination of fluorescein solutions, Am. J. Ophthalmol. **39**(1):55-61, 1955.

Vidal, F.L.: Medical complications of contact lenses, Int. Ophthalmol. Clin. **1**(2):495-504, 1961.

Wechsler, S., and Wilson, G.: Changes in hydrogel contact lens power due to flexure, Am. J. Optom. Physiol. Opt. **55:**78-83, 1978.

Weidt, A.R., and Cunin, B.M.: The bifocal alternative, Contact Intraocular Lens Med. J. **7**(3):250-251, July-Sept. 1981.

Weinberg, R.J.: Corneal vascularization in aphakia, Am. J. Ophthalmol. **83**(1):121, Jan. 1977.

Weis, D.R.: Contact lenses for athletes, Int. Ophthalmol. Clin. **21**(4):139-148, Winter 1981.

Weissman, B.A., Fatt, I., and Rasson, J.: Diffusion of oxygen in human corneas in vivo, Invest. Ophthalmol. Vis. Sci. **20**(1):123-125, Jan. 1981.

Welsh, R.C.: Contact lenses in aphakia, Int. Ophthalmol. Clin. **1**(2):401-440, 1961.

Welsh, R.C.: The moving ring scotoma: with its jack-in-the-box phenomenon of strong-plus (aphakic) spectacle lenses, Am. J. Ophthalmol. **51**(6):1277-1281, 1961.

Welsh, R.C.: Experimental simulation of aphakia, Br. J. Ophthalmol. **49**(2):84-86, 1965.

Wesley, N.K.: The Sphercon bifocal contact lens, Optom. Weekly **49:**586, 1958.

Westheimer, G.A.: Aberrations of contact lenses, Am. J. Optom. Arch. Am. Acad. Optom. **38**(8):445-448, 1961.

Westheimer, G.A.: A method of photoelectric keratoscopy, Am. J. Optom. **42**(5):315-320, 1965.

Wilson, L.A., Schlitzer, R.L., and Ahearn, D.G.: *Pseudomonas* corneal ulcers associated with soft contact lens wear, Am. J. Ophthalmol. **92**(4):546-554, Oct. 1981.

Winkler, C.H., and Dixon, J.M.: Bacteriology of the eye. Part III: A. Effect of contact lenses on the normal flora. B. Flora of the contact lens, Arch. Ophthalmol. **72**(6):817-819, 1964.

Woodworth, H.W.: Monocular correction of presbyopia with contact lenses, Presented at annual meeting, Contact Lens Society of America, St. Louis, 1961.

Wulfing, B.: The need of soft contact lenses for older aphakics: a pilot study, Contact Intraocular Lens Med. J. **1**(1-2):40-41, Jan.-June 1975.

Zekman, T.N., and Krimmer, B.M.: The treatment of conical cornea: introduction of a new multicurve fluidless corneal contact lens. Arch. Ophthalmol. **54**(2):481-488, 1955.

Zekman, T.N., and Sarnat, L.A.: Clinical evaluation of the silicone corneal contact lens, Am. J. Ophthalmol. **74**(3):534, Sept. 1972.

Zantos, S.G., and Holden B.A.: Research techniques and materials for continuous wear of contact lenses, Aust. J. Optom. **60:**86-95, March 1977.

APPENDIXES

THICKNESS CONVERSION TABLE

Inches	mm	Inches	mm
0.001	0.025	0.021	0.525
0.002	0.050	0.022	0.550
0.003	0.075	0.023	0.575
0.004	0.100	0.024	0.600
0.005	0.125	0.025	0.625
0.006	0.150	0.026	0.650
0.007	0.175	0.027	0.675
0.008	0.200	0.028	0.700
0.009	0.225	0.029	0.725
0.010	0.250	0.030	0.750
0.011	0.275	0.031	0.775
0.012	0.300	0.032	0.800
0.013	0.325	0.033	0.825
0.014	0.350	0.034	0.850
0.015	0.375	0.035	0.875
0.016	0.400	0.036	0.900
0.017	0.425	0.037	0.925
0.018	0.450	0.038	0.950
0.019	0.475	0.039	0.975
0.020	0.500	0.040	1.000

From Hartstein, J.: Questions and answers on contact lens practice, ed. 2, St. Louis, 1973, The C.V. Mosby Co.

CONVERSION TABLES FOR DIOPTERS TO MILLIMETERS OF RADIUS

Diopter conversion table

Diopters	mm	Diopters	mm	Diopters	mm	Diopters	mm
20.00	16.875	36.00	9.375	39.00	8.653	42.00	8.035
22.00	15.340	36.12	9.343	39.12	8.627	42.12	8.012
24.00	14.062	36.25	9.310	39.25	8.598	42.25	7.988
26.00	12.980	36.37	9.279	39.37	8.572	42.37	7.965
27.00	12.500	36.50	9.246	39.50	8.544	42.50	7.941
28.00	12.053	36.62	9.216	39.62	8.518	42.62	7.918
29.00	11.638	36.75	9.183	39.75	8.490	42.75	7.894
29.50	11.441	36.87	9.153	39.87	8.465	42.87	7.872
30.00	11.250	37.00	9.121	40.00	8.437	43.00	7.848
30.50	11.065	37.12	9.092	40.12	8.412	43.12	7.826
31.00	10.887	37.25	9.060	40.25	8.385	43.25	8.803
31.50	10.714	37.37	9.031	40.37	8.360	43.37	7.781
32.00	10.547	37.50	9.000	40.50	8.333	43.50	7.758
32.50	10.385	37.62	8.971	40.62	8.308	43.62	7.737
33.00	10.227	37.75	8.940	40.75	8.282	43.75	7.714
33.50	10.075	37.87	8.912	40.87	8.257	43.87	7.693
34.00	9.926	38.00	8.881	41.00	8.231	44.00	7.670
34.25	9.854	38.12	8.853	41.12	8.207	44.12	7.649
34.50	9.783	38.25	8.823	41.25	8.181	44.25	7.627
34.75	9.712	38.37	8.795	41.37	8.158	44.37	7.606
35.00	9.643	38.50	8.766	41.50	8.132	44.50	7.584
35.25	9.574	38.62	8.738	41.62	8.109	44.62	7.563
35.50	9.507	38.75	8.708	41.75	8.083	44.75	7.541
35.75	9.440	38.87	8.682	41.87	8.060	44.87	7.521

From Stein, H.A., and Slatt, B.J.: The ophthalmic assistant, ed. 4, St. Louis, 1982, The C.V. Mosby Co.

Diopters	mm	Diopters	mm	Diopters	mm	Diopters	mm
45.00	7.500	48.00	7.031	51.00	6.617	54.00	6.250
45.12	7.480	48.12	7.013	51.12	6.602	54.12	6.236
45.25	7.458	48.25	6.994	51.25	6.585	54.25	6.221
45.37	7.438	48.37	6.977	51.37	6.569	54.37	6.207
45.50	7.417	48.50	6.958	51.50	6.553	54.50	6.192
45.62	7.398	48.62	6.941	51.62	6.538	54.62	6.179
45.75	7.377	48.75	6.923	51.75	6.521	54.75	6.164
45.87	7.357	48.87	6.906	51.87	6.506	54.87	6.150
46.00	7.336	49.00	6.887	52.00	6.490	55.00	6.136
46.12	7.317	49.12	6.870	52.12	6.475	55.12	6.123
46.25	7.297	49.25	6.852	52.25	6.459	55.25	6.108
46.37	7.278	49.37	6.836	52.37	6.444	55.37	6.095
46.50	7.258	49.50	6.818	52.50	6.428	55.50	6.081
46.62	7.239	49.62	6.801	52.62	6.413	55.62	6.068
46.75	7.219	49.75	6.783	52.75	6.398	55.75	6.054
46.87	7.200	49.87	6.767	52.87	6.383	55.87	6.041
47.00	7.180	50.00	6.750	53.00	6.367	56.00	6.027
47.12	7.162	50.12	6.733	53.12	6.353	56.50	5.973
47.25	7.142	50.25	6.716	53.25	6.338	57.00	5.921
47.37	7.124	50.37	6.700	53.37	6.323	57.50	5.869
47.50	7.105	50.50	6.683	53.50	6.308	58.00	5.819
47.62	7.087	50.62	6.667	53.62	6.294	58.50	5.769
47.75	7.068	50.75	6.650	53.75	6.279	59.00	5.720
47.87	7.050	50.87	6.634	53.87	6.265	60.00	5.625

SPECTACLE LENS POWER WORN AT VARIOUS DISTANCES TO EQUIVALENT CONTACT LENS POWER

Vertex conversion table

Spectacle lens power	Effective power at corneal plane of spectacles at designated distance from cornea (vertex distance/millimeters)							
	Plus lenses							
	8 mm	*9 mm*	*10 mm*	*11 mm*	*12 mm*	*13 mm*	*14 mm*	*15 mm*
4.00	4.12	4.12	4.12	4.12	4.25	4.25	4.25	4.25
4.50	4.62	4.75	4.75	4.75	4.75	4.75	4.75	4.87
5.00	5.25	5.25	5.25	5.25	5.25	5.37	5.37	5.37
5.50	5.75	5.75	5.75	5.87	5.87	5.87	6.00	6.00
6.00	6.25	6.37	6.37	6.37	6.50	6.50	6.50	6.62
6.50	6.87	6.87	7.00	7.00	7.00	7.12	7.12	7.25
7.00	7.37	7.50	7.50	7.62	7.62	7.75	7.75	7.75
7.50	8.00	8.00	8.12	8.12	8.25	8.25	8.37	8.50
8.00	8.50	8.62	8.75	8.75	8.87	8.87	9.00	9.12
8.50	9.12	9.25	9.25	9.37	9.50	9.50	9.62	9.75
9.00	9.75	9.75	9.87	10.00	10.12	10.25	10.37	10.37
9.50	10.25	10.37	10.50	10.62	10.75	10.87	11.00	11.12
10.00	10.87	11.00	11.12	11.25	11.37	11.50	11.62	11.75
10.50	11.50	11.62	11.75	11.87	12.00	12.12	12.25	12.50
11.00	12.00	12.25	12.37	12.50	12.75	12.87	13.00	13.12
11.50	12.62	12.87	13.00	13.12	13.37	13.50	13.75	13.87
12.00	13.25	13.50	13.62	13.87	14.00	14.25	14.50	14.62
12.50	13.87	14.12	14.25	14.50	14.75	15.00	15.25	15.37
13.00	14.50	14.75	15.00	15.25	15.50	15.62	16.00	16.12
13.50	15.12	15.37	15.62	15.87	16.12	16.37	16.62	16.87
14.00	15.75	16.00	16.25	16.50	16.75	17.12	17.50	17.75
14.50	16.50	16.75	17.00	17.25	17.50	17.87	18.25	18.50
15.00	17.00	17.37	17.75	18.00	18.25	18.62	19.00	19.37
15.50	17.75	18.00	18.25	18.75	19.00	19.37	19.75	20.25
16.00	18.25	18.75	19.00	19.37	19.75	20.25	20.50	21.00
16.50	19.00	19.37	19.75	20.25	20.50	21.00	21.50	21.87
17.00	19.75	20.25	20.50	21.00	21.00	22.00	22.25	22.87
17.50	20.50	20.75	21.25	21.75	22.25	22.75	23.25	23.75
18.00	21.00	21.50	22.00	22.50	23.00	23.50	24.00	24.62
18.50	21.75	22.25	22.75	23.25	23.75	24.50	25.00	25.62
19.00	22.50	23.00	23.50	24.00	24.75	25.25	26.00	26.50

From Stein, H.A., and Slatt, B.J.: The ophthalmic assistant, ed. 4, St. Louis, 1982, The C.V. Mosby Co.

Effective power at corneal plane of spectacles at designated distance from cornea (vertex distance/millimeters)

Minus lenses

8 mm	9 mm	10 mm	11 mm	12 mm	13 mm	14 mm	15 mm
3.87	3.87	3.87	3.87	3.87	3.75	3.75	3.75
4.37	4.37	4.25	4.25	4.25	4.25	4.25	4.25
4.75	4.75	4.75	4.75	4.75	4.75	4.62	4.62
5.25	5.25	5.25	5.12	5.12	5.12	5.12	5.12
5.75	5.62	5.62	5.62	5.62	5.50	5.50	5.50
6.12	6.12	6.12	6.00	6.00	6.00	6.00	5.87
6.62	6.62	6.50	6.50	6.50	6.37	6.37	6.37
7.12	7.00	7.00	6.87	6.87	6.87	6.75	6.75
7.50	7.50	7.37	7.37	7.25	7.25	7.25	7.25
8.00	7.87	7.87	7.75	7.75	7.62	7.62	7.50
8.37	8.37	8.25	8.25	8.12	8.00	8.00	8.00
8.87	8.75	8.62	8.62	8.50	8.50	8.37	8.37
9.25	9.12	9.12	9.00	8.87	8.87	8.75	8.75
9.62	9.62	9.50	9.37	9.37	9.25	9.12	9.12
10.12	10.00	9.87	9.75	9.75	9.62	9.50	9.50
10.50	10.37	10.37	10.25	10.12	10.00	9.87	9.87
11.00	10.87	10.75	10.62	10.50	10.37	10.25	10.12
11.37	11.25	11.12	11.00	10.87	10.75	10.62	10.50
11.75	11.62	11.50	11.37	11.25	11.12	11.00	10.87
12.25	12.00	11.87	11.75	11.62	11.50	11.37	11.25
12.62	12.50	12.25	12.12	12.00	11.87	11.75	11.50
13.00	12.75	12.62	12.50	12.37	12.25	12.00	11.87
13.37	13.25	13.00	12.87	12.75	12.50	12.37	12.25
13.75	13.62	13.50	13.25	13.00	12.87	12.75	12.62
14.25	14.00	13.75	13.62	13.50	13.25	13.00	12.87
14.50	14.37	14.12	14.00	13.75	13.62	13.50	13.25
15.00	14.75	14.50	14.25	14.12	14.00	13.75	13.50
15.37	15.12	14.87	14.75	14.50	14.25	14.00	13.87
15.75	15.50	15.25	15.00	14.75	14.62	14.37	14.12
16.12	15.87	15.62	15.37	15.12	14.87	14.75	14.50
16.50	16.25	16.00	15.75	15.50	15.25	15.00	14.75

TABLE OF SAGITTAL VALUES

Diameter of CPC (mm)	Radius of curvature of central posterior curve (CPC) (mm)								
	8.44 mm 40.00 D	8.33 mm 40.50 D	8.23 mm 41.00 D	813. mm 41.50 D	8.04 mm 42.00 D	7.94 mm 42.50 D	7.85 mm 43.00 D	7.76 mm 43.50 D	7.67 mm 44.00 D
5.4	0.444	0.450	0.455	0.461	0.467	0.473	0.479	0.485	0.491
5.6	0.478	0.485	0.491	0.497	0.503	0.510	0.516	0.523	0.529
5.8	0.514	0.521	0.528	0.535	0.541	0.549	0.555	0.562	0.569
6.0	0.554	0.559	0.566	0.574	0.581	0.589	0.596	0.603	0.611
6.2	0.590	0.598	0.606	0.614	0.622	0.630	0.638	0.646	0.654
6.4	0.630	0.639	0.648	0.656	0.664	0.673	0.682	0.691	0.699
6.6	0.672	0.682	0.691	0.700	0.708	0.718	0.727	0.737	0.746
6.8	0.715	0.725	0.735	0.745	0.754	0.765	0.775	0.785	0.795
7.0	0.760	0.771	0.781	0.792	0.802	0.813	0.823	0.834	0.845
7.2	0.806	0.818	0.829	0.840	0.851	0.863	0.874	0.886	0.897
7.4	0.854	0.867	0.879	0.891	0.902	0.915	0.927	0.939	0.951
7.6	0.904	0.917	0.930	0.943	0.955	0.968	0.981	0.994	1.008
7.8	0.955	0.969	0.983	0.996	1.009	1.024	1.037	1.051	1.066
8.0	1.098	1.023	1.037	1.052	1.066	1.081	1.096	1.110	1.126
8.2	1.063	1.079	1.094	1.110	1.124	1.140	1.156	1.172	1.188
8.4	1.119	1.136	1.152	1.169	1.184	1.202	1.218	1.235	1.252
8.6	1.178	1.196	1.213	1.230	1.247	1.265	1.282	1.300	1.319
8.8	1.238	1.257	1.275	1.294	1.311	1.331	1.349	1.368	1.388
9.0	1.300	1.320	1.339	1.359	1.377	1.398	1.418	1.438	1.459
9.2	1.364	1.385	1.406	1.427	1.446	1.468	1.489	1.510	1.533
9.4	1.430	1.453	1.474	1.496	1.517	1.541	1.563	1.585	1.609
9.6	1.498	1.522	1.545	1.568	1.590	1.615	1.639	1.663	1.669

From Creighton, C.P.: Contact lens fabrication tables, Tonawanda, New York, 1964, Creighton Publishers.

Diameter of CPC-POZ* (mm)	Radius of curvature of central posterior curve (CPC) (mm)							
	7.59 mm 44.50 D	7.50 mm 45.00 D	7.42 mm 45.50 D	7.34 mm 46.00 D	7.26 mm 46.50 D	7.18 mm 47.00 D	7.11 mm 47.50 D	7.03 mm 48.00 D
5.4	0.496	0.503	0.509	0.515	0.521	0.527	0.533	0.539
5.6	0.535	0.542	0.549	0.555	0.562	0.568	0.575	0.582
5.8	0.576	0.583	0.590	0.597	0.604	0.612	0.618	0.626
6.0	0.618	0.626	0.634	0.641	0.649	0.657	0.664	0.672
6.2	0.662	0.671	0.679	0.687	0.695	0.704	0.711	0.720
6.4	0.708	0.717	0.725	0.734	0.743	0.753	0.761	0.771
6.6	0.755	0.765	0.774	0.784	0.793	0.803	0.812	0.823
6.8	0.804	0.815	0.825	0.835	0.845	0.856	0.866	0.877
7.0	0.855	0.867	0.877	0.888	0.899	0.911	0.921	0.933
7.2	0.908	0.920	0.932	0.943	0.955	0.968	0.979	0.992
7.4	0.963	0.976	0.988	1.001	1.014	1.027	1.039	1.052
7.6	1.020	1.034	1.047	1.060	1.074	1.088	1.101	1.116
7.8	1.079	1.094	1.108	1.122	1.136	1.152	1.165	1.188
8.0	1.140	1.156	1.170	1.186	1.201	1.217	1.232	1.249
8.2	1.203	1.220	1.236	1.252	1.269	1.286	1.301	1.319
8.4	1.268	1.286	1.303	1.320	1.338	1.357	1.373	1.393
8.6	1.336	1.355	1.373	1.391	1.410	1.430	1.448	1.468
8.8	1.405	1.426	1.445	1.465	1.485	1.506	1.525	1.547
9.0	1.478	1.500	1.520	1.541	1.563	1.585	1.605	1.629
9.2	1.553	1.576	1.598	1.620	1.643	1.667	1.689	1.714
9.4	1.630	1.655	1.678	1.702	1.727	1.752	1.775	1.802
9.6	1.711	1.737	1.762	1.787	1.813	1.840	1.865	1.894

*POZ, Peripheral optic zone.

CONVERSION TABLE RELATING DIOPTERS OF CORNEAL REFRACTING POWER TO MILLIMETERS OF RADIUS OF CURVATURE

Diopters	Radius (mm)	
	Curvature	
Drum reading	Convex	Concave
52.00	6.49	6.51
51.87	6.50	6.53
51.75	6.52	6.54
51.62	6.54	6.56
51.50	6.55	6.57
51.37	6.57	6.59
51.25	6.58	6.61
51.12	6.60	6.62
51.00	6.62	6.64
50.87	6.63	6.66
50.75	6.65	6.67
50.62	6.66	6.69
50.50	6.68	6.71
50.37	6.70	6.72
50.25	6.73	6.75
50.12	6.73	6.75
50.00	6.75	6.77
49.87	6.76	6.79
49.75	6.80	6.82
49.62	6.80	6.82
49.50	6.82	6.84
49.37	6.83	6.85
49.25	6.85	6.87
49.12	6.87	6.89
49.00	6.89	6.91
48.87	6.90	6.93
48.75	6.92	6.95
48.62	6.94	6.96
48.50	6.96	6.98
48.37	6.97	7.00
48.25	6.99	7.02
48.12	7.01	7.03
48.00	7.03	7.05

Conversion table relating diopters of corneal refracting power to millimeters of radius of curvature for an assumed index of refraction of 1.3375. The column under convex curvature should be used when the keratometer is used to measure the cornea, and the third column is used to measure concave surfaces such as the CPC of a corneal contact lens in terms of its equivalent corneal refracting power in diopters.

Diopters	*Radius (mm)*		*Diopters*	*Radius (mm)*		*Diopters*	*Radius (mm)*	
Drum reading	*Curvature*		*Drum reading*	*Curvature*		*Drum reading*	*Curvature*	
	Convex	*Concave*		*Convex*	*Concave*		*Convex*	*Concave*
47.87	7.05	7.07	43.87	7.67	7.72	39.87	8.47	8.50
47.75	7.07	7.09	43.75	7.72	7.74	39.75	8.49	8.52
47.62	7.08	7.11	43.62	7.74	7.77	39.62	8.52	8.55
47.50	7.10	7.13	43.50	7.76	7.79	39.50	8.54	8.58
47.37	7.12	7.15	43.37	7.78	7.81	39.37	8.57	8.61
47.25	7.14	7.17	43.25	7.80	7.84	39.25	8.60	8.63
47.12	7.16	7.19	43.12	7.83	7.86	39.12	8.63	8.66
47.00	7.18	7.21	43.00	7.85	7.88	39.00	8.65	8.69
46.87	7.20	7.23	42.87	7.88	7.90	38.87	8.68	8.72
46.75	7.22	7.25	42.75	7.90	7.92	38.75	8.71	8.75
46.62	7.24	7.27	42.62	7.92	7.95	38.62	8.74	8.78
46.50	7.26	7.29	42.50	7.95	7.97	38.50	8.77	8.80
46.27	7.28	7.31	42.37	7.97	8.00	38.37	8.80	8.84
46.25	7.30	7.33	42.25	8.00	8.02	38.25	8.82	8.86
46.12	7.32	7.35	42.12	8.01	8.05	38.12	8.85	8.89
46.00	7.34	7.37	42.00	8.04	8.07	38.00	8.88	8.92
45.87	7.36	7.39	41.87	8.06	8.10	37.87	8.91	8.95
45.75	7.38	7.41	41.75	8.09	8.12	37.75	8.94	8.98
45.62	7.40	7.43	41.62	8.11	8.15	37.62	8.97	9.01
45.50	7.42	7.45	41.50	8.13	8.17	37.50	9.00	9.04
45.37	7.44	7.47	41.37	8.16	8.19	37.37	9.03	9.07
45.25	7.46	7.49	41.25	8.18	8.22	37.25	9.06	9.10
45.12	7.48	7.51	41.12	8.20	8.24	37.12	9.09	9.13
45.00	7.50	7.53	41.00	8.23	8.27	37.00	9.12	9.16
44.87	7.52	7.55	40.87	8.26	8.29	36.87	9.14	9.19
44.75	7.55	7.57	40.75	8.28	8.32	36.75	9.19	9.23
44.62	7.57	7.58	40.62	8.31	8.34	36.62	9.22	9.26
44.50	7.59	7.60	40.50	8.34	8.37	36.50	9.25	9.29
44.37	7.61	7.62	40.37	8.36	8.39	36.37	9.28	9.32
44.25	7.63	7.65	40.25	8.39	8.42	36.25	9.31	9.35
44.12	7.65	7.67	40.12	8.41	8.44	36.12	9.35	9.38
44.00	7.67	7.70	40.00	8.44	8.47	36.00	9.38	9.42
						34.00	9.93	9.97

COMPENSATION FOR EFFECT OF VERTEX DISTANCES (USED WHEN PLUS LENS IS MOVED FROM THE EYE)

Rx power (D)	Distance moved (mm)									
	1	2	3	4	5	6	7	8	9	10
7.00	6.95	6.90	6.86	6.81	6.76	6.72	6.67	6.63	6.59	6.54
7.25	7.20	7.15	7.10	7.05	7.00	6.95	6.90	6.85	6.81	6.76
7.50	7.44	7.39	7.33	7.28	7.23	7.18	7.13	7.08	7.03	6.98
7.75	7.69	7.63	7.57	7.52	7.46	7.41	7.35	7.30	7.24	7.19
8.00	7.94	7.87	7.81	7.75	7.69	7.63	7.58	7.52	7.46	7.41
8.25	8.18	8.12	8.05	7.99	7.92	7.86	7.80	7.74	7.68	7.62
8.50	8.43	8.36	8.29	8.22	8.15	8.09	8.02	7.96	7.90	7.83
8.75	8.67	8.60	8.53	8.45	8.38	8.31	8.24	8.18	8.11	8.05
9.00	8.92	8.84	8.76	8.69	8.61	8.54	8.47	8.40	8.33	8.26
9.25	9.17	9.08	9.00	8.92	8.84	8.76	8.69	8.61	8.54	8.47
9.50	9.41	9.32	9.24	9.15	9.07	8.99	8.91	8.83	8.75	8.68
9.75	9.66	9.56	9.47	9.38	9.30	9.21	9.13	9.04	8.96	8.88
10.00	9.90	9.80	9.71	9.62	9.52	9.43	9.35	9.26	9.17	9.09
10.25	10.15	10.04	9.94	9.85	9.75	9.66	9.56	9.47	9.38	9.30
10.50	10.39	10.28	10.18	10.08	9.98	9.88	9.78	9.69	9.59	9.50
10.75	10.64	10.52	10.41	10.31	10.20	10.10	10.00	9.90	9.80	9.71
11.00	10.88	10.76	10.65	10.54	10.43	10.32	10.21	10.11	10.01	9.91
11.25	11.12	11.00	10.88	10.77	10.65	10.54	10.43	10.32	10.22	10.11
11.50	11.37	11.24	11.12	10.99	10.87	10.76	10.64	10.53	10.42	10.31
11.75	11.61	11.48	11.35	11.22	11.10	10.98	10.86	10.74	10.63	10.51
12.00	11.86	11.72	11.58	11.45	11.32	11.19	11.07	10.95	10.83	10.71
12.25	12.10	11.96	11.82	11.68	11.54	11.41	11.28	11.16	11.03	10.91
12.50	12.35	12.20	12.05	11.90	11.76	11.63	11.49	11.36	11.24	11.11
12.75	12.59	12.43	12.28	12.13	11.99	11.84	11.71	11.57	11.44	11.31
13.00	12.83	12.67	12.51	12.36	12.21	12.06	11.92	11.78	11.64	11.50
13.25	13.08	12.91	12.74	12.58	12.43	12.27	12.13	11.98	11.84	11.70
13.50	13.32	13.15	12.97	12.81	12.65	12.49	12.33	12.18	12.04	11.89
13.75	13.56	13.38	13.21	13.03	12.87	12.70	12.54	12.39	12.24	12.09
14.00	13.81	13.62	13.44	13.26	13.08	12.92	12.75	12.59	12.43	12.28
14.25	14.05	13.86	13.67	13.48	13.30	13.13	12.96	12.79	12.63	12.47

Rx power (D)	Distance moved (mm)									
	1	*2*	*3*	*4*	*5*	*6*	*7*	*8*	*9*	*10*
14.50	14.29	14.09	13.90	13.70	13.52	13.34	13.16	12.99	12.83	12.66
14.75	14.54	14.33	14.12	13.93	13.74	13.55	13.37	13.19	13.02	12.85
15.00	14.78	14.56	14.35	14.15	13.95	13.76	13.57	13.39	13.22	13.04
15.25	15.02	14.80	14.58	14.37	14.17	13.97	13.78	13.59	13.41	13.23
15.50	15.26	15.03	14.81	14.60	14.39	14.18	13.98	13.79	13.60	13.42
15.75	15.51	15.27	15.04	14.82	14.60	14.39	14.19	13.99	13.79	13.61
16.00	15.75	15.50	15.27	15.04	14.81	14.60	13.39	14.18	13.99	13.79
16.25	15.99	15.74	15.49	15.25	15.03	14.81	14.59	14.38	14.18	13.98
16.50	16.23	15.97	15.72	15.48	15.24	15.01	14.79	14.57	14.37	14.16
16.75	16.47	16.21	15.95	15.70	15.45	15.22	14.99	14.77	14.56	14.35
17.00	16.72	16.44	16.18	15.92	15.67	15.43	15.19	14.96	14.74	14.53
17.25	16.96	16.67	16.40	16.44	15.88	15.63	15.39	15.16	14.93	14.71
17.50	17.20	16.91	16.63	16.36	16.09	15.84	15.59	15.35	15.12	14.89
17.75	17.44	17.14	16.85	16.57	16.30	16.04	15.79	15.54	15.31	15.07
18.00	17.68	17.37	17.08	16.79	16.51	16.25	15.99	15.73	15.49	15.25
18.25	17.92	17.61	17.30	17.01	16.72	16.45	16.18	15.92	15.68	15.43
18.50	18.16	17.84	17.53	17.23	16.93	16.65	16.38	16.11	15.86	15.61
18.75	18.40	18.07	17.75	17.44	17.14	16.85	16.57	16.30	16.04	15.79
19.00	18.65	18.30	17.98	17.66	17.35	17.06	16.77	16.49	16.23	15.97
19.25	18.89	18.54	18.20	17.87	17.56	17.26	16.96	16.68	16.41	16.14
19.50	19.13	18.77	18.42	18.09	17.77	17.46	17.16	16.87	16.59	16.32
19.75	19.37	19.00	18.65	18.30	17.97	17.66	17.35	17.06	16.77	16.49
20.00	19.61	19.23	18.87	18.52	18.18	17.86	17.54	17.24	16.95	16.67
20.25	19.85	19.46	19.09	18.73	18.39	18.06	17.74	17.43	17.13	16.84
20.50	20.09	19.69	19.31	18.95	18.59	18.25	17.93	17.61	17.31	17.01
20.75	20.33	19.92	19.53	19.16	18.80	18.45	18.12	17.80	17.48	17.18
21.00	20.57	20.15	19.76	19.37	19.00	18.65	18.31	17.98	17.66	17.36
21.25	20.81	20.38	19.98	19.59	19.21	18.85	18.50	18.16	17.84	17.53
21.50	21.05	20.61	20.20	19.80	10.41	19.04	18.69	18.34	18.01	17.70
21.75	21.29	20.84	20.42	20.01	19.62	10.24	18.88	18.53	18.19	17.87

COMPENSATION FOR EFFECT OF VERTEX DISTANCES (USED WHEN PLUS LENS IS MOVED TOWARD THE EYE)

Rx power (D)	Distance moved (mm)									
	1	2	3	4	5	6	7	8	9	10
7.00	7.05	7.10	7.15	7.20	7.25	7.31	7.36	7.42	7.47	7.53
7.25	7.30	7.36	7.41	7.47	7.52	7.58	7.64	7.70	7.76	7.82
7.50	7.56	7.61	7.67	7.73	7.79	7.85	7.92	7.98	8.04	8.11
7.75	7.81	7.87	7.93	8.00	8.06	8.13	8.19	8.26	8.33	8.40
8.00	8.06	8.13	8.20	8.26	8.33	8.40	8.47	8.55	8.62	8.70
8.25	8.32	8.39	8.46	8.53	8.60	8.68	8.76	8.83	8.91	8.99
8.50	8.57	8.56	8.72	8.80	8.88	8.96	9.04	9.12	9.20	9.29
8.75	8.83	8.91	8.99	9.07	9.15	9.23	9.32	9.41	9.50	9.59
9.00	9.08	9.16	9.25	9.34	9.42	9.51	9.61	9.70	9.79	9.89
9.25	9.34	9.42	9.51	9.61	9.70	9.79	9.89	9.99	10.09	10.19
9.50	9.59	9.68	9.78	9.88	9.97	10.07	10.18	10.28	10.39	10.50
9.75	9.85	9.94	10.04	10.15	10.25	10.36	10.46	10.58	10.69	10.80
10.00	10.10	10.20	10.31	10.42	10.53	10.64	10.75	10.87	10.99	11.11
10.25	10.36	10.46	10.58	10.69	10.80	10.92	11.04	11.17	11.29	11.42
10.50	10.61	10.73	10.84	10.96	11.08	11.21	11.33	11.46	11.60	11.73
10.75	10.87	10.99	11.11	11.23	11.36	11.49	11.62	11.76	11.90	12.04
11.00	11.12	11.25	11.38	11.51	11.64	11.78	11.92	12.06	12.21	12.36
11.25	11.38	11.51	11.64	11.78	11.92	12.06	12.21	12.36	12.52	12.68
11.50	11.63	11.77	11.91	12.05	12.20	12.35	12.51	12.67	12.83	12.99
11.75	11.89	12.03	12.18	12.33	12.48	12.64	12.80	12.97	13.14	13.31
12.00	12.15	12.30	12.45	12.61	12.77	12.93	13.10	13.27	13.45	13.64
12.25	12.40	12.56	12.72	12.88	13.05	13.22	13.40	13.58	13.77	13.96
12.50	12.66	12.82	12.99	13.16	13.33	13.51	13.70	13.89	14.08	14.29
12.75	12.91	13.08	13.26	13.44	13.62	13.81	14.00	14.20	14.40	14.61
13.00	13.17	13.35	13.53	13.71	13.90	14.10	14.30	14.51	14.72	14.94
13.25	13.43	13.61	13.80	13.99	14.19	14.39	14.60	14.82	15.04	15.27
13.50	13.68	13.87	14.07	14.27	14.48	14.69	14.91	15.13	15.37	15.61
13.75	13.94	14.14	14.34	14.55	14.77	14.99	15.21	15.45	15.69	15.94
14.00	14.20	14.40	14.61	14.83	15.05	15.28	15.52	15.77	16.02	16.28
14.25	14.46	14.67	14.89	15.11	15.34	15.58	15.83	16.09	16.35	16.62

R_x power (D)	Distance moved (mm)									
	1	*2*	*3*	*4*	*5*	*6*	*7*	*8*	*9*	*10*
14.50	14.71	14.93	15.16	15.39	15.63	15.88	16.14	16.41	16.88	16.96
14.75	14.97	15.20	15.43	15.67	15.92	16.18	16.45	16.73	17.01	17.30
15.00	15.23	15.46	15.71	15.96	16.22	16.48	16.76	17.05	17.34	17.65
15.25	15.49	15.73	15.98	16.24	16.51	16.79	17.07	17.37	17.68	18.00
15.50	15.74	16.00	16.26	16.52	16.80	17.09	17.39	17.69	18.01	18.35
15.75	16.00	16.26	16.53	16.81	17.10	17.39	17.70	18.02	18.35	18.70
16.00	16.26	16.53	16.81	17.09	17.39	17.70	18.02	18.35	18.69	19.05
16.25	16.52	16.80	17.08	17.38	17.69	18.01	18.34	18.68	19.03	19.40
16.50	16.78	17.06	17.36	17.67	17.98	18.31	18.65	19.01	19.38	19.76
16.75	17.04	17.33	17.64	17.95	18.28	18.62	18.97	19.34	19.72	20.12
17.00	17.29	17.60	17.91	18.24	18.58	18.93	19.30	19.68	20.07	20.48
17.25	17.55	17.87	18.19	18.53	18.88	19.24	19.62	20.01	20.42	20.85
17.50	17.81	18.13	18.47	18.82	19.18	19.55	19.94	20.35	20.77	21.21
17.75	18.07	18.40	18.75	19.11	19.48	19.86	20.27	20.69	21.12	21.58
18.00	18.33	18.67	19.03	19.40	19.78	20.18	20.59	21.03	21.48	21.95
18.25	18.59	18.94	19.31	19.69	20.08	20.49	20.92	21.37	21.84	22.32
18.50	18.85	19.21	19.59	19.98	20.39	20.81	21.25	27.71	22.20	22.70
18.75	19.11	19.48	19.87	20.27	20.69	21.13	21.58	22.06	22.56	23.08
19.00	19.37	19.75	20.15	20.56	20.99	21.44	21.91	22.41	22.92	23.46
19.25	19.63	20.02	20.43	20.86	21.30	21.76	22.25	22.75	23.28	23.81
19.50	19.89	20.89	20.71	21.15	21.61	22.08	22.58	23.10	23.65	24.22
19.75	20.15	20.56	20.99	21.44	21.91	22.40	22.92	23.46	24.02	24.61
20.00	20.41	20.83	21.28	21.74	22.22	22.73	23.26	23.81	24.39	25.00
20.25	20.67	21.10	21.56	22.03	22.53	23.05	23.59	24.16	24.76	
20.50	20.82	21.38	21.84	22.33	22.84	23.38	23.93	24.52		
20.75	20.91	21.65	22.13	22.63	23.15	23.70	24.28			
21.00	21.45	21.92	22.41	22.93	23.46	24.03				
21.25	21.71	22.19	22.70	23.22	23.78					
21.50	21.97	22.47	22.98	23.52						
21.75	22.23	22.74	23.37							

OPTICAL CONSTANTS OF THE EYE

Optical constants of the eye are summarized as follows:

1. The curvature of the anterior face of the cornea is 7.5 mm.
2. The index of refraction of the corneal tissue, the aqueous humor, and the vitreous equals 1.332.
3. The distance separating the anterior pole of the cornea from the posterior pole of the crystalline lens is 3.6 mm.
4. The curvature of the anterior face of the crystalline lens measures 10.0 mm.
5. The curvature of the posterior face of the crystalline lens is 6.0 mm.
6. The distance separating the anterior pole of the crystalline lens from the posterior pole of the crystalline lens is 4.0 mm.
7. The main refraction index of the crystalline lens equals 1.40.

From Hartstein, J.: Basics of contact lenses manual, Rochester, Minn., 1979, American Academy of Ophthalmology.

8. The dioptric power of the cornea equals 44.26 D.
9. The dioptric power of the crystalline lens alone, when both of its surfaces are immersed in a medium having an index of 1.332, equals 17.82 D.
10. The total power of the eye equals 58.53 D.
11. The distance of the first principal plane of the crystalline lens back of the anterior pole of the crystalline lens is 2.4 mm.
12. The distance of the second principal plane of the crystalline lens ahead of the posterior pole of the crystalline lens is 1.4 mm.
13. The distance separating these two planes is 0.2 mm.
14. The distance of the principal plane of the whole eye behind the anterior pole of the whole cornea is 1.370 mm.
15. The distance of the second principal plane of the whole eye behind the anterior pole of the whole cornea is 1.664 mm.
16. The distance separating these two planes is 0.294 mm.

SAGITTAL RELATIONSHIP OF VARIOUS BASE CURVES AND DIAMETERS

Diameter (mm)	Radius (mm)	Diameter (mm)	Radius (mm)
Flatter			
13.0	8.7	15.0	8.7
13.0	8.4	14.0	7.8
13.5	8.7	14.5	8.1
13.0	8.1	15.0	8.4
13.5	8.4	15.5	8.7
14.0	8.7	13.5	7.2
13.0	7.8	14.0	7.5
13.5	8.1	14.5	7.8
14.0	8.4	15.0	8.1
13.0	7.5	15.5	8.4
14.5	8.7	14.0	7.2
13.5	7.8	14.5	7.5
14.0	8.1	15.0	7.8
13.0	7.2	15.5	8.1
14.5	8.4	15.0	7.5
13.5	7.5	15.5	7.8
		Steeper	

DIOPTRIC CURVES FOR EXTENDED RANGE OF KERATOMETER

High power (with +1.25 D lens over aperture)				Low power (with −1.00 D lens over aperture)			
Drum reading (D)	True dioptric curvature (D)	Drum reading (D)	True dioptric curvature (D)	Drum reading (D)	True dioptric curvature (D)	Drum reading (D)	True dioptric curvature (D)
52.00	61.00	46.87	55.87	42.00	36.00	36.87	30.87
51.87	60.87	46.75	55.75	41.87	35.87	36.75	30.75
51.75	60.75	46.62	55.62	41.75	35.75	36.62	30.62
51.62	60.62	46.50	55.50	41.62	35.62	36.50	30.50
51.50	60.50	46.37	55.37	41.50	35.50	36.37	30.37
51.37	60.37	46.25	55.25	41.37	35.37	36.25	30.25
51.25	60.25	46.12	55.12	41.25	35.25	36.12	30.12
51.12	60.12	46.00	55.00	41.12	35.12	36.00	30.00
51.00	60.00			41.00	35.00		
		45.87	54.87				
50.87	59.87	45.75	54.75	40.87	34.87		
50.75	59.75	45.62	54.62	40.75	34.75		
50.62	59.62	45.50	54.50	40.62	34.62		
50.50	59.50	45.37	54.37	40.50	34.50		
50.37	59.37	45.25	54.25	40.37	34.37		
50.25	59.25	45.12	54.12	40.25	34.25		
50.12	59.12	45.00	54.00	40.12	34.12		
50.00	59.00			40.00	34.00		
		44.87	53.87				
49.87	58.87	44.75	53.75	39.87	33.87		
49.75	58.75	44.62	53.62	39.75	33.75		
49.62	58.62	44.50	53.50	39.62	33.62		
49.50	58.50	44.37	53.37	39.50	33.50		

Courtesy Bausch & Lomb, Inc.

High power (with +1.25 D lens over aperture)				Low power (with −1.00 D lens over aperture)			
Drum reading (D)	*True dioptric curvature (D)*	*Drum reading (D)*	*True dioptric curvature (D)*	*Drum reading (D)*	*True dioptric curvature (D)*	*Drum reading (D)*	*True dioptric curvature (D)*
49.37	58.37	44.25	53.25	39.37	33.37		
49.25	58.25	44.12	53.12	39.25	33.25		
49.12	58.12	44.00	53.00	39.12	33.12		
49.00	58.00			39.00	33.00		
		43.87	52.87				
48.75	57.75	43.75	52.75	38.87	32.87		
48.62	57.62	43.62	52.62	38.75	32.75		
48.50	57.50	43.50	52.50	38.62	32.62		
48.37	57.37	43.37	52.37	38.50	32.50		
48.25	57.25	43.25	52.25	38.37	32.37		
48.12	57.12	43.12	52.12	38.25	32.25		
48.00	57.00	43.00	52.00	38.12	32.12		
				38.00	32.00		
47.87	56.87						
47.75	56.75			37.87	31.87		
47.62	56.62			37.75	31.75		
47.50	56.50			37.62	31.62		
47.37	58.37			37.50	31.50		
47.25	56.25			37.37	31.37		
47.12	56.12			37.25	31.25		
47.00	56.00			37.12	31.12		
				37.00	31.00		

EDGE-THICKNESS* CHANGES AS A FUNCTION OF LENS POWER† (FOR BASE CURVE 7.6 MM)‡

Power (D)	Lens diameter (chord diameter in mm)										
	6.0	6.5	7.0	7.5	8.0	8.5	9.0	9.5	10.0	10.5	11.0
1.00	0.010	0.013	0.015	0.018	0.021	0.024	0.028	0.033	0.038	0.045	0.052
2.00	0.020	0.025	0.029	0.035	0.041	0.047	0.055	0.064	0.075	0.088	0.102
3.00	0.031	0.037	0.044	0.053	0.062	0.071	0.083	0.097	0.113	0.132	0.153
4.00	0.041	0.049	0.059	0.070	0.081	0.094	0.110	0.128	0.149	0.173	0.201
5.00	0.051	0.062	0.074	0.087	0.102	0.118	0.138	0.160	0.186	0.216	0.251
6.00	0.062	0.074	0.088	0.104	0.122	0.141	0.164	0.191	0.221	0.257	0.298
7.00	0.071	0.086	0.102	0.120	0.141	0.163	0.190	0.220	0.255	0.297	0.344
8.00	0.082	0.099	0.117	0.138	0.161	0.187	0.217	0.252	0.291	0.337	0.390
9.00	0.092	0.110	0.131	0.154	0.180	0.209	0.242	0.281	0.324	0.375	0.433
10.00	0.102	0.122	0.145	0.171	0.199	0.231	0.268	0.310	0.357	0.413	0.476
11.00	0.112	0.134	0.159	0.187	0.218	0.253	0.293	0.339	0.391	0.451	0.520
12.00	0.122	0.146	0.173	0.204	0.238	0.276	0.319	0.369	0.425	0.490	0.564
13.00	0.132	0.158	0.187	0.220	0.257	0.296	0.344	0.397	0.457	0.527	0.605
14.00	0.142	0.170	0.201	0.237	0.276	0.319	0.369	0.426	0.490	0.563	0.647
15.00	0.152	0.181	0.215	0.252	0.294	0.340	0.393	0.453	0.521	0.598	0.687
16.00	0.162	0.193	0.229	0.269	0.313	0.362	0.418	0.482	0.553	0.635	0.728
17.00	0.171	0.205	0.242	0.285	0.331	0.383	0.442	0.509	0.584	0.670	0.767
18.00	0.181	0.216	0.256	0.300	0.349	0.404	0.466	0.536	0.615	0.704	0.806
19.00	0.191	0.228	0.270	0.317	0.368	0.426	0.491	0.564	0.646	0.740	0.846
20.00	0.200	0.239	0.282	0.331	0.385	0.445	0.512	0.589	0.674	0.771	0.881

*Edge thickness is measured perpendicularly to the chord diameter of the lens.

†For minus-powered lenses, values shown serve to increase the edge thickness of the lens over the center thickness. For minus lenses, increase thickness by the following amount for each 0.1 mm of center thickness: 0.002 0.003 0.004 0.005 0.006 0.007 0.008 0.009 0.011 0.013. For plus-powered lenses, values shown serve to decrease the edge thickness of the lens over the center thickness. For plus lenses, do not modify values given for center thickness as is done for minus lenses—this chart for plus lenses is based upon the minimum lens thickness for the powers and diameters shown.

‡This chart was calculated for a base curve of 7.6 mm. However, there is only a small change in values as the base curve is changed; therefore the chart is valid for base curves 7.2 to 8.0 mm. As the base curve is made steeper, the values shown increase; as the base curve is made flatter, the values shown decrease.

ESTIMATING VISUAL LOSS

Loss of central vision in one eye

Visual acuity for distance (Snellen)	Snellen	Meters (D)	Jaeger	Percent visual efficiency*	Percent visual loss
20/20	14/14	0.35	1 –	100	0
20/25	14/18	0.44	2 –	96	4
20/30	14/21	0.59	—	91	9
20/40	14/28	0.71	3	84	16
20/50	14/35	0.88	6	77	23
20/60	14/42	1.08	—	70	30
20/70	14/49	1.30	7	64	36
20/80	14/56	—	8	59	41
20/100	14/70	1.76	11	49	51
20/160	14/112	—	14 –	29	71
20/200	14/140	3.53	—	20	80
20/400	14/280	7.06	—	3	97

*The percentage of visual efficiency of the two eyes may be determined by the following formula:

$$\frac{(3 \times \% \text{ visual efficiency of better eye}) + \% \text{ visual efficiency of poorer eye}}{4} = \% \text{ binocular visual efficiency}$$

Estimating loss of visual field. A visual field test is performed on the perimeter with a 3 mm test object in each of the eight 45-degree meridians. The sum of each of these meridians is added and the percentage of visual efficiency is arrived at when one divides by 485, the total of a normal field. For example:

Normal field	Degrees
Temporally	85
Down and temporally	85
Down	55
Nasally	55
Up and nasally	55
Down and nasally	50
Up	45
Up and temporally	55
TOTAL	485

Constricted field	Degrees
Temporally	45
Down and temporally	25
Down	30
Down and nasally	25
Nasally	25
Up and nasally	25
Up	25
Up and temporally	35
TOTAL	235

% visual efficiency $\dfrac{235 \times 100}{485} = 46\%$

Estimating loss of muscle function. To determine the degree of visual efficiency lost from diplopia, diplopia fields are measured on the perimeter at 33 cm or on the tangent screen to

From Stein, H.A., and Slatt, B.J.: The opththalmic assistant, ed. 4, St. Louis, 1982, The C.V. Mosby Co.

determine the disability from the double vision.

Diplopia within the central 20 degrees in the straight-ahead position represents 100% loss of visual efficiency of one eye. In the regions beyond 20 degrees the loss of visual efficiency is dependent on the position of gaze. Looking straight down in an area between 20 and 30 degrees would represent a loss of 50%, whereas looking up in the same area between 20 and 30 degrees (a region not commonly used for visual activity) would represent only a 10% loss of vi-

sual efficiency. Looking to the sides between 20 and 30 degrees would repesent a 20% loss of visual efficiency of the eye.

In more peripheral zones, where the eyes normally do not function, visual loss from diplopia would be less. For example, looking down between 30 and 40 degrees would represent a 30% loss of visual efficiency, and looking to the sides between 30 and 40 degrees would represent only a 10% loss of visual efficiency.

DRUGS COMMONLY USED IN OPHTHALMOLOGY

Drug	Strength	Container size
Glaucoma medications to improve outflow		
Adsorbocarpine	1%, 2%, 4%	15 ml plastic dropper bottle
Carcholin Powder		0.5 g bottles
Cellucarpine Solution		15 ml bottles
E-Carpine Solution	1%, 2%, 3%, 4%, 6%	15 ml dropper bottle
E-Pilo Solution	1%, 2%, 3%, 4%, 6%	10 ml plastic dropper bottles
Floropryl Solution and Ointment	0.1%	3.5 g tubes
Humorsol Solution	0.125%, 0.25%	5 ml vials with dropper
Isopto Carpine Solution	0.5%, 1%, 2%, 3%, 4%, 6%	15 and 30 ml plastic Drop-Tainer
Isopto Carbachol Solution	0.75%, 1.5%, 2.25%, 3%	15 ml Drop-Tainer
Isopto Eserine Solution	0.25%, 0.5%	15 ml Drop-Tainer
Isopto P-ES Solution		15 ml Drop-Tainer
Miocarpine Solution	0.5%, 1%, 2%, 3%, 4%, 6%	15 and 30 ml plastic bottles
Ocusert Pilo 20		Packages of 8 units
Ocusert Pilo 40		Packages of 8 units
P_2E_1 and P_4E_1 Solutions	2%, 4%	10 and 12.5 ml plastic drops vials
P.V. Carpine Liquifilm Solution	0.5%, 1%, 2%, 3%, 4%, 6%	15 ml plastic dropper
Phospholine Iodide Solution	0.06%, 0.125%, 0.25%	
Pilocar Solution	0.5%, 1%, 2%, 3%, 4%, 6%	15 ml plastic dropper bottles
Pilocel Solution	0.25%, 0.5%, 1%, 2%, 3%, 6%	15 ml plastic container
Pilofrin Solution	0.5%, 1%, 2%, 3%, 4%, 6%	15 ml plastic dropper bottles
Propine	0.1%	10 ml plastic dropper bottles
Glaucoma medications to decrease inflow and improve outflow		
Epifrin Solution	0.25%, 0.5%, 1%, 2%	5 and 15 ml plastic dropper bottles
Epinal Solution	0.25%, 0.5%, 1%	7.5 ml Drop-Tainer
Eppy/N Solution	½%, 1%	7.5 ml dropper bottles
Glaucon Solution	½%, 1%, 2%	10 ml dropper bottles
Propine	0.1%	10 ml dropper bottles
Timoptic	0.25%, 0.5%	5 and 10 ml dispenser

From Stein, H.A., and Slatt, B.J.: The ophthalmic assistant, ed. 4, St. Louis, 1982, The C.V. Mosby Co.

Drug	Strength	Container size
Hyperosmotic agents		
Glycerol (50%)	1 to 1.5 g/kg body weight	
Mannitol (20%)	1 to 2 g/kg body weight	
Urea (30%)	1 to 2 g/kg body weight	
Solutions and ointments to dilate the pupil		
Atropine Sulfate Ointment	0.5%, 1%	3.5 g tubes
Atropine Sulfate Solution	1%, 2%	15 ml plastic dropper bottles
Atropisol Aqueous and Oil Solution	0.5%, 1%, 2%, 3%, 4%	5 ml dropper bottles
Cyclogyl Solution	0.5%, 1%, 2%	15 ml dropper bottles
Cyclomydril Solution	2%	2 and 7.5 ml bottles
Homatropine	2%, 5%	15 ml plastic dropper bottles
Isopto Atropine Solution	0.5%, 1%, 2%	5 and 15 ml Drop-Tainer
Isopto Homatropine Solution	2%, 5%	5 and 15 ml Drop-Tainer
Isopto Hyoscine Solution	0.25%	5 and 15 ml Drop-Tainer
Mydplegic Solution	1%	15 ml plastic dropper bottles
Mydriacyl Solution	0.5%, 1%, 2%	15 ml dropper bottles
Mydfrin	2.5%	5 ml dropper bottles
Neo-Synephrine	2.5%, 10%	30 ml and 5 ml bottles
Paredrine Solution	1%	15 ml dropper bottles
Phenoptic	5%, 10%	5 ml plastic bottles
Scopolamine Ointment	0.2%	⅛ oz tubes
Scopolamine Solution	0.25%	15 ml plastic dropper bottles
Decongestants		
Albalon A		15 ml plastic dropper bottles
Degest 2		15 ml plastic dropper bottles
Isopto Frin Solution	0.12%	15 ml Drop-Tainer
Neo-Propisol Solution		15 ml Steri-Tainer
Neo-Synephrine Solution	0.125%, 2.5%, 10%	15 ml plastic container
Neozin Solution	0.125%	15 ml plastic container
Prefrin-A Solution		15 ml bottle
Prefrin Liquifilm Solution		15 ml plastic dropper bottles
Prefrin-Z Liquifilm		15 ml plastic dropper bottles
Privine Solution	0.1%	15 ml dropper bottles
Soothe Solution	0.125%	15 ml plastic dropper bottle
Tear-Efrin Solution	0.12%	15 ml Lacrivials
Vasoclear		15 ml dropper bottles
Vasocon Regular Solution		15 ml plastic squeeze bottles
Visine Solution	0.05%	15 ml dropper bottles
Zincfrin A Solution	0.25%	15 ml Drop-Tainer
Antihistaminics		
Albalon A		15 ml dropper bottles
Antistine Solution		15 ml dropper bottles
Prefrin-A Solution		15 ml plastic dropper bottles
Vasocon-A Solution		15 ml plastic dropper bottles
Vernacel Solution		15 ml plastic containers
Zincfrin A Solution		15 ml dropper bottles
Steroids		
Cortamed Solution	2.5%	10 ml bottle
Cortril Ointment	0.5%, 2.5%	⅛ oz ophthalmic tipped tubes
Decadron Solution and Ointment		2.5 and 5 ml bottles
Econopred Solution	⅛%, 1%	5 ml bottle
FML Liquifilm Suspension		5, 10, 15 ml plastic dropper bottle
HMS Liquifilm Suspension		5 and 10 ml plastic dropper bottle

Drug	Strength	Container size
Hydeltra Ointment and Solution		Ointment: 3.5 g tubes Solution: 2.5 and 5 ml dropper bottles
Hydrocortone Ointment and Suspension	1.5%, 0.5%, 0.25%	Ointment: 3.5 g tubes Suspension: 5 ml dropper bottles
Inflamase Forte Solution	1%	5 ml dropper bottles
Inflamase Solution	⅛%	5 ml dropper bottles
Isopto Hydrocortisone Suspension	0.5%, 2.5%	5 ml Drop-Tainer
Maxidex Suspension	1%	5 ml plastic Drop-Tainer
Medrysone Solution	1%	5 and 10 ml plastic bottles
Penthasone Solution	0.1%	5 ml bottle
Pred Forte Suspension	1%	5 and 10 ml plastic dropper bottles
Pred Mild Solution	0.12%	5 and 10 ml plastic dropper bottles

Combinations of steroids with sulfonamides or antibiotics

Drug	Strength	Container size
Blephamide Liquifilm Suspension	5 and 10 ml plastic dropper bottles	
Blephamide ointment		3.5 g tubes
Celestone-S		2.5 and 5 ml dropper bottles
Cetapred Ointment		3.5 g tubes
Chloromycetin hydrocortisone suspension		5 ml bottle with droppers
Chloroptic-P ointment		3.5 g tube
Cortisporin ointment and suspension		Ointment: ⅛ oz tubes Suspension: 5 ml dropper bottles
Isopto Cetapred suspension		5 and 15 ml Drop-Tainer
Maxitrol suspension and ointment		Suspension: 5 ml plastic bottles Ointment: 3.5 g tubes
Metimyd with neomycin ointment		⅛ oz tubes
Metimyd suspension		5 ml dropper bottles
Metreton suspension		5 ml dropper bottles
Neo-Aristocort ointment		⅛ oz tubes
Neo-Cortef drops and ointment	0.5%, 1.5%	Drops: 0.5% in 5 ml dropper bottles 1.5% in 2.5 and 5 ml dropper bottles
Neo-Decadron ointment and solution		Ointment: 3.5 g tubes Solution: 2.6 and 5 ml dropper bottles
Neo-Deltef solution		2.5 ml plastic dropper bottles
Neo-Medrol ointment	0.1%	⅛ oz tubes
PolyPred		5 ml plastic dropper bottles
Predmycin solution		5 ml plastic dropper bottles
Sulfapred suspension		5 ml plastic containers
Terra-Cortril suspension		5 ml dropper bottles
Vasocidin solution		5 ml plastic dropper-tipped vials

Sulfonamides

Drug	Strength	Container size
Bleph-10 and Bleph-30 Liquifilm solutions	10%, 30%	5 and 15 ml plastic dropper bottles
Bleph 10 ointment	10%	3.5 g tubes
Cetamide ointment	10%	3.5 g tubes
Gantrisin solution and ointment	4%	Solution: 5 and 15 ml dropper bottles Ointment: ⅛ oz applicator tubes

Drug	Strength	Container size
Isopto Cetamide solution	15%	5 ml dropper bottles and 15 ml Drop-Tainer
Suladrin ointment		3.5 g tubes
Sulamyd ointment and solution	10%, 30%	Solution: 15 ml dropper bottles
		Ointment: ⅛ oz tubes
Sulfacidin solution	10%	7.5 ml Lacrivials
Vasosulf solution	15%	15 ml plastic dropper bottles

Antibiotics

Drug	Strength	Container size
Aureomycin ointment and solution	0.5%, 1%	Ointment: ⅛ oz tubes
		Solution: 5 ml bottles
Achromycin suspension	1.0%	4 ml plastic bottles
Chloromycetin drops and ointment		Solution: 15 ml dropper bottles
		Ointment: ⅛ oz tube
Chloromycetin-polymyxin ointment		⅛ oz tubes
Chloroptic solution and ointment		Solution: 0.5% in 10 ml plastic bottles
		Ointment: 1% in 3.5 g tubes
Fenicol ointment	1%	3.5 g tubes
Garamycin solution and ointment		Solutin: 5 ml dropper bottles
		Ointment: ⅛ oz tubes
Genoptic solution		5 ml plastic dropper bottles
Genoptic ointment		3.5 g tubes
Ilotycin ointment		⅛ oz tubes
Isopto Fenicol solution	0.25%	5 ml dropper bottles
Neo-Polycin ointment and solution		Solution: 10 ml dropper bottles
		Ointment: ⅛ oz tubes
Neosporin ointment and solution		Solution: 10 ml bottle with dropper
		Ointment: ⅛ oz tubes
Pentamycetin solution and ointment		Solution: 10 ml dropper bottle
		Ointment: ⅛ oz tube
Polyspectrin Liquifilm		10 ml dropper bottles
Polyspectrin ointment		⅛ oz tubes
Polysporin ointment		⅛ oz tubes
Spectrocin ointment		⅛ oz tubes
Statrol solution		5 ml dropper bottles
Sulfacidin solution		10 ml Lacrivials and 1 ml Droperettes
Terramycin solution		5 ml dropper vials
Terramycin-polymixin ointment		⅛ oz tubes
Tobrex solution		5 ml dropper vials

Antivirals

Drug	Strength	Container size
Dendrid solution	0.1%	15 ml dropper bottles
Herplex solution and ointment	0.1%	Solution: 15 ml plastic dropper bottles
		Ointment: ⅛ oz tubes
Stoxil solution	0.1%	15 ml dropper bottles
Viroptic (trifluridine)	1%	5 ml dropper bottles

Antifungal

Drug	Strength	Container size
Natacyn	5%	15 ml glass bottles

Antibacterial and steroid combinations

Drug	Strength	Container size
Achromycin ointment		⅛ oz tubes
Blephamide Liquifilm Suspension		5 ml and 10 ml plastic dropper bottles

Drug	Strength	Container size
Belphamide ointments		3.5 g tubes
Celestone-S suspension		5 ml dropper bottles
Chloromycetin hydrocortisone suspension		5 ml dropper bottles and 5 ml vials
Chloroptic-P ointment		3.5 g tubes
Cortisporin ointment and suspension		Ointment: ⅛ oz tubes
		Suspension: 5 ml dropper bottles
Isopto Cetapred suspension		5 and 15 ml Drop-Tainer
Maxitrol suspension and ointment		Suspension: 5 ml plastic bottles
		Ointment: 3.5 g tubes
Metamyd suspension		5 ml dropper bottles
Metimyd with neomycin ointment		⅛ oz tubes
Neo-Aristocort ointment		⅛ oz tubes
Neo-Cortef drops and ointment	0.5%, 1.5%	Drops: 5 ml dropper bottles
		Ointment: ⅛ oz tubes
Neo-Decadron ointment and solution		Ointment: 3.5 g tubes
		Solution: 2.5 and 5 ml dropper bottles
Neo-Deltef solution		2.5 ml plastic dropper bottles
Neo-Hydeltrasol ointment and solution		Ointment: 3.5 g tubes
		Solution: 2.5 and 5 ml dropper bottles
Ophthocort ointment		⅛ oz tubes
Pentamycetin/hydrocortisone solution and ointment		Solution: 10 ml bottle
		Ointment: ⅛ oz tube
Sulfapred suspension		5 ml plastic containers
Terra-Cortril suspension		5 ml dropper bottles
Vasocidin solution		5 ml plastic dropper vials

Anesthetic, topical

Alcaine	0.5%	15 ml plastic bottles
Cocaine	0.25%, 0.5%	Special preparation
Dibucaine	0.1%	15 ml bottles
Ophthaine solution	0.5%	15 ml plastic bottles
Ophthetic solution	0.5%	15 ml plastic bottles
Pontocaine solution	0.5%	15 ml plastic bottles
Proparacaine solution	0.5%	

Carbonic anhydrase inhibitors

Cardrase		125 mg tablets
Daranide		50 mg tablets
Diamox		250 mg tablets
Ethamide		125 mg tablets
Hydrazol		250 mg tablets
Naptazane		50 mg tablets
Oratrol		50 mg tablets

Miscellaneous

Adsorbonac solution	2%, 5%	15 ml plastic dropper bottle
Adsorbotear solution		15 ml plastic dropper bottle
Balanced salt solution		15 ml bottles
Blinx liquid solution		30 ml bottles
Carbachol, intraocular		5 ml bottles
Catarase suspension		3 ml vials
Dacriose irrigating solution		120 ml irrigating bottles
Degest-2		0.5 ml bottles
Duratears		3.5 g tubes
Enuclene solution		15 ml plastic dropper bottles
Estivin solution		¼ oz dropper bottles

Drug	Strength	Container size
Fluorescite solution	5%	10 ml ampules
Fulgo (sodium fluorescein strips)		
Fluress solution		5 ml bottles
Gonio-gel	2.5%	3.5 g tubes
Hypotears		14 ml dropper bottles
Isopto tears	0.5%, 1%	15 ml Drop-Tainer
Lacril artificial tears	0.5%	15 ml plastic dropper bottles
Lacri-Lube ointment		⅛ oz tube
Liquifilm Forte Solution		15 ml dropper bottle
Liquifilm tears	1.4%	15 and 30 ml plastic dropper bottles
Lyteers drops		15 ml dropper bottles
Methisol solution		15 ml plastic bottles
Methulose solution		15 ml plastic bottles
Murocel	1%	15 and 30 ml plastic dropper bottles
Muro 128	5%	15 and 30 ml plastic dropper bottles
Miochol		3 ml vials
Neotears		15 ml bottles
Normal solution		30 ml bottles
Tearisol solution		15 ml Lacrivials
Tears naturale		15 ml plastic dropper bottles
Tears plus		15 ml plastic dropper bottles
Vas-I-Zinc solution		15 ml plastic bottles
Zolyse solution		Unit cartons

SHORT FORMS IN CLINICAL USE

Acc.	accommodation	RH	right hyperphoria
add	addition	LH	left hyperphoria
o.d., OD	right eye (*oculus dexter*)	P.D. or IPD	interpupillary distance
o.s., OS	left eye (*oculus sinister*)	NPA	near point of accommodation
o.u., OU	each eye, both eyes (*oculus uterque*)	NPC	near point of convergence
RE	right eye	MR	medial rectus (muscle)
LE	left eye	LR	lateral rectus (muscle)
NV	near vision	SR	superior rectus (muscle)
PH	pinhole	IR	inferior rectus (muscle)
V	vision or visual acuity	SO	superior oblique (muscle)
mm	millimeter	IO	inferior oblique (muscle)
mg	milligram	BO	base out
SC	without correction	BI	base in
CC	with correction	BD	base down
HM	hand movements	BU	base up
LP	light perception	NRC	normal retinal correspondence
MR	Maddox rod	ARC	abnormal retinal correspondence
L & A	light and accommodation	J1, J2, J3, etc.	test types for reading vision
EOMB	extraocular muscle balance	N5, N6, etc.	test types for near vision
EOM	extraocular movements	b.i.d., b.d.	twice daily
CF	counting fingers	t.i.d., t.d.	three times daily
XP	exophoria	q.i.d.	four times daily
XT	exotropia	a.c.	before meals
W	wearing	p.c.	after meals
IOP	intraocular pressure	i.c.	between meals
T	tension	ne rep. or non rep.	do not repeat
ung	ointment	oculent	eye ointment
A	applanation tensions	per os	orally, by mouth
KP	keratitic precipitates	p.r.n.	when required, as necessary
PSC	posterior subcapsular cataract	q.h.	every hour
ASC	anterior subcapsular cataract	q.2h.	every 2 hours
ET	esotropia	q.s.	quantity sufficient
°	degree	stat.	at once
Δ	prism diopter		
D	diopter		

From Stein, H.A., and Slatt, B.J.: The ophthalmic assistant, ed. 4, St. Louis, 1982, The C.V. Mosby Co.

The following abbreviations may be found on ophthalmic charts:

VA	visual acuity	S or sph	spheric lens
VAc or VAcc	visual acuity with correction	C or cyl	cylinder lens
		⌣	combined with
VAs̄ or VAsc	visual acuity without correction	∞	infinity
		E_1	esophoria for distance
VA=	visual acuity with the unaided eye	E^1	esophoria for near range
OT	ocular tension	ET_1	esotropia for distance
AT or Appl	applanation tension	ET^1	esotropia for near range
		X_1	exophoria for distance
ST	Schiøtz tension	X^1	exophoria for near range
EOM	extraocular muscle	E(T)	intermittent esotropia
Pr	presbyopia	X(T)	intermittent exotropia
PRRE	pupils round, regular, and equal	dd	disc diameters

APPENDIX O

VISION AND DRIVING

Good vision is essential for the proper and safe operation of a motor vehicle. Generally, available vision-testing instruments can be used to ascertain if a person has adequate vision to meet specific standards set by the various state licensing jurisdictions. Because of the increasing injury and death toll resulting from traffic crashes, many of which may be related to visual impairment, physicians should consider it a medical obligation to diagnose visual deficiencies and to inform the patient of potential hazards involved in driving with such deficiencies.

There is no practical way of testing alertness or cerebral perception of what the eye focuses on, but it is important for drivers to have their eyes periodically examined for defects that can be evaluated. This is particularly important for those drivers with significant progressive visual deterioration.

In general, if any doubt exists about a person's visual ability to operate an automobile safely, the physician should not hesitate to recommend road tests for specific evaluation of visual skills.

Visual acuity. Automobile drivers with corrected central visual acuity of 20/40 or better generally read traffic signs and note obstructions, vehicles, and pedestrians while driving at usual speeds, whereas those with optimally corrected vision of 20/70 or less in the better eye have a serious limitation and should not drive.

Adapted from the American Medical Association: Physician's guide for determining driver limitation, Chicago, 1968, The Association.

Drivers with visual acuity between 20/40 and 20/70 should be referred to an ophthalmologist to ascertain if their vision can be improved. The physician, in serving the best interests of patients, should consider the conditions under which each patient drives and the presence or absence of associated defects. The physician is then in a position to advise the patient against driving under certain conditions, such as congested traffic, hazardous road conditions, bad weather, high speed, or at night. It is hoped that continuing research will more exactly define the criteria on which to advise patients.

One-eyed drivers and spectacle-corrected aphakic drivers have visual field limitations and present an increased risk of intersectional crashes. Most postoperative aphakic patients, particularly those in advanced years, also have increased difficulty with night vision and dynamic visual responses. They require special evaluation. Preoperative cataract patients, with early to moderate changes in the lenses of the eye, similarly have night-driving limitations (glare intolerance and reduced night vision) that generally preclude night driving. Patients requiring pupil-constricting medication, as in the control of chronic glaucoma, also have limitation for night operation.

Visual fields. Visual fields are obviously important for safe driving, since a driver must of necessity possess some breadth or lateral awareness to pass approaching vehicles safely and to be aware of vehicles or pedestrians approaching from the side.

Although visual form fields of 140 degrees generally are considered adequate for drivers of private motor vehicles, that figure should be considered as the absolute minimum for drivers of commercial and passenger-carrying vehicles. Such drivers also must have coordinate use of both eyes, as well as a corrected acuity of at least 20/30 in the better eye and no worse than 20/40 in the poorer eye. Persons with lesser fields have driver limitation and must be evaluated for the driving of private vehicles on the basis of the conditions under which they drive, the amount of lateral vision retained, and underlying ocular pathologic condition.

Persons with greatly constricted fields, such as those from advanced glaucoma or retinitis pigmentosa, have distinct driver limitation and should be so advised.

Ocular muscle imbalance. Ocular muscle imbalance (heterophoria) is an indirect cause of automotive crashes in that it may cause driver fatigue. If sudden diplopia occurs, the crash may be directly attributable to the diplopia. Therefore, patients with uncontrolled or intermittent diplopia have definite driver limitation.

Color blindness. Impaired or defective color vision has been considered a potential cause of highway accidents. However, most traffic lights have been standardized, at least regionally; and it is doubtful if this deficiency is too hazardous, except in severe cases. A completely color-blind, or achromatic, individual has very poor vision and should not drive under any circumstance. This also applies to the very limited number of individuals who have severe protanopia, or red deficiency.

Dark adaptation. Dark adaptation and susceptibility to glare are of great importance in night driving, but testing procedures and standards are still largely empiric and not a component of routine eye tests. Dark glasses should never be worn for night driving, and windshield tinting should be limited to the upper one third.

Depth perception. Current testing techniques in the near range do not have significant correlation with distance visual requirements in driving but are adequate for determining visual ability for such tasks as parking. The road test, however, is still the best and most practical guide in this area.

AMERICAN ACADEMY OF OPHTHALMOLOGY'S POLICY REGARDING THE USE OF CONTACT LENSES IN AN INDUSTRIAL ENVIRONMENT

POLICY

Except for unusual situations in which there exists significant risk of ocular damage, individuals should not be disqualified from industrial employment because they wear contact lenses.

BACKGROUND

Patients who wear contact lenses (either for cosmetic or medical reasons) have been disqualified from industrial employment.

Some individuals must wear contact lenses for medical reasons to obtain their best visual performance. An example would be a young monocular aphakic who needs to wear a contact lens in order to obtain binocular vision.

EVALUATION

Recognizing this problem, to assist industry, the Contact Lens Association of Ophthalmologists, and the National Society to Prevent Blindness, have adopted a position paper which defines a reasonable policy, based on current scientific information.

POSITION

Safety and/or medical personnel should not disqualify an employee who can achieve visual rehabilitation by contact lenses, either in job placement or return to a job category. Rather,

employees whose central and peripheral vision can be increased by the wearing of contact lenses, as contrasted to spectacle lenses, should be encouraged to wear contact lenses in industrial environments, in combination with appropriate industrial safety eyewear,* except where there is likelihood of injury from intense heat, massive chemical splash, highly particulate atmosphere, or where federal regulations‡ prohibit such use. Safety and/or medical personnel should determine on an individual basis the advisability of wearing contact lenses in jobs which require unique visual performance, based on consideration of Occupational Safety and Health Administration (OSHA) and National Institute of Occupational Safety and Health (NIOSH) recommendations.†

Employees who do wear contact lenses should be identified and known to their employer. All first aid personnel should be trained in the proper removal of contact lenses. Employees wearing contact lenses should be required to keep a spare pair of contacts and/or prescription spectacles in their possession on the job to avoid an inability to function if they should damage or lose a contact lens while working.

*ANSI, Z80.1, 1979, or as subsequently amended.
†Federal Register, Vol. 36, No. 106, Part II 1910. 134(e)(5)(ii) page 10591, Saturday, May 29, 1971. NIOSH/OSHA Pocket Guide to Chemical Hazards. (DHEW, Publication No. 78210.)

Developed by Ophthalmic Contact Lenses Subcommittee, Ophthalmic Instruments and Devices Committee. Approved by Board of Directors, Nov. 1, 1980.

CANADIAN OPHTHALMOLOGICAL SOCIETY'S POLICY ON CONTACT LENSES IN THE WORK ENVIRONMENT

Contact lenses may be worn in any work environment if proper forward safety eye wear is utilized in conjunction with contact lens. Exception, however, may be in chemical or fume environments where individual considerations should apply.

CANADIAN OPHTHALMOLOGICAL SOCIETY'S CONTACT LENS POLICY

1. Contact lens fitting is a medical problem.
2. It is ethical and proper for a medical practitioner to fit contact lenses and to charge a fee for his professional services.
3. It is considered ethical and proper for the medical practitioner to be involved with the supply and the nonprofit dispensing of contact lenses and their ancillary equipment as a part of the complete contact lens prescription procedure.
4. The use of contact lenses by patients is a potential hazard. Their use necessitates continuing medically orientated care, as provided by an ophthalmologist, to deal with possible complications.
5. The major component of the contact lens fitting fee to the patient is for professional services. This fact emphasizes that contact lenses are not to be grouped with glasses as optical appliances.
6. Those medical practitioners who carry out supervision of patients who are to be, are being, or have been fitted with contact lenses by someone other than themselves, shall charge only a fee commensurate with their professional services.
7. There are clear medical indications for the prescription and fitting of contact lenses as in aphakia, keratoconus, irregular astigmatism, bullous keratopathy and other pathological eye conditions.

INDEX